Sandra Smith's Review for NCLEX-RN

Eighth Edition

Sandra Smith's Review for NCLEX-RN

Eighth Edition

Sandra F. Smith, RN, MS

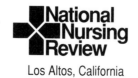

National Nursing Review

Los Altos, California

International Standard Book Number: 0-917010-58-2

In the writing of this text, the authors and publisher have made every attempt to follow current nursing practice and to ensure that suggested diets, drug selection and dosages, and nursing procedures are up to date and conform with current recommendations and practices at time of publication. However, in view of new research conclusions, technological advancements, and government regulations, it is the responsibility of the nurse to be aware of any changes that may alter suggested drug and diet therapies or nursing protocols. The authors recommend that nurses and nursing students be aware of hospital and school policies regarding their role and responsibilities in performing nursing actions. The authors and publisher disclaim any liability, loss or damage incurred as a result of direct or indirect use of this book.

Copies of this book may be obtained from:
National Nursing Review
342 State Street, Suite 6, Los Altos, CA 94022
1-800-950-4095
4   3   2   1

CONTRIBUTING AUTHORS

Chapter Contributors

Barbara Devine Bode, RN, MN
University of Illinois—Doctoral Program

Juliet Marie Corbin, RN, DNSc
University of California, San Francisco

Donna Johnson Duell, RN, MS
Cabrillo College

Dolores Hilden, RN, MS, PhD
Marycrest College

Beverly Smith Meyer, RN, MS
Oregon Health Sciences University

Sandra Fucci Smith, RN, MS
Stanford University—Doctoral Candidate

Section Contributors

Lida G. Chase, RN, MS, PhD
University of Hawaii

Lori Costa, RN, JD
L.C. Associates, San Francisco

Kathleen Dooley, RN, AHNP, MBA
V.A. Hospital, San Francisco

Joan Frommhagen, RN, MA, MN
Cabrillo College

Barbara Martin, RN, MS
Tulsa University

Susan D. North, RN, MS, ScD
Johns Hopkins Medical Center

Virgil Parsons, RN, DNSc
San Jose State University

Kate De Clue Schejbal, RN, PhD
St. Louis University

JoAnn Rupert Behm, RN, MS, CCRN
President, Applied Medical Training

Judith A. Yanda, RN, MS
West Valley College

Editorial Advisors

Loretta Higgins, RN, MS, EdD
Boston College

Andrea Hollingsworth, RN, PhD
University of Pennsylvania

Kyra Hubis, RN, MSN
Evergreen Valley College

Leslie Mancuso, RN, MSN
Project Hope, Nursing Director

PREFACE

Passing the National Council Licensure Examination (NCLEX) is a milestone in your nursing career. You have entered a profession that requires years of preparation. This education culminates with passing the licensing examination which will enable you to begin practicing as a professional nurse. The purpose of NCLEX is to determine if you can practice safe and effective entry-level nursing care. NCLEX, while only a test, actually determines whether or not you will be allowed to function in a professional role. ***Sandra Smith's Review for NCLEX-RN*** was written with the explicit purpose of assisting you to prepare for and pass NCLEX. Years of education, experience and teaching have enabled me to identify the essential nursing content that you must know to successfully pass NCLEX. Adequate preparation, using this book as a guide, will increase your confidence and enable you to review essential nursing concepts.

The best way to prepare for NCLEX is to thoroughly review the material most likely to be covered on the exam and to take practice tests that simulate NCLEX. With this objective in mind, ***Sandra Smith's Review for NCLEX-RN*** is organized into nine chapters. To keep pace with nursing education and the NCLEX Test Plan, we have presented each chapter's content in terms of the Nursing Process. The outline format is designed to help you review quickly, as well as to emphasize significant content. The selection and presentation of content in this review text are directed toward minimizing your review time and maximizing your test results.

The practice tests serve a dual purpose—to acquaint you with the type and format of questions to expect on the examination and to give you an opportunity to test and improve your knowledge of concepts and expertise in realistic nurse-client situations. The answers and rationale sections are intended to discourage rote memorization and to reinforce learning by describing the underlying principles which tell you why the answers are right or wrong.

Acknowledgments

I wish to extend my thanks to all of the contributing authors and to the many other people who helped with the development and production of this book. Because of their valuable assistance, this review book is available to help nursing students prepare for the current RN Licensure Examination.

Sandra L. Smith

CONTENTS

INTRODUCTION

Sandra Smith's Review for NCLEX-RN is designed to assist candidates for registered nurse licensure to prepare for the National Council Licensure Examination-RN. This text focuses on nursing skills, the nurse's responsibilities, major disease processes, and nursing care related to common health problems within the framework of the nursing process and client needs. The nursing content in this book is presented in outline format to help you focus your review on the most important information and utilize your review time most effectively.

A thorough review of the material in this book will enable you to recognize your areas of expertise. You can then concentrate on studying the less familiar content. The review questions at the end of the book will assist you to test your mastery of basic nursing principles and their application to clinical situations.

The following sections in this chapter provide general background information on RN licensure, the NCLEX Test Plan, and Computer Adaptive Testing, followed by helpful techniques for studying and achieving positive test results.

RN Licensure Procedures

The NCLEX-RN measures the licensure candidate's competence to perform safe and effective entry-level nursing practice. The boards of nursing in all 50 states, the District of Columbia, and the U.S. territories of Guam, the Virgin Islands, American Samoa, Puerto Rico, and the Northern Marina Islands administer this screening test as developed by the National Council of State Boards of Nursing (NCSBN). This system of licensure provides protection for health care consumers and defines common entry-level standards throughout the U.S. In order to take the NCLEX, the candidate for licensure applies to the board of nursing in the state or jurisdiction in which the candidate plans to practice nursing.

The NCLEX-RN Test Plan Framework

The NCSBN is responsible to provide its member boards of nursing with a psychometrically sound and legally defensible licensure examination. The purpose of the NCLEX-RN is to separate licensure candidates into two groups: those who can demonstrate minimal competence to perform safe and effective entry-level nursing care, and those who cannot. Although administration of the test via computerized adaptive testing (CAT) is a new procedure implemented in 1994, the basic test plan that provides the framework for presenting the questions has remained essentially unchanged since 1987. The NCSBN contracts with clinical nurses and nurse educators to write questions (referred to as test items) that test your ability to apply your nursing knowledge. The test questions focus on job tasks normally performed by entry-level RNs during their first 6 to 12 months on the job. The NCSBN identifies these tasks by conducting extensive surveys, called job analyses, about every three years. It is entirely possible that your RN program may have included instruction on certain tasks that are not considered to be entry level by the NCSBN's job surveys. It is also possible that your RN program may not have provided you with instruction on some of the tasks about which questions have been included in the current test pool.

The job analysis studies are also used to help validate the test plan and to provide the basis for the proportional distribution of questions among the various subjects covered by the test. The test's two most significant conceptual areas are the Nursing Process and Client Needs. The following sections describe each step in the Nursing Process, define the four broad categories of Client Needs, and list the 17 subcategories of Client Needs.

According to the National Council, "The purpose of the test plan is to guide the selection of content and behaviors to be tested" on NCLEX-RN. To accomplish this, the test plan requires knowledge of:

- The Nursing Process
- Management and coordination of safe, effective care
- Client's physiological needs
- Client's psychosocial needs
- Maintenance and promotion of health

The above five categories of nursing knowledge integrate the following elements in the NCLEX.

- Accountability
- Mental health concepts
- Pharmacology
- Nutrition
- Body structure and function

- Pathophysiology
- Principles of asepsis
- Growth and development
- Documentation
- Communication and teaching

Additional areas of content you can expect to be included on NCLEX that will test your knowledge, skills, and abilities are basic principles of management; continuity of care; psychodynamics of behavior; treatment modalities including group dynamics; response to therapies; environmental and personal safety measures; client's rights; confidentiality; infectious agents; immunity; routine nursing measures; ADLs; managing emergencies; comfort measures; reproduction and human sexuality; birthing and parenting; effects of immobility; use of special equipment; and cultural and religious influences.

The Nursing Process

The phases of the Nursing Process that are measured by NCLEX include Assessment, Analysis, Planning, Implementing, and Evaluating. Nursing Diagnosis is included as an essential step in the Analysis phase. The candidate for licensure can expect 15% to 25% of the questions to focus on each phase of the Nursing Process. While NCLEX questions are unlikely to test knowledge of nursing process definitions, the questions will be phrased in terminology reflecting the five phases. For example, a question will ask which assessment is the most important for a particular circumstance (the specific clinical situation that is presented), then the four answer options will be phrased as assessment (observation) parameters. If a question focuses on nursing implementation, the four alternatives will be phrased as nursing actions or interventions.

Client Needs

The basic health needs of patients are grouped under four broad categories and 17 subcategories that are weighted according to the results of the job analysis studies conducted by the NCSBN. The emphasis on each category is summarized by the percentage breakdown of questions on NCLEX as follows:

Safe, Effective Care Environment	25–31%
Physiological Integrity	42–48%
Psychosocial Integrity	9–15%
Health Promotion and Maintenance	12–18%

Safe, Effective Care Environment

To meet the client's needs in this area, the nurse must be able to provide and direct nursing care in the following areas:

- Coordinated Care
- Quality Assurance
- Goal-oriented Care
- Environmental Safety
- Preparation for Treatments and Procedures
- Safe and Effective Treatments and Procedures

Physiological Integrity

To meet the client's needs for physiological integrity—which includes potentially life-threatening conditions and/or chronically recurring physiological conditions, and potential complications or untoward effects of treatments of management modalities—the nurse must be able to provide and direct nursing care in the following areas:

- Physiological Adaptation
- Reduction of Risk Potential
- Mobility
- Comfort
- Provision of Basic Care

Psychosocial Integrity

To meet the client's needs for psychosocial integrity during periods of stress or crisis-related situations, the nurse must be able to provide and direct nursing care in the following areas:

- Psychosocial Adaptation
- Coping/Adaptation

Health Promotion and Maintenance

To meet the client's needs for health promotion and maintenance throughout the life cycle, the nurse must be able to provide and direct nursing care for clients and their significant others in the following areas:

- Continued Growth and Development
- Self-Care
- Integrity of Support Systems
- Prevention and Early Treatment of Disease

Adapted from *The National Council Licensure Examination for Registered Nurses.* National Council of State Boards of Nursing, Chicago, 1988.

Computerized Adaptive Testing

With the introduction of Computerized Adaptive Testing (CAT) in 1994, the procedures for taking the NCLEX changed radically from prior protocol. The major new elements include:

(1) Locating test sites throughout the U.S. where each candidate makes an appointment to take the test on an individual basis.

(2) Presenting the test on a computer screen rather than in a printed test booklet. Answer selections are made by pressing keys on a computer keyboard instead of marking an answer sheet with a pencil.

(3) Each candidate's test is unique because the computer selects each subsequent question based upon the candidate's prior answers.

The Advantages of CAT

CAT is described as providing a more comfortable and convenient way to take NCLEX. The testing environment at a Sylvan Technology Center will be similar to a small classroom or learning laboratory in contrast to a large hall or convention center with the distractions and tension associated with a large group of candidates taking the test simultaneously. From a procedural standpoint, the advantages of CAT are defined as:

(1) A more efficient way to test and measure competency than the prior pencil and paper test format.

(2) Reduction of testing time to a maximum of five hours in one test session.

(3) Greater security and the avoidance of inconvenience to candidates if security measures break down.

(4) Year-round testing schedules that provide applicants with greater flexibility and convenience than the prior twice-per-year system.

(5) Substantial reduction in the time required between applying to take NCLEX and receiving one's results.

The Administrative Organizations for NCLEX-CAT

Three organizations are involved with administering NCLEX: (1) boards of nursing from each state or jurisdiction, (2) the Educational Testing Service (ETS), and (3) Sylvan Learning Systems. As a candidate for licensure, it will help you to know the role of each organization.

As described earlier in this section, the NCSBN designs the test plan, conducts the job analysis, and sets the passing standard. The Educational Testing Service formulates the test questions to conform to the National Council's Test Plan. ETS maintains a test pool of several thousand questions written by specially selected item writers approved by the state boards of nursing. All NCLEX questions are drawn from this test pool. You will make an appointment with and physically take the NCLEX at a Sylvan Technology Center. Approximately 200 of these centers are available throughout the U.S. for NCLEX testing.

Application Procedures for the NCLEX-CAT

After the state (jurisdiction) in which you plan to practice accepts your application and verifies your eligibility to take the NCLEX, you will receive an Authorization to Test and other information that includes the locations and telephone numbers of the Sylvan Technology Centers. You will then contact a test center of your choice to make an appointment to take the test. The test center does not need to be located in the state to which you have applied for licensure. As a first time test taker, you should be able to schedule your appointment within 30 days of your call. Read all instructions carefully, especially noting the items that you must bring to the test center.

Taking the NCLEX-CAT

Upon arriving at the Sylvan Technology Center, you will present your Authorization to Test and two forms of identification, both signed and one with a photo. A driver's license, school or employee I.D., and passport are the most accepted forms. A social security card is an example of an unacceptable proof of identity. At check-in, you will be photographed and thumb printed. Before commencing the test questions, you will complete a brief computer tutorial to make certain that you are comfortable with the keyboard procedures. The National Council advises that no prior computer experience is necessary for CAT.

Two types of questions appear on NCLEX. The real questions test your competency and safety and provide the basis for your pass or fail score. The tryout questions are items being field tested for future NCLEX exams. You have no way of knowing the difference between real and tryout.

The minimum number of questions for each RN licensure candidate will be 60 real and 15 tryout for a total of 75. The National Council maintains that the essential Test Plan categories can be covered by 60 carefully selected questions. The maximum number of real questions will be 250, so by adding the 15 tryouts, you could answer a total of 265 items.

Because the number of questions will vary from candidate to candidate, there is no maximum time you should spend per question. However, because you won't know how long it will take you to reach the 95% confidence level, it is not wise to spend several minutes on many individual questions. If you don't know the answer, guess and move on, rather than spend five minutes and risk becoming immobilized.

CAT does not allow you to skip questions, change answers, or go back to look at questions already answered. Each question has an assigned degree of difficulty. Based on your prior answers—correct or incorrect—the computer selects the next question. Therefore, you must answer each question as it is presented. Because the computer draws from a large pool of questions, each candidate's test is unique. There is no absolute passing score in terms of the number or percent of questions that you must answer correctly in order to pass.

After you have answered the minimum number of questions, your test continues until the computer calculates with a 95% degree of confidence that you fall into the safe/competent group or that you do not. Although there is no minimum amount of time for your test, the maximum allowable test duration is five hours, including your computer tutorial and rest breaks. A mandatory rest break of 10 minutes is required after two hours of testing and an optional break is available after the next 1-1/2 hours.

The results of your test will be electronically transmitted from the Sylvan Technology Center where you take the test to Educational Testing Service in Princeton, New Jersey, for processing. Within 48 hours, ETS will forward your results to the board of nursing to which you applied for licensure. Your results—pass or fail—will be sent to you by the board of nursing. A failure report will be accompanied by a diagnostic analysis to help you identify your specific areas of weakness. The time required for the board of nursing to notify the candidate will vary from state to state.

Guidelines for NCLEX Review

Familiarize Yourself with the Organization of Material in This Book

Sandra Smith's Review for NCLEX-RN summarizes extensive nursing content to which you have been introduced during your RN training. The material is organized into nine chapters and presented in outline format for your review. Nursing theory and practical applications of this theory are included for each major subject area. Nursing theory includes pathophysiology, signs and symptoms of diseases, diagnosis and treatment of medical conditions, and the appropriate nursing care. The tables, appendices and glossaries are distributed throughout the book to assist you to efficiently review factual material. Familiarize yourself with how the contents are organized chapter by chapter and how the Nursing Process is integrated throughout the book.

The multiple-choice questions that follow the content review are similar in format, subject matter, length, and degree of difficulty to those contained in the NCLEX-RN. The answer and rationale sections provide you with an added learning experience; if you understand the basic principles of nursing content, you can transfer that knowledge to the clinical situations and questions on the NCLEX.

Your Personal Review Program

Ideally, you will begin your review process several months prior to NCLEX; but if, like most students, you allocate only a few weeks to prepare for this exam, it is important that you conduct the review process in an efficient manner. The following recommendations are offered to help you achieve maximum results for the amount of time invested.

A. Schedule regular periods for your study and review.
   1. Arrange to study when mentally alert. Studying during periods of mental and physical fatigue reduces your efficiency.
   2. Allow short breaks at relatively frequent intervals. Breaks used as rewards for hard study serve as incentives for continued concentrated effort. A 10 to 15 minute break is recommended after each hour of concentrated study.
B. Analyze your strengths and weaknesses.
   1. Consider past performance on classroom tests and written clinical applications of factual material. Learn from your past errors on tests by looking up and studying the correct material in this book.
   2. Analyze your results on practice questions. Identify topics where your knowledge or understanding is weak. These areas will require a more thorough review on your part.

3. Allow sufficient time for repeated review in this book of subject areas that continue to be difficult for you.

C. Familiarize yourself with the examination format.
   1. Review the NCLEX Test Plan description so that you understand the Nursing Process and Client Needs categories. Notice which areas have the greater number of questions and allocate more review time to these topics.
   2. Study the format used for NCLEX questions. You must know how to read, evaluate and respond to multiple-choice questions similar to the ones at the end of this book.

D. Systematically study the material contained in each chapter of this book.
   1. First, gain a general impression of the content unit to be reviewed. Skim over the entire section and identify the main ideas.
   2. Then, read and study the tables, glossaries, and appendices carefully.
   3. Mark key material that is not thoroughly understood.

E. Follow up on your priority areas.
   1. Set priorities on the material that is to be learned or reviewed. Identify the most crucial sections and underline the essential thoughts.
   2. Review what you have read. Think of examples that illustrate the main points you have studied.
   3. To be sure that you have learned the material, write down the main ideas or explain the major points to another person.

F. Test yourself on what you have learned.
   1. Complete the practice questions at the end of this book. You can either mark your answers in the book or use the computer disk enclosed inside the back cover. If you use "paper and pencil," correct each question and read the rationale. If you utilize the disk, the computer will score the test for you, identify the questions that you missed, and provide you with a helpful Performance Summary. Reading the rationale will enable you to understand the underlying principle for each answer. These principles will apply to NCLEX-RN questions that focus on the same topics.
   2. Acquire the flexibility to answer questions that are phrased in different ways but cover the same wide range of content. You will find additional practice questions in Review Questions for NCLEX-RN by Sandra F. Smith, RN, MS.

Test-Taking Strategies

The following test-taking strategies can provide you with useful guidelines when answering questions. These strategies are neither absolute nor fool-proof; they are intended to guide you to choose the best response for each question.

A. Carefully read each question. Determine what the question is really asking. Some details may not be important. Mentally note important factors; pay attention to key terms and phrases. For example, do not misread grams as milligrams.

B. When answering multiple-choice questions, an effective strategy is to first eliminate the answers that you know are wrong, and then spend time deciding among the remaining answers. If you are not sure about any of the four possible answers, you will have to make an educated guess. Remember, you are not allowed to skip a question, nor will you be able to change any of the answers you have selected on earlier questions.

C. A first "hunch" is usually correct. Many candidates have a first impression, choose an answer, and, upon reflection, change their mind. Sensing that a particular alternative is correct has some basis. Your brain has made rapid connections. You came to an immediate conclusion based on your knowledge and experience. The fact that you did not go through the logical steps of arriving at the correct solution does not indicate that your choice is incorrect.

D. Be alert for a question that requires you to identify which answer is not correct. Read the question as it is stated, not as you would like it to be stated.

E. The most comprehensive answer is often the best choice. For example, if two alternatives seem reasonable but one answer includes the other (i.e., it is more detailed, extends the first answer, or is more comprehensive), then this answer may be the best choice.

F. Eliminate answers that focus on medical knowledge. Remember, this is an RN test, and the questions are designed to test your competency and safety. It is unlikely that a question would require a medical action for the correct answer; it may, however, offer these actions as distractors.

G. Evaluate the answers in relation to the stem (the question), not to other answers. Choose the answer that best fits the question rather than an answer that appears to be a correct statement but may not fit the question.

H. Eliminate answers that are obviously different from what is logically right, such as an answer given in grams when other choices are given in milligrams.

I. Do not look for a pattern to the answers. The questions are chosen at random, and the same number may possibly and correctly answer several consecutive questions.

J. Be on guard for answers that contain qualifiers such as always and never. They rarely fit within a logical framework. However, some situations may be true only when a qualifier is added.

K. If a clinical situation precedes a question, read the situation very carefully. Identify the essential ideas. Be careful of answer selections that divert your attention from key ideas.

L. Scratch paper will be available for you to use when making or checking calculations. This will assist you to determine the correct answer before entering your selection on the computer.

Final Preparation

A. The night before the test.
   1. Assemble the materials needed for the test as specified in your instructions from the Sylvan Technology Center.
   2. Get a good night's sleep. Do not stay up all night trying to learn new material.
   3. Avoid the use of stimulants or depressants, either of which may affect your ability to think clearly during the test.

4. Approach the test with confidence and the determination to do your best. Think positively and concentrate on all that you do know rather than on what you think you do not know.

B. The day of the test.
   1. Eat a good breakfast. Do not rush.
   2. Allow ample time to travel to your testing site, including time to park, and to present your Authorization to Test, two proofs of identity, and any other required documents.
   3. If possible, choose a station in the testing room where you are least likely to be distracted by other people taking tests.

The Importance of a Confident Attitude

Anxiety, a forceful deterrent to test-taking success, interferes with your ability to think clearly. Anxiety blocks the search and retrieval process so that you cannot access the knowledge held in your "memory bank." Fear of the unknown is a major source of anxiety. This fear can be overcome by diligent review. As you gain mastery over the nursing content, your self-confidence increases. It is also important to understand test construction and test-taking strategies. This introduction is designed to reduce many of the unknowns associated with NCLEX-RN and to provide you with review guidelines and test-taking techniques.

These strategies are guidelines, not absolutes. Always use your own judgment, knowledge, and nursing experience. These personal assets will serve you well when taking the NCLEX-RN. Be confident that you will pass, and, in fact, you will.

Practice Computer Disk

A vinyl envelope containing a computer disk is attached inside the back cover of this book. This 3.5-inch disk, which will operate on IBM and IBM-compatible personal computers, contains the same questions that are printed at the back of the book. After completing the questions on the disk, you can obtain your Performance Summary in terms of Nursing Process, Client Needs, and Clinical Area. You will also be able to obtain a list of questions you answered incorrectly. We recommend that you refer to the rationales printed at the back of the book to understand the principles underlying the answers for all of the practice questions.

1

NURSING THROUGH THE LIFE CYCLE

General aspects of stress are discussed in the first section of this chapter. The body's responses to stress and Dr. Selye's primary principles of stress are included. Since all phases of illness are accompanied by stress, the nurse should have an understanding of the basic concepts.

Growth and development from infancy to old age are discussed in the next section. The concepts of grief, death and dying are presented to assist the nurse to intervene therapeutically and to support the dying child and the client through the dying process. A fourth section, human sexuality, has been added in recognition of today's emphasis on holistic nursing.

HOMEOSTASIS: STRESS AND ADAPTATION

HOMEOSTASIS

Definition: The maintenance of a constant state in the internal environment through self-regulatory techniques that preserve the organism's ability to adapt to stresses.

A. Dynamics of homeostasis.
1. Danger or its symbols, whether internal or external, result in the activation of the sympathetic nervous system and the adrenal medulla.
2. The organism prepares for flight or fight.
B. Adaptation factors.
1. Age—adaptation is greatest in youth and young middle life, and least at the extremes of life.
2. Environment—adequate supply of required materials is necessary.
3. Adaptation involves the entire organism.
4. The organism can more easily adapt to stress over a period of time than suddenly.
5. Organism flexibility influences survival.
6. The organism usually uses the adaptation mechanism that is most economical in terms of energy.
7. Illness decreases the organism's capacity to adapt to stress.
8. Adaptation responses may be adequate or deficient.
9. Adaptation may cause stress and illness, i.e., ulcers, arthritis, allergy, asthma, and overwhelming infections.

STRESS

A. Definitions of stress.
1. A physical, a chemical, or an emotional factor that causes bodily or mental tension and that may be a factor in disease causation; a state resulting from factors that tend to alter an existing equilibrium.
2. Selye's definition of stress.
a. The state manifested by a specific syndrome that consists of all the nonspecifically induced changes within the biologic system.
b. The body is the common denominator of all adaptive responses.
c. Stress is manifested by the measurable changes in the body.
d. Stress causes a multiplicity of changes in the body.
B. General aspects of stress.
1. Body responses to stress are a self-preserving mechanism that automatically and immediately becomes activated in times of danger.
a. Caused by physical or psychological stress: disease, injury, anger, or frustration.
b. Caused by changes in internal and/or external environment.
2. There are a limited number of ways an organism can respond to stress (for example, a cornered amoeba cannot fly).

Selye's Theory of Stress

A. General adaptive syndrome (GAS).
1. Alarm stage (call to arms).
a. Shock: the body translates as sudden injury, and the GAS becomes activated.
b. Countershock: the organism restored to its pre-injury condition.
2. Stage of resistance: the organism is adapted to the injuring agent.
3. State of exhaustion: if stress continues, the organism loses its adaptive capability and goes into exhaustion, which is comparable to shock.
B. Local adaptive syndrome (LAS).
1. Selective changes within the organism.
2. Local response elicits general response.
3. Example of LAS: a cut, followed by bleeding, followed by coagulation of blood, etc.
4. Ability of parts of the body to respond to a specific injury is impaired if the whole body is under stress.

C. Whether the organism goes through all the phases of adaptation depends both upon its capacity to adapt and the intensity and continuance of the injuring agent.
   1. Organism may return to normal.
   2. Organism may overreact; stress decreases.
   3. Organism may be unable to adapt or maintain adaptation, a condition that may lead to death.
D. Objective of stress response.
   1. To maintain stability of the organism during stress.
   2. To repair damage.
   3. To restore body to normal composition and activity.

Psychological Stress

Definition: All processes that impose a demand or requirement upon the organism, the resolution or accommodation of which necessitates work or activity of the mental apparatus.

Characteristics

A. May involve other structures or systems, but primarily affects mental apparatus.
   1. Anxiety is a primary result of psychological stress.
   2. Causes mental mechanisms to attempt to reduce or relieve psychological discomfort.
      a. Attack/fight.
      b. Withdrawal/flight.
      c. Play dead/immobility.
B. Causes of psychological stress.
   1. Loss of something of value.
   2. Injury/pain.
   3. Frustrations of needs and drives.
   4. Threats to self-concept.
   5. Many illnesses cause stress.
      a. Disfigurement.
      b. Venereal disease.
      c. Long-term or chronic diseases.
      d. Cancer.
      e. Heart disease.
   6. Conflicting cultural values, i.e., the American values of competition and assertiveness vs. the need to be dependent.
   7. Future shock: physiological and psychological stress resulting from an overload of the organism's adaptive systems and decision-making processes brought about by too rapidly changing values and technology.
   8. Cultural shock: stress developing in response to transition of the individual from a familiar environment to unfamiliar one.
      a. Involves unfamiliarity with communication, technology, customs, attitudes, and beliefs.
      b. Examples: individual moving to new area from foreign country or individual placed in hospital environment.

Assessment

1. Assess increased anxiety, anger, helplessness, hopelessness, guilt, shame, disgust, fear, frustration, or depression.
2. Evaluate behaviors resulting from stress.
   a. Apathy, regression, withdrawal.
   b. Crying, demanding.
   c. Physical illness.
   d. Hostility, manipulation.
   e. Senseless violence, acting out.

Implementation

A. Gather information about client's internal and external environment.
B. Modify external environment so that adaptation responses are within the capacity of client.
C. Support the efforts of client to adapt or to respond.
D. Provide client with the materials required to maintain constancy of internal environment.
E. Understand body's mechanisms for accommodating stress.
F. Prevent additional stress.
G. Reduce external stimuli.
H. Reduce or increase physical activity depending on the cause of and response to stress.

Table 1. SELYE'S STRESS ADAPTATION SYNDROME

STAGE	GENERAL FUNCTION	INTERPERSONAL	BEHAVIORAL	AFFECTIVE	COGNITIVE	PHYSIOLOGICAL
1 Alarm reaction	Mobilization of body defenses	Interpersonal communication effectiveness decreases	Task oriented Increased restlessness Apathy, regression Crying	Feelings of anger, suspiciousness, helplessness Anxiety level increases	Alert Thinking becomes narrow and concrete Symptoms of thought blocking, forgetfulness, and decreased productivity	Muscle tension Increase in epinephrine and cortisone Stimulation of adrenal cortex and lymph glands Increase in blood pressure, heart rate, blood glucose
2 Stage of resistance	Adaptation to stresses Resistance increases	Interpersonal communication self-oriented Uses interpersonal relationships to meet own needs	Automatic behaviors Self-oriented behaviors Fight or flight behavior apparent	Increased use of defense mechanisms Emotional responses may be automatic or exaggerated	Thought processes more habitual than problem solving oriented	Hormonal levels return to pre-alarm stage All physiological responses return to normal or are channeled into psychosomatic symptoms
3 Stage of exhaustion	Depletion or exhaustion of organs and resources Loss of ability to resist stress	Disintegration of personal interactions Communication skills ineffective and disorganized Self-oriented	Restless, withdrawn, agitated; may become violent or self-destructive Diminished productivity	Depressed, flat, or inappropriate Exaggerated or inappropriate use of defense mechanisms Decreased ability to cope	Thought disorganization, hallucinations, preoccupation Reduced intellectual processes	Exhaustion, with increased demands on organism Adrenal cortex hormone depletion Death, if stress is continuous and excessive

GROWTH AND DEVELOPMENT THROUGH THE LIFE CYCLE

CHILDREN

One Month

A. Physical and motor development.
1. Follows with eyes to midline.
2. Follows bright, moving objects with eyes.
3. Lifts head slightly from prone.
4. Lies awake on back with head averted.
5. Keeps fists clenched.
6. Responds to sharp sounds, i.e., bell, etc.
7. Does not grasp objects.
B. Language and social development.
1. Regards face, may smile.
2. Responds to voice.
3. Makes throaty noises.
4. Is alert about one out of every ten hours.
C. Parent counseling guidelines for play.
1. Smile and talk to infant.
2. Touch, stroke, cuddle.
3. Talk and sing to infant.
4. Play soft music.
5. Play with infant.
6. Hold infant while feeding.
7. Provide toys such as colorful, hanging mobiles.

Two Months

A. Physical and motor development.
1. Ceases activity to listen for a bell.
2. Follows better vertically and horizontally with jerky eye movements.
3. Moves arms and legs vigorously.
4. Lifts head to 45 degrees when prone on abdomen.
5. Turns from side to back.
6. Grasp becomes voluntary.
7. No longer exhibits crossed extensor reflex.

B. Language and social development.
1. Vocalizes and smiles responsively.
2. Visually follows moving person.
3. Makes single vowel sounds such as "ah," "eh," "uh."
4. Differentiates by crying.
5. Begins social smile.
6. Exhibits tactile and oral stimulation, not social.
C. Parent counseling guidelines for play.
1. Smile and talk to infant.
2. Use cradle gym and infant seat.
3. Allow infant the freedom of kicking with clothes off.
4. Place infant in prone position on floor or in bed.
5. Expose infant to different textures.
6. Exercise infant's arms and legs.
7. Provide bright pictures and hanging objects that move.

Three Months

A. Physical and motor development.
1. Lifts head and chest when prone.
2. Brings objects to mouth.
3. Displays nimble and busy fingers.
4. Rotates head from side to side.
5. Improves convergence.
6. Discovers and stares at hands.
7. Briefly holds toy in hand.
B. Language and social development.
1. Babbles, pronounces initial vowels, and coos.
2. Smiles more readily.
3. Ceases to cry when mother enters room or caresses him or her.
4. Enjoys playing during feeding.
5. Stays awake longer without crying.
6. Turns head to follow familiar person.
C. Parent counseling guidelines for play.
1. While infant prone on abdomen, move bright object upward to encourage head movement.
2. Bounce infant on bed.
3. Continue to introduce new sounds.
4. Provide social stimulation (important).
5. Play with infant during feeding.
6. Provide rattles, large soft animals.

Four Months

A. Physical and motor development.
  1. Infant lifts head and shoulders to a 90-degree angle.
  2. Looks ahead while in prone position on abdomen.
  3. Can follow object 180 degrees.
  4. Can move from side to side; tries to roll over.
  5. Grasps for toy with whole hand.
  6. Brings hands or toys to mouth.
  7. Sucks thumb or fist.
  8. Begins teething.
B. Language and social development.
  1. Coos, gurgles, and laughs aloud.
  2. Begins babbling.
  3. Knows mother.
  4. Imitates mother.
  5. Demands attention by fussing.
  6. Begins to respond to "no."
  7. Enjoys being placed in sitting position with support.
  8. Responds to and enjoys being handled.
C. Parent counseling guidelines for play.
  1. Show child his or her reflection in mirror.
  2. Increase sensory stimulation.
  3. Give frequent baths as infant enjoys splashing in tub.
  4. Play music as child is quieted by it.
  5. Move mobile out of reach; child may grab it and injure self.
  6. Repeat child's sounds to him or her.
  7. Provide soft, colorful squeeze toys; rattles; mirror; toys whose parts cannot be removed.

Five to Six Months

A. Physical and motor development.
  1. Visually pursues lost object.
  2. Holds block in each hand.
  3. Exhibits hand-eye coordination.
  4. Sits for short periods leaning forward on hands.
  5. Creeps and rocks.
  6. Reaches for objects beyond grasp.
  7. Rolls from back to stomach and stomach to back.
  8. Weighs twice as much as at birth.
B. Language and social development.
  1. Begins to recognize strangers.
  2. Shows fear and anger.

  3. Vocalizes vowel sounds and well-defined syllables.
  4. Shows anticipation; waves and raises arms to be picked up.
  5. Expresses protest.
  6. Understands name.
C. Parent counseling guidelines for play.
  1. Play sitting-up games.
  2. Encourage reaching for objects.
  3. Provide teething toys, soft blocks and squeeze toys, metal cup and wooden spoon for banging.

Seven to Nine Months

A. Physical and motor development.
  1. Reaches for objects unilaterally.
  2. Can transfer a toy.
  3. Exhibits complete thumb opposition.
  4. Sits alone steadily with good coordination.
  5. Advances from creeping to crawling.
  6. Can pull self to feet with assistance.
  7. Feeds self a cracker.
  8. Develops eye-to-eye contact while talking.
  9. Engages in social games.
B. Language and social development.
  1. Begins imitative expressions.
  2. Shows fear of strangers.
  3. Makes polysyllable vowel sounds.
  4. Play is self-contained.
  5. Laughs out loud.
  6. Listens to conversations.
C. Parent counseling guidelines for play.
  1. Play social games such as peek-a-boo and pat-a-cake.
  2. Allow child to drop and retrieve toys.
  3. Allow child to play with spoon at feeding.
  4. Give child soft finger-foods.
  5. Take safety precautions as child puts everything into mouth.
  6. Show excitement at child's achievements.
  7. Provide squeeze toys in bath, toys that make noise, large nesting toys, crumpled paper.

Ten to Eleven Months

A. Physical and motor development.
  1. Sits without support indefinitely.
  2. Pulls self to feet.
  3. Stands on toes with support.

4. Creeps and cruises very well.
5. Can pick up objects fairly well.
6. Uses index finger and thumb to grasp.
7. Can hold own bottle or cup.
8. Shows interest in tiny objects.

B. Language and social development.
   1. Vocabulary of one to two words ("Mama," "Dada").
   2. Recognizes meaning of "no."
   3. Shows moods; looks hurt, sad.
   4. Is very aware of environment.
   5. Responds to own name.
   6. Imitates gestures, facial expressions, sounds.
   7. Begins to test parental reaction during feeding and at bedtime.
   8. Entertains self for long periods of time.

C. Parent counseling guidelines for play.
   1. Use plastic bottle.
   2. Protect child from dangerous objects.
   3. Have child with family at mealtime.
   4. Allow exploration outdoors.
   5. Provide new objects (blocks); toys that stimulate; containers (milk cartons); toys that can be filled, emptied, knocked down, and stacked up; fabric books.

Twelve to Eighteen Months

A. Physical and motor development.
   1. Stands and walks alone.
   2. Puts objects in and out of containers; can release objects at will.
   3. Points to indicate wants.
   4. Holds a cup with both hands.
   5. Throws a ball.
   6. Looks at pictures with interest.
   7. Triples birth weight at 12 months; has closed anterior fontanel.
   8. Begins to develop fine muscle coordination.
   9. Has protruding abdomen.

B. Language and social development.
   1. Is aware of expressive function of language; uses jargon, imitates sounds.
   2. Cooperates in dressing; removes socks.
   3. Likes an audience and will repeat performance.
   4. Shows anxiety about strangers.
   5. Distinguishes self from others.
   6. Has a vocabulary of ten meaningful words.

7. Finds security in a blanket, favorite toy, or thumb sucking.
8. Plays alone but near others (parallel play).
9. Is dependent upon parents but shows first signs of desire for autonomy.

C. Parent counseling guidelines for play.
   1. Make no attempt to change from use of left to right hand.
   2. Provide frequent changes of environment.
   3. Allow self-directed play rather than adult-directed play.
   4. Continue to expose child to different foods.
   5. Show affection and encourage child to reciprocate.
   6. Create safe environment (medications locked up and harmful items out of reach).
   7. Provide pull and push toys, Teddy bears, pots and pans, musical toys, telephone, sand box and fill toys, cloth picture books with colorful, large pictures.

Eighteen Months to Two Years

A. Physical and motor development.
   1. Exhibits well developed eye accommodation.
   2. Walks up and down stairs one at a time with pauses.
   3. Turns door knobs; climbs on furniture.
   4. Chews more effectively.
   5. Walks and runs with a stiff gait and wide stance.
   6. Uses a spoon without spilling.
   7. Builds tower of six cubes.
   8. Kicks a ball in front of him or her without support.
   9. Has daytime bladder and bowel control; occasional accidents; nighttime control not complete.

B. Language and social development.
   1. Displays receptive vocabulary of 200 to 300 words; speaks vowels correctly.
   2. Begins to use short sentences.
   3. Has fear of parents leaving.
   4. Helps to undress; tries to button.
   5. Wants to hoard and not share; "snatch and grab stage."
   6. Violently resists having toys taken away.
   7. Begins to have feelings of autonomy.

8. Begins process of identification; uses "no" as assertion of self.
9. Begins cooperation in toilet training.

C. Parent counseling guidelines for play.
   1. In toilet training, allow child to follow own pattern.
   2. Provide peer companionship.
   3. Allow child to eat with family.
   4. Provide role-modeling for positive behavior (important for child).
   5. Provide building blocks, wagons, pull toys, pounding toys like a drum, books with pictures.

Two and One-Half Years

A. Physical and motor development.
   1. Pushes and pulls large toys.
   2. Jumps; squats to play.
   3. Builds tower of eight blocks.
   4. Copies horizontal and vertical strokes.
   5. Feeds self; uses fork.
   6. Pours from pitcher.
   7. Can undress.
   8. Begins to use scissors.
   9. Has full set (20) of baby teeth.

B. Language and social development.
   1. Knows full name.
   2. Refers to self by pronoun "I."
   3. Shows negativism, has temper tantrums, and is ritualistic.
   4. Learns power of "yes" and "no."
   5. Shows poorly developed judgment.
   6. Can tolerate short periods of separation from parents.
   7. Begins to identify sex (gender) roles.
   8. Explores environment outside the home.
   9. Engages in associative play.

C. Parent counseling guidelines for play.
   1. Allow child his or her preferences.
   2. Control temper tantrums.
   3. Allow ritualism, especially at night.
   4. Be aware that negativism and ritualism is normal behavior at this age.
   5. Provide discipline as a way of socializing and educating child. Discipline simply for the sake of establishing authority is counterproductive.
   6. Use firmness and consistency.

7. Read simple book to child to help develop language and memory skills.
8. Provide manipulative toys for muscle coordination, crayons and paper, simple games.

Three Years

A. Physical and motor development.
   1. Goes up and down stairs, alternating feet.
   2. Rides tricycle.
   3. Stands momentarily on one foot.
   4. Swings, climbs.
   5. While running, can stop suddenly or turn corners.

B. Language and social development.
   1. Begins to cooperate but is still self-centered.
   2. Begins imaginative and make-believe play.
   3. Wants to please.
   4. Knows own age and sex, and the concept of *one.*
   5. Verbalizes toilet needs and goes to toilet by self (needs help wiping).
   6. Uses "I," "me," "you" speech.
   7. Has vocabulary of 900 words.
   8. Begins to understand what it means to take turns.
   9. Can remember and repeat three numbers.

C. Parent counseling guidelines for play.
   1. Encourage and promote social contacts and imaginative outlets.
   2. Alternate group activity with solitary play.
   3. Listen to child's conversations and narratives.
   4. Base expectations within child's limitations.
   5. Provide climbing apparatus, keys, tricycle, wagons, dump trucks, simple puzzles, music, record player.

Three to Four Years

A. Physical and motor development.
   1. Has 20/20 vision.
   2. Races up and down steps.
   3. Skips, hops, performs stunts; has good balance.
   4. Draws man with two to four parts besides the head.
   5. Cuts on line with scissors.
   6. Feeds self.
   7. Dresses self; laces shoes but cannot tie; buttons.

8. Brushes teeth.
B. Language and social development.
1. Asks abundant questions: What? Why? How?
2. Recites nursery rhyme or poem, or sings a song.
3. Gives full name.
4. Shows interest in world: nurses, firemen, police, doctors.
5. Begins to share; seeks peer relationships.
6. Exhibits excessive imaginative and make-believe play.
7. Displays less negative behavior.
8. Can tolerate separation from mother longer.
C. Parent counseling guidelines for play.
1. Encourage widening horizon and exploration of environment, imagination, peer relationships.
2. Encourage pretending, story telling, expressing.
3. Give simple explanation as to cause and effect.
4. Provide alternate periods of active and quiet play.
5. Provide books, puzzles, drawing materials, puppets.

Four to Five Years

A. Physical and motor development.
1. Exhibits improved muscle coordination; is more agile and graceful; jumps, hops, skips on alternate feet.
2. Draws recognizable pictures.
3. Is quieter and less restless; has greater concentration.
4. Draws triangle and square from copy.
5. Names four colors, the heavier of two weights, and the longer of two lines.
6. Builds steps.
7. Exhibits good posture; carries arms near body; narrows stance.
8. Transports objects in trucks and cars.
9. Dresses and undresses with skill but still needs some supervision.
B. Language and social development.
1. Exhibits improved concept and language development.
2. Asks questions about the meaning of words.
3. Prints simple words.
4. Is cooperative, has poise, and controls behavior.

5. Is creative.
6. Is capable of longer attention span; completes activities; shows imaginative, dramatic play.
7. Displays planning, space, depth, expression, and creativity in drawing.
8. Begins to develop an elementary conscience.
9. Displays high energy during play.
C. Parent counseling guidelines for play.
1. Give kind but unmistakable discipline.
2. Build self-confidence.
3. Provide consistent control.
4. Encourage responsibility for putting things away.
5. Widen and vary experiences in reading and music.
6. Enroll child in kindergarten.
7. Encourage group play and cooperation and sharing in projects.

Five to Six Years

A. Physical and motor development.
1. Improves balance.
2. Begins to ride two-wheel bicycle.
3. Runs skillfully and plays games at the same time.
4. Is able to wash without wetting clothing.
5. Begins to lose baby teeth.
6. Exhibits good control with small motor movements.
7. Catches a ball.
8. Shows little awareness of dangers, but has good motor development.
9. Uses hands as manipulative tools in cutting, pasting, hammering.
B. Language and social development.
1. Has well-developed vocabulary.
2. Repeats sentence of 10 syllables or more.
3. Talks constantly.
4. Is cooperative.
5. Does simple chores at home.
6. Begins to take responsibility for actions.
7. Understands units such as a week or month.
8. Knows right and left hand.
9. Still requires parental support but pulls away from overt signs of affection.
C. Parent counseling guidelines for play.
1. Provide family atmosphere conducive to child's emotional development.

2. Give guidance and limits, but avoid humiliating punishment.
3. Provide sufficient exercise to stimulate motor and psychosocial development.
4. Include other children for stimulation during play.
5. Provide books, games, bicycle.

Six to Seven Years

A. Physical and motor development.
   1. Begins growth spurt.
   2. Is very active, impulsive.
   3. Dresses self.
B. Language and social development.
   1. Defines words by use.
   2. Shows more independence in play.
   3. Enjoys group play in small groups.
   4. Begins to accept authority outside home.
   5. Considers ideas of teachers important.
   6. Learns to read.
   7. Knows number combinations to 10.
C. Parent counseling guidelines for play.
   1. Provide opportunity for collecting various items.
   2. Provide imaginary dramatic play: "dress up," school, firemen, soldiers; table games (tiddlywinks, marbles); dolls.

Seven to Eight Years

A. Physical and motor development.
   1. Has fully developed eyes.
   2. Is less impulsive and boisterous in activities.
   3. Frequently develops nervous habits such as nail-biting.
   4. Is more coordinated.
   5. Is capable of fine hand movements.
B. Language and social development.
   1. Is more competitive.
   2. Recognizes differences between his or her home and others.
   3. Wishes to be like his or her friends.
   4. Tells time; knows days of the week.
   5. Shows curiosity about sex differences.
   6. May have periods of shyness.
C. Parent counseling guidelines.
   1. Recognize child's periods of shyness as normal behavior.

2. Give reassurance and understanding if and when nightmares occur.
3. Provide table games and card games; magic tricks; games that develop physical and mental skill.

Eight to Nine Years

A. Physical and motor development.
   1. Exhibits long arms in proportion to body.
   2. Shows good coordination of fine muscles.
   3. Engages in active play.
   4. May begin secondary sex characteristics (females).
   5. Learns to use script.
B. Language and social development.
   1. Is more self-assured in environment.
   2. Likes group projects, clubs.
   3. Has increased modesty.
   4. Recognizes property rights.
   5. Needs help accepting defeat in games.
   6. Begins to have sense of humor.
   7. Through play, learns new ideas and independence: competition, compromise, cooperation, and beginning collaboration.
C. Parent counseling guidelines.
   1. Give child opportunity to obtain adult approval.
   2. Give small household responsibilities.
   3. Answer child's questions regarding sex in simple, honest words.
   4. Do not become overly concerned with common problems such as teasing and quarreling, as they are usually temporary.
   5. Provide sports, books (geography and adventure), erector sets, comics and funny papers.

Nine to Ten Years

A. Physical and motor development.
   1. Shows skill in manual activities because hand-eye coordination is developed.
   2. Exhibits decreased growth in height.
   3. Is very active physically.
   4. Cares completely for own physical needs.
B. Language and social development.
   1. Shows sex differences in play.
   2. Likes to have secrets.
   3. Displays antagonism between the sexes.

4. Grasps easy multiplication and division.

5. Has special friend to confide in.

C. Parent counseling guidelines.

1. Determine cause if lying and stealing occur.

2. Provide parental understanding.

3. Provide opportunity to enroll in clubs and organizations.

4. Provide books, musical instruments, TV, records, practical projects.

Ten to Eleven Years

A. Physical and motor development.

1. Shows onset of major secondary sex characteristics (males).

2. Attempts perfection of physical skills.

B. Language and social development.

1. Enjoys companionship more than play.

2. Needs privacy occasionally.

3. Exhibits increased ability to discuss problems.

4. Has growing capacity for thought and conceptual organization.

5. Sees physical qualities as constant despite changes in size, shape, weight, volume.

6. Shows group conformity.

C. Parent counseling guidelines.

1. Continue sex education and preparation for adolescent body changes.

2. Encourage participation in organized clubs, youth groups.

Eleven to Twelve Years

A. Physical and motor development.

1. Begins puberty; physical changes appear in both males and females.

2. Begins menstruation (females).

3. May require more sleep due to body changes.

B. Social development.

1. Participates in community and school affairs.

2. Tends toward segregation of the sexes.

3. Likes to be alone occasionally.

4. Exhibits interest in world affairs.

5. Comprehends world of possibility and abstraction.

6. Begins to question parental values.

C. Parent counseling guidelines.

1. Provide help in school and sports to channel energy in proper direction.

2. Provide guidance during dependence/independence conflict.

3. Set realistic limits.

4. Give adequate explanation of body changes.

5. Provide special consideration for child who lags behind in physical development.

Table 1. PIAGET'S COGNITIVE DEVELOPMENT

Age	Developmental Level
Infancy to two years	Sensorimotor Development of intellect through sensory-motor apparatus Simple problem-solving
Two to seven years	Preoperational Thought
Two to four years	Preconceptual Phase Use of symbols—language Imitative play to understand the world
Four to seven years	Intuitive Phase Egocentric and stage of "moral realism" Beginning use of symbols for cognition Asks questions
Seven to twelve years	Concrete Operational Thought Wide use of symbols Observes relationships between objects Understands cause and effect Visualizes conclusions
Twelve-plus years	Formal Operational Thought Abstract thinking processes Conceptualization Ability to test hypotheses

EARLY ADOLESCENCE

A. Physical development.

1. Exhibits further development of secondary sex characteristics.

2. Shows poor posture.

3. Exhibits rapid growth and becomes awkward and uncoordinated.

4. Shows changes in body size and development.

B. Social development.
1. Needs social approval of peer group.
2. Strives for independence from family.
3. Has one or two very close friends in peer group.
4. Becomes more interested in opposite sex.
5. Period of upheaval: displays confusion about body image.
6. Must again learn to control strong feelings (love, aggression).

C. Counseling guidelines.
1. Provide adult understanding when adolescent deals with social, intellectual, and moral issues.
2. Allow some financial independence.
3. Provide limits to ensure security.
4. Provide necessary assurance to help adolescent accept changing body image.
5. Show flexibility in adjusting to emotional and erratic mood swings.
6. Be calm and consistent when dealing with an adolescent.

D. Developmental tasks.
1. Finds identity; moves out of role diffusion.
   a. Integrates childhood identifications with basic drives.
   b. Expands concept of social roles.
2. Moves toward heterosexuality.
3. Begins separation from family.
4. Integrates personality.

Table 2. ERIKSON'S STAGES OF PERSONALITY DEVELOPMENT

Stage	Approx. Age	Psychological Crises	Significant Persons	Accomplishments
Infant	0–1	Basic trust vs. mistrust	Mother or maternal figure	Tolerates frustration in small doses Recognizes mother as separate from others and self
Toddler	1–3	Autonomy vs. shame and doubt	Parents	Begins verbal skills Begins acceptance of reality vs. pleasure principle
Preschool	3–6	Initiative vs. guilt	Basic family	Asks many questions Explores own body and environment Differentiates between sexes
School	6–12	Industry vs. inferiority	Neighborhood school	Gains attention by accomplishments Explores things Learns to relate to own sex
Puberty and adolescence	12–?	Identity vs. role diffusion	Peer groups External groups	Moves toward heterosexuality Begins separation from family Integrates personality (altruism, etc.)
Adolescence and young adult	—	Intimacy and solidarity vs. isolation	Partners in friendship, sex	Is able to form lasting relationships with others Learns to be creative and productive

Based on Erikson: *Childhood and Society*

ADOLESCENCE TO YOUNG ADULTHOOD

A. Physical development.
1. Completes sexual development.
2. Exhibits signs of slowing down of body growth.
3. Is capable of reproduction.
4. Shows more energy after growth spurt tapers off.
5. Exhibits increased muscular ability and coordination.
B. Menstruation.
1. Menstruation is the sloughing off of the endometrium that occurs at regular monthly intervals if conception fails to take place. The discharge consists of blood, mucus, and cells, and it usually lasts for four to five days.
2. Menarche—onset of menstruation—usually occurs between the ages of eleven and fourteen.
3. Discomforts associated with menstruation.
   a. Breast tenderness and feeling of fullness.
   b. Tendency toward fatigue.
   c. Temperament and mood changes—because of hormonal influence and decreased levels of estrogen and progesterone.
   d. Discomfort in pelvic area, lower back, and legs.
   e. Retained fluids and weight gain.
4. Abnormalities of menstruation.
   a. Dysmenorrhea (painful menstruation).
      (1) May be caused by psychological factors: tension, anxiety, preconditioning (menstruation is a "curse" or should be painful).
      (2) Physical examination is usually done to rule out organic causes.
   b. Treatment.
      (1) Oral contraceptives—produce anovulatory cycle.
      (2) Mild analgesics such as aspirin.
      (3) Urge client to carry on normal activities to occupy her mind.
      (4) Dysmenorrhea may subside after childbearing.
   c. Amenorrhea (absence of menstrual flow).
      (1) Primary—over the age of seventeen and menstruation has not begun.
         (a) Complete physical necessary to rule out abnormalities.

      (b) Treatment aimed at correction of underlying condition.
      (2) Secondary—occurs after menarche—does not include pregnancy and lactation.
         (a) Causes include psychological upsets or endocrine conditions.
         (b) Evaluation and treatment by physician is necessary.
   d. Menorrhagia (excessive menstrual bleeding)—may be due to endocrine disturbance, tumors, or inflammatory conditions of the uterus.
   e. Metrorrhagia (bleeding between periods)—symptom of disease process, benign tumors, or cancer.
5. Counseling guidelines.
   a. Provide education about the physiology of normal menstruation and correct misinformation.
   b. Provide education about abnormal conditions associated with menstruation—absence of menstruation, bleeding between menstrual periods, etc.
   c. Provide education related to normal hygiene during menstruation.
      (1) Importance of cleanliness.
      (2) Use of perineal pads and tampons.
      (3) Continuance of normal activities.
C. Social development.
1. Is less attached to peers.
2. Shows increased maturity.
3. Exhibits more interdependence with family.
4. Begins romantic love affairs.
5. Increases mastery over biologic drives.
6. Develops more mature relationship with parents.
7. Values fidelity, friendship, cooperation.
8. Begins vocational development.
D. Counseling guidelines.
1. Assist adolescent in vocational choice.
2. Provide safety education, especially regarding driving.
3. Encourage good attitudes toward health in issues of nutrition, drugs, smoking, and drinking.
4. Attempt to understand own (parental) difficulties in accepting transition of adolescent to independence and adulthood.
E. Developmental tasks.
1. Intimacy and solidarity versus isolation.

a. Moves from security of self involvement to insecurity of building intimate relationships with others.

b. Becomes less dependent and more self-sufficient.

2. Able to form lasting relationships with others.
3. Learns to be productive and creative.
4. Handles hormonal changes of developmental period.

ADULTHOOD

Developmental Tasks

A. Achieves goal of generativity versus stagnation or self-absorption.
1. Shows concern for establishing and guiding next generation.
2. Exhibits productiveness, creativity, and an attitude of looking forward to the future.
3. Stagnation results from the refusal to assume power and responsibility of the goals of middle age.
   a. Suffers pervading sense of boredom and impoverishment.
   b. Undergoes but does not resolve midlife crisis.
B. Has relaxed sense of competitiveness.
C. Opens up new interests.
D. Shifts values from physical attractiveness and strength to intellectual abilities.
E. Shows productivity (may be most productive years of one's life).
F. Has more varied and satisfying relationships.
G. Exhibits no significant decline in learning abilities or sexual interests.
H. Shifts sexual interests from physical performance to the individual's total sexuality and need to be loved and touched.
I. Assists next generation to become happy, responsible adults.
J. Achieves mature social and civic responsibility.
K. Accepts and adjusts to physiological changes of middle life.
L. Uses leisure time satisfactorily.
M. Failure to complete developmental tasks may cause the individual to approach old age with resentment and fear.

1. Neurotic symptoms may appear.
2. Increased psychosomatic disorders develop.

Values of Adulthood

A. Becomes more introspective.
B. Shows less concern as to what others think.
C. Identifies self as successful even though all life goals may not be achieved.
D. Shows less concern for outward manifestations of success.
E. Lives more day-to-day and values life more deeply.
F. Has faced one's finiteness and eventual death.

Parenting in Adulthood

A. Characteristics.
1. Tendency toward smaller families.
2. Career-oriented women who limit family size or who do not want children.
3. Early sexual experimentation, necessitating sexual education, contraceptive information.
4. Tendency toward postponement of children.
   a. To complete education.
   b. Economic factors.
5. High divorce rates.
6. Alternate family designs.
   a. Single parenthood.
   b. Communal family.
B. Family planning.
1. General concepts.
   a. Dealing with individuals with particular ideas regarding contraception.
   b. No perfect method of birth control.
   c. Method must be suited to individual.
   d. Individuals involved must be thoroughly counseled on all available methods and how they work—including advantages and disadvantages. This includes not only female but also sexual partner (if available).
   e. Once a method is chosen both parties should be thoroughly instructed in its use.
   f. Individuals involved must be motivated to succeed.
2. Effectiveness depends upon:
   a. Method chosen.
   b. Degree to which couple follows prescribed regimen.

c. Thorough understanding of method.

d. Motivation on part of individuals concerned.

Physiological Changes

Menopause

A. Characteristics.
1. The cessation of menstruation caused by physiologic factors; ovulation no longer occurs.
2. Menopause usually occurs between the ages of forty to fifty.

B. Mechanisms in menopause.
1. Ovaries lose the ability to respond to pituitary stimulation and normal ovarian function ceases.
2. Gradual change due to alteration in hormone production.
    a. Failure to ovulate.
    b. Monthly flow becomes smaller, irregular, and gradually ceases.
3. Menopause is accompanied by changes in reproductive organs—the vagina gradually becomes smaller; uterus, bladder, rectum, and supporting structures lose tone, leading to uterine prolapse, rectocele, and cystocele.
4. Atherosclerosis and osteoporosis are more likely to develop at this time.

Assessment

A. Assess presence of symptoms—varies with individuals and may be mild to severe.

B. Assess feelings of loss as children grow and leave home and aging process continues.

C. Assess presence of physiological symptoms.
1. Hot flashes.
2. Headache.
3. Depression.
4. Insomnia.
5. Weakness.
6. Dizziness.

Implementation

A. Monitor estrogen therapy—usually given on cyclic basis: one pill daily except for five days during the month when medication is not taken.

B. Evaluate need for treatment of psychological problems.

Major Health Problems

A. Heart disease in both male and female.

B. Diabetes.

C. Hypertension.

D. Accidents.

E. Confrontation with the most acute psychological problems of any age group.
1. Depression.
2. Involutional psychosis.

F. Cancer.

Psychosocial Changes

Midlife Crisis

A. A normal stage in the ongoing life cycle in which the middle-aged person reevaluates his or her total life situation in relation to youthful achievements and actual accomplishments.
1. Struggles to maintain physical attractiveness in relation to younger people.
2. Partner or lover critical self-definition.
3. Feels he or she has peaked in ability.
4. Blames environment or others for failure to succeed.
5. Displays increased interest in sexuality.
6. Exhibits competitiveness in career plans.

B. Unresolved crisis.
1. May result in stagnation, boredom, and decreased self-esteem and depression.
2. Age for crisis varies.
    a. Women pass through it between 35 to 40 years old.
    b. Men experience the crisis between 40 to 45 years old.

Major Causes of Psychological Problems

A. Fears losing job.

B. Competition with younger generation.

C. Loss of job.

D. Loss of nurturing functions.

E. Loss of spouse, particularly females. (Forty-five percent of women over sixty-five are widowed.)

F. Realization that person is not going to accomplish some of the things that he or she wanted to do.

G. Changes in body image.

H. Illness.

I. Role change within and outside of family.
J. Fear of approaching old age.
K. Physiological changes.

THE AGED

Developmental Tasks

A. Maintains ego integrity versus despair.
   1. Integrity results when an individual is satisfied with his or her own actions and lifestyle, feels life is meaningful, remains optimistic, and continues to grow.
   2. Despair results from the feeling that he or she has failed and that it is too late to change.
B. Continues a meaningful life after retirement.
C. Adjusts to income level.
D. Makes satisfactory living arrangements with spouse.
E. Adjusts to loss of spouse.
F. Maintains social contact and responsibilities.
G. Faces death realistically.
H. Provides knowledge and wisdom to assist those at other developmental levels to grow and learn.
I. There will be approximately 20 million people over the age of sixty-five in the United States by 1980.

Physiological Changes

A. Decrease in ability to maintain homeostasis.
   1. Decrease in physical strength and endurance.
   2. Decrease in muscular coordination and strength.
B. Changes in bone composition.
   1. Loss of density and increased brittleness.
   2. Spine curvatures increase.
C. Tendency to gain weight.
D. Loss of pigment in hair and elasticity of skin
E. Diminution of sensory faculties.
   1. Vision decreases.
   2. Loss of hearing.
   3. Smell and taste become dull.
   4. Greater sensitivity to temperature changes with low tolerance to cold.
F. Decreased resistance to infection and disease.
G. Degenerative changes in the cardiovascular system.
   1. Heart pump action diminishes.
      2. Blood flow decreases—may be due to fat deposits in arteries.
      3. Vascular changes result in less effective oxygenation.
H. Changes in respiratory system.
   1. Blood flow decreases to lungs: contributes to decrease in function.
   2. Less oxygen diffusion so tolerance is less.
I. Changes in gastrointestinal system.
   1. Absorption function impaired.
      a. Body absorbs less nutrients.
      b. Decrease in gastric enzymes affects absorption.
   2. Peristalsis weakens and constipation is common.
J. Changes in urinary system.
   1. Structural and functional changes occur in kidney through degeneration.
   2. Decreased musculature ability leads to atonic bladder.

Major Health Problems

A. All systems are more vulnerable due to the aging process; degeneration can be affected.
   1. Chronic disease and disability.
   2. Nutritional deprivation.
   3. Sensory impairment: blindness and deafness.
   4. Organic brain changes.
      a. Not all persons become senile.
      b. Most people have memory impairment.
      c. The change is gradual.
B. Impact of disease on aged.
   1. Diseases may be multiple and chronic (over 40 percent have more than one illness concurrently).
   2. Disability results more readily when an aging person becomes ill.
   3. Response to treatment is diminished.
   4. Resistance is lower due to the aging process so person is more susceptible to disease.
   5. The aged have less resistance to stressors: mental, environmental, and physical.
   6. Changes in the neurological system make the aged person more prone to organic brain changes.

Psychosocial Changes

A. Developmental process retrogresses.

1. Exhibits increasing dependency.
2. Concerns focus increasingly on self.
3. Displays narrower interests.
4. Needs tangible evidence of affection.

B. Major fears of the aged.
1. Physical and economic dependency.
2. Chronic illness.
3. Loneliness.
4. Boredom resulting from not being needed.

C. Major problems of the aged.
1. Alteration in living style, i.e., nursing home, moving in with children.
2. Economic deprivation.
   a. Increased cost of living on a fixed income.
   b. Increased need for costly medical care.
3. Chronic disease and disability.
4. Social isolation loneliness.
5. Sensory deprivation (blindness and deafness).
6. Senility, confusion and lack of awareness.
7. Nutritional deprivation.
8. Series of losses, i.e., relationships, friends, family.
9. Loss of physical strength and agility.

D. Sexuality and aging.
1. Older people are sexual beings also.
2. There is no particular age at which a person's sexual functioning ceases.
3. Frequency of genital sexual behavior (intercourse) may tend to decline gradually in later years, but capacity for expression and enjoyment continue far into old age.
4. Touching and companionship are of importance for older people and should be encouraged.

DEATH, DYING, AND GRIEF PROCESS

THE GRIEF PROCESS

Definition: A process that an individual goes through in response to the loss of a significant or loved person. The grieving process follows certain predictable phases—classic description originally done by Dr. Eric Lindeman. The normal grieving process is described by George Engle, M.D., in "Grief and Grieving," *American Journal of Nursing,* September 1964.

A. First response is shock and refusal to believe that the loved one is dead.
1. Displays inability to comprehend the meaning of loss.
2. Attempts to protect self against painful feelings.

B. As awareness increases, the bereaved experiences severe anguish.
1. Crying is common in this stage.
2. Anger directed toward those people or circumstances thought to be responsible.

C. Mourning is the next stage where the work of restitution takes place.
1. Rituals of the funeral help the bereaved accept reality.
2. Support from friends and spiritual guidance comfort the bereaved.

D. Resolution of the loss occurs as the mourner begins to deal with the void.

E. Idealization of the deceased occurs next where only the pleasant memories are remembered.
1. Characterized by the mourner's taking on certain qualities of the deceased.
2. This process takes many months as preoccupation with the deceased diminishes.

F. Outcome of the grief process takes a year or more.
1. Indications of successful outcome are when the mourner remembers both the pleasant and unpleasant memories.

2. Eventual outcome influenced by:
   a. Importance of the deceased in the life of mourner.
   b. The degree of dependence in the relationship.
   c. The amount of ambivalence toward the deceased.
   d. The more hostile the feelings that exist, the more guilt that interferes with the grieving process.
   e. Age of both mourner and deceased.
   f. Death of a child is more difficult to resolve than that of an aged loved one.
   g. Number and nature of previous grief experiences.
   h. Degree of preparation for the loss.

Counseling Guidelines

A. Recognize that grief is a syndrome with somatic and psychological symptomatology.
   1. Weeping, complaints of fatigue, digestive disturbance, and insomnia.
   2. Guilt, anger, and irritability.
   3. Restless, but unable to initiate meaningful activity.
   4. Depression and agitation.
B. Be prepared to support the family as they learn of the death.
   1. Know the general response to death by recognizing the stages of the grief process.
   2. Understand that the behavior of the mourner may be unstable and disturbed.
C. Use therapeutic communication techniques.
   1. Encourage the mourner to express feelings, especially tears.
   2. Attempt to meet the needs of the mourner for privacy, information, and support.
   3. Show respect for the religious and social customs of the family.

DEATH AND DYING

Impact of Dying Process for Adults

A. Physical symptoms of dying.
   1. Cardiovascular collapse.
   2. Renal failure.

3. Decreased physical and mental capacity.
   4. Gradual loss of consciousness.
B. Stages of dying.
   1. The dying process is ably protrayed in *Death and Dying,* by Elisabeth Kübler-Ross, New York, Macmillan Publishing Company, Inc., 1970.
   2. Individual is stunned at the knowledge he or she is dying and denies it.
   3. Anger and resentment usually follow as the individual questions, "Why me?"
   4. With the beginning of acceptance of impending death comes the bargaining stage, that is, bargaining for time to complete some situation in his or her life.
   5. Full acknowledgment usually brings depression; individual begins to work through feelings and to withdraw from life and relationships.
   6. Final stage is full acceptance and preparation for death.
   7. Throughout the dying process, hope is an important element that should be supported but not reinforced unrealistically.
C. Psychosocial clinical manifestations.
   1. Depression and withdrawal.
   2. Fear and anxiety.
   3. Focus is internal.
   4. Agitation and restlessness.

The Concept of Death in the Aging Population

A. In American culture, death is very distasteful.
B. The elderly may see death as an end to suffering and loneliness.
C. Death is not feared if the person has lived a long and fulfilled life, having completed all developmental tasks.
D. Religious beliefs and/or philosophy of life important.

Death and Children

A. Understanding of death for the young child.
   1. Death is viewed as a temporary separation from parents, sometimes viewed synonymously with sleep.

2. Child may express fear of pain and wish to avoid it.
3. Child's awareness is lessened by physical symptoms if death comes acutely.
4. Gradual terminal illness may simulate the adult process: depression, withdrawal, fearfulness, and anxiety.

B. Older children's concerns.
1. Death is identified as a "person" to be avoided.
2. Child may ask directly if he or she is going to die.
3. Concerns center around fear of pain, fear of being left alone, and fear of leaving parents and friends.

C. Adolescent concerns.
1. Death is recognized as irreversible and inevitable.
2. Adolescent often avoids talking about impending death, and staff may enter into this "conspiracy of silence."
3. Adolescents have more understanding of death than adults tend to realize.

Nursing Management for Dying Client

Nursing Management of the Adult

A. Minimize physical discomfort.
1. Attend to all physical needs.
2. Make client as comfortable as possible.

B. Recognize crisis situation.
1. Observe for changes in client's condition.
2. Support client.

C. Be prepared to give the dying client the emotional support needed.

D. Encourage communication.
1. Allow client to express feelings, to talk, or to cry.
2. Pick up cues that client wants to talk, especially about fears.
3. Be available to form a relationship with client.
4. Communicate honestly.

E. Prepare and support the family for their impending loss.

F. Understand the grieving process of client and family.

Nursing Management for Dying Child

A. Always elicit the child's understanding of death before discussing it.

B. Before discussing death with child, discuss it with parents.

C. Parental reactions include the continuum of grief process and stages of dying.
1. Reactions depend on previous experience with loss.
2. Reactions also depend on relationship with the child and circumstances of illness or injury.
3. Reactions depend on degree of guilt felt by parents.

D. Assist parents in expressing their fears, concerns, and grief so that they may be more supportive to the child.

E. Assist parents in understanding siblings' possible reactions to a terminally ill child.
1. Guilt: belief that they caused the problem or illness.
2. Jealousy: demand for equal attention from the parents.
3. Anger: feelings of being left behind.

HUMAN SEXUALITY

Overview of Human Sexuality

A. Biological sexuality is determined at conception.
   1. Male sperm contributes an X or a Y chromosome.
   2. Female ovum has an X chromosome.
   3. Fertilization results in either an XX (female) or an XY (male).
B. Preparation for adult sexuality originates in the sexual role development of the child.
   1. Significant differences between male and female infants are observable even at birth.
   2. Biological changes are minimal during childhood, but parenting strongly influences a child's behavior and sexual role development.
   3. Anatomical and physiological changes occur during adolescence which establish biological sexual maturation.
C. Human sexuality pervades the whole of an individual's life.
   1. More than a sum of isolated physical acts.
   2. Functions as a purposeful influence in human nature and behavior.
   3. Observable in everyday life in endless variations.
D. Each society develops a set of normative behaviors, attitudes, and values in respect to sexuality which are considered "right" and "wrong" by individuals.
E. Freud described the bisexual (androgynous) nature of the person.
   1. Each person has components of maleness-femaleness, masculinity-femininity, and heterosexuality-homosexuality.
   2. These components are physiological and psychological in nature.
   3. All components influence an individual's sexuality and sexual behavior.
F. Gender identity (identified at birth) refers to whether a person is male or female.
   1. Cases of "ambiguous genitalia" are rare (1/3000 births), and require special care for the infant and parents.
   2. Ambiguous genitalia is a clinical label similar to slang term "morphodite," or biological term "hermaphrodite."
G. Sexual object choice is the selection of a mode of outlet for sexual desire, usually with another person.
   1. Generally occurs during adolescence and beyond.
   2. Includes heterosexuality, homosexuality, bisexuality, celibacy, and narcissism/onanism.
H. Sexual object choice has strong influence on a person's lifestyle.
   1. Individual must establish patterns of intimacy and sexual behavior that are acceptable to self, to significant others, and to society to a certain extent.
   2. Psychological demands and expectations throughout life influence an individual's sexual interest, activity, and functional capacity.
   3. Sexual object choice can affect a person's choices in life such as whether to be a parent, where to live, and what career to maintain.

Sexual Behavior

A. Sexual behavior is a composite of developed patterns of intimacy, psychological demands and expectations, and sexual object choice.
   1. Can be genital (sexual intercourse), intimate (holding, hugging), or social (dating, choice of clothing).
   2. Beyond the obvious examples, one never stops "behaving sexually."
   3. Dress, communication, and activity are all expressions of sexuality.
   4. Every person exhibits sexual behavior continually; no one is sexless.
B. "Transvestite" and "transsexual" are two terms that often cause confusion and need definition and differentiation.
   1. Transvestite refers to one who enjoys wearing clothing of the opposite sex; may or may not be homosexual.
   2. Transsexual is a person who chooses sexual reassignment: a complex physical (surgical), psychological, and social process of taking on the gender identity, sex role, sexual object choice, and sexual behavior of the opposite sex.

C. Sexuality, although difficult to define, is pervasive from birth to death, and nurses need to look beyond the framework of reproduction and procreation to understand the influence of sexuality on clients' health and illness.

Characteristics

A. Difficult to define precisely, human sexuality is considered to be a pervasive life force and includes a person's total feelings, attitudes, and behavior.
B. It is related to gender identity, sex-role identity, and sexual motivation.
C. Touching, intimacy, and companionship are factors that have unique meaning for each person's sexuality.
D. Sex role describes whether a person assumes masculine or feminine behaviors, usually a combination of both.
   1. This role generally considered to be fairly established by age five.
   2. Usually referred to by the concepts boy/girl and man/woman.

Assessment

A. If necessary, obtain a full sexual history.
B. Include consideration of each client's sexuality in assessing health and illness status.
C. Assess primary sexual concerns.
D. Listen for nonverbal cues of sexual problems.
E. Elicit verbalization of underlying concerns.
F. Identify major problem area.
   1. Be aware that most common problem is the need for sexual recognition of each client.
   2. Allow sexual expression within appropriate limits.
   3. Assess whether client has correct information or misconceptions about sexuality.
   4. Assess the relationship between each client's health problems and his or her sexuality needs.

Planning and Analysis

A. Client feels free and comfortable enough to verbally express concerns.
B. Client understands effect of illness on sexual behavior.
C. Client finds resolution of problem.

Implementation

A. Provide sex education and counseling.
   1. Clients consider nurses to be experts in sexuality.
   2. Intervention requires knowledge and skill.
   3. Nurses need to know referral sources for interventions beyond their ability.
B. Give clients "permission" or acceptance to maintain sexuality and sexual behavior.
C. Be aware of the effect of medications on clients' sexuality and sexual functioning.
   1. Oral contraceptives are considered by some to have played a major role in creating a sense of sexual freedom in contemporary society.
   2. Drugs that decrease sexual drive or potency may act directly on the physiological mechanisms or may decrease interest through a depressant effect on the central nervous system.
   3. Drugs with an adverse effect on sexual activity include antihypertensive drugs, antidepressants, antihistamines, antispasmodics, sedatives and tranquilizers, ethyl alcohol, and some hormone preparations and steroids.
   4. There are no known drugs that specifically increase libido or sexual performance; those that seem to enhance sexual behavior do so indirectly through transient relaxation of tensions, alleviation of discomfort, or release of inhibitions.
   5. Long-term use of any drug or medicine will likely have a negative effect on sexual interest and capability.
D. Be aware of the problems to which nursing personnel should direct themselves in relation to the area of human sexuality.
   1. Attitudes.
      a. Nurses should increase their self-awareness of their own attitudes and the effect of these attitudes on the sexual health care of their clients.
      b. Nurses should suppress negative biases and prejudices and/or make appropriate referrals when they cannot give effective sexual health care.
   2. Knowledge.
      a. May have to be actively sought although nursing programs are increasing the sexuality content in their curricula.
      b. Also available through books, journal articles, classes and workshops, and preparation for sexuality therapy on the graduate level.

3. Skills.
  a. Primary skills needed are interpersonal techniques such as therapeutic communication, interviewing, and teaching.
  b. As with any skill, practice is needed for proficiency in sexual-history taking, education, and counseling.

Evaluation

A. Client freely expresses concerns related to sexuality.
B. Client verbalizes understanding of the effect of his or her illness on sexual behavior and functioning.
C. Client resolves problem and learns to live with decision of sexual behavior.

Common Problems and Implications for Nursing

A. Masturbation.
  1. A common sexual outlet for many people.
  2. For clients requiring long-term care, masturbation may be only means for gratifying sexual needs.
  3. Nurses frequently react negatively to any type of masturbatory activity, especially by male clients.
  4. Clients should be allowed privacy; if nurse walks in on a client masturbating, he or she should leave with an apology for having intruded on the client's privacy.
  5. Frequent or inappropriate masturbation may be harmful to the client's health.
    a. Nurse should use team planning to identify what need the client is attempting to meet.
    b. Limits need to be set to protect client and other clients if behavior is inappropriate.
B. Homosexuality
  1. Homosexuality is accepted by many as a viable life style.
  2. Nurses have tended to have negative attitudes and incorrect knowledge about homosexuality.
  3. A client's homosexual (gay) life style should be accepted and respected.
  4. As with any client, visitors should be encouraged as appropriate for the health/illness status, and these people should not be embarrassed or ridiculed.

5. For chronically ill clients, such as in a nursing home, it is essential that sexuality needs be considered in the total care plan and special efforts be made to have these needs met.
D. Inappropriate sexual behavior.
  1. Difficult to precisely define "inappropriate" sexual behavior.
  2. Sometimes sexual behavior is in reaction to unintentional "seductive" behavior of nurses.
  3. Specific nursing interventions.
    a. Set limits to unacceptable behavior immediately.
    b. Interact without rejecting client.
    c. Help client express feelings in an appropriate manner.
    d. Teach alternative behaviors that are acceptable.
    e. Provide acceptable outlets to sexual feelings.
E. Venereal disease.
  1. Based on reported cases, the incidence of gonorrhea and syphilis is increasing slowly.
  2. Both syphilis and gonorrhea can be cured with appropriate antibiotic therapy. (Recently there has occurred a strain of syphilis resistant to antibiotic therapy, so prevention is an important teaching concept.)
  3. Treatment and care should be given without stigma.
  4. Case finding and treatment are still very difficult, especially for adolescents who may need parental consent to obtain health services.
F. Contraception.
  1. Nurses are considered experts on forms of birth control.
  2. Nurses should be familiar with different methods and relative effectiveness of each one.
  3. Clients should be assisted to make their own choices as to whether to use contraception and what method is best for them.
  4. More detailed outline of contraception appears in maternity chapter.
G. Therapeutic abortion.
  1. Clients need information about resources for and procedures of therapeutic abortions.
  2. Clients should be given nonjudgmental assistance and support in decision-making process.
  3. If nurse cannot in good conscience assist the client, referral should be made to someone who can.

4. More detailed outline of abortion appears in maternity chapter.

H. Rape.

1. Rape is basically an act of violence and is only secondarily a sex act.

2. Treatment should consist of both medical and psychological intervention.

3. Sexual assault can have a long-term impact on the victim.

4. Victims may need encouragement and support to report rape occurrences to authorities.

5. Female nurses especially can play a valuable role in giving assistance and support to female rape victims.

6. Many communities have "hot-lines" that offer telephone information and crisis counseling to victims of sexual assault and to professionals.

I. Child sexual abuse.

1. There is only a beginning awareness of this problem area.

2. Most child sexual abuse involves a male adult and female child, but male children can also be victims of female or male sexual abusers.

3. The child may need special protection or temporary placement outside the home, but often the family unit can be maintained.

4. Child sexual abuse is a form of child abuse, and nurses should know local regulations and procedures for case finding and reporting.

J. Sexuality and disability.

1. Physically and developmentally disabled persons are sexual beings also.

2. Developmentally disabled persons should be given sexuality education and counseling in preparation for responsible sexual expression and behavior.

3. After spinal cord injury, the level of the lesion and degree of interruption of nerve impulses influence sexual functioning; adaptation of previous sexual practices may be needed after the injury.

4. Fertility and the ability to bear children are usually not compromised in women with spinal cord injury.

5. Nurses working with disabled clients must make special effort to include sexuality in total health care and services.

2

NUTRITION
AND
PHARMACOLOGY

This chapter presents nutrition and pharmacology as they relate to nursing. These subjects play important roles throughout the health care process. The nutrition section reviews general nutritional concepts and emphasizes therapeutic diet management. The pharmacology section provides the reader with an overview of drugs and their administration.

Current trends in holistic health have increased the public awareness of diets and health supplements. This interest continues to carry throughout the health care field. Another trend with important implications for nurses is the frequency of malpractice suits throughout the medical and nursing profession. It is essential that nurses are sufficiently knowledgeable regarding pharmacology for the protection of both their clients and themselves.

NUTRITION

Nutrition is the nourishment of the body by food. Essential nutrients, necessary for growth and development through the life cycle, are carbohydrates, fats, proteins, vitamins, minerals, and water. When these are supplied to the body in proper balance, the body utilizes them for energy, growth and development, tissue repair, and regulation and maintenance of body processes.

ESSENTIAL NUTRIENTS

Carbohydrates

A. Carbohydrates are the chief source of energy and contain carbon, hydrogen, and oxygen.
   1. Carbohydrates include sugars, starches, and cellulose.
   2. Simple sugars, such as fruit sugar, are easily digested.
   3. Starches, which are more complex, require more sophisticated enzyme processes to be reduced to glucose.
   4. Glucose, which is converted sugar or starch, appears in the body as blood sugar.
      a. It is "burned" as fuel by the tissues.
      b. Some glucose is processed by the liver, converted to glycogen, and stored by the liver for later use.
B. Ingesting too many carbohydrates is unhealthy.
   1. Too many carbohydrates crowd out other important foods.
   2. They prevent the body from receiving the necessary nutrients for healthy maintenance.
C. Too few carbohydrates are also unhealthy.
   1. Too few carbohydrates lead to loss of energy, depression, ketosis.
   2. They also lead to a breakdown of body protein.
D. The amount and kind of carbohydrates that should be consumed for optimal health are determined by several factors.

   1. Differences in body structure.
   2. Energy expenditure.
   3. Basal metabolism rate.
   4. General health status.

Fats

A. Fats or lipids are the second important group of nutrients.
   1. They provide energy.
   2. When oxidized, they are the most concentrated sources of energy.
   3. They furnish the calories necessary for survival.
B. Fats also act as carriers for the fat-soluble vitamins, A, D, E, and K.
C. Consuming too much fat is unhealthy.
   1. Too much fat leads to weight problems.
   2. It causes poor metabolism of food products because the digestive and absorption processes are affected.
D. Fatty acids are the basic components of fat and comprise two main groups.
   1. Saturated fatty acids usually come from animal sources.
   2. Unsaturated fatty acids primarily come from vegetables, nuts, or seed sources.
      a. This group contains three essential fatty acids.
      b. These acids are called "essential" because they are necessary to prevent a specific deficiency disease.
      c. The body cannot manufacture these acids. They are obtained only from the diet.
      d. These acids are called linoleic acid, arachidonic acid, and linolenic acid.
      e. A deficiency in this group would lead to skin problems, illness, and unhealthy blood and arteries.

Proteins

A. Proteins are complex organic compounds that contain amino acids.
B. Protein is critical to all aspects of growth and development of body tissues.
C. This substance is necessary for the building of muscles, blood skin, internal organs, hormones, and enzymes.

D. Protein is also a source of energy.
  1. When there is insufficient carbohydrate or fat in the diet, protein is burned.
  2. When protein is spared, it is either used for tissue repair and maintenance or converted by the liver and stored as fat.
E. When proteins are digested and broken down, they form 22 amino acids.
  1. Amino acids are absorbed from the intestine into the bloodstream.
  2. They are carried to the liver for synthesis into the tissues and organs of the body.
F. Amino acids are the chemical basis for life, and if just one is missing, protein synthesis will decrease or even stop.
G. All but eight can be produced by the body.
  1. These eight must be obtained from the diet.
  2. If all eight are present in a particular food, the food is a "complete protein."
  3. Foods that lack one or more are called "incomplete proteins."
  4. Most meat and dairy products are complete proteins.
  5. Most vegetables and fruits are incomplete proteins.
  6. When several incomplete proteins are ingested, they should be combined carefully so that the result will be a balance yielding complete protein. For example, the combination of beans and rice is a complete protein food.
H. The National Research Council recommends that 0.42 grams of protein be consumed per day per 0.4 kg of body weight.
  1. Recent research shows that this amount can be decreased by about one-third without negative results.
  2. As long as the essential amino acids are included in the diet, the total grams of protein can be reduced.
I. Protein deficiency can affect the entire body—organs, tissues, skin, and muscles, as well as certain body processes.

Water

A. While not specifically a nutrient, water is essential for survival.
  1. Water is involved in every body process from digestion and absorption to excretion.
  2. It is a major portion of circulation and is the transporter of nutrients throughout the body.
B. Body water performs three major functions.
  1. Water gives form to the body, comprising from 50 to 75 percent of the body mass.
  2. It provides the necessary environment for cell metabolism.
  3. It maintains a stable body temperature.
C. Almost all foods contain water that is absorbed by the body.
D. The average adult body contains 59 liters of water and loses about 3 liters a day.
  1. If a person suffers severe water depletion, dehydration and salt depletion can result and can eventually lead to death.
  2. A person can survive longer without food than without water.

Vitamins

A. Vitamins are organic food substances and are essential in small amounts for growth, maintenance, and the functioning of body processes.
B. Vitamins are found only in living things—plants and animals—and usually cannot be synthesized by the human body.
C. Vitamins can be grouped according to the substance in which they are soluble.
D. The fat-soluble group includes vitamins A, D, E, and K.
E. The water-soluble vitamins include the B-complex vitamins, vitamin C, and the bioflavonoids.
F. Vitamins have no caloric value, but they are as necessary to the body as any other basic nutrient.
  1. Currently, there are about 20 substances identified as vitamins.
  2. Recent research is concerned with identifying even more of these substances since they are so essential to survival.
G. The most commonly used are the listings of the Recommended Dietary Allowances (RDA), based on standards established by the National Academy of Sciences.

Table 1. FOODS RICH IN FAT- AND WATER-SOLUBLE VITAMINS

Foods rich in fat-soluble vitamins

Vitamin A—liver, egg yolk, whole milk, butter, fortified margarine, green and yellow vegetables, fruits

Vitamin D—fortified milk and margarine, fish oils

Vitamin E—vegetable oils and green vegetables

Vitamin K—egg yolk, leafy green vegetables, liver, cheese

Foods rich in water-soluable vitamins

Vitamin C—citrus fruits, tomatoes, broccoli, cabbage

Thiamine (B_1)—lean meat such as beef, pork, liver; whole grain cereals and legumes

Riboflavin (B_2)—milk, organ meats, enriched grains

Niacin—meat, beans, peas, peanuts, enriched grains

Pyridoxine (B_6)—yeast, wheat, corn, meats, liver, and kidney

Cobalamin (B_{12})—lean meat, liver, kidney

Folic acid—leafy green vegetables, eggs, liver

Minerals

A. Minerals are inorganic substances, widely prevalent in nature, and essential for metabolic processes.

B. Minerals are grouped according to the amount found in the body.

C. Major minerals include calcium, magnesium, sodium, potassium, phosphorus, sulfur, and chlorine, all of which have a known function in the body.

D. Trace minerals are iron, copper, iodine, manganese, cobalt, zinc, and molybdenum and their function in the body remains unclear.

E. There remains another group of trace minerals found in scanty amounts in the body and whose function is also unclear.

F. Minerals form 60 to 90 percent of all inorganic material in the body, and are found in bones, teeth, soft tissue, muscle, blood, and nerve cells.

G. Minerals act on organs and in metabolic processes.

1. They serve as catalysts for many reactions such as controlling muscle responses, maintaining the nervous system, and regulating acid-base balance.

2. They assist in transmitting messages, maintaining cardiac stability, and regulating the metabolism and absorption of other nutrients.

H. Even though they are considered separately, all minerals work synergistically with other minerals, and their actions are interrelated.

1. A deficiency in one mineral will affect the action of others in the body.

2. Adequate minerals must be ingested because a mineral deficiency can result in severe illness.

3. Excessive amounts of minerals can throw the body out of balance.

I. Adequate diet can supply sufficient minerals.

Table 2. ESSENTIAL BODY NUTRIENTS

Carbohydrates	Monosaccharides
	  Glucose, fructose, galactose
	Disaccharides
	  Sucrose, lactose, maltose
	Polysaccharides
	  Starch, dextrin, glycogen, cellulose, hemicellulose

Fats	Linoleic acid, linolenic acid, arachidonic acid
Proteins	Amino acids Phenylalanine, lysine, isoleucine, leucine, methionine, valine, tryptophan, threonine

Vitamins	Fat-soluble
	  Vitamins A, D, E, and K
	Water-soluble
	  Vitamins B_1, B_2, B_6, B_{12}, niacin, pantothenic acid, folacin, biotin, choline, mesoinositol, para-aminobenzoic acid, and vitamin C

Minerals	Major elements Calcium, chlorine, iron, magnesium, phosphorus, potassium, sodium, sulfur Trace elements
Water	

ASSIMILATION OF NUTRIENTS

Gastrointestinal Tract

A. The main functions of the gastrointestinal system consist of the following.
1. Secretion of enzymes and electrolytes to break down raw materials that are ingested.
2. Movement of ingested products through the system.
3. Complete digestion of nutrients.
4. Absorption of nutrients into the blood.
5. Storage of nutrients.
6. Excretion of the end products of digestion.
B. When nutrients reach the stomach, both mechanical and chemical digestive processes occur.
1. Nutrients are churned, and peristaltic waves move the material through the stomach.
2. At intervals, with relaxation of the pyloric sphincter, they move into the duodenum.
3. This chemical action creates hydrochloric acid, which provides a medium for pepsin to split protein into proteoses and peptones.
4. The digestive process produces other chemical actions.
   a. Lipase, a fat-splitting enzyme.
   b. Rennin, an enzyme that coagulates the protein of milk.
   c. The intrinsic factor, which acts on certain good components to form the antianemic factor.
C. Nutrients then move into the duodenum and the jejunum.
1. Intestinal juices provide a large number of enzymes.
   a. These break down protein into amino acids.
   b. They form and convert maltase to glucose.
   c. They split nucleic acids into nucleotides.
2. The large intestine provides for the absorption of nutrients and the elimination of waste products.
   a. Vitamins K and B_{12}, riboflavin, and thiamin are formed.
   b. Water is absorbed from the fecal mass.

The Accessory Organs

A. The accessory organs of the gastrointestinal tract play an important role in the utilization of nutrients.
B. The liver plays a major role in the metabolism of carbohydrates, fats, and proteins.
1. Liver converts glucose to glycogen and stores it.
2. It reconverts glycogen to glucose when the body requires higher blood sugar.
3. The process of releasing carbohydrates (end products) into the bloodstream is called glycogenolysis.
4. Fats are metabolized through the process of oxidation of fatty acids and the formation of acetoacetic acid.
5. Lipoproteins, cholesterol, and phospholipids are formed, and carbohydrates and protein are converted to fats.
6. Proteins are metabolized in the liver, and deamination of amino acids takes place.
7. The formation of urea and plasma proteins is completed.
8. The interconversions of amino acids and other compounds occur in the liver.
C. The gallbladder's primary function is to act as a reservoir for bile.
1. Bile emulsifies fats through constant secretion.
2. Secretion rate is 500 to 1000 ml every 24 hours.
D. The pancreas secretes pancreatic juices that contain enzymes for the digestion of carbohydrates, fats, and proteins.
1. Enzymes are secreted as inactive precursors that do not become active until secreted into the intestine.
2. In the intestine, the enzyme trypsin acts on proteins to produce peptones, peptides, and amino acids.
3. Pancreatic amylase acts on carbohydrates to produce disaccharides.
4. Pancreatic lipase acts on fats to produce glycerol and fatty acids.

NUTRITIONAL CONCEPTS

Normal and Therapeutic Nutrition

A. Normal nutrition.
1. A guide for determining adequate nutrition is the U.S. Department of Agriculture recommended daily dietary allowances (see Appendix 1).

a. The guide is scientifically designed for the maintenance of healthy people in the United States.

b. The values of the caloric and nutrient requirements given in the guide are used in assessing nutritional states.

c. Stress periods in the life cycle, which require alterations in the allowances, should be considered during the planning of menus.

2. The basic four food groups are described in *A Daily Food Guide: the Basic Four* (see Appendix 3).

a. Choices in four food groups are offered to meet the nutrient recommendations during the life cycle. (Caloric requirement is not included.)

b. Basic nutrients in each food group should be related to dietary needs during the life cycle when menus are planned for each age group.

Table 3. RECOMMENDED NUTRIENT REQUIREMENTS

Total calories
2800 for tissue repair; 6000 for extensive repair

Protein
50 to 75 g/day early in postoperative period.
100 to 200 g/day if needed for new tissue synthesis.

CHO—sufficient in quantity to meet calorie needs and allow protein to be used for tissue repair

Fat—not excessive as it leads to poor tissue healing and susceptibility to infection

Vitamins
Vitamin C—up to 1 g/day
Vitamin B—increased above normal
Vitamin K—normal amounts

B. Therapeutic nutrition.

1. The therapeutic or prescription diet is a modification of the nutritional needs based on the disease condition and/or the excess or deficit nutrition state.

2. Combination diets, which include alterations in minerals, vitamins, proteins, carbohydrates, and fats, as well as fluid and texture, are prescribed in therapeutic nutrition.

3. Although not all such diets will be included in this review, study of the selected diet concepts will enable you to combine two or more diets when necessary.

C. Normal and therapeutic nutrition considerations.

1. Cultural, socioeconomic, and psychological influences, as well as physiological requirements, must be considered for effective nutrition.

2. In any given situation, the nutrition requirements must be considered within the context of the bio-psycho-social needs of an individual.

THERAPEUTIC DIET MANAGEMENT

Nutritional Problems in the Hospital

A. Nutrition is frequently neglected as a viable component of client management.

B. For clients who seem to be stable on admission and give no history of nutritionally related food problems, the usual hospital diet is adequate.

1. These clients must be reassessed periodically to prevent nutritional problems from developing.

2. A periodical assessment is especially important for clients hospitalized for a long period of time.

3. Studies conducted at various medical centers support the claim that clients become more malnourished the longer they remain in a hospital.

C. For clients identified as having a nutritional problem, a client care plan must be developed.

1. First, cause of depletion must be determined.

2. Research indicates that poor food intake is the leading cause of malnutrition.

3. Reasons for poor food intake include the following.

a. The client may feel fear, anxiety, or depression prior to or during hospitalization.

b. Some clients may not be capable of feeding themselves or may have poor fitting dentures.

c. Treatment and therapy may limit the capability of a client to eat or interfere with a client's appetite.

d. Although the desire for food is present, shortly after eating a certain food, a client may have cramps, pain, gas, or diarrhea or feel nauseous and/or vomits.

D. As clients become more and more malnourished, they lose the ability to handle foodstuffs metabolically.

1. As intake decreases below nutritional requirements, the body cannot generate the epithelium of the gastrointestinal tract from the crypt cells.

2. The villi and microvilli needed to metabolize and absorb food flatten and become ineffective.

3. This condition leads to malabsorption, with resulting malnutrition.

Instituting Therapeutic Regimens

A. Institute therapeutic procedures that meet the needs of the client.

B. Evaluate the status of the client's gastrointestinal tract to determine if modifications in nutrients are necessary.

1. Can the client split intact protein into the peptides and amino acids needed for absorption?

2. Can the client tolerate the osmotic load of monosaccharides or disaccharides?

3. Is the client fat intolerant, or does the client need special fat? Is the client lactose intolerant?

C. Check that therapeutic diet is ordered.

D. Be aware of compliance by the client.

1. The nurse can best determine the client's actual intake.

2. The nurse should ensure that the client is not receiving inappropriate foods from other sources.

3. The nurse should check that the client is actually eating the foods prescribed.

E. If the prescribed diet is not meeting the client's needs, consider an alternative method of feeding.

1. If oral feedings prove inadequate, then alternative methods such as nasogastric, nasoduodenal, or nasojejunal tube feeding should be considered.

2. A variety of delivery systems and methods of enteral feeding are now available for adequate care of the client.

3. When other methods have failed, parenteral nutrition may be the management of choice.

a. This can be administered peripherally, using isotonic concentrations of glucose, crystalline amino acids, and fats.

b. It can be administered through a central, high-flow vein in which hypertonic glucose is given, supplemented with crystalline amino acids, fats, electrolytes, vitamins, and trace elements.

F. Be alert to clients' nutritional needs so that no client becomes or remains malnourished nor develops any kind of nutritional problem.

1. As a health professional, the nurse is responsible for meeting the client's needs.

2. Among these needs are adequate nutritional requirements to maintain status and to be able to successfully deal with or overcome the medical problems for which the client is being treated.

Providing Appropriate Nutrition

Assessment

A. Appropriate dietary order.

B. Nutritional needs of client.

C. Sociocultural orientation of client.

D. Diet history, eating habits, and food preferences of client.

E. Ability of client to comply with diet regime.

F. Analysis of appropriate diagnostic tests.

G. Alterations in health status that indicate need for therapeutic vs. regular diet.

H. Status of gastrointestinal tract, including digestion and/or absorption.

1. Ability of the client to split intact protein into peptides and amino acids needed for absorption.

2. Ability of the client to tolerate osmotic load of monosaccharides or disaccharides.

3. Ability of the client to tolerate lactose.

4. Assessment of client's fluid intake needs.

I. Recommended daily dietary allowances.

J. Essential body nutrients.

Planning and Analysis

A. Diet is nutritious and appropriate for the client's needs.
B. The client complies with the diet.
C. Diet is tolerated physiologically and emotionally by the client.

Implementation

A. Assist physician in determining a diet appropriate for the client's needs.
B. Elicit food preferences of the client.
C. Send request to the diet kitchen for the specific diet and keep diet sheets or diet rands up to date.
D. Check all diet trays before serving to ensure the diet provided is the one ordered.
E. Ensure that hot food is hot and cold food is cold.
F. Keep food trays attractive. Avoid spilling liquids on tray.
G. Position the client in a chair or up in bed (unless otherwise ordered) to assist in feeding.
H. Assist the client with cutting meat and opening milk cartons as needed.
I. Feed the client if necessary.

Evaluation

A. Client receives adequate diet, fluids, electrolytes, vitamins, minerals, and trace elements.
B. Reasonable compliance to diet is maintained.
C. Diet is tolerated physiologically and emotionally by client.
D. Client is able to assimilate foods metabolically.

Nutritional Guidelines for Managing Clients

A. An adequate diet must include carbohydrates, fats, proteins, vitamins and minerals.
  1. Carbohydrates are the chief source of energy, and diets not sufficient in carbohydrates lead to a low energy level, use of protein for energy, and ketosis.
  2. Fats provide the most concentrated source of energy and are carriers for fat-soluble vitamins.
  3. Proteins are essential for building body tissue and are necessary for tissue repair.
  4. Vitamins are essential for growth, maintenance, and functioning of body processes.
  5. Minerals are essential for metabolic processes.

B. Digestion takes place throughout the gastrointestinal tract.
  1. The gastrointestinal system breaks down raw materials through the secretion of enzymes and electrolytes.
  2. Mechanical and chemical digestive processes are necessary for nutritional synthesis.
  3. Nutrients are absorbed through the large intestine.
  4. The liver plays a major role in nutritional metabolism.

C. Nutritional needs are based on a client's disease condition and excess or deficit of a nutritional state.
  1. Therapeutic diets are used to alter health status.
  2. Combination diets, which include alteration of all the major nutrients, are prescribed for certain disease conditions.

D. Alternative methods of providing nutrients must be instituted when clients are unable to ingest or assimilate foods orally.
  1. Enteral feedings provide life-sustaining nutrients when other oral methods cannot be utilized.
  2. Parenteral nutrition may be administered peripherally, using isotonic concentrations, or centrally with intravenous catheter placement.

Administering Therapeutic Diets

Assessment

A. Total condition of client—physical, emotional, and mental status.
B. Appropriateness of prescribed therapeutic diet as related to altered state of health.
C. Ability of client to tolerate diet.
D. Mental state of client in regard to compliance to diet regimen.
E. Refer to general assessment steps in maintaining normal nutritional status (see Appendix 2).

Planning and Analysis

A. Prescribed diet is appropriate for the client's needs.
B. Diet is tolerated by client.
C. Client complies with diet regimen.

Implementation

Carbohydrates

A. Hypoglycemia occurs when the supply of insulin is so high that most of the glucose moves from the blood into the cells and leaves an inadequate supply for the brain.
  1. Foods prescribed are high protein, high fat, and moderate-complex carbohydrates.
  2. Foods not allowed are simple carbohydrates, for example, sugar, syrup, candy. Complex carbohydrates or starches have higher nutritional values and more fiber.

B. A diabetic diet modifies the insulin disorder and controls sugar intake.
  1. Foods included on the diet are usually found on the food exchange list.
  2. Foods not allowed are refined sugars.

Diabetic Guidelines

A. Diet is the cornerstone of disease management.
  1. Normal weight must be maintained and may dramatically reduce symptoms.
  2. Diet together with insulin supplement or oral medication and exercise complete the regimen.
  3. Goal of dietary therapy is to have a well-balanced diet with controlled calories.
  4. Diabetics do not have to give up their favorite foods; they must learn the amounts that are allowed and substitutions permitted.

B. Calories divided into:
  Carbohydrate 45–55% or 50%
  Fat 30–35% or 30%
  Protein 15–20% or 20%

C. Level of activity must be assessed to determine energy requirements.
  1. Increased activity uses more carbohydrates.
  2. Most adults require 30 calories/kg of ideal body weight.

DIABETIC EXCHANGE DIETS

Food Group	Unit of Exchange	Calories	Food Allowed
Milk			
Whole	1 cup	170	1 cup whole milk = 1 cup skim milk and 2 fat exchanges
Skim	1 cup	80	
Fruit	Varies according to allotted calories	40	Fresh or canned without sugar or syrup
Vegetables			
A	1 cup	Varies	Green, leafy vegetables; tomatoes
B	½ cup	35	Vegetables other than above
Bread	1 slice	70	Can exchange cereals, starch items, some vegetables
Meat	31 grams	75	Lean meats, egg, cheese, seafood
Fat	1 teaspoon	45	1 teaspoon butter or mayonnaise; bacon, oil, olives, avocado
Unlimited foods			Coffee, tea, bouillon, spices

Protein

A. A low-protein diet is utilized for renal impairment since protein is processed through the kidneys.
  1. End products of protein metabolism are controlled by limiting protein intake.

2. Protein processing uses up calcium reserves.

3. Conditions utilizing low-protein diets.
   a. Pyelonephritis.
   b. Glomerulonephritis, if oliguria present.
   c. Uremia.
   d. Kidney failure.
   e. Dialysis management.

B. A high-protein diet is necessary for tissue building and body growth. Protein intake should average 40–60 gm/day for women and men respectively.

1. By increasing intake of high-quality protein food sources, protein loss is corrected.

2. Suggest protein supplements (usually ordered by physician), such as Sustagen, Meritene, and Proteinum.

3. Conditions that require a high-protein diet include:
   a. Burns.
   b. Ulcerative colitis.
   c. Nephrotic syndrome.
   d. Addison's disease.
   e. Hyperthyroidism.
   f. Anemia.
   g. Postoperative.
   h. Malabsorption syndromes.
   i. Tissue building and correction of protein deficiency.
   j. Oncology clients.
   k. Pregnancy.
   l. Malnutrition.

C. Amino acid metabolism abnormality diet is utilized for phenylketonuria (PKU), galactosemia, and lactose intolerance.

1. Reduce and/or eliminate the offending enzyme in the food intake of protein and utilize substitute nutrient foods.

2. Avoid milk and milk products as they constitute the main source of enzymes for the three diseases.

3. Employ substitutes to meet daily allowances.

HIGH PROTEIN FOODS

Food	Protein (Grams)
Dairy and eggs	
Cottage cheese, 1/2 cup	14.0
Milk, 1 cup	8.5
Cheddar cheese, 1 oz.	7.1
Egg, 1 medium	6.1
Ice cream, 1/2 cup	2.4
Meat and fish	
Tuna, canned, drained, 4 oz.	32.0
Chicken, 4 oz. cooked	31.2
Hamburger, 4 oz. cooked	30.7
Sirloin steak, 4 oz. cooked	26.7
Grains	
Whole-wheat flour, 1/2 cup	8.0
Spaghetti, 1 cup cooked	6.0
Cornmeal, 1/2 cup	5.5
Rice, brown, 1 cup cooked	5.0
Rice, white, 1 cup cooked	4.0
Legumes	
Soybeans, 1/2 cup cooked	12.0
Peanut butter, 1 oz.	7.1
Lima beans, 1/2 cup cooked	6.1
Cashews, 1 oz.	4.8

Protein Management in Renal Disease

A. A low-protein diet and essential amino acid diet (modified Giovannetti diet) is comprised of 20 gm of protein and 1500 mg of potassium.

1. Prevent electrolytes and by-products of metabolism from accumulating to a fatal level between artificial kidney treatments.

2. Allow foods such as one egg daily, 6 ounces of milk, low-protein bread, fruit, vegetables, butter, oil, jelly, candy, tea, and coffee.

3. Restrict foods such as meat, chicken, fish, peanuts, and high-protein bread.

B. A low-calcium diet is utilized to prevent formation of renal calculi.
  1. Decrease the total daily intake of calcium to prevent further stone formation. Total calcium intake is 400 mg per day instead of 800 mg (normal).
  2. Allow foods such as milk (one cup daily), juices, tea, coffee, eggs, and fresh fruits and vegetables.
  3. Restrict foods such as rye and whole grain breads and cereals, dried fruits and vegetables, fish, shellfish, cheese, chocolate, and nuts.
C. An acid ash diet is utilized to prevent precipitation of stone elements.
  1. Establish a well-balanced diet in which the total acid ash is greater than the total alkaline ash daily.
  2. Allow foods such as breads and cereals of any type, fats, fruits (one serving), vegetables, meat, eggs, cheese, fish, fowl (two servings), and spices.
  3. Restrict foods such as carbonated beverages, dried fruits, bananas, figs, raisins, dried beans, carrots, chocolate, nuts, olives, and pickles.
D. A low-purine diet is utilized to prevent uric acid stones; also utilized for gout clients.
  1. Restrict purine, which is the precursor of uric acid; four percent of urinary stones are composed of uric acid.
  2. Allow foods such as milk, tea, fruit juices, carbonated beverages, breads, cereals, cheese, eggs, fat, and most vegetables.
  3. Restrict foods such as glandular meats, gravies, fowl, fish, and high meat quantities.

FOODS HIGH IN CALCIUM

Milk, cream

Cottage cheese

Mustard greens, turnip greens

Kale

Shrimp, clams and oysters

Salmon

Cheese

Ice cream

FOODS HIGH IN ACID ASH

Cranberries

Eggs

Fish

Gelatin

Meat

Plums, prunes

FOODS HIGH IN ALKALI ASH

Citrus fruits

Milk

Milk products

Vegetables

FOODS HIGH IN PURINE

Meat extracts

Shellfish

Liver and other organ meats

Sardines, mussels, anchovies

Chicken, turkey

Beans, lentils

Peas

Spinach

Cauliflower

Asparagus

Fat

A. A restricted cholesterol diet is utilized for cardiovascular diseases, diabetes mellitus, and high serum cholesterol levels.
  1. Blood cholesterol level is reduced and/or maintained at a normal level by restricting foods high in cholesterol.
  2. The average person should consume 250–300 mg of cholesterol a day. (One egg has 275 mg of

cholesterol; one three ounce serving of hamburger has 50 mg of cholesterol).

3. Encourage low-cholesterol foods, such as vegetable oils, raw or cooked vegetables, fruits, lean meats, and fowl.

B. A modified fat diet is utilized according to individual tolerance in specific diseases and conditions and for those wishing to lose weight.

1. Attempt to lower fat content in diet to reduce irritation of diseased organs and to reduce fat content where there is inadequate absorption.
2. Low-fat diet: Avoid such foods as gravies, fatty meat and fish, cream, fried foods, rich pastries, whole milk products, cream soups, salad and cooking oils, nuts and chocolate. Allow eggs (2 to 3 per week), lean meat, and small amount of butter or margarine.
3. Fat-free diet: Allow vegetables, fruits, lean meats, fowl, fish, bread, and cereal and restrict all fatty meats and fat.
4. Conditions utilizing or restricting low-cholesterol diets in their management.
   a. Cardiovascular diseases.
   b. Diabetes.
   c. Cholecystitis.
   d. Cholelithiasis.
   e. Pancreatitis.
   f. High serum cholesterol levels.
5. Modified fat diets are appropriate for the following conditions.
   a. Malabsorption syndromes.
   b. Cystic fibrosis.
   c. Obstructive jaundice.
   d. Liver disease.

C. A high-polyunsaturated fat diet is utilized primarily for cardiovascular diseases.

1. Reduce intake of saturated fats and increase intake of foods rich in polyunsaturated fats. (Physician usually prescribes caloric level as well as restrictions.)
2. Avoid foods originating from animal sources and selected peanuts, olives, avocado, coconuts, chocolate, and cashew nuts.
3. Allow foods originating from vegetable sources (except for those named above), margarine, corn/soybean/safflower oil, fresh ground peanut butter, and nuts (except cashews).

FOODS HIGH IN CHOLESTEROL

Beef liver	Chicken
Organ meats	Lobster
Eggs	Turkey
Sardines	Ice cream
Veal	Hot dogs
Lamb	White fish
Beef	
Pork	
Bacon	

SECRET HIGH FAT SOURCES

Foods High in Fat	Grams of Fat Per Serving
Avocados, 1/2	19
Chocolate, 1 bar	10
Cheddar cheese, 2 oz.	18
Swiss cheese, 2 oz.	16
Ice cream, 1/2 cup	7
Fatty meats	
Bacon, 2 slices	8
Hot dogs, beef, 1	13.5
Bologna, 2 slices	17
Chicken, with skin, 3 oz.	13
Ground beef, lean, 3 oz.	17
French fries, regular size	11.5
Granola, 3 oz.	12–18
Whole milk	8
Peanuts, 1/4 cup	18
Peanut butter, 2 Tbsp.	16
Pizza, 1/4 large	17
Potato chips, 1 oz.	10

MAJOR FOOD SOURCES OF VITAMINS

Vitamin A	Vitamin B Group	Vitamin C	Vitamin D	Vitamin E	Vitamin K
Dairy products (milk)	Pork, beef, fish, liver, organ meats	Fruits and vegetables: citrus (oranges, grapefruit, lemons), strawberries, tomatoes, bell peppers, cantaloupe, broccoli, greens	Foods fortified with vitamin D-milk	Vegetable oils	Meats
Liver	Eggs		Egg yolk	Nuts, seeds	Egg yolks
Egg	Peanuts, nuts		Fish	Green vegetables, especially leafy vegetables	Liver
Dark green and dark yellow vegetables & fruits: carrots, sweet potato, spinach, cantaloupe, broccoli, watermelon, leaf lettuce	Enriched whole grains			Wheat germ; whole grain products	Vegetable oils
	Legumes, beans, spinach				Tomatoes
	Green, leafy vegetables				Cauliflower
	Yeast				Peas
	Oatmeal				Potatoes
					Cheese

Vitamins

A. An increased vitamin diet is necessary for treatment of specific vitamin deficiencies.
   1. Provide high-vitamin diet for clients with burns, healing wounds, raised temperatures, and infections. Also used for pregnant clients. *See* vitamin chart.
   2. Evaluate diseases, such as cystic fibrosis and liver disease, that require water-soluble vitamins. *See* chart for water-soluble vitamins.
B. Total low-vitamin diets are not generally prescribed—although specific vitamins might be decreased for periods of illness.

Minerals

A. Sodium restriction.
   1. Correct and/or control the retention of sodium and water in the body by limiting sodium intake. May be done by restriction of salt in the diet or in combination with medications.
   2. Restrict salt in cooking or at the table. In clients requiring dietary modification in salt intake any product containing sodium, such as soda bicarbonate, may be prohibited.
   3. Explain sodium restrictions in diet.
      Mild: 2 to 3 gm sodium
      Moderate: 1000 mg sodium
      Strict: 500 mg sodium
      Severe: 250 mg sodium
   4. Conditions utilizing low sodium in their management.
      a. Meniere's disease.
      b. Congestive heart failure.
      c. Right ventricular failure.
      d. Hypertension.
      e. Cirrhosis with edema.
      f. Portal hypertension.
      g. Uremia.
      h. Dialysis management.
      i. Pregnancy induced hypertension.

DEFINITIONS OF SODIUM RESTRICTIONS

- Mild: 2 to 3 g sodium
- Moderate: 1000 mg sodium
- Strict: 500 mg sodium
- Severe: 250 mg sodium

Foods High in Sodium

Table salt and all prepared salts, such as celery salt
Smoked meats and salted meats
Most frozen or canned vegetables with added salt
Butter, margarines, and cheese

44

Quick-cooking cereals
Shellfish and frozen or salted fish
Seasonings and sauces
Canned soups
Chocolates and cocoa
Beets, celery, and selected greens (spinach)
Foods with salt added, such as potato chips,
    popcorn

Foods High in Potassium
Fruit juices such as orange, grapefruit, banana,
    apple
Instant, dry coffee powder
Egg, legumes, whole grains
Fish, especially fresh halibut and codfish
Pork, beef, lamb, veal, chicken
Milk, skim and whole
Dried dates, prunes
Bouillon and meat broths

B. Potassium management.

   1. Replace potassium loss from the body with specific foods high in potassium or a potassium supplement. (Severe loss is managed with intravenous therapy.)

   2. Avoid no specific foods unless there is a sodium restriction because some foods high in potassium are also high in sodium.

   3. Conditions utilizing low potassium in their management.
      a. Glomerulonephritis.
      b. Dialysis management.

   4. Conditions utilizing increased potassium in their management.
      a. Diabetic acidosis.
      b. Burns, after the first 48 hours.
      c. Vomiting
      d. Extended high temperature.
      e. Use of diuretic drugs.

C. Iron supplements.

   1. Replace a deficit of iron caused by inadequate intake or chronic blood loss. Women especially tend to be low in iron.

   2. Suggested iron intake is 18 mg/day.

   3. Conditions utilizing high iron in their management.
      a. Peptic ulcer disease.
      b. Diverticulosis.
      c. Ulcerative colitis.
      d. Anemias: nutritional, pernicious.
      e. Hemorrhage.
      f. Postgastrectomy syndrome.
      g. Malabsorption syndrome.
      h. Crohn's disease.
      i. Increased for pregnancy and lactation.

FOODS HIGH IN IRON

Organ meats, especially beef liver

Red meat, turkey, chicken

Fish, shellfish

Blackstrap molasses

Egg yolk

Lima beans, legumes

Sunflower seeds

Almonds, pecans, cashews

Dried fruits, apricots, prunes, raisins

Leafy vegetables, broccoli, brussel sprouts

Peas

Kidney beans

Brewer's yeast

Cheese—Swiss, ricotta, roquefort

Wild rice

Yogurt

Wheat germ

Bananas

MAJOR FOOD SOURCES OF MINERALS

Magnesium	Potassium	Sodium	Zinc	Iodine	Calcium
Nuts	Veal, chicken, pork, turkey, beef, liver	Table salt and all prepared salts, such as celery salt	Beans	Marine fish and shellfish	Milk products
Peanut butter			Seeds and nuts		Dark green vegetables
Beans	Fish: halibut, codfish, salmon	Smoked meats and salted meats	Legumes	Dairy products	Canned salmon, sardines
Avocado			Milk	Iodized salt	
Cheese	Molasses		Wheat bran	Most vegetables	Dried beans
Bitter chocolate	Peanut butter	Most frozen or canned vegetables with added salt	Shellfish		Tofu
Green leafy vegetables	Almonds, cashews, etc.				Almonds
Instant coffee	Dried fruit: apricots, dates, prunes	Butter, margarines, and cheese			
Bran					
Tofu	Avocados	Quick-cooking cereals			
	Bananas				
	Lima beans				
		Shellfish and frozen or salted fish			
	Brussels sprouts	Seasonings and sauces			
	Bitter chocolate	Canned soups			
	Instant powdered coffee	Chocolates and cocoa			
	Eggs	Beets, celery, and selected greens (spinach)			
	Wheat germ, bran				
	Catsup	Foods with salt added, such as potato chips, popcorn			
		Catsup			
		Green olives			
		Whole grains, breads			
		Salad dressings (bottled)			

Fiber Control

A. A high-fiber (roughage) diet is an important constituent of our diet. The average person eats 20 gm of fiber per day; 30–40 gm is recommended.
   1. High fiber foods help you lose weight, keep the heart healthy, and lower the risk of developing cancer of the colon
   2. Foods low in carbohydrates are usually high in residue.
B. A low-residue diet is utilized for certain diseases and conditions such as diarrhea and diverticulitis (when inflammation decreases, diet may revert to high residue).
   1. Low-residue foods are ground meat, fish, broiled chicken without skin, creamed cheeses, limited fat, warm drinks, refined strained cereals, and white bread.
   2. Foods high in carbohydrates are usually low in residue.
   3. Conditions that require a low-residue diet.
      a. Crohn's disease.
      b. Postoperative colon and rectal surgery.
      c. Diverticulitis–while inflammatory period lasts.
      d. Rheumatic fever.
      e. Diarrhea and enteritis.
      f. Oncology clients.
      g. Intestinal tumors.

Calorie Control

A. A restricted calorie diet reduces the caloric intake of food below the energy demands of the body so weight loss will occur.
   1. Provide psychological support and exercise.
   2. Restrict such foods as carbohydrates and fats.
B. An increased calorie diet is utilized to meet the increased metabolic needs of the body. There is usually an increase in protein and vitamins when increased calories are ordered.
C. Conditions utilizing high calorie intake in their management.
      a. Viral hepatitis.
      b. Pyelonephritis.
      c. Nephrotic syndrome.
      d. Leukemia.
      e. Pheochromocytoma.

Bland Food Diets

A. A bland diet is utilized to promote the healing of the gastric mucosa by eliminating food sources that are chemically and mechanically irritating.
   1. Bland diets are presented in stages with the gradual addition of certain foods.
   2. Frequent, small feedings during active stress periods are important.
B. Move from bland to regular diet and establish regular meals and food patterns when condition permits.
C. Bland diets are appropriate for the following conditions.
      a. Duodenal and gastric ulcers.
      b. Chronic pancreatitis.
      c. Prostate surgery, postoperative.
      d. Stomach surgery, postoperative.

BLAND DIET ALLOWANCES

Foods allowed

Milk, butter, eggs (not fried), custard, vanilla ice cream, cottage cheese

Cooked refined or strained cereal, enriched white bread

Jello; homemade creamed, pureed soups

Baked or broiled potatoes

Examples of foods that are eliminated

Spicy and highly seasoned foods

Raw foods

Very hot and very cold foods

Gas-forming foods (varies with individuals)

Coffee, alcoholic beverages, carbonated drinks

High-fat contents (some butter and margarine allowed)

Pre- and Postoperative Diets

A. A high-protein preoperative diet is essential for the maintenance of normal serum protein levels during and following surgery. This diet also restores nitrogen balance if protein-depleted for burn victims, the elderly, and severely debilitated clients.

1. Provide adequate carbohydrates to maintain liver glycogen and adequate amino acids to promote wound healing.
2. Provide a 2500-calorie diet that is high in carbohydrates, moderate in protein with high-protein supplements.
3. Instruct client that an elemental diet is low in residue and contains a synthetic mixture of CHO, amino acids, and essential fatty acids with added minerals and vitamins. It is bulk free and easily assimilated and absorbed.

B. A special postoperative surgical diet is necessary to promote wound healing, avoid shock from decreased plasma proteins and circulating red blood cells, prevent edema, and promote bone healing.
   1. Provide 2800 total calories for tissue repair and 6000 calories for extensive repair.
   2. Fluid intake is 2000 to 3000 cc/day for uncomplicated surgery and 3000 to 4000 cc/day for sepsis or renal damage. Seriously ill clients with drainage can require up to 7000 cc/day.

C. A postoperative diet protocol progresses from nothing by mouth the day of surgery to a general diet within a few days following surgery. Foods allowed in each phase of the progressive diet include:
   1. A clear-liquid diet is 1000 to 1500 cc/day and is comprised of water, tea, broth, jello, and juices (apple, cranberry or 7-up. Avoid juices with pulp).
   2. A full-liquid diet is clear liquids, milk and milk products, custard, puddings, creamed soups, sherbet, ice cream and any fruit juice.
   3. A surgical soft diet is full liquid and, in addition, pureed vegetables, eggs (not fried), milk, cheese, fish, fowl, tender beef, veal, potatoes, and cooked fruit. Do not include gas-formers.
   4. General diet: Take into consideration specific alterations necessary for client's health status.

Mechanical Soft Diet

A. A mechanical soft diet is used when clients are edentulous, have poorly fitted dentures, have difficulty chewing or do not chew food thoroughly.
B. Any food that can be easily broken down can be included in this diet. It allows patients variations in taste that are not allowed on a soft diet (chili beans).

Puree Diet

A. A puree diet provides food that has been blenderized to a smooth consistency.
   1. Mainly used for clients with dysphagia or who are unable to chew.
   2. Often used with small babies.
   3. Some hospitals provide this type of diet for gastrostomy feedings.
B. When assisting clients with this type of diet, talk with them about the meal, describing the different foods; when the texture is all the same, distinguishing between foods is difficult.
C. Do not mix all pureed food together or feed out of one bowl or dish. Try to keep foods separate and feed alternately with dessert last.

SUMMARY OF DIETARY CONTROL FOR DISORDERS

Malabsorption syndromes

Cystic fibrosis: high calorie, high protein, low fat, with vitamin and mineral supplements.

Ulcerative colitis: high protein, high calorie, low lactase, low residue.

Crohn's disease: low residue, high protein, and vitamin mineral supplements.

Diverticulosis: high fiber.

Constipation: high fiber with liquids.

Diarrhea: low residue.

Liver, biliary and pancreatic problems

Liver involvement: high calories, high protein, high carbohydrates, low to moderate fat intake.

Gall bladder: low fat and exclude any foods that cause problems (fatty foods, gas-forming vegetables).

Pancreatitis: high protein, high carbohydrate, low fat and decreased alcohol intake.

Genitourinary problems

Urinary tract infection: increase acid ash, reduce alkali ash (citrus, milk, vegetables).

Renal failure: high carbohydrates, limited protein, low potassium.

Chronic renal failure: low protein, low salt, restricted fluids.

Renal calculi: acid ash diet for stones formed of exalate or phosphate and alkali ash when stones formed of uric acid or cystine. Force fluids.

Specific disorders

Gout: restrict foods high in purine, increase fluid intake, high carbohydrate and control of calories.

Hyperthyroidism: high carbohydrate and high protein, restrict caffeine.

Phenylketonuria (PKU): restrict phenylalanine. (Phenylalanine is found in all natural protein foods; meat, milk, etc., are eliminated.)

Obesity: restrict calories but nutritionally sound with adequate protein, complex carbohydrates, and limited fat. (Fat and carbohydrates are retained to ensure protein utilization.)

Providing Nutrients Through Enteral Feeding

Assessment

A. Assess overall status:
1. Weight change/loss.
2. Temperature.
3. Presence of sepsis.
4. Trauma.
5. Mental state.
6. Other medically related nutritional problems, e.g., diabetes, hyperlipidemia, alcoholism.
B. Evaluate oral intake.
C. Assess nutritional requirements.
D. Assess status of GI tract.
E. Assess capacity to chew and swallow.
F. Check for presence of gag reflex.
G. Evaluate respiratory or thoracic conditions.
H. Check for renal complications.
I. Check for vomiting and/or diarrhea.
J. With high-protein diets, assess for fluid and electrolyte imbalance.

Planning and Analysis

A. The necessary nutrients are provided to sustain normal weight.

B. The client complies and is able to tolerate method of ingesting nutrients.
C. The equipment functions efficiently and the correct volume is given to the client.
D. The fluid and electrolyte balance is maintained.

Implementation

A. Inserting a nasogastric tube.
1. Check order for tube feeding.
2. Warm feeding to room temperature.
3. Discuss procedure with the client.
4. Demonstrate and display items to be used in order to allay the client's fear and to gain cooperation.
5. Wash your hands.
6. Position the client at 45-degree angle or more.
7. Examine nostrils and select the most patent nostril by having the client breathe through each one.
8. Measure from tip of nose to earlobe to xiphoid process of sternum to determine appropriate length for tube insertion. If tube is to go below stomach, add additional 15 to 25 cm. Mark point on tube with tape.
9. Lubricate first 10 cm of tube with watersoluble lubricant and stylet if used.
10. Insert tube through nostril to back of throat and ask the client to swallow. Sips of water may aid in pushing tubing past oropharynx.
11. Continue advancing tube until taped mark is reached.
12. Check position of tube.
    a. It is no longer considered safe practice to place proximal end of NG tube in a glass of water and observe for bubbling.
    b. Inject 10 ml of air through NG tube and listen with the stethoscope over stomach for a rush of air (whoosh sound).
    c. The most accurate method is to aspirate gastric contents, sometimes difficult with small bore tubes, and check the pH. If pH is acidic (below 3 with litmus paper red) tube is in the stomach.
    d. X-ray confirmation. If nasoduodenal or nasojejunal feedings required, client should have x-ray to confirm correct placement.
13. Tape securely to nose and cheek.
14. Remain with and talk with client until anxiety is decreased and client is comfortable.

B. Irrigating a nasogastric tube.
  1. Obtain a disposable irrigation set or emesis basin for irrigation solution, a 20-cc syringe, and a normal saline irrigation solution.
  2. Wash your hands.
  3. Place client in a semi-Fowler's position.
  4. Check for nasogastric tube placement by instilling air and listening for "woosh" sound.
  5. Draw up 20-cc normal saline into the irrigating syringe.
  6. Gently instill the normal saline into the nasogastric tube. Do not force the solution.
  7. Withdraw the 20-cc irrigation solution and empty into basin.
  8. Repeat the procedure twice.
  9. Record on I&O sheet the irrigation solution that has not been returned.
C. Administering a tube feeding.
  1. Obtain order from the physician for appropriate formula (calories and/or amount).
  2. Send requisition for formula to diet kitchen.
  3. Check early in shift to ensure adequate formula is available.
  4. Warm formula to room temperature using a microwave or set formula in basin of hot water.
  5. Assemble feeding equipment. If using bag, fill with ordered amount of formula.

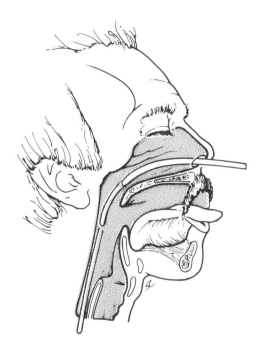

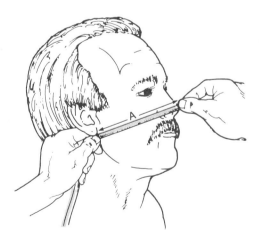

A—Tip of Nose to Ear Lobe
B—Tip of Ear Lobe to Xiphoid

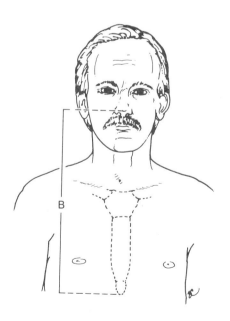

6. Explain procedure to the client and assure privacy.
7. Place the client on right side in high-Fowler's position.
8. Aspirate stomach contents to determine amount of residual.
9. Return aspirated contents to stomach to prevent electrolyte imbalance.
10. Pinch the tubing to prevent air from entering stomach.
11. Attach syringe to nasogastric tube.
12. Fill syringe with formula. (If using feeding bag, adjust drip rate to infuse over 30 minutes.)
13. Hold tubing no more than 39 cm above client.
14. Allow formula to infuse slowly (between 20 to 35 minutes) through the tubing.
15. Follow tube feeding with water in amount ordered.
16. Clamp end of the tube.
17. Wash tray and return it to client's bedside.
18. Give water in between feedings if tube feeding is the sole source of nutrition.

D. Procedure for continuous tube feedings (Dubbhoff, Keofeed tubes).
1. Insert tube (tubes are weighted at the distal end with mercury or tungsten) or check patency of existing tube.
2. Irrigate feeding tube with sterile water or saline at least every eight hours.
3. Administer formula at prescribed infusion rate. Infusion pumps are used to maintain continuous flow.

4. Avoid keeping formula at room temperature for longer than four hours to prevent spoilage and bacterial contamination.
5. Routinely assess the abdomen for abdominal distention and bowel sounds.
6. Keep client in semi-Fowler's position.
7. Turn off flow when placing client supine.

E. Procedure for gastrostomy feeding.
1. Assess gastric contents to determine amount per intermittent feeding. Hold feeding if more than 50–100 cc.
2. Feed slowly for intermittent feeding or keep at prescribed rate for continuous feeding.
3. Observe gastrostomy tube insertion site for signs of dislodging or infection.
4. Provide site care; wash area with warm water and soap.
5. Apply skin protective barrier. Cover area with sterile dressing.

Evaluation

A. Client tolerates feeding well, and weight is maintained or increased.
B. Appropriate residual is obtained from aspiration of stomach contents.
C. Client complies with feeding procedure.
D. Intake and output balance is maintained.
E. Fluid and electrolyte balance is maintained.
F. Nasogastric tube functions efficiently.
    1. Tube remains patent.
    2. No aspiration or vomiting occurs.
G. Client does not develop stress ulcer from permanent tube placement.

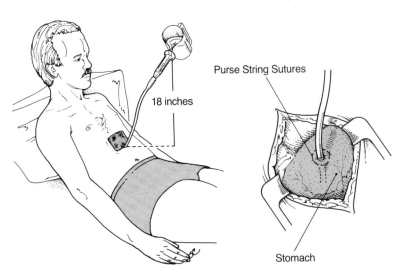

18 inches

Purse String Sutures

Stomach

Total Parenteral Nutrition

Assessment

A. Assess nutritional needs of clients unable to ingest calories normally.

B. Identify the caloric intake necessary to promote positive nitrogen balance, tissue repair, and growth.

C. Observe for correct additives in each hyperalimentation bottle.

D. Check label of solution against physician's orders.

E. Check rate of infusion on physician's orders.

F. Assess ability of client to understand instructions during procedure.

G. Ensure patency of central venous line following insertion.

H. Observe catheter insertion site for signs of infection, thrombophlebitis, or possible infiltration.

I. Inspect dressing over central line to ensure a dry, noncontaminated dressing.

Planning and Analysis

A. A nitrogen source is provided for clients unable to ingest protein normally.

B. Adequate calories provided for clients unable to tolerate oral feedings.

C. Nutrients are provided for clients requiring bypass of the gastrointestinal tract.

D. Increased calories are given when regular IV solutions are insufficient.

E. A contamination-free mode of delivering the hyperalimentation solution is provided.

Implementation

A. Teach the Valsalva's maneuver if client does not have a cardiac disorder. This maneuver prevents air from entering the catheter during catheter insertion or tubing changes.

1. Ask client to take a deep breath and bear down.

2. Apply gentle pressure to the abdomen.

B. Review physician's order for correct hyperalimentation solution additives.

1. TPN bottles come directly from the pharmacy and are numbered sequentially.

2. Each TPN bottle label will include client's name, room, number, additives, IV number, start time, date, and stop time.

3. Inspect TPN bottle for cracks, turbidity or precipitates.

C. Position client in head-down position with head

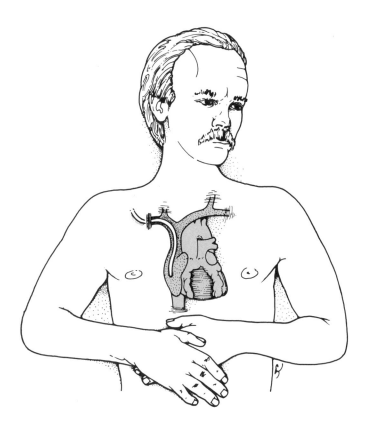

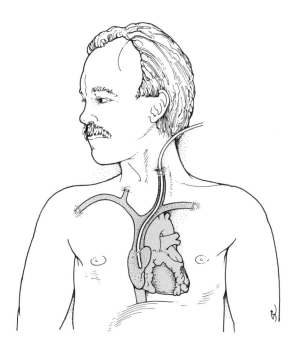

turned to opposite direction of catheter insertion site. Place a small roll between client's shoulders to expose insertion site.

D. Cleanse insertion area with acetone and then Betadine solution.

E. Don mask and sterile gloves and assist physician as needed during catheter insertion.

F. Instruct client in Valsalva's maneuver when stylet is removed from catheter and when IV tubing is connected to catheter.
   1. After tubing is connected, instruct client to breathe normally.
   2. Tape area between tubing and catheter hub.

G. Turn on IV infusion pump, using normal saline solution, at slow rate, 10 drops/minute, until x-ray ensures accurate catheter placement.

H. Apply 4 × 4 sterile gauze pad over IV site and occlude dressing with micropore or plastic tape.

I. Confirm catheter placement via x-ray and change IV solution to hyperalimentation solution.
   1. Store hyperalimentation solution in refrigerator until 30 minutes before use. This prevents growth of organisms, but should be warmed to room temperature prior to use.
   2. Change solution every 12 hours if dextrose is used.

J. Time tape the bottle after adjusting flow rate. Be prepared to document on IV hourly infusion record.

K. Observe for signs of air embolism, subcutaneous bleeding, pneumothorax, or allergic responses to protein (chills, increased temperature, nausea, headache, urticaria, dyspnea).

L. Take vital signs every four hours.

M. Maintain central vein infusion.
   1. Change IV tubing, filter, and infusion pump cassette (if used) every 24 hours.
   2. Change extension tubing every 48 hours. Change should accompany IV fluid bottle change.
   3. Maintain IV flow rate at prescribed rate.
      a. If rate is too rapid, hyperosmolar diuresis occurs (excess sugar will be excreted); if severe enough, intractable seizures, coma, and death can occur.
      b. If rate is too slow, little benefit will be derived from the calories and nitrogen.
      c. Do not correct an overload or deficit in flow, as doing so could result in complications for the client. Notify physician if this occurs.
   4. Monitor IV flow rate every 30 to 60 minutes even though you are using an IV pump.

N. Check urine specific gravity, sugar, and acetone every four hours.
   1. If necessary, administer insulin according to prescribed rainbow coverage.
   2. Notify physician of urine sugars of 3+ or 4+ and positive urine acetone. Most clients will show

a sugar level as high as 2+ during the first few days of treatment.

O. Maintain accurate I&O. Record on special total parenteral nutrition (TPN) sheet at least every four hours.

P. Weigh daily and record on graphic sheet and TPN sheet.

Dressing and Tubing Change

A. Maintain sterile technique for both procedures.
   1. Use sterile gloves, drape and equipment.
   2. Goal is to prevent contamination of site and prevent infection.
B. Observe insertion site for erythema, drainage, etc., then cleanse with hydrogen peroxide.
C. Defat skin around catheter and apply povidone-iodine.
D. Apply dressing every 24 hours.
E. Change tubing every 24 hours.
   1. Loosen tubing at catheter hub.
   2. Tell client to hold breath and bear down while new tubing is inserted to prevent air from entering catheter causing air embolism.
   3. Observe for signs of respiratory distress: air embolism, pneumothorax.
      a. Cyanosis.
      b. Hypotension.
      c. Rapid, weak pulse.
      d. Alterations in heart sounds.
      e. Elevated CVP.

4. Check vital signs frequently, including temperature.
5. If respiratory distress occurs—suspected air embolism.
   a. Place client in Trendelenburg's position with right chest uppermost and left chest down.
   b. Inform physician.
   c. Administer oxygen at 6 l/ minute via nasal prongs.

Hyperalimentation for Children

A. Examine solution.
   1. Generally, there is a higher concentration of calcium, phosphorus, magnesium, and vitamins.
   2. Usually, a 10 percent solution of dextrose is started—it can be increased to 25 percent if tolerated.
B. Monitor patency of catheter (usually placed through internal or external jugular or scalp veins). Stopcocks are never used. Monitor constant infusion pump and filter.
C. Obtain urine sugar and acetone samples. Sugar level will rise, but usually exogenous insulin is not required as the pancreas adapts to high glucose loads.
D. Change the dressing every 48 hours and the tubing every 24 hours using aseptic technique.
   1. Stockinette can be used to keep scalp dressing secure.
   2. Tight-fitting T-shirt can keep chest site secure.

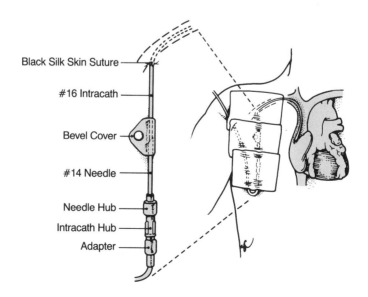

Black Silk Skin Suture
#16 Intracath
Bevel Cover
#14 Needle
Needle Hub
Intracath Hub
Adapter

Composition of Hyperalimentation Solutions

Amino acid—Freamine or Aminosol
Carbohydrates
Vitamins
Minerals
Hypertonic glucose/dextrose (20% to 50%)—
    calories (1000 to 2000 cal/liter)
Electrolytes
Water
Hyperalimentation solution is prepared in the pharmacy under a laminar flow hood.

E. Monitor for accurate rate of infusion.
  1. Do not "catch up" if infusion is behind.
  2. Positive pressure pumps can be used to maintain infusion rates, particularly when small amounts of solution are being infused.
F. Observe the child when ambulating for accidents such as twisting or kinking the tubing, getting the tubing caught in the crib, or stepping on it.

Evaluation

A. Catheter is placed correctly with no infiltration.
B. Solution is infused at prescribed flow rate and tolerated by client.
C. Dressing remains dry and intact during interval between changes.
D. Insertion site remains free of infection and inflammation.
E. Client receives nutrients necessary for tissue repair and sustenance.

Appendix 1. RECOMMENDED DAILY DIETARY ALLOWANCES

Designed for the maintenance of good nutrition of practically all healthy people in the U.S.A.

	Age (years)	Weight (kg)	Weight (lbs)	Height (cm)	Height (in)	Protein (g)	Fat-Soluble Vitamins Vitamin A (μg R.E.)[b]	Vitamin D (μg)[c]	Vitamin E (mg α T.E.)[d]	Water-Soluble Vitamins Vitamin C (mg)	Thiamin (mg)	Riboflavin (mg)
Infants	0.0–0.5	6	13	60	24	kg × 2.2	420	10	3	35	0.3	0.4
	0.5–1.0	9	20	71	28	kg × 2.0	400	10	4	35	0.5	0.6
Children	1–3	13	29	90	35	23	400	10	5	45	0.7	0.8
	4–6	20	44	112	44	30	500	10	6	45	0.9	1.0
	7–10	28	62	132	52	34	700	10	7	45	1.2	1.4
Males	11–14	45	99	157	62	45	1000	10	8	50	1.4	1.6
	15–18	66	145	176	69	56	1000	10	10	60	1.4	1.7
	19–22	70	154	177	70	56	1000	7.5	10	60	1.5	1.7
	23–50	70	154	178	70	56	1000	5	10	60	1.4	1.6
	51+	70	154	178	70	56	1000	5	10	60	1.2	1.4
Females	11–14	46	101	157	62	46	800	10	8	50	1.1	1.3
	15–18	55	120	163	64	46	800	10	8	60	1.1	1.3
	19–22	55	120	163	64	44	800	7.5	8	60	1.1	1.3
	23–50	55	120	163	64	44	800	5	8	60	1.0	1.2
	51+	55	120	163	64	44	800	5	8	60	1.0	1.2
Pregnant						+30	+200	+5	+2	+20	+0.4	+0.3
Lactating						+20	+400	+5	+3	+40	+0.5	+0.5

	Water-Soluble Vitamins Niacin (mg N.E.)[e]	Vitamin B$_6$ (mg)	Folacin[f] (μg)	Vitamin B$_{12}$ (μg)	Minerals Calcium (mg)	Phos- phorus (mg)	Magne- sium (mg)	Iron (mg)	Zinc (mg)	Iodine (μg)
Infants	6	0.3	30	0.5[g]	360	240	50	10	3	40
	8	0.6	45	1.5	540	360	70	15	5	50
Children	9	0.9	100	2.0	800	800	150	15	10	70
	11	1.3	200	2.5	800	800	200	10	10	90
	16	1.6	300	3.0	800	800	250	10	10	120
Males	18	1.8	400	3.0	1200	1200	350	18	15	150
	18	2.0	400	3.0	1200	1200	400	10	15	150
	19	2.2	400	3.0	800	800	350	10	15	150
	18	2.2	400	3.0	800	800	350	10	15	150
	16	2.2	400	3.0	800	800	350	10	15	150
Females	15	1.8	400	3.0	1200	1200	300	18	15	150
	14	2.0	400	3.0	1200	1200	300	18	15	150
	14	2.0	400	3.0	800	800	300	18	15	150
	13	2.0	400	3.0	800	800	300	18	15	150
	13	2.0	400	3.0	800	800	300	10	15	150
Pregnant	+2	+0.6	+400	+1.0	+400	+400	+150	[h]	+5	+25
Lactating	+5	+0.5	+100	+1.0	+400	+400	+150	[h]	+10	+50

Food and Nutrition Board, National Academy of Sciences—National Research Council

Appendix 2. BASIC NUTRITIONAL ASSESSMENT

Assessment	Normal	Abnormal
Appetite	Remains unchanged	Recently increased or decreased Particular cravings
Weight	Previous weight maintained Normal for client Appropriate for age and body build	Changed—recently increased or decreased Rapid or slow changes
Nutritional Intake	Adequate foods and fluids to supply body nutrients Nonallergic response to major food groups No pattern of fad diets Absence of drugs, chemicals, or other substances that influence appetite or metabolism	Elimination of certain food categories that results in limited nutrients Emphasis on some food groups (sugar) to the exclusion of others (vegetables) Allergic response to certain foods Constant use of fad diets to lose weight Use of drugs or chemicals that interferes with appetite nutrient assimilation Presence of emotional disorder (depression, anorexia, manic response) that interferes with food ingestion
Meal Patterns	Three to six home-prepared meals per day Adequate time and calm atmosphere for meals	Fast-food or packaged foods Missed meals, constant snacking, or over-eating Eating "on the run" or hurried
Physical Factors	Adequate chewing and swallowing capability Mouth and gums healthy so food can be ingested Physical exercise adequate for calorie intake	Teeth and/or gums in poor condition or ill-fitting dentures Swallowing impairs ingestion Inadequate physical exercise to burn calories
Presence of Disease	No disease process that interferes with nutrient assimilation No congenital condition or postsurgery condition that interferes with nutrient assimilation	Disease present that interferes with ingestion, digestion, assimilation, or excretion Congenital condition, rehabilitation phase, or postsurgery that interferes with food assimilation
Sociocultural-Religious Factors	Ability to afford adequate foods in all food categories Cultural beliefs that do not eliminate whole food groups Religious beliefs that do not eliminate whole food groups Food does not lose all nutrient value in preparation	Economic position that precludes purchase of adequate foods Religious or cultural beliefs that interfere with receiving balanced diet (macrobiotic diets) Inadequate knowledge, experience, or intelligence to prepare healthy meals
Elimination Schedule	Regular, adequate elimination of foods Absence of constant flatus, discharge, or mucus	Irregular and/or painful elimination Presence of constant flatus Presence of discharge, blood, or mucus

Appendix 3. THE BASIC FOUR FOOD GROUPS

Dairy Products

Foods Included:

- Milk: whole, evaporated, skim, dry, buttermilk
- Cheese: cottage, cream, cheddar, natural or processed
- Ice cream

Contribution to Diet: Milk is a leading source of calcium, which is needed for bones and teeth. It also provides high-quality protein, riboflavin, vitamin A, vitamin D (if milk is whole or fortified).

Amounts Recommended: 2 servings. Recommended amounts are given below in terms of whole fluid milk.

	8-ounce cups—237 ml
Children under 9	2 to 3
Children 9 to 12	3 or more
Teenagers	4 or more
Adults	2 or more
Pregnant women	3 or more
Nursing mothers	4 or more

Part or all of the milk may be fluid skim milk, buttermilk, evaporated milk, or dry milk.

Cheese and ice cream may replace part of the milk. To substitute, figure the amount on the basis of calcium content. Common portions of various kinds of cheese and ice cream and their milk equivalents in calcium are:

2.5-cm cube cheddar-type cheese	=	1/2 cup milk
1/2 cup cottage cheese	=	1/3 cup milk
2 tablespoons cream cheese	=	1 tablespoon milk
1/2 cup ice cream or ice milk	=	1/3 cup milk

Protein

Foods Included:

- Beef; veal; lamb; pork; variety meats, such as liver, heart, kidney
- Poultry and eggs
- Fish and shellfish
- Alternates: dry beans, dry peas, lentils, nuts, peanuts, peanut butter

Contribution to Diet: Foods in this group are valued for their protein, which is needed for growth and repair of body tissues—muscle, organs, blood, skin, and hair. These foods also provide iron, thiamin, riboflavin, and niacin.

Amounts Recommended: Choose two servings every day.

Count as a serving: 62 to 93 gm (not including bone weight) cooked lean meat, poultry, or fish. Count as alternates for 1/2 serving meat or fish: 1 egg, 1/2 cup cooked dry beans, dry peas, or lentils; or 2 tablespoons peanut butter.

Vegetable-Fruit Group

Foods Included: All vegetables and fruit. This guide emphasizes those that are valuable as sources of vitamin C and vitamin A.

Sources of Vitamin C

Good sources: grapefruit or grapefruit juice, orange or orange juice, cantaloupe, guava, mango, papaya, raw strawberries, broccoli, brussels sprouts, green pepper, sweet red pepper

Fair sources: honeydew melon, lemon, tangerine or tangerine juice, watermelon, asparagus tips, raw cabbage, cauliflower, collards, garden cress, kale, kohlrabi, mustard greens, potatoes and sweet potatoes cooked in the jacket, rutabagas, spinach, tomatoes or tomato juice, turnip greens

Sources of Vitamin A

Dark-green and deep-yellow vegetables and a few fruits, namely, apricots, broccoli, cantaloupe, carrots, chard, collards, cress, kale, mango, persimmon, pumpkin, spinach, sweet potatoes, turnip greens and other dark-green leaves, winter squash.

Contribution to Diet: Fruits and vegetables are valuable chiefly because of the vitamins and minerals they contain. In this plan, this group is counted on to supply nearly all the vitamin C needed and over half of the vitamin A. Vitamin C is needed for healthy gums and body tissues. Vitamin A is needed for growth, normal vision, and healthy condition of skin and other body surfaces.

Appendix 3. THE BASIC FOUR FOOD GROUPS (continued)

Amounts Recommended: Choose five or more servings every day, including:

- One serving of a good source of vitamin C or two servings of a fair source

- One serving, at least every other day, of a good source of vitamin A. If the food chosen for vitamin C is also a good source of vitamin A, the additional serving of vitamin A food may be omitted.

- The remaining three or more servings may be of any vegetable or fruit, including those that are valuable for vitamin C and vitamin A.

Count as one serving: $1/2$ cup of vegetable or fruit; or a portion as ordinarily served, such as one medium apple, banana, orange, or potato, half a medium grapefruit, a slice of cantaloupe, or the juice of one lemon.

Complex Carbohydrates

Foods Included: All breads and cereals that are whole grain, enriched, or restored; check labels to be sure. Specifically, this group includes bread, cooked cereal, ready-to-eat cereal, cornmeal, crackers, flour, grits, pasta, noodles, rolled oats, grains (wheat, corn, millet, oats, rice), whole-grain or enriched flour, beans, potatoes, and nuts (preferably unsalted).

Contribution to Diet: Foods in this group furnish worthwhile amounts of protein, iron, several of the B vitamins, and food energy.

Amounts Recommended: Choose six or more servings daily. Or, if no cereals are chosen, include an extra serving of bread or baked goods, which will make at least five servings from this group daily.

Count as one serving: one slice of bread; 31 gm ready-to-eat cereal; $1/2$ to $3/4$ cup cooked cereal, cornmeal, grits, macaroni, noodles, rice, or spaghetti.

Other Foods

To round out meals and meet energy needs, almost everyone will use some foods not specified in the four food groups. Such foods include unenriched, refined bread, cereal, flour; sugar; butter, margarine, other fats. Often these are ingredients in a recipe, or are added to other foods during preparation or at the table. Include some vegetable oil among the fats used.

Appendix 4. NUTRITIONAL GUIDELINES FOR INFANTS AND CHILDREN

Nutrition for the Infant

A. Calories.
   1. Birth to three months—give 50 to 55 calories per pound per day.
   2. Three months to one year—give 45 calories per pound per day.
B. Fluids.
   1. First six months—two to three ounces per pound per day.
   2. Requirements increase in hot weather.
C. Number of feedings.
   1. First week—six to ten per day.
   2. One week to one month—six to eight per day.
   3. One to three months—five to six per day.
   4. Three to seven months—four to five per day.
   5. Four to nine months—three to four per day.
   6. Eight to twelve months—three per day.
D. Vitamins.
   1. Breast-fed infants—if mother's source adequate, infant adequate.
   2. Formula-fed infants—vitamin supplements depend on type of formula and what vitamins are already included in it.
E. Solid foods—recent trends suggest introducing solid foods at four to six months of age.
   1. Cereal—infants are least allergic to rice.
   2. Fruits and vegetables.
      a. New foods should be introduced once a day in small amounts until the child becomes accustomed to them.
      b. Introduce only one new food per week.
      c. Bananas and applesauce are well tolerated.
      d. Orange juice is usually not well tolerated, initially. It can be introduced, diluted with water, when the child is six months old.
      e. Green and yellow vegetables can be introduced at about four months of age.
   3. Eggs
      a. Introduce yolks after child is six months old.
      b. Usually yolks are well tolerated, but sometimes there are allergic reactions to egg whites.
   4. Meat.
      a. May be introduced at six months.
      b. Usually more palatable if mixed with fruits or vegetables.
   5. Starchy foods.
      a. May be introduced during the second six months.
      b. Should not be given in place of green vegetables or fruit.
      c. Chief value is caloric.
      d. Zweiback and other crackers are good for the gumming infant.
   6. Avoid 2% milk, skim milk, whole milk.
F. Diarrhea—temporary.
   1. Usually caused by incorrect formula preparation, contaminated food, or viral infection.
   2. Review feeding preparation and storage of formula with caretaker.
   3. Usually corrected by withholding all solids and milk for two or three feedings and giving boiled, cooled, sugar water or balanced electrolyte solution.
G. Constipation.
   1. Increase fluid and sugar intake.
   2. In child three months old or older, increase cereal, fruit, and vegetable intake.
   3. On occasion, prune juice (half an ounce) may be given.

Nutrition for the Second Year

A. Rate of growth is slowing down; thus there is a decreased caloric need.
B. Self-selection—children usually select over a period of several days a diet that is balanced.
   1. Serve small amount of food so child can finish it.
   2. Don't mix food on plate.
C. Child should be feeding him or herself, with some assistance.
D. Assess food intake by associated findings.
   1. Weight, growth normal for age.
   2. Level of activity.
   3. Assess condition of skin, eyes, hair.
   4. Assess elimination problems.
   5. Assess emotional state: is child happy and content, fussy or unhappy?
E. Avoid baby bottle syndrome: sweet formula or milk bottle at night leads to destruction of teeth.

Appendix 4. NUTRITIONAL GUIDELINES FOR INFANTS AND CHILDREN (continued)

Nutrition for the Preschooler

A. Child begins to imitate family's likes and dislikes.
B. Finger foods are popular.
C. Single foods are preferable to a combination.
D. Counsel mothers—they express concerns about poor eating habits, which are common at this age.

Nutrition for the School-Age Child

A. Patterns of good eating habits are established at this time.
B. Avoid snacks—except fruits.
C. Appetite increases due to increased calorie needs for growth.
D. Child's appetite at a meal is influenced by the day's activity level.
E. Boys require more calories than girls.
F. Both boys and girls need more iron in prepuberty than in seven to ten year old age group.
G. Tendency toward obesity at this age.
H. Every child needs daily exercise.

Adolescent Eating Patterns

A. Period of rapid growth and appetite increases.
B. Adolescents frequently gain weight easily and use fad diets.
C. Girls adapt themselves to fashionable weight goals, which may be unhealthy.
D. There is social eating of nonnutritious foods.
E. One form of rebellion against parents is to refuse to eat "healthy" foods.
F. Adolescent girls are often deficient in iron, calcium, vitamins C and A.
G. Important teaching for adolescents is that they must not just fill stomachs with food, but nutritious food necessary for growth.

Malnutrition Disorders

A. Kwashiorkor—caused by a lack of protein; frequently seen in ages one to three, when high-protein intake is necessary.
B. Nutritional marasmus—a disease caused by a deficiency of food intake. It is a form of starvation.
C. Vitamin A deficiency—night blindness may progress to xerophthalmia and, finally, keratomalacia.
D. Vitamin C deficiency: scurvy—symptoms begin with muscle tenderness as walls of capillaries become fragile. Hemorrhage of vessels results.
E. Vitamin D deficiency: rickets—caused because vitamin D is necessary for adequate calcium absorption by the bones.
F. Thiamine deficiency: beriberi—primarily a disease of rice-eating people; symptoms include numbness in extremities and exhaustion.
G. Niacin deficiency: pellagra—symptoms include dermatitis, diarrhea, dementia, and, finally, death.
H. Iodine deficiency—leads to hyperplasia of the thyroid gland, or goiter.

Appendix 5. RECOMMENDED DAILY DIETARY ALLOWANCES FOR PREGNANCY AND LACTATION

	Pregnancy		Lactation		Function	Sources
	14 to 18	Adult	14 to 18	Adult		
Calories	2400	2300	2600	2500	Meet increased nutritional needs as well as body maintenance.	All foods. Important to emphasize food values of foods and avoid empty calories.
Protein	78	76	68	66	Augment maternal tissues—breasts, uterus, blood. Growth and development of placenta and fetal tissue. Constant repair and maintenance of maternal tissue.	All essential amino acids may be found in milk, meat, eggs, and cheeses. Other sources, though not complete protein by themselves: tofu, whole grains, legumes, nuts, peanut butter.
Iron mg	30+	30+	*	*	Essential constituent of hemoglobin. Part of various enzymes. Fetal development and storage, especially later part of pregnancy.	Good sources: liver, kidney, heart, cooked dry beans, lean pork and beef, dried fruits such as apricots, peaches, prunes, and raisins. Fair sources: spinach, mustard greens, eggs.
Calcium mg	1200	1200	1200	1200	Skeletal tissue. Bones; teeth. Blood coagulation. Neuromuscular irritability. Myocardial function. Fetal stores, especially last months.	Good sources: milk, cheese, ice cream, yogurt. Fair sources: broccoli, canned salmon with bones, dried beans, dark leafy vegetables.
Phosphorus mg	1200	1200	1200	1200	90 percent compounded with calcium. Rest distributed throughout cells—involved in energy production, building and repairing tissue, buffering.	Whole grain items: cereals, whole wheat bread, brown rice; milk.
Sodium	0.5 g	0.5 g	0.5 g	0.5 g	Metabolic activities. Fluid balance and acid-base balance. Cell permeability. Muscle irritability.	Table salt, meat, eggs, carrots, celery, beets, spinach, salted nuts, carbonated beverages.
Iodine μg	125	125	125	125	Necessary for health: mother and fetus; prevents goiter in mother; decreases chance of cretinism in infants.	Iodized table salt, cod liver oil.
Vitamin A IU	5000	5000	6000	6000	Tooth formation and skeletal growth. Cell growth and development. Integrity of epithelial tissue. Vision—light/dark adaptation. Fat metabolism.	Good sources: butter, egg yolk, fortified margarine, whole milk, cream, kidney, and liver. Fair sources: dark green and yellow vegetables such as sweet potatoes, pumpkins, mustard greens, collards, kale, bok choy, carrots, cantaloupe, apricots.
Riboflavin mg	1.7	1.5	1.9	1.7	Enzyme systems. Tissue functioning. Tissue oxygenation and respiration. Energy metabolism. Excreted in breast milk.	Good sources: kidney, liver, heart, milk. Fair sources: cheese, ice cream, dark leafy vegetables, lean meat, poultry.
Thiamine mg	1.4	1.3	1.4	1.3	Carbohydrate metabolism. Normal appetite and digestion. Health of nervous system.	Good sources: enriched and whole grain products—bread and cereals, dried peas, beans, liver, heart, kidney, nuts, potatoes, lean pork. Fair sources: eggs, milk, poultry, fish, vegetables.

* Iron needs during lactation are not different from those of a non-pregnant female (18 mg/day taken with vitamin C to increase assimilation), but continued supplementation following birth is important to replenish iron stores depleted by pregnancy.

Appendix 5. RECOMMENDED DAILY DIETARY ALLOWANCES (continued)

	Pregnancy		Lactation		Function	Sources
	14 to 18	Adult	14 to 18	Adult		
Niacin mg	16	15	18	17	Cell metabolism.	Good sources: fish, lean meat, poultry, liver, heart, peanuts, peanut butter. Fair sources: enriched and whole grain cereals and bread, milk, potatoes.
Folic acid B_{12} mg	4.0	4.0	4.0	4.0	Cell growth. Reproduction and formation of heme. Enzyme activities in production of protein. Deficiency results in megaloblastic anemia.	Dark green and leafy vegetables.
Pyridoxine B_6 mg	2.5	2.5	2.5	2.5	Essential coenzyme with amino acids. Deficiency may lead to hypochromic microcytic anemia.	Animal and vegetable protein such as meat, fish, beans, nuts and seeds, milk and milk products.
Vitamin D IU	400	400	400	400	Influences absorption, retention and utilization of calcium and phosphorus. Formation of bones, teeth and other tissue.	Good sources: fortified milk, butter, egg yolk, liver, fish oils.
Vitamin C Ascorbic acid mg	60	60	80	80	Production of intracellular substances necessary for development and maintenance of normal connective tissue in bones, cartilage and muscles. Role in metabolic processes involving protein and tissues. Increases absorption of iron.	Good sources: citrus fruits and juice, broccoli, cantaloupe, collards, mustard and turnip greens, peppers. Fair sources: asparagus, raw cabbage, other melons, spinach, prunes, tomatoes, canned or fresh chilis.

Appendix 6. NUTRITIONAL GUIDELINES FOR PREGNANCY

A. Influences upon dietary habits and nutrition.
1. Food—many emotional connotations originating in infancy.
2. Eating habits influenced by:
   a. Emotional factors.
   b. Cultural factors.
   c. Religious beliefs.
   d. Nutritional information.
   e. Age—especially adolescent and aged.
   f. Physical health.
   g. Personal preferences.

B. Nutritional needs in pregnancy.
1. Influenced by above factors.
2. Must supply caloric and nutritional needs of mother as well as promote optimum fetal growth.
3. May be complicated by:
   a. Poor maternal nutrition before pregnancy.
   b. Medical complications prior to pregnancy (diabetes, anemia).
   c. Complications resulting from pregnancy (toxemia, anemia).
   d. Pica (cravings).

C. Weight gain in pregnancy.
1. Average weight gain recommended (even for obese patients)—24 pounds.
   a. 1st trimester—3 to 4 pounds.
   b. 2nd trimester—10 pounds.
   c. 3rd trimester—10 pounds.
2. Weight gain accounted by:
   a. Product of conception.

Fetus—average size	7.5 pounds
Placenta	1.5
Amniotic fluid	2
Uterus	2.5
Breasts	1
Extracellular fluid	3
Blood volume	3
	20.5 pounds

   b. Rest of weight gain deposited as fat stores or fluid representing energy stored for lactation.

D. Revised daily food guide.
1. This revised daily guide meets R.D.A. standards for daily nutrients except for:
   a. Iron and folacin—cannot be ingested in sufficient quantities by dietary means. Must be supplemented during pregnancy.
   b. 300 additional calories needed to meet recommended allowances.
2. Protein intake includes both animal and vegetable protein.
   a. Vegetable protein may be omitted in those whose income will allow by increasing animal servings to three 3-oz. servings.
   b. One serving at least should be red meats.
3. Whole grain items are better choices than enriched breads and cereals. They contain more magnesium, zinc, folacin, and vitamin B_6.
4. At least two tablespoons of fat or oils should be consumed daily for vitamin E and essential fatty acids.

E. Special diets.
1. Adolescents.
   a. Have high proportion of low-birth-weight infants.
   b. Dietary habits often poor.
   c. Plan menu to include necessary items around foods they like.
   d. Stress balanced diet—avoid empty calories.
2. Low sodium.
   a. Presently sodium restriction is *deemphasized*.
   b. Sodium essential in maintaining increased body fluids needed for adequate placental flow, increased tissue requirements, and renal blood flow.
   c. If moderate salt intake is necessitated, avoid highly salted foods such as canned soups, potato chips, soda pop.
3. Weight control.
   a. Presently, weight loss in pregnancy is discouraged.
   b. Even obese client should gain 24 pounds to insure adequate nutrition for fetal growth.
   c. Strict dieting may lead to ketosis which has proven harmful to fetal brain development.
   d. Stress careful dietary planning to include essential nutrients and avoid empty calories.
   e. Weight reduction program should begin *after* lactation only.
4. Vegetarians.
   a. Sound nutritional planning to include those combinations of foods which, when combined, include all essential amino acids.

64

DRUG-NUTRIENT INTERACTIONS

THERAPEUTIC CLASS	DRUG NAME PROPRIETARY EXAMPLES	GENERIC/ ACTIVE COMPOUND	RECOMMENDED DAILY VITAMIN/MINERAL SUPPLEMENT OR RESTRICTION DURING DRUG THERAPY*
Dermatological preparation	Accutane®	isotretinoin	Avoid vitamin A supplement
Antibiotics	Panmycin® Achromycin® Other	tetracycline	Riboflavin (B$_2$), 5 mg Ascorbic acid, 100-200 mg Calcium, 0.8-1.5 gm**
	Aureomycin®	chlortetracycline	
Anticonvulsants	Dilantin®	phenytoin	Vitamin D, 400-800 IU† Vitamin K, 1-5 mg Folic acid, 0.4-1.0 mg (not > 2.0 mg/day)
	Mysoline®	primidone	Vitamin K, 1-5 mg†
Anti-inflammatory	Azulfidine®	sulfasalazine	Folic acid, 0.4-1.0 mg
	Bayer aspirin® Bufferin® Other aspirin	aspirin	Ascorbic acid, 50-100 mg Folic acid, 0.4-1.0 mg Iron, 20-50 mg
	Indocin®	indomethacin	Iron, 20-50 mg
Antilipemic	Questran® Colestid®	cholestyramine colestipol	Vitamin A, 2000-5000 IU Vitamin D, 200-800 IU Vitamin K, 2-25 mg‡ Folic acid, 0.4-1.0 mg
Antituberculous	INH Rifamate®	isoniazid rifampin-isoniazid	Vitamin B$_6$, 25-50 mg Niacin, 15-25 mg Vitamin D, 400-800 IU
Anticoagulant	Coumadin®	coumarin anticoagulants	Avoid vitamin K
Diuretic	Dyrenium® Dyazide®	triamterene	Folic acid, 0.4-1.0 mg
Gastrointestinal	Agoral®	mineral oil	Vitamin A, 5000-10,000¹¹ IU Vitamin D, 400-800 IU
	Soda mint	antacids	Folic acid, 0.4-0.8 mg
Hypotensive	Apresoline®	hydralazine	Vitamin B$_6$, 25-100 mg
Oral contraceptives	Norinyl® Demulen® Ovral® Ortho-Novum® Modicon® and others	estrogen/progestin	Vitamin B$_6$, 1.5-5 mg Folic acid, 0.4-1.0 mg Avoid high doses of vitamin C (i.e. ≥ 1000 mg)
Tranquilizer	Thorazine® Mellaril®	chlorpromazine thioridazine other phenothiazines	Riboflavin, 2-5 mg
Other	Larodopa®	levodopa	Vitamin B$_6$, restrict supplement < 5 mg
	Depen®	penicillamine	Vitamin B$_6$, 25-100 mg

ROCHE Prepared by Daphne Roe, M.D., Professor of Nutrition, Cornell University, Ithaca, New York, as a service to the health profession by Hoffmann-La Roche Inc.

PHARMACOLOGY

Therapeutic agents are drugs or medications which, when introduced into a living organism, modify the physiological functions of that organism. The term "therapeutic agent" usually refers to a chemical compound, although a vitamin, mineral, herb, or a natural food can have a therapeutic effect. In this chapter, therapeutic agents refer to drugs and their actions.

DRUG METABOLISM

Stages of Metabolism

Definition: Drug metabolism in the human body is accomplished in four basic stages—absorption, transportation, biotransformation, and excretion. In order for a drug to be completely metabolized, it must first be given in sufficient concentration to produce the desired effect on body tissues. When this critical drug concentration level is achieved, body tissues change.

A. Absorption.
1. The first stage of metabolism refers to the route a drug takes from the time it enters the body until it is absorbed in the circulating fluids.
2. Drugs are absorbed by the mucous membranes, the gastrointestinal tract, the respiratory tract, and the skin.
   a. The mucous membranes are one of the most rapid and effective routes of absorption because they are highly vascular.
   b. Drugs are absorbed through these membranes by diffusion, infiltration, and osmosis.
3. Drugs given by mouth are absorbed in the gastrointestinal tract.
   a. Portions of these drugs dissolve and absorb in the stomach.
   b. The rate of absorption depends on the pH of the stomach's contents, the food content in the stomach at the time of ingestion, and the presence of disease conditions.
   c. Most of the drug concentrate dissolves in the small intestine where the large vascular surface and moderate pH level enhance the process of dissolution.
4. Methods of administration include intradermal, subcutaneous, intravenous, and intra-arterial injections.
   a. Parenteral methods are the most direct, reliable, and rapid route of absorption.
   b. The actual administration site will depend on type of drug, its action, and the client.
5. Another route of administration is inhalation or nebulization through the respiratory system.
   a. This method is not as rapid as parenteral injections but faster than the gastrointestinal tract.
   b. Drugs administered through the respiratory tract must be made up of small particles that can pass through to the alveoli in the lungs.
6. The final mode of absorption is the skin.
   a. Most drugs, when applied to the skin, produce a local rather than a systemic effect.
   b. The degree of absorption will depend on the strength of the drug as well as where it is applied on the body surface.
B. Transportation.
1. The second stage of metabolism refers to the way in which a drug is transported from the site of introduction to the site of action.
2. First, a drug enters or is absorbed by the body.
   a. The drug binds to plasma protein in the blood.
   b. Then the drug is transported through circulation to all parts of the body.
3. As a drug moves from the circulatory system, it crosses cell membranes and enters the body tissues.
   a. Some of the drug is distributed to and stored in fat and muscle.
   b. Greater masses of tissue (such as fat and muscle) attract the drug.
4. The amount of drug that is distributed to body tissues depends on the permeability of the membranes and the blood supply to the absorption area.

5. A drug that first accumulates in the brain may move into fat and muscle tissue and then back to the brain because the drug is still chemically active.
   a. The drug is released in small quantities from the tissues and travels back to the brain.
   b. Equal drug and blood concentration levels in the body are maintained.

C. Biotransformation.
   1. The third stage of metabolism takes place as the drug, a foreign substance in the body, is converted by enzymes into a less active and harmless agent that can be easily excreted.
   2. Most of this conversion occurs in the liver.
      a. Both synthetic and biochemical reactions take place.
      b. Some conversion does take place in the kidney, plasma, and intestinal mucosa.
   3. Synthetic reactions: liver enzymes conjugate the drug with other substances to make it less harmful for the body.
   4. Biochemical reactions: drugs are oxidized, reduced, hydrolyzed, and synthesized so they become less active and more easily eliminated from the body.

D. Excretion.
   1. The final stage in metabolism takes place when the drug is changed into an inactive form or excreted from the body.
   2. The kidneys are the most important route of excretion.
   3. The kidneys eliminate both the pure drug and the metabolites of the parent drug.
      a. During excretion these two substances are filtered through the glomeruli.
      b. They are then secreted by the tubules.
      c. Finally, they are reabsorbed through the tubules or directly excreted.
   4. Other routes of excretion include the lungs (which exhale gaseous drugs), feces, saliva, tears, and mother's milk.

Factors That Affect Drug Metabolism

A. Personal attributes.
   1. Body weight.
   2. Age.
   3. Sex.
B. Physiological factors.
   1. State of health.
   2. Disease processes.
C. Acid-base and fluid and electrolyte balance.
D. Permeability.
E. Diurnal rhythm.
F. Circulatory capability.
G. Genetic and immunologic factors.
H. Drug tolerance.
I. Cumulation effect of drugs.
J. Other factors.
   1. Psychological.
   2. Emotional.
   3. Environmental.
K. Responses to drugs vary.
   1. Responses depend on the speed with which the drug is absorbed into the blood or tissues.
   2. Responses depend on the effectiveness of the body's circulatory system.

ORIGIN AND NOMENCLATURE OF DRUGS

Common Sources

A. Plant sources.
   1. Roots, bark, sap, leaves, flowers, and seeds from medicinal plants can be used as drug components.
   2. Component substances.
      a. Alkaloid.
         (1) Alkaline (base) in reaction.
         (2) Bitter in taste.
         (3) Physiologically powerful in activity.
      b. Glycoside: a compound containing a carbohydrate molecule.
      c. Resin: soluble in alcohol; insoluble in water.
      d. Gum.
         (1) Mucilaginous (gelatin-like) excretion.
         (2) Used in bulk laxatives; may absorb water.
         (3) Used in skin preparations as a soothing effect, e.g., Karaya gum.
      e. Oil.
         (1) Fixed oil: does not evaporate on warming; occurs as a solid, semisolid, or liquid, e.g., castor oil.
         (2) Volatile oil: evaporates readily; occurs in aromatic plants, e.g., peppermint.

B. Animal sources.
1. Processed from an organ, from organ secretion, or from organ cells.
2. Insulin, as an example, is a derivative from the pancreas of sheep, cattle, or hogs.
C. Mineral sources.
1. Inorganic elements occurring in nature, but not of plant or animal origin; may be metallic or nonmetallic.
2. Usually form a base or acid salt in food.
3. Dilute hydrochloric acid (HCl), as an example, is diluted in water and then taken through a straw to prevent damage to teeth by acid.
D. Synthetic sources.
1. A pure drug made in a laboratory from chemical, not natural, substances.
2. Many drugs, sulfonamides for example, are synthetics.

Methods of Naming Drugs

A. Chemical name.
1. Precise description of chemical constituents with the exact placement of atom groupings.
2. "N-Methyl-4-carbethoxypiperidine hydrochloride" is an example of a chemical name.
B. Generic name.
1. Reflects chemical name to which drug belongs, but is simpler.
2. It is never changed and used commonly in medical terminology.
3. The synthetic narcotic meperidine is an example of a generic name.
C. Trademark name (brand name, proprietary name).
1. Appears in literature with the sign ®, e.g., Demerol ®.
2. The sign indicates the name is registered; use of the name is restricted to the manufacturer who is the legal owner.
3. Trademark name is capitalized or shown in parentheses if generic name stated.

DRUG CLASSIFICATION

Classification by Action

A. Anti-infectives.
1. Antiseptics.
   a. Action—inhibit growth of microorganisms (bacteriostatic).
   b. Purpose—application to wounds and skin infections, sterilization of equipment, and hygienic purposes.
2. Disinfectants.
   a. Action—destroy microorganisms (bactericidal).
   b. Purpose—destroy bacteria on inanimate objects (not appropriate for living tissue).
B. Antimicrobials.
1. Sulfonamides.
   a. Action—inhibit the growth of microorganisms.
   b. Reduce or prevent infectious process especially for urinary tract infections.
2. Antibiotics (e.g., penicillin).
   a. Action—interfere with microorganism metabolism.
   b. Usage—reduce or prevent infectious process.
   c. Specific drug and dosage based on culture and sensitivity of organism.
C. Metabolic drugs.
1. Hormones obtained from animal sources, found naturally in foods and plants.
2. Synthetic hormones.
D. Diagnostic materials.
1. Action—dyes and opaque materials ingested or injected to allow visualization of internal organs.
2. Purpose—to analyze organ status and function.
E. Vitamins and minerals.
1. Action—necessary to obtain healthy body function.
2. Found naturally in food or through synthetic food supplements.
F. Vaccines and serums.
1. Action—prevent disease or detect presence of disease.
2. Types.
   a. Antigenics produce active immunity.
      (1) Vaccines—attenuated suspensions of microorganisms.
      (2) Toxoids—products of microorganisms.
   b. Antibodies—stimulated by microorganisms or their products.
      (1) Antitoxins.
      (2) Immune serum globulin.

c. Allergens—agents for skin immunity tests.
   (1) Extracts of materials known to be allergenic.
   (2) Can be used to relieve allergies.
d. Antivenins—substances which neutralize venom of certain snakes and spiders.

G. Antifungals—check growth of fungi.

H. Antihistaminics.
  1. Action—prevent histamine action.
  2. Purpose—relieve symptoms of allergic reaction.

I. Antineoplastics—prevent growth and spread of malignant cells.

Classification by Body Systems

Central Nervous System

A. Drugs affect CNS by either inhibiting or promoting the actions of neural pathways and centers.
  1. Action promoting drug groups (stimulants).
    a. Antidepressants—psychic energizers used to treat depression.
    b. Caffeine—increases mental activity and lessens drowsiness.
    c. Ammonia—used as revival from fainting spell (client smells cap, not contents of bottle).
  2. Action inhibiting drug groups (depressants).
    a. Analgesics—reduce pain by interfering with conduction of nerve impulses.
      (1) Narcotic analgesics—opium derivatives may depress respiratory centers; must be used with caution and respiratory rate above 12.
        (a) A narcotic antagonist drug counteracts depressant drugs.
        (b) Such antagonist drugs are Lorfan, Narcan, and Nalline.
      (2) Nonnarcotic antipyretics—reduce fever and relieve pain.
      (3) Antirheumatics—analgesics given to relieve arthritis pain; may reduce joint inflammation.
    b. Alcohol—stimulates appetite when given in small doses but classified as a depressant.
    c. Hypnotics—sedatives that induce sleep; common form is the barbiturates.
    d. Antispasmotics—relieve skeletal muscle spasms; anticonvulsants prevent muscle spasms or convulsions.
    e. Tranquilizers.
      (1) Relieve tension and anxiety, preoperative and postoperative apprehension, headaches, menstrual tension, chronic alcoholism, skeletal muscle spasticity, and other neuromuscular disorders.
      (2) Tranquilizers and analgesics frequently given together (in reduced dosage); the one drug enhances the action of the other (synergy).
    f. Anesthetics—produce the state of unconsciousness painlessly.

B. Precautions to be taken with CNS drugs.
  1. Drugs which act on CNS may potentiate other CNS drugs.
  2. Client may be receiving other medications; find out drug name and dosage.
  3. Dependence on CNS drugs may occur.

Autonomic Nervous System

A. This system governs several body functions so that drugs that affect the ANS will at the same time affect other system functions.

B. The ANS is made up of two nerve systems—the sympathetic and parasympathetic.
  1. Parasympathetic is the stabilizing system.
  2. Sympathetic is the protective emergency system.

C. Each system has a separate basic drug group acting on it.
  1. Adrenergics—mimic the actions of sympathetic system.
    a. Vasoconstrictors—stimulants such as Adrenalin.
      (1) Action is to constrict peripheral blood vessels thereby increasing blood pressure.
      (2) Dilate bronchial passages.
      (3) Relax gastrointestinal tract.
    b. Vasodilators—depressants such as nicotinic acid.
      (1) Antagonists of epinephrine and similar drugs.
      (2) Vasodilate blood vessels.

(3) Increase tone of GI tract.

(4) Reduce blood pressure.

(5) Relax smooth muscles.

(6) *Caution:* If drug is to be stopped, reduce dosage gradually over a period of a week; do not stop it suddenly.

2. Cholinergics—mimic actions of parasympathetic system.

a. Cholinergic stimulants (e.g., Prostigmin or neostigmine).

(1) Decrease heart rate.

(2) Contract smooth muscle.

(3) Contract pupil in eye.

(4) Increase peristalsis.

(5) Increase gland secretions.

b. Cholinergic inhibiters (anticholinergics).

(1) Decrease gland secretion.

(2) Relax smooth muscle.

(3) Dilate pupil in eye.

(4) Increase heart action.

Gastrointestinal System

A. Drugs affecting GI system act upon muscular and glandular tissues.

B. Drug groups and actions.

1. Antacids—counteract excess acidity.

a. Have alkaline base.

b. Used in the treatment of ulcers.

c. Neutralize hydrochloric acid in the stomach.

d. Given frequently (two hour intervals or more often).

e. May be given with water.

f. May cause constipation, depending on type of medication.

g. Baking soda is a systemic antacid which disturbs the pH balance in the body. Most other antacids coat the mucous membrane and neutralize hydrochloric acid.

2. Emetics—produce vomiting (emesis).

C. H_2 receptor antagonists (block gastric acid secretion) e.g., cimetidine, ranitidine.

D. Antiulcer drugs—sucralfate; give 1 hour a.c. and at HS; nonsystemic.

E. Digestants—relieve enzyme deficiency by replacing secretions in digestive tract.

F. Antidiarrheics—prevent diarrhea.

G. Cathartics—affect intestine and produce defecation.

a. Provide temporary relief for constipation.

b. Rid bowel of contents before surgery, and prepare viscera for diagnostic studies.

c. Counteract edema.

d. Treat diseases of GI tract.

e. Are contraindicated when abdominal pain is present.

f. Classifications.

(1) By degree of action.

(a) Laxative—mild action.

(b) Cathartic—moderate action.

(c) Purgative—severe action.

(2) By method of action.

Respiratory System

A. Drugs act on respiratory tract, tissues, and cough center.

B. Action is to suppress, relax, liquefy, and stimulate.

1. Respiratory stimulants stimulate depth and rate of respiration.

C. Bronchodilators (relax smooth muscle of trachea and bronchi).

1. Sympathomimetics.

(1) Taken p.o. or inhaled (fewer side effects).

(2) Beta$_2$ agonists preferred (e.g., albuterol, metaproterenol).

2. Anticholinergics (e.g., atropine sulfate by nebulizer or metered dose inhaler).

3. Theophyllines.

(1) Monitor serum levels.

(2) Examples: theophylline p.o., aminophylline IV.

4. Anti-inflammatory agents (reduce bronchospasm).

(1) Antimediators (e.g., chromolyn sodium).

(2) Corticosteroids (p.o., IV, or inhaled).

Urinary System

A. Drugs that act on kidneys and urinary tract.

B. Action is to increase urine flow, destroy bacteria, and perform other important body functions.

1. Diuretics.

a. Rid body of excess fluid and relieve edema.

b. Some drugs that act on the GI tract and circulatory system also are diuretic in action.

2. Urinary antiseptics.

3. Acidifiers and alkalinizers—certain foods will also increase body acids or alkalies.

Circulatory System

A. Drugs that act on heart, blood, and blood vessels.
B. Action is to change heart rhythm, rate, and force and to dilate or constrict vessels.
  1. Cardiotonics used for heart-strengthening.
    a. Direct heart stimulants that speed heart rate, e.g., caffeine, Adrenalin.
    b. Indirect heart stimulants, e.g., digitalis.
      (1) Stimulate vagus nerve.
      (2) Slow heart rate and stengthen it.
      (3) Improve heart action, thereby improving circulation.
      (4) Do not administer if apical pulse below 60.
  2. Cardioprotective drugs.
    a. Beta adrenergic blockers.
    b. Calcium entry blockers.
  3. Antiarrhythmic drugs used clinically to convert irregularities to a normal sinus rhythm.
  4. Drugs that alter blood flow.
    a. Anticoagulants (inhibit blood clotting action; e.g., heparin, coumadin).
    b. Thrombolytic agents (streptokinase, urokinase).
    c. Platelet inhibiting agents (aspirin, dipyridamole).
    d. Vasodilators.
    e. Hemorrheologic agent, e.g., pentoxifyline (trental).
  5. Blood replacement.

DOSAGE AND PREPARATION FORMS

Solids

A. Extract—obtained by dissolving drug in water or alcohol and allowing solution to evaporate; residue is the extract.
B. Powder—finely ground drugs.
C. Pills—common term for tablet; made by rolling drug and binder into a sphere.
D. Suppository.
  1. Contains drugs mixed with a firm base.
  2. Liquefies at body temperature when inserted into orifice.
  3. Releases drug to produce a local or systemic effect.
E. Ointment—semisolid mixture of drugs with a fatty base.

F. Lozenge—flavored flat tablet that releases drug slowly when held in mouth.
G. Capsule.
  1. Drugs in small, cylindrical gelatin containers that disguise the taste of the drug.
  2. Capsule can be opened and drug mixed with food or jam to mask taste.
H. Tablets
  1. Dried, powdered drugs that are compressed into a small disk which easily disintegrates in water.
  2. Enteric coated—tablet does not dissolve until reaching intestines, where release of drug occurs.

Liquids

A. Fluid extract.
  1. Concentrated fluid preparation of drugs produced by dissolving crude plant drug in a solvent.
  2. Strength of extract is such that 1 cc (about ¼ teaspoon or 15 to 16 gtt) represents 1 gram of the drug at 100 percent strength.
B. Tincture.
  1. Diluted alcoholic extract of a drug.
  2. Varies in stength from 10 to 20 percent.
C. Spirit—preparation of volatile (easily vaporized) substances dissolved in alcohol.
D. Syrup—drug contained in a concentrated sugar solution.
E. Elixir—solution of drug made with alcohol, sugar, and some aromatic or pleasant-smelling substance.
F. Suspension.
  1. Undissolved, finely divided particles of drug dispersed in a liquid.
  2. Gels and magma are other forms of suspensions.
  3. Shake all bottles of suspension well before giving.
G. Emulsion—suspension of unmixed oils, fats, or petrolatum in water.
H. Liniment and lotion—liquid suspension of medication applied to the skin.

Packaging Methods and Dispensing

A. Unit dosage package method.

1. Package contains premeasured amount of drug in proper form for administering.
2. Pharmacy may deliver the daily needs for each client to the floor.
3. Procedures for delivery and storage vary from hospital to hospital.
4. Nurse administers the medication to the client.

B. Traditional method.
  1. Nurse prepares medication on the unit.
  2. Supplies come from stock or bulk on the ward or from a multiple dose bottle of client's.

C. The nurse is responsible for accuracy of the medication given, regardless of the packaging or dispensing method used.

ROUTES OF ADMINISTRATION

Oral Route

A. Ingested (swallowed).
B. Sublingual (under tongue).
C. Buccal (on mucous membrane of cheek or tongue).

Rectal Route

A. Suppository.
B. Liquid (retention enema).

Parenteral Route

A. Intravenous.
  1. The response is fast and immediate.
  2. Over 5 cc medication can be given.
  3. Drug *must be* given slowly and usually in diluted form.
  4. Check medication leaflets to determine if medication route is IM or IV.

B. Intradermal.
  1. Injected into skin; usual site is inner aspect of forearm or scapular area of back.
  2. A short bevel 26-gauge, 1-cm needle is used.
  3. Needle should be inserted with bevel up.
  4. This route is usually used to inject antigens for skin or tuberculin tests.
  5. Amount injected ranges from 0.01 to 0.1 cc.

C. Subcutaneous.
  1. A 25-gauge, 1.3- to 1.6-cm needle is used.
  2. Injection site is the fatty layer under skin.
    a. Abdomen at navel.
    b. Lateral upper arm or thigh.
  3. This route usually used for injecting medication that is to be absorbed slowly with a sustained effect.
  4. Amount injected ranges from 0.5 to 1.5 cc.
  5. If repeated doses are necessary, as with insulin for a diabetic person, rotate the injection sites.

D. Intramuscular.
  1. Needle gauge and length will vary with site.
    a. Deltoid—located by having client raise arm.
      (1) A 23- to 25-gauge, 1.6- to 2.5-cm needle is used.
      (2) Administer no more than 2 cc.
    b. Thigh and buttock.
      (1) Needle must be long enough to reach muscle; may vary from 2 to 8 cm.
      (2) Needle gauge depends upon substance of medication.
      (3) Oil bases require 20 gauge; water bases require 22 gauge.
  2. Absorption rate of IM medication dependent upon circulation of person injected.
  3. This route usually used for systemic effect of an irritating drug.
  4. Amount of medication must not be over 5 cc, as absorption would be difficult and painful.
  5. Techniques for lessening pain for the client receiving an IM medication:
    a. Encourage relaxation of area to be injected; request client to lie on side with flexed knee or out flat on abdomen, if giving injection in buttock.
    b. Reduce puncture pain by "darting" needle.
    c. Prevent antiseptic from clinging to needle during insertion by waiting until skin antiseptic is dry.
    d. If medication must be drawn through a rubber stopper, use a new needle for injection.
    e. Avoid sensitive or hardened body areas.
    f. After needle is under skin, aspirate to be certain that needle is not in a blood vessel.
    g. Inject slowly.
    h. Maintain grasp of syringe.
    i. Withdraw needle quickly after injection.
    j. Massage relaxed muscle gently to increase circulation and to distribute medication.
  6. Observe for side effects of medication following injection.

Other Routes

A. Inhalation route.
B. Topical route.

ADMINISTRATION OF MEDICATIONS

Basic Guidelines for Medication Administration

A. Determine the correct dosage, actions, side effects, and contraindications of any medication before administration.
B. Determine if medications ordered by the physician are appropriate for client's condition. This is part of the nurse's professional responsibility.
C. Question the physician about any medication orders that are incomplete, illegible, or inappropriate for the client's condition.
   1. Remember, the nurse may be liable if a medication error is made.
   2. Report every medication error to the physician and nursing administrator.
   3. Complete a medication incident report.
D. Check to determine if the medication ordered is compatible with the client's condition and with other medications prescribed.
E. Ascertain what the client has been eating or drinking before administering a medication.
   1. Determine what effect the client's diet has on the medication.
   2. Do not administer medication if contraindicated by diet. For example, do not give an MAO inhibitor to a client who has just ingested cheddar cheese or wine.
F. Check that calculated drug dosage is accurate for young children, elderly people, or for very thin or obese clients. These age and weight groups require smaller or larger dosages.

Safety Rules

A. The five rights.
   1. Right medication.
      a. Compare drug card with drug label three times.
      b. Know general purpose, dosage, method of administration.
      c. Know side effects of drug.
   2. Right client: check ID band and door number.
   3. Right time.
   4. Right method of administration.
   5. Right amount.
      a. Check all calculations of divided dosages with another nurse.
      b. Check heparin, insulin, and IV digitalis doses with another nurse.
B. The five rights should be practiced each and every time a medication is given.

DOCUMENTATION OF MEDICATIONS

Medication Orders

A. Medication administered to client must have a physician's order or prescription before it can be legally administered.
B. Physician's order is a verbal or written order, recorded in a book or file or in client's chart.
C. If order is given verbally over the telephone, nurse must write a verbal order in client's chart for the physician to sign at a later date.
D. Written orders are safer—they leave less room for potential misunderstanding or error.
E. Drug order should consist of seven parts:
   1. Name of the client.
   2. Date the drug was ordered.
   3. Name of the drug.
   4. Dosage.
   5. Route of administration and any special rules of administration.
   6. Time and frequency the drug should be given.
   7. Signature of the individual who ordered the drug.

Types of Medication Schedules

A. Routine orders.
   1. Administered according to instructions until it is cancelled by another order.

2. Can also be used for p.r.n. drugs.
   a. Administered when client needs the medication.
   b. Not given on a routine time schedule.
3. Continued validity of any routine order should be assessed—physicians occasionally forget to cancel an order when it is no longer appropriate for client's condition.

B. One-time orders.
   1. Administered as stated, only one time.
   2. Given at a specified time or "stat," which means immediately.

Medication Errors

A. Nurse who prepares a medication must also give it to client and chart it.
   1. If client refuses drug, chart that medication was refused—report this information to the physician.
   2. When charting medications, use the correct abbreviations and symbols.
B. If error in a drug order is found, it is nurse's responsibility to question the order.
   1. If order cannot be understood or read, verify with the physician.
   2. Do not guess at the order as this constitutes gross negligence.
   3. In many hospitals it is the pharmacist's responsibility to contact physicians when medication orders are unclear.
C. Always report medication errors to the physician immediately.
   1. This action minimizes potential danger to the client.
   2. Measures can be taken immediately to assess and evaluate the client's status.
   3. A plan of action can be implemented to reverse the effects of the medication.
D. Errors in medication are documented in a medication incident report and on the client's record.
   1. This action is necessary for both legal reasons and nursing audits.
   2. Nursing audits are conducted to determine problems in medication administration:
      a. A particular source of problems.
      b. A range of problems that seem to have no connection.

Legal Issues in Drug Administration

A. Nurse must not administer a specific drug unless allowed to do so by the particular state's Nurse Practice Act.
B. Nurse is to take every safety precaution in whatever he or she is doing.
C. Nurse is to be certain that employer's policy allows him or her to administer a specific drug.
D. A drug may not lawfully be administered unless all the above items are in effect.
E. General rules.
   1. Never leave tray with prepared medicines unattended.
   2. Always report errors immediately.
   3. Send labeled bottles that are unintelligible back to pharmacist for relabeling.
   4. Store internal and external medicines separately if possible.

ADMINISTERING MEDICATIONS

Administering Oral Medication

Assessment

A. Assess that oral route is the most efficient means of medication administration.
B. Check medication orders for their completeness and accuracy.
C. Assess client's physical ability to take medication as ordered.
   1. Swallow reflex present.
   2. State of consciousness.
   3. Signs of nausea and vomiting.
   4. Uncooperative behavior.
D. Check to make sure you have the correct medication for the client.
E. Assess correct dosage when calculation is needed.

Planning and Analysis

A. Client is able to ingest and metabolize medication without feelings of nausea or vomiting.
B. Client emotionally accepts medication.
C. Client experiences a sustained action of drug and a positive effect on his or her body.

Implementation

A. Preparing oral medications.

1. Obtain client's medication record. Medication record may be a drug card, medication sheet, or drug Kardex, depending on the method of dispensing medications in the hospital.
2. Compare the medication record with the most *recent* physician's order.
3. Wash your hands.
4. Gather necessary equipment.
5. Remove the medication from the drug box or tray on medication cart.
6. Compare the label on the bottle or drug package to the medication record.
7. Correctly calculate dosage if necessary and check the dosage to be administered.
8. Pour the medication from the bottle into the lid of the container and then into the medicine cup. With unit dosage, take drug package from medication cart tray and place in medication cup. Do not remove drug from drug package.
9. Check medication label again to ensure correct drug and dosages if drug is not prepackaged.
10. Place medication cup on a tray, if not using medication cart.
11. Return the multidose vial bottle to the storage area. If medication to be given is a narcotic, sign out the narcotic record sheet with your name.

B. Administering oral medications to adults.
1. Take medication tray or cart to client's room; check room number against medication card or sheet.
2. Place client in sitting position, if not contraindicated by his or her condition.
3. Tell the client what type of medication you are going to give and explain the actions this medication will produce.
4. Check the client's Identaband and ask client to state name so that you are sure you have correctly identified him or her.
5. If prepackaged medication is used, read label, take medication out of package, and put into medication cup.
6. Give the medication cup to the client.
7. Offer a fresh glass of water or other liquid to aid swallowing, and give assistance with taking medications.
8. Make sure the client swallows the medication.
9. Discard used medicine cup.
10. Position client for comfort.
11. Record the medication on the appropriate forms.

C. Administering oral medications to children.
1. Follow the procedures for the previous intervention, keeping the following guidelines in mind:
   a. Play techniques may help to elicit a young child's cooperation.
   b. Remember, the smaller the quantity of dilutent (food or liquid), the greater the ease in eliciting the child's cooperation.
   c. Never use a child's favorite food or drink as an enticement when administering medication because the result may be the child's refusal to eat or drink anything.
   d. Be honest and tell the child that you have medicine, not candy.
2. Assess child for drug action and possible side effects.
3. Explain medication action and side effects to parents.

Evaluation

A. Client is able to ingest and metabolize medication without feeling nauseated or vomiting.
B. Client emotionally accepts medication.
C. Client experiences a sustained action of drug and a positive effect on the body.
D. Client does not have an allergic or anaphylactic response to the medication.

Narcotic Administration

A. Check medication card or sheet for narcotic orders.
B. Check time frame since last narcotic administered.
C. Open narcotic box or cupboard and find appropriate narcotic container.
D. Count number of pills, ampules or injectable cartridges in container.
E. Check narcotic sign-out sheet and check that number of narcotics matches number of sign-out sheets.
F. Rectify situation before proceeding with narcotic administration if narcotics and sign-out sheets do not coincide.
G. Sign out for narcotic on narcotic sheets, after taking narcotic out of drawer or cupboard.
H. Lock drawer or cupboard after taking out medication.
I. Sign out narcotics on medication record according to usual procedure.

J. Check narcotics every 8 hours.
1. One off-going and one on-going nurse check the narcotics.
2. Number of sign-out sheets must match remaining number of narcotics.
3. Each narcotic sheet is checked for accuracy.
K. Return counter (if used) to pharmacy with completed narcotic sign-out sheet when sheet is filled.
1. A new narcotic supply and narcotic check sheet are signed out in pharmacy.
2. The nurse receiving narcotics signs drug record receipt.

Administering Parenteral Medications

Assessment

A. Determine appropriate method for administration of drug:
1. Intradermal (intracutaneous): injection is made below surface of the skin.
2. Subcutaneous: small amount of fluid is injected beneath the skin in the loose connective tissues.
3. Intramuscular: larger amount of fluid is injected into large muscle masses in the body.
4. Intravenous: medication is injected or infused directly into a vein—route used when immediate drug effect is desired.
B. Evaluate condition of administration site for presence of lesions, rash, inflammation, lipid dystrophy, ecchymosis, etc.
C. Assess for tissue damage from previous injections.
D. Assess client's level of consciousness.
1. For client in shock: certain methods (subcutaneous) will not be used.
2. For presence of anxiety: make sure client is allowed to express his or her fear of injections and offer explanations of ways in which injections will be less frightening.
E. Check client's written and verbal history for past allergic reactions. Do *not* rely solely on client's chart.
F. Review client's chart noting previous injection sites, especially insulin and heparin administration sites.
G. Check label on medication bottle to determine if medication can be administered via route ordered.

Planning and Analysis

A. Injection process is completed without technical complications.
B. Injection is as painless as possible.
C. Medication enters bloodstream promptly and is actively utilized by the tissues.

Implementation

A. Preparing medications.
1. Wash your hands.
2. Obtain equipment for injection: needle and syringe, alcohol wipes, medication tray (medication container if needed).
3. Assemble the needle and syringe. Select the appropriate size needle, considering the size of the client's muscle mass and the viscosity of the medication.
4. Open the alcohol wipe and cleanse the top of the vial or break top of ampule.
5. Remove the needle guard and place on alcohol wipe or medication tray.
6. Pull back on barrel of syringe to markings where medication will be inserted.
7. Pick up vial, insert needle into vial, and inject air in an amount equal to the solution to be withdrawn by pushing barrel of syringe down. If using an ampule, break off top at colored line, insert syringe, but do not inject air into ampule as it causes a break in the vacuum and possible loss of medication through leakage.
8. Extract the desired amount of fluid. Remove needle from container and cover needle with guard. Needle should be changed to prevent tracking medication on skin and subcutaneous tissue.
9. Double-check drug and dosage against drug card or medication sheet and vial or ampule.
10. Place syringe on tray.
11. Check label and drug card or medication sheet for accuracy before returning multidose vial to correct storage area.
12. Return multidose vial to correct storage area or discard used vial or ampule.
B. Administering intradermal injections.
1. Take medication to client's room. Check room number against medication card or sheet.
2. Explain the medication's action and the procedure for administration to client.

3. Check client's Identaband and ask client to state name.
4. Wash your hands.
5. Select the site of injection.
6. Cleanse the area with an alcohol wipe, wiping in circular area from inside to outside.
7. Take off needle guard and place on tray.
8. Grasp client's forearm from underneath and gently pull the skin taut.
9. Insert the needle at 10- to 15-degree angle with the bevel of needle facing up.
10. Inject medication slowly. Observe for wheals and blanching at the site.
11. Withdraw the needle, wiping the area gently with a dry 2 × 2 bandage to prevent dispersing medication into the subcutaneous tissue.
12. Return the client to a comfortable position.
13. Discard supplies in appropriate area.
14. Chart the medication and site used.

C. Administering subcutaneous (sub q) injections.
1. Take medication to client's room.
2. Set tray on a clean surface, not the bed.
3. Check client's Identaband and ask client to state name.
4. Explain action of medication and procedure of administration.
5. Provide privacy when injection site is other than on the arm.
6. Wash your hands.
7. Select site for injection by identifying anatomical landmarks. Remember to alternate sites each time injections are given.
8. Cleanse area with alcohol wipe. Using a circular motion cleanse from inside outward.
9. Take off needle guard.

10. Express any air bubbles from syringe.
11. Insert the needle at a 45-degree angle.
12. Pull back on the plunger.
13. Inject the medication slowly.
14. Withdraw needle quickly and massage area with alcohol wipe to aid absorption and lessen bleeding. Put on Bandaid if needed.
15. Return client to a position of comfort.
16. Discard used supplies in proper areas. Remember to break needle from syringe and discard needle in safety container.
17. Chart the medication and site used.

D. Administering insulin injections.
1. Gather equipment and check medication orders, injection site, and rotation chart. Insulin does not need to be refrigerated.
2. Wash your hands.
3. Obtain specific insulin syringe for strength of insulin being administered (U100).
4. Rotate insulin bottle between hands to bring solution into suspension.
5. Wipe top of insulin bottle with alcohol.
6. Take off needle guard.
7. Pull plunger of syringe down to desired amount of medication and inject that amount of air into the insulin bottle.
8. Draw up ordered amount of insulin into syringe.
9. Expel air from syringe.
10. Replace needle guard.
11. Check medication card, bottle, and syringe with another RN for accuracy.
12. Take medications to client's room.
13. Double-check site of last injection with client.
14. Provide privacy.

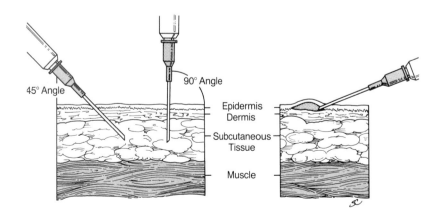

45° Angle

90° Angle

Epidermis
Dermis

Subcutaneous
Tissue

Muscle

Insert needle at 45- or 90-degree angle into tissue for subcutaneous injection.

Insert needle at 15-degree angle just under the epidermis for intradermal injection.

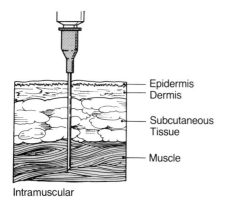

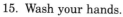

Intramuscular

Insert needle at 90-degree angle for intramuscular injections.

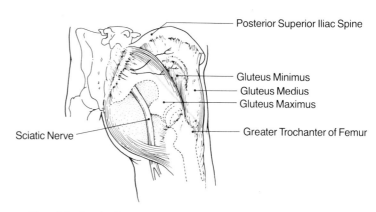

Place injection in gluteus medius above and outside the diagonal line for
intramuscular injections.

15. Wash your hands.
16. Follow protocol for administration of medica-
    tions by subcutaneous injections.
E. Administering intramuscular (IM) injections.
  1. Take medication to client's room. Check room
     number against medication card or sheet.
  2. Set tray on a clean surface, not the bed.
  3. Explain the procedure to client.
  4. Check client's Identaband and have client state
     name.
  5. Provide privacy for client.
  6. Wash your hands.
  7. Select the site of injection by identifying ana-
     tomical landmarks. Remember to alternate
     sites each time injections are given.
  8. Cleanse the area with alcohol wipe. Using a
     circular motion, cleanse from inside outward.
  9. Hold the syringe; take off needle cover.
 10. Express air bubbles from syringe. Some clini-
     cians suggest leaving a small air bubble at the
     tip so that all medicine will be expelled.
 11. Insert the needle at 90-degree angle.
 12. Pull back on plunger. If blood returns, you
     know you have entered a blood vessel and need
     to reposition the needle and aspirate again.
 13. Inject the medication slowly.
 14. Withdraw the needle and massage the area
     with an alcohol wipe. Put on a Bandaid, if
     needed.
 15. Return client to a comfortable position.
 16. Discard supplies in appropriate area.
 17. Chart the medication and site used.

Evaluation

A. Injection process is completed without technical
   complications.
B. Injection is as painless as possible.
C. Medication enters bloodstream promptly and is
   effectively utilized by the tissues.

SYSTEMS OF MEASUREMENT

Apothecary System

A. Older system based on unrelated, arbitrary units
   of measure; gradually being replaced by metric
   system.
  1. Portions of a unit of measurement designated
     by common fractions, e.g., one-fourth grain,
     written as gr¼.
  2. Symbols for ounces and drams are similar in
     form and must be written clearly (e.g., ℥ is
     dram; ℥ is ounce).
  3. Symbols and abbreviations are placed before
     roman numerals (5 grains written as gr v).
B. Common apothecary measures and symbols.

drop	gtt
minim	m
dram	℥
ounce	℥
pint	0
grain	gr

C. Equivalents.

1 drop	= 1 minim
15 drops	= 1 grain
60 minims	= 1 fluid dram
8 fluid drams	= 1 fluid ounce
16 fluid ounces	= 1 pint

Metric System

A. French-invented system based on rationally and related derived units.
  1. Developed in the eighteenth century.
  2. Basic units of measure used in drug administration are the gram and liter.
  3. Other units are decimal, fractions, and Arabic numerals.
  4. Number and fraction placed before symbol.
B. Common metric measures and symbols.

gram	g, gm, *or* G
kilogram	kg
milligram	mg
milliliter	ml
liter	L *or* l

C. Weight and volume equivalents with corresponding symbols.

1 gram = 1,000 milligrams	1 g = 1,000 mg
1 liter = 1,000 milliliters	1 l = 1,000 ml

Household System

A. System based on familiar measures used in the home.
  1. Most measures not sufficiently accurate for measure of medicines.
  2. Pints and quarts also used in apothecary system.
B. Common household measures and their abbreviations.

pint	pt	tablespoon	T
teaspoon	t	quart	qt

MATHEMATIC CONVERSIONS

Approximate Equivalents

A. The metric system is the universal system of weights and measures.

B. Apothecary and metric do not use same size units; denominations of one system not compatible with the other.
C. Equivalency tables established to list measurement denominations of one system in terms of another. (See Appendix 2.)
  1. Conversion from one system to another can be computed, but is not equivalent in absolute terms.
  2. If there is occasion to compute, have computations checked by another licensed nurse.
    a. Do not compute unless allowed to do so by your state's Nurse Practice Act.
    b. Check hospital policy for further guidelines.

Computation

A. Drugs are not always labeled clearly as to number of tablets to administer so computation may be necessary. Always have your computation checked by another licensed nurse.
B. Method.
  1. Both desired (ordered) dose and dose on hand must be in same unit of measurement, e.g., grains, grams, milligrams.
  2. If not same, convert so that unit of measure is the same.
    a. Refer to conversion table. (Appendix 1.)
    b. To convert one measure unit to another, basic equivalencies must be memorized.
  3. After converting, divide desired dose by dose on hand to find amount to administer.

Calculation of Dosages

A. Using equivalent tables to calculate drug dosages.
  1. To convert milligrams to grains, use the following formula:

     Example: Convert 180 milligrams to grains.

     $$\frac{1 \text{ gr}}{\text{mg in gr}} = \frac{\text{dose desired}}{\text{dose on hand}}$$

     $$\frac{1}{60} = \frac{x}{180}$$

     $$60x = 180$$

     $$x = 3 \text{ grains}$$

2. You may also make this conversion as a ratio:

1 gr:60 mg: :x gr:180 mg   60x = 180

x = 3 grains

3. Check equivalency tables in the drug supplement.

B. Calculating oral dosages of drugs.

1. To calculate oral dosages, use the following formula:

$$\frac{D}{H} = X$$

where D = dose desired

H = dose on hand

X = dose to be administered

Example: Give 500 mg of ampicillin when the dose on hand is in capsules containing 250 mg.

$$\frac{500 \text{ mg}}{250 \text{ mg}} = 2 \text{ capsules}$$

2. To calculate oral dosages of liquids, use the following formula:

$$\frac{D}{H} \times Q = X$$

where Q = quantity

Example: Give 375 mg of ampicillin when it is supplied as 250 mg/5 ml.

$$\frac{375 \text{ mg}}{250 \text{ mg}} \times 5$$

1.5 × 5 = 7.5 ml

You can also set up a direct proportion and following the algebraic principle, cross multiply:

$$\frac{375 \text{ mg}}{x} = \frac{250 \text{ mg}}{5 \text{ ml}}$$

250x = 1875

x = 7.5 ml (of strength 250 mg/5 ml)

C. Calculating parenteral dosages of drugs.

1. To calculate parenteral dosages, use the following formula:

$$\frac{D}{H} \times Q = X$$

Example: Give client 40 mg gentamicin. On hand is a multidose vial with a strength of 80 mg/2 ml.

$$\frac{40}{80} \times 2 = 1 \text{ ml}$$

2. Check your calculations before drawing up medication.

Calculation of Solutions

A. Types of solutions.

1. Volume to volume (v/v): a given volume of solute is added to a given volume solvent.

2. Weight to weight (w/w): a stated weight of solute is dissolved in a stated weight of solvent.

3. Weight to volume (w/v): a given weight of solute is dissolved in a given volume of solvent which results in the proper amount of solution.

B. Preparing solutions.

1. Liquid to drug solutions.

a. Determine the strength of the solution, the strength of the drug on hand, and the quantity of solution required.

b. Use this formula for preparing solutions:

$$\frac{D}{H} \times Q = X$$

where D = desired strength

H = strength on hand

Q = quantity of solution desired

X = amount of solute

Example: You have a 100% solution of hydrogen peroxide on hand. You need a liter of 50% solution.

$$\frac{50}{100} \times 1000 \text{ ml} = 500 \text{ ml}$$

If the strength desired and strength on hand are not in like terms, you need to change one of the terms.

Example: You have 1 liter of 50% solution on hand. You need a liter of 1:10 solution. 1:10 solution is the same as 10%.

$$\frac{10\%}{50\%} \times 1000 \text{ ml} = 200 \text{ ml}$$

Add 200 ml of the drug to 800 ml of the solvent to make a liter of 10% solution.

2. Volume to volume solutions.

Use the formula:

$$\frac{D}{H} \times Q = X$$

where X = amount of stock solution used

Example: Prepare a liter of 5% solution from a stock solution of 50%.

$$\frac{5\%}{50\%} \times 1000 \text{ ml} = 100 \text{ ml}$$

Add 100 ml to 900 ml of diluent to make 1 liter of 5% solution.

3. Solutions from tablets.
  a. Use the formula:

$$\frac{D}{H} \times Q = X$$

where X = amount/number of tablets used

Example: Prepare 1 liter of a 1:1000 solution, using 10 grain tablets.

$$\frac{1/1000}{10 \text{ gr}} \times 1000 \text{ ml} = X$$

  b. First convert 10 grains to grams so the numerator and denominator are in the same unit of measure. 1 gm = 15 gr; therefore, 10 gr = ⅔ gm. Now substitute the new numbers in the formula and solve for X.

$$\frac{1/1000}{2/3} \times \frac{1000}{1} \text{ ml} = X$$

$$\frac{3}{2000} \times \frac{1000}{1} = X$$

X = ³⁄₂, or 1½ tablets

Place 1½ tablets into the 1 liter of solution and dissolve.

GOVERNING LAWS

Federal Food, Drug, and Cosmetic Act of 1938

A. The act is an update of the Food and Drug Act first passed in 1906.
B. It designates *United States Pharmacopeia* and *National Formulary* as official standards.
C. The federal government has the power to enforce standards.
D. Provisions of the act.
  1. Drug manufacturer must provide adequate evidence of drug's safety.
  2. Correct labeling and packaging of drugs.
E. Amended in 1952 to include control of barbiturates by restricting prescription refills.
F. Amended in 1962 to require substantial investigation of drug and evidence that drug is effective in terms of labeling claims.

Harrison Narcotic Act of 1914

A. Provisions of the act.
  1. Regulates manufacture, importation, and sale of opium, cocaine, and their derivatives.
  2. Amendments have added addictive synthetic drugs to the regulated drug listing.
B. Applications of the act.
  1. Individuals who produce, sell, dispense (pharmacists), and prescribe (dentists, physicians) these drugs must be licensed and registered; prescriptions must be in triplicate.
  2. Hospitals order drugs on special blanks that bear hospital registry number. The following information is recorded for each dose:
    a. Name of drug.
    b. Amount of drug.
    c. Date and time drug obtained.
    d. Name of physician prescribing drug.
    e. Name of client receiving drug.
    f. Nurse's signature and type of license (RN, LVN, or LPN).

The Controlled Substance Act of 1970

A. Provisions of the act.
  1. Regulates potentially addictive drugs as to prescription, use, and possession.
    a. Regulations refer to use in hospital, office, research, and emergency situations.
    b. Regulations cover narcotics, cocaine, amphetamines, hallucinogens, barbiturates, and other sedatives.
  2. Controlled drugs are placed in five different schedules or categorical listings, each governed by different regulations.
    a. The regulations govern manufacture, transport, and storage of the controlled drugs.
    b. The use of the drugs is controlled as to prescription, authorization, the mode of dispensation, and administration.
B. Application of the act for use of controlled drugs in hospital.
  1. The nurse is to keep the stock supply of controlled drugs under lock and key.
    a. Nurse must sign for each dose (tablet, cc) of drug.

b. Key is held by the nurse responsible for administration of medication.

c. At the end of each shift, nurse must account for all controlled drugs in the stock supply.

2. Violations of the Controlled Substance Act.

a. Violations are punishable by fine, imprisonment, or both.

b. Nurses, upon conviction of violation, are subject to losing their licenses to practice nursing.

Prescription and Medication Orders

A. Prescription is a written order for dispensation of drugs that can be used only under physician's supervision.

B. Prescriptions outside the hospital.

1. Formula to pharmacist for dispensing drugs to client.

2. Consists of four parts.

a. Superscription (symbolized by Rx, meaning "take").

(1) Client's name.

(2) Client's address (required only for controlled drugs).

(3) Age (required only if age is factor in dose preparation).

(4) Date (must *always* be included).

b. Inscription.

(1) Specifies ingredients and their quantities.

(2) May specify other ingredients necessary to specific drug form.

c. Subscription—directions to pharmacist as to method of preparation.

d. Signature—consists of two parts.

(1) Accurate instructions to client as to when, how, and in what quantities to take medication; typed on label.

(2) Physician's signature and refill instructions.

C. Orders inside the hospital.

1. Physician writes medication order in book, file, or client's chart; if given over phone, nurse writes verbal order which physician later signs.

2. Order consists of six parts.

a. Name of drug.

b. Dosage.

c. Route of administration with time drug was given.

d. Reason drug required (not always included).

e. Length of time client is to receive drug (not always included).

f. Signature of individual who ordered drug.
Example: Aspirin gr xPO q3h for pain for 3 days.

D. Smith, M.D.

Informational Resources

Official Publications

A. A drug listed in the following publications is designated as official by the Federal Food, Drug, and Cosmetic Act (FDC).

1. *The United States Pharmacopeia* (USP).

2. *National Formulary* (NF).

3. *Homeopathic Pharmacopeia of the United States.*

B. These publications establish standards of purity and other criteria for product acceptability; these standards are binding according to law.

C. Publications contain information on each drug entry.

1. Source.

2. Chemical and physical composition.

3. Method of storage.

4. General type or category.

5. Range of dosage and usual therapeutic dosage.

Other Publications

A. *American Hospital Formulary* is a publication indexed by generic and proprietary names.

B. *Physicians' Desk Reference* (PDR).

1. Annual publication with quarterly supplements.

2. Handy source of information about dosage and drug precautions.

Miscellaneous Resources

A. Package inserts from manufacturers that accompany the product.

B. Pharmacist.

C. Physician.

D. Nursing journals.

E. Pharmaceutical and medical treatment texts.

Appendix 1. ABBREVIATIONS AND SYMBOLS FOR ORDERS, PRESCRIPTIONS, AND LABELS

aa	of each		os	mouth
ac	before meals		oz or ʒ	ounce
ad lib	freely, as desired		pc	after meals
Ba	barium		per	by, through
bid	twice each day		p.r.n.	whenever necessary
c̄	with		qh	every hour
C	carbon		q.i.d.	four times each day
Ca	calcium		qs	as much as required
Cl	chlorine		q2h	every two hours
dr or ʒ	dram		q3h	every three hours
et	and		q4h	every four hours
GI	gastrointestinal		R_x	treatment, "take thou"
gt or gtt	drop(s)		s̄	without
H_2O	water		s̄s̄	one-half (½)
H_2O_2	hydrogen peroxide		stat	immediately
IM	intramuscular		t.i.d.	three times a day
in.	inch		tsp	teaspoon
K	potassium		WBC	white blood cell
lb or #	pound		°	degree
m	minimum (a minim)		−	minus, negative, alkaline reaction
Mg	magnesium		+	plus, positive, acid reaction
N	nitrogen, normal		%	percent
Na	sodium		v	roman numeral five
n.p.o.	nothing by mouth		vii	roman numeral seven
o.d.	everyday		ix	roman numeral nine
o.o.b.	out of bed		xiii	roman numeral thirteen

Appendix 2. CONVERSION TABLES

Table A. HOUSEHOLD EQUIVALENTS (VOLUME)

Metric	Apothecary	Household
0.06 ml	1 minim	1 drop
5 (4) ml	1 fluidram	1 teaspoonful
15.0 ml	4 fluidrams	1 tablespoonful
30.0 ml	1 fluidounce	2 tablespoonfuls
180.0 ml	6 fluidounces	1 teacupful
240.0 ml	8 fluidounces	1 glassful

Table B. APOTHECARY EQUIVALENTS (VOLUME)

Metric	Apothecary
1.0 ml/1.0 cc	15 minims
0.06 ml	1 minim
4.0 ml	1 fluidram
30.0 ml	1 fluidounce
500.0 ml	1 pint
1000.0 ml (1 L)	1 quart

Table C. APOTHECARY EQUIVALENTS (WEIGHT)

Metric	Apothecary		Metric			Apothecary
4 gm	1 dr		0.2	gm	" 200 mg	gr iii
30 gm	1 oz		0.1	gm	" 100 mg	gr 1½
1 kg	2.2 lbs		0.06	gm	" 60 mg	gr 1
			0.05	gm	" 50 mg	gr ¾
1.0 gm or 1000 mg	gr xv		0.03	gm	" 30 mg	gr ½
0.6 gm " 600 mg	gr x		0.015 gm		" 15 mg	gr ¼
0.5 gm " 500 mg	gr viiss		0.010 gm		" 10 mg	gr ⅙
0.3 gm " 300 mg	gr v		0.008 gm		" 8 mg	gr ⅛

UNIVERSAL PRECAUTIONS

The following guidelines are recommended for use with all clients whether identified as infectious or not, to prevent transmission of infections. Please follow these guidelines when caring for clients.

- Wear gloves if there is a possibility of direct contact with blood or bodily secretions (pus, sputum, urine, feces, blood, saliva, etc.). This includes a neonate before first bath. Wash as soon as possible if unanticipated contact with these body substances occurs.

- Protect clothing with gowns or plastic aprons if there is a possibility of being splashed.

- Wear masks and/or goggles to avoid being splashed; includes during suctioning, irrigations and deliveries.

- Wash hands thoroughly and before and after all client contact.

- Do not break needles into receptacles; rather, discard them intact and uncapped into containers.

- Place all contaminated articles and trash in leak-proof bags. Check hospital policy regarding labeling bags.

- Handle laboratory specimens with care. All specimens are potentially infected.

- Place soiled linen in a laundry bag, then in a plastic bag to prevent leakage.

- Clean spills quickly with bleach or hydrogen peroxide.

- Incineration is preferred method of disposal of infectious waste and should be used whenever possible.

Precautions to Prevent Transmission of HIV

Many hospitals expand the concept of universal precautions to include precautions that extend from gloves to gown, mask and goggles. The CDC suggests further guidelines for prevention of HIV transmission.

1. Gloves should be worn for contact with blood and body fluids, mucous membranes, or nonintact skin of *all* clients. Gloves should be worn for handling items or surfaces soiled with blood or body fluids and for performing venipuncture or other vascular access procedures.
2. Gloves should be changed after contact with each client.
3. Masks and protective eyewear should be worn during procedures that could generate blood droplets or other body fluids to prevent exposure of mucous membranes of mouth, eyes, and nose.
4. Gowns should be worn during procedures that are likely to involve blood or other body fluids splashed on clothing.
5. Hands and other skin surfaces should be washed immediately and thoroughly if contaminated with blood or other body fluids. Hands should also be washed immediately after gloves are removed.
6. Health care workers should take precautions to prevent injuries caused by needles, scalpels, or other sharp instruments or devices. To prevent needlestick injuries, needles should *not* be recapped, purposely bent or broken by hand, removed from disposable syringes, or otherwise handled. All such instruments should be placed in puncture-resistant containers for disposal.
7. Emergency mouth-to-mouth mouthpieces, resuscitation bags, or other ventilation devices should be available for use to minimize direct contact between client and health care worker even though saliva has not been implicated in HIV transmission.
8. Health care workers who have open lesions or weeping dermatitis should refrain from all direct client contact and from handling client care equipment.
9. All health care workers who participate in invasive procedures must routinely use appropriate barrier precautions to prevent skin and mucous membrane contact with blood and other body fluids. These precautions include gloves and surgical masks, protective eyewear, or face shields for any procedure that may result in splashing of blood or body fluids. Gowns or aprons should also be used when splashing is likely to occur.
10. Because of the risk of transmission of HIV from mother to fetus, pregnant health care workers should be especially familiar with and strictly adhere to precautions to minimize the risk of HIV transmission. At this time, pregnant health care workers are not known to be at greater risk of contracting HIV than other workers.
11. All health care workers who perform or assist in vaginal or cesarean deliveries should wear gloves and gowns when handling the placenta or the infant until blood and amniotic fluid have been removed from the infant's skin; they should also wear gloves during post-delivery care of the umbilical cord.

Selection of Gloves

The Center for Devices and Radiological Health, a section of the FDA, has responsibility for regulating the medical glove industry. There are no reported differences in barrier effectiveness between latex and vinyl gloves, so the type of gloves selected should be appropriate for the procedure that is being performed. The CDC suggests the following guidelines.

1. Use sterile gloves for procedures involving contact with normally sterile areas of the body.
2. Use examination gloves for procedures involving contact with mucous membranes, unless otherwise indicated, and for client care or procedures that do not require use of sterile gloves.
3. Change gloves between client contact.
4. Do not wash, disinfect, or reuse surgical or examination gloves.
5. Use general-purpose utility gloves (rubber household gloves) for housekeeping tasks that involve potential blood contact and for instrument cleaning and decontamination procedures.

Material from this section was adapted from the Centers for Disease Control, MMWR, June 1988: "Update: Universal Precautions for Prevention of Transmission of Human Immunodeficiency Virus, Hepatitis B Virus, and Other Bloodborne Pathogens in Health Care Settings."

COMMON DRUGS THAT MAY BE TESTED ON NCLEX-RN

MEDICAL-SURGICAL

ONCOLOGY

Chemotherapy (page 93–96)
Antimetabolites
Mitotic inhibitors
Alkylating agents
Antitumor antibiotics
Mitrosoureas
Hormones
Miscellaneous: Procarbizine

NEUROLOGICAL SYSTEM

Drugs affecting CNS and ANS (page 68)

Intracranial Pressure (page 110)
Steroids (Decadron)
Osmotic diuretics (Mannitol)

Epilepsy (page 113–114)
Dilantin
Valium
Phenobarbital
Tegretol
Clonopin

Myasthenia Gravis (page 123)
Neostigmine
Tensilon

Parkinson's (page 124–125)
Amantadine
Anticholinergics (Ethopropazine)
Levodopa
Sinemet
Bromocriptine
Antihistamines
Antispasmodics (Artane, Kemadrin)

Cataract (page 131)
Miotics
Mydriatics
Beta blockers
Carbonicanhydrase
   Inhibitors

Glaucoma (page 132)
Miotic drugs (Pilocarpine)
Beta blocker (Timolol maleate)
Epinephrine
Acetazolamide
Cycloplegic drops (post-op)

CARDIOVASCULAR SYSTEM

Drugs affecting CV system (page 70)

Angina (page 141–142)
Nitroglycerin sublingual
Nitroglycerin IV (Tridil)
Long-acting nitrite (Isordil)
Beta blocker (Inderal)
Ca blocking agent (Cardizem)

Congestive Heart Failure (page 146)
Digitalis
Nitrates
Diuretics
Vasodilators

Anticoagulants (page 159–160)
Heparin
Coumadin

Thrombolytic Agents (page 159)
Streptokinase
Urokinase

Cardiac drugs (page 162–165)
Digitalis
Calcium Blocking Agents
Coronary Vasodilators
Antiarrhythmic Drugs
   Norpace
Antihypertensive Drugs
Diuretics
Afterload Drugs

RESPIRATORY SYSTEM

Respiratory Drugs (page 69)

Tuberculosis (page 174)
Tuberculin skin test (PPD)
Isoniazid (INH)
Rifampin (RIF)
Ethambutol
Pyrazinamide (PYZ)
Streptomycin

Asthma (page 179)
Bronchodilators
(see also page 189)
   Epinephrine
   Aminophylline
   Isupril
   Ephedrine

Pulmonary Medications (page 189–190)
Sympathomimetic Bronchodilators
Methylxantine Bronchodilators
Anticholinergic Bronchodilators
Antimediators/Anti-inflammatory agents
Mucokinetic agents

GASTROINTESTINAL SYSTEM

Drugs affecting GI system (page 69)

Esophageal Varices (page 202)
Pitressin
Vitamin K

Peptic Ulcer (page 205–206)
Antacids
   Calcium carbonate
   Magnesium oxide
Cimetidine (Tagamet)

Sucralfate (Carafate)

Ulcerative Colitis (page 212)
Steroids
Anti-infectives
Tranquilizers
Anticholinergics

Diverticulitis/Diverticulosis (page 212)
Anticholingeric
   Donnatal
   Pro-Banthine

Hepatic Coma (page 220)
Bile salts
Lactulose

Cholecystitis and Cholelithiasis (page 221)
Chenodeoxy
Cholic acid
Nitroglycerin
Papaverine
Questran

Pancreatitis (page 223)
Antacids (Maalox)
Histamine antagonists (Zantac, Tagamet)
Anticholinergics (Atropine, Pro-Banthine)
Pancreatic enzymes (Viokase, Cotazym)

GENITOURINARY SYSTEM

Urinary Antiseptics (page 239)
   Gantrisin
   Furadantin
   NegGram

MUSCULOSKELETAL SYSTEM

Prostatic Surgery (page 249)
Estrogen Therapy
Anticholinergics

Arthritis (page 259)
Salicylates
NSAIDS (Phenylbutazone, Motrin)
Anti-inflammatory
   Gold Salts
   Antimetabolics
   Corticosteroids

Gout (page 260)
Antiflammatory agents
   Colchicine
   Phenylbutazone
   Indomethacin
   Corticosteroids
Allopurinol

INTEGUMENTARY SYSTEM

Herpes (page 271)
Acyclovir Cream

Note: To assist you in reviewing for the NCLEX, we have listed drugs by condition, disorder or disease. This drug list is not all inclusive, nor are the drugs only used for conditions noted.

COMMON DRUGS THAT MAY BE TESTED ON NCLEX-RN (CONTINUED)

Burns (page 275–276)
Mafenide (Sulfamylon)
Silvadene
Silver nitrate

Iron Deficiency Anemia (page 282)
Ferrous sulfate
Imferon

Pernicious Anemia (page 283)
Vitamin B$_{12}$ (IM)

BLOOD AND SPLEEN

Leukemia (page 285)
Antimetabolites (5-FU, Methotrexate)
Alkylating agents (Cytoxan)
Antibiotic agents
Plant alkaloids (Vincristine)

Hodgkin's Disease (page 288)
Cytoxin
Nitrogen Mustard
Thiotepa

ENDOCRINE SYSTEM

Graves Disease (page 300)
Antithyroid
    Trapezol
    Iodine (SSKI, Lugol's solution)

Diabetes (page 305–306)
Insulin types:
    Short acting: regular, semilente, humulin
    Intermediate acting: NPH, lente, humulin
    Long acting: PZI, ultralente
Tolbutamide (Orinase)
Chlorpropamide (Diabinese)
Tolazamide (Tolinase)

Preoperative Medications (page 313)
Barbiturates
Belladonna Alkaloids
Hypnotics

Anesthetic Agents (page 314)

Postoperative Medications (page 315–316)
Analgesics (page 68)
    Opiates: Morphine sulfate; Dilaudid;
        Numorphan, Codeine sulfate
    Synthetic opiate-like drugs: Demerol
        (meperidine); Talwin (pentazocine)
    Nonnarcotic pain relievers:
        Salicylates (aspirin)
        Nonsalicylate analgesics
            (acetaminophen)
        Nonsteroid antiinflammatory (NSAIDS)
Antiemetics
    Compazine (prochlorperazine)
    Phenergan (promethazine)

Dramamine (dimenhydrinate)
Tigan (trimethobenzamide)

OBSTETRICS & GYNECOLOGY

Newborn (page 414)
Erythromycin
Silver nitrate (eyedrops)

Pregnancy (page 429)
RhoGam

Common Maternity Drugs
(page 437–438)
Oxytocin
Syntocinon
Pitocin
Methergine
Apresoline (hydralazine
    hydrochloride)
Magnesium sulfate
Vasodilan (isoxsuprine)
Ritodrine (improved analog of
    isoxsuprine)
Terbutaline, B$_2$

PEDIATRICS

Epilepsy (page 462)
Tegretol
Dilantin
Mephenytoin
Ethosoximide

Congestive Heart Failure (page 467)
Digoxin
Diuretics

Asthma (page 477)
Epinephrine
Ephedrine sulfate
Aminophylline

Cystic Fibrosis (page 480)
Pancreatic enzymes: Viokase, Cotazym
Antibiotics: ampicillin, penicillin, Keflin

Poisoning (page 483)
Syrup of ipecac or apomorphine

Parasitic Worms (page 490)
Piperazine citrate (pin or round worms)
Mebendazole, Pyrantel Pamoate, (pin worms)

Giardiasis (page 490)
Furazolidone, Guinacrine

Oncology (page 511)
Predisone
6-Mercaptopurine
Methotrexate

Cytoxin
Vincristine

Lead Poisoning (page 520)
Calcium disodium edetate (EDTA)
BAL

Immunizations (page 521)
DPT—diphtheria and tetanus toxoids and
    pertussis vaccine
TOPV—trivalent oral polio virus vaccine
MMR—measles, mumps, and rubella vaccine;
    may be combined or separate
TD—combined tetanus and diphtheria toxoids

PSYCHIATRIC DRUG CLASSIFICATION

Antipsychotic (page 564)
    Phenothiazines
        Stelazine
        Trilafon, Vesprin
        Prolixin
        Haldol
        Clozaril

Antianxiety (page 564–565)
    Benzodiazepines
        Atarax
        Librium, Serax, Xanax
        Valium
    Nonbenzodiazepines
        Vistaril, Equanil

Antidepressants-Mood Elevators
(page 565)
    Tricyclics
        Tofranil
        Elavil
        Sinequan
    MAO Inhibitors
        Marplan
        Niamid
        Nardil
        Parnate
    Desyrel
    Prozac

Antimanic (page 565)
    Lithium carbonate

Antiparkinson (page 566)
    Cogentin
    Artane
    Benedryl

GERONTOLOGICAL NURSING

Medications for the Elderly
(page 604–640)

Note: To assist you in reviewing for the NCLEX, we have listed drugs by condition, disorder or disease. This drug list is not all inclusive, nor are the drugs only used for conditions noted.

3

ONCOLOGY NURSING

Oncology is the area of nursing that focuses on the client with cancer. Cancer is second only to cardiovascular disease as the leading cause of death in the United States. As such, it is an area that will demand more nursing care and involvement in the future. This chapter focuses on cancer as a disease, its treatment, and the concepts of oncology nursing. Specific oncological diseases are included in the Medical-Surgical chapter and in the Pediatric chapter.

ONCOLOGICAL NURSING

Cancer Incidence and Trends

A. Cancer—a definition.
  1. Term represents a group of more than 100 neoplastic diseases that involve all body organs.
  2. One or more cells lose their normal growth-controlling mechanism and continue to grow uncontrolled.
B. Second leading cause of death in U.S. after heart disease.
  1. Ranks fourth for males and first for females as cause of death; second after accidents as cause of death for children.
  2. Greatest increase seen in lung cancer—consistent with smoking patterns.
C. Incidence rate:
  1. Five million in U.S. diagnosed with cancer.
  2. Number of cancer deaths increased by 11% during past 40 years.

Identified Causes and Risk Factors

A. Multiplicity theory: multiple factors lead to the development of cancer; 60–90% thought to be related to environmental factors.
B. Carcinogens: agents known to increase susceptibility to cancer.
  1. Chemical carcinogens: asbestos, benzene, vinyl chloride, by-products of tobacco, etc.
  2. Iatrogenic chemical agents: DES; chemotherapy; hormone treatment; immunosuppressive agents.
  3. Radiation carcinogens: x-rays; sunlight (ultraviolet light); nuclear radiation.
  4. Viral factors: herpes simplex; Epstein-Barr; Hepatitis B and Retroviruses.
  5. Genetic factors: hereditary or familial tendencies.
  6. Demographic and geographic factors.
  7. Dietary factors: obesity; high-fat diet; diets low in fiber; diets high in smoked or salted foods; preservatives and food additives; alcohol.
  8. Psychological factors: stress.

Comparison of Benign and Malignant Tumors		
	Malignant	Benign
Cell type	Abnormal from those of original tissues	Close to those of original tissues
Growth	Rapid; infiltrates surrounding tissues in all directions	Slow and noninfiltrating
Encapsulated	Infrequent	Frequent
Metastasis	Through blood, lymph, or new tumor sites	Remains localized
Effect	Terminal without treatment	Can become malignant or obstruct vital organs

Preventive Measures

A. Optimal Dietary Patterns.*
  1. Avoid obesity (at 40% overweight, there is a 55% increased risk of cancer in females and 33% in males).
  2. Decrease fat intake of both saturated and unsaturated fats—maximum 30% of total calories.
  3. Increase total fiber in diet—decreases risk of colon cancer.
  4. Increase Vitamin A—reduced incidence of larynx, esophagus, and lung cancers.
  5. Increase Vitamin C—aids tumor encapsulation and promotes longer survival time.
  6. Increase Vitamin E—inhibits growth of brain tumors, melanomas, and leukemias.
  7. Decrease alcohol consumption.
  8. Avoid salt-cured, smoked, or nitrate-cured foods.

* Core curriculum for Oncology Nursing.

B. Minimize exposure to carcinogens.
  1. Avoid smoking—thought to be a cause of 75% lung cancers in U.S.
  2. Avoid oral tobacco—increases incidence of oral cancers.
  3. Avoid exposure to asbestos fibers and constant environmental dust.
  4. Avoid exposure to chemicals.

5. Avoid radiation exposure and excessive exposure to sunlight.

C. Obtain adequate rest and exercise to decrease stress.
   1. Chronic stress associated with decreased immune system functioning.
   2. Strong immune system responsible for destruction of malignant cells as they develop.

Early Detection Methods

A. Risk Assessment (see Risk Factors).
B. Health history and physical assessment.
C. Screening methods.
   1. Tests such as a mammography, Pap test, sigmoidoscopy, etc.
   2. Self-care practices: breast self-examination (BSE); testicular self-examination (TSE); skin inspection.
D. Teaching the seven early warning signs of cancer.
   1. Change in bowel or bladder habits.
   2. Any sore that does not heal.
   3. Bleeding or unusual discharge.
   4. Lump or thickening in breast or elsewhere.
   5. Indigestion or difficulty swallowing.
   6. Obvious change in wart or mole.
   7. Nagging cough or hoarseness.

Characteristics

A. Benign Neoplasms: usually encapsulated, remain localized, and are slow-growing.
B. Malignant Neoplasms; not encapsulated, will metastasize and grow, and exert negative effects on host.
C. Categories of malignant neoplasms:
   1. Carcinomas—grown from epithelial cells; usually solid tumors (skin, stomach, colon, breast, rectal tumors).
   2. Sarcomas—arise from muscle, bone, fat, or connective tissue—may be solid.
   3. Lymphomas—arise from lymphoid tissue (infection-fighting organs).
   4. Leukemias and myelomas—grow from blood-forming organs.
D. Mechanisms of metastases.
   1. Metastases occur via lymphatics—spreads along lymph channels to mass in lymphs nodes (e.g., breast to axillary nodes) or spread diffusely.

2. The bloodstream may carry cells form one site to another (e.g., liver to bone, etc.).
3. Direct spread of cancer cells (seeding) where there are no boundaries to stop the growth (e.g., ovary and stomach).
4. Transplantation is the transfer of cells from one site to another.

Diagnosis

A. Laboratory and radiologic tests often identify a problem first.
   1. Radiographic procedures (e.g., tomography, CT, contrast studies).
   2. Ultra sonography.
   3. Radioisotopic Scanning Studies (e.g., brain scan, Gallium imaging).
   4. Magnetic Resonance Imaging (MRI).
   5. Biologic response markers (useful for diagnosing primary tumors).
   6. Other laboratory tests (enzyme tests, such as acid phosphatase).
B. Biopsy: definitive diagnosis of cancer.
   1. Excisional biopsy—removes all suspicious tissue.
   2. Incisional biopsy—removes a sample of tissue from a mass.
   3. Needle aspiration—aspiration of small amount of core tissue from a suspicious area.
   4. Exfoliative cytology—cells in tissue or secretions are evaluated by PAP method.
C. Tissue specimens are evaluated by frozen or permanent sections by a pathologist.
D. Results from biopsy and other diagnostic procedures (blood tests, x-ray studies, endoscopic procedures) will determine extent of disease-staging.

Staging: How Cancer is Classified

A. Staging describes the extent or metastasis of a malignant tumor; also quantifies severity of disease.
B. A useful system of staging for carcinomas is the TNM system.
   1. T: Primary tumor.
   2. N: Regional nodes.
   3. M: Metastasis.
C. The extent to which malignancy has increased in size:
   1. TO: no evidence of primary tumor.
   2. TIS: carcinoma in situ.

3. T_1, T_2, T_3 T_4: progressive increase in tumor, size, and involvement.
4. TX: tumor cannot be assessed.
D. Involvement of regional nodes.
   1. NO: regional lymph nodes not abnormal.
   2. N_1 N_2, N_3, N_4: increasing degree of abnormal regional lymph nodes.
   3. NX: regional lymph nodes cannot be assessed clinically.
E. Metastatic development.
   1. MO: no evidence of distant metastasis.
   2. M_1 to M_3: increasing degree of distant metastasis.

Treatment Methods

A. Broad goals.
   1. Goal of therapy is to cure the client—eradicate the tumor.
   2. When cure is not possible, controlling or arresting tumor growth becomes the goal—to prolong survival.
   3. Palliation or alleviation of symptoms is a third goal.
B. The major forms of cancer treatment include surgery, radiation therapy, chemotherapy, and combined approaches.

Surgery

A. Useful as primary treatment for localized cancer (breast, colon, melanoma of skin, etc.).
   1. Highest rate of cure for localized disease.
   2. Disadvantage—deforming or debilitating to client.
B. Types of treatment.
   1. Local excision: simple surgery with small margin of normal tissue surrounding tumor.
   2. En bloc dissection or wide excision: removal of tumor, tissues, and any contiguous structures.
   3. Surgery on cancer in situ.
      a. Electrosurgery—application of electrical current to cancerous cells.
      b. Cryosurgery—deep freezing with liquid nitrogen.
      c. Chemosurgery—applied chemotherapeutic agents layer by layer with surgical excision.
      d. CO_2 laser—use of laser for local excision.
   4. Palliative surgery—promotes comfort and quality of life without cure.

Implementation

A. Preoperative care.
   1. Promote health status prior to surgery.
      a. Malnourished client is at risk for infection, delayed wound healing, and dehiscence.
      b. Mental status may impact surgery results.
   2. Provide emotional support prior to surgery.
      a. Encourage talking about fears and anxieties.
      b. Provide accurate information—clarify levels of knowledge.
      c. Assess family needs and provide information and support.
B. Postoperative care.
   1. Provide traditional post-op care (see page 311).
   2. Provide for physical comfort.
      a. Enteral feeding.
      b. Pain relief.
      c. Positioning and activity.
      d. Wound care and healing.
   3. Provide emotional support.
      a. Allow for grief process—encourage expression of fears.
      b. Discuss change in body image—support increase in self-esteem.
      c. Provide accurate information.
   4. Support rehabilitation process.
      a. Encourage family involvement.
      b. Make referrals to appropriate resources.
      c. Complete discharge planning.

Radiation Therapy

A. Definition: use of high energy moving through space or medium to treat disease.
B. Indications.
   1. Used to treat solid tumors—ionizing radiation transfers energy to molecules present in cancer cell.
   2. Different tissues have different radiosensitivities—rapidly dividing tissues (testes, ovaries, lymphoid tissues, and bone marrow) are more sensitive.
C. Types of radiation.
   1. Electromagnetic—radiation in wave form.
      a. X-rays—linear accelerators.
      b. Electrons—delivered by machines.
      c. Gamma rays—delivered by machines that contain radioactive sources (Cobalt-60,

Cesium-137) or radioactive substances (seeds, threads, or liquids).

2. Particulate—radiation in the form of heavy particles.
   a. Beta particles—high speed electrons (Phosphorus-32; Strontium-90).
   b. Neutrons and Pions—currently used experimentally.

External Radiation

A. Teletherapy—external source of radiation. (Machine is a distance from client.)
B. Types.
   1. Natural radioactive source—gamma rays delivered via machine to lesion.
   2. Machine is the linear accelerator—high voltage electric current delivers electrons to client.
C. Side effects: fatigue—major systemic effect; headache; nausea and vomiting; skin irritation or injury; scaling, erythema; dryness.

Implementation

A. Offer psychological support and teaching.
   1. What to expect from treatment.
   2. Explanation of radiotherapy room.
   3. Possible side effects and ways to minimize them.
B. Promote diet: high protein, high carbohydrate, fat free, and low residue.
   1. Foods to avoid: tough, fibrous meat; poultry; shrimp; all cheeses (except soft); coarse bread; raw vegetables; irritating spices.
   2. Foods allowed: soft-cooked eggs, ground meat, pureed vegetables, milk, cooked cereal.
   3. Increase fluids.
   4. Diet supplement to increase calorie and fluid intake.
   5. Do not eat several hours before treatment.
C. Administer medications.
   1. Compazine—nausea.
   2. Lomotil—diarrhea.
D. Provide skin care—radiodermatitis occurs three to six weeks after start of treatment.
   1. Avoid creams, lotions, perfume to irradiated areas.
   2. Wash with lukewarm water, pat dry (some physicians allow mild soap).
   3. Avoid exposure to sunlight or artificial heat such as heating pad.

4. Baby oil may be ordered t.i.d.
E. Observe for "wet" reaction.
   1. Weeping of skin due to loss of upper layer.
   2. Promote rest after therapy.
   3. Cleanse area with warm water and pat dry b.i.d.
   4. Apply antibiotic lotion or steroid cream if ordered.
   5. Expose site to air.

Internal Radiation/Brachytherapy

A. Implantation of radioactive substance within a client.
B. Types.
   1. Unsealed sources: isotopes (^{131}I and ^{32}p.).
      a. Liquid and administered orally.
      b. Half-life generally short but varies with isotope.
      c. Precautions important during high risk period (usually first four days).
   2. Sealed sources: radium needles, radon seeds, and ^{137}Cs.
      a. Radioactive substance encased in metal capsule placed in body cavity.
      b. Delivers radiation directly to tumor.
      c. Even though implant is sealed, special precautions are instituted.
C. Side effects.
   1. Occur when normal cells are damaged.
   2. Acute side effects occur during or shortly after radiation therapy; chronic effects occur months or years following therapy.
   3. Common side effects from radiation therapy: alopecia; mouth dryness; mucositis; esophagitis; nausea and vomiting; diarrhea; cystitis; erythema; and dry and wet desquamation.
   4. Factors influencing degree of side effects.
      a. Body site irradiated.
      b. Radiation dose—higher dose given, the more potential side effects.
      c. Extent of body area treated (larger area, more potential for side effects).
      d. Method of radiation therapy.

Implementation

A. Maintain bed rest when radiation source in place.
   1. Restrict movement to prevent dislodging radiation source.

2. Do not turn or position client except on back (when cesium needle in tongue or cervix).

B. Administer range-of-motion exercise q.i.d.

C. Avoid direct contact around implant site; avoid washing areas, etc.

D. Take vital signs every four hours (report temperature over 100°F).

E. Observe for dehydration or paralytic ileus (if cervical implant).

F. Observe and report skin eruption, discharge, abnormal bleeding.

G. Provide clear liquid diet (low residue is sometimes ordered) and force fluids.

H. Insert Teflon Foley catheter (radiation decomposes rubber) to avoid necessity of bedpan.

I. Observe frequently for dislodging of radiation source (especially linen and dressings).
   1. When radiation source falls out, do not touch with hands. Pick up source with foot-long applicator.
   2. Put source in lead container and call physician.
   3. If unable to locate source, call physician immediately and bar visitors from room.

J. After source is removed.
   1. Administer Betadine douche if cervical implant.
   2. Give Fleets enema.
   3. Client may be out of bed.
   4. Avoid direct sunlight to radiation areas.
   5. Administer cream to relieve dryness or itching.

K. Instruct that client may resume sexual intercourse within seven to ten days.

L. Notify physician if nausea, vomiting, diarrhea, frequent urination or bowel movements, or temperature above 100°F is present.

Radiation Safety Measures

A. General guidelines for radiation safety measures.
   1. Wear radiation badges to monitor total amount of radiation exposure. Cumulative dose (measured in millirems) not to exceed 1,250 every 3 months.
   2. Observe for displacement or dislodgement of radiation source every 4 to 6 hours.
   3. Check that sealed lead container is kept in client's room in case of accidental dislodgement.
   4. Collect body waste until it can be determined radiation source is not dislodged.
   5. Radiation source removed at prearranged time—after removal, client is no longer radioactive.

6. Do not allow persons under 18 or pregnant women to visit or care for clients with radioactive implant.

7. Never touch a dislodged sealed source—use long-handled tongs or contact radiation safety personnel.

8. Mark client's room and chart with radiation safety precautions.

B. Follow special principles of time, distance, and shielding.
   1. Minimize time.
      a. Radiation exposure proportional to amount of time spent with client.
      b. Care planned to be delivered in shortest amount of time to meet goals—be efficient with time.
      c. Review procedures before beginning them.
   2. Maximize distance.
      a. Intensity of radiation related to distance from client.
      b. Duration of safe exposure increases as distance is increased; work as far away from source as possible.
   3. Utilize shielding.
      a. Use lead shields or other equipment to reduce transmission of radiation.
      b. Store radioactive material in lead-shielded container when not in use.

C. Follow radiation precautions for isotope implant.
   1. All body secretions considered contaminated—use special techniques for disposal.
   2. If client vomits within first 4 hours—everything vomitus touches is considered contaminated.
   3. Use disposable gown, dishes, etc.
   4. Limit contact with hospital personnel and visitors.

Chemotherapy

Characteristics

A. The medical management of cancer includes the use of chemotherapy. First used in the early 50s, there are now more than 80 effective drugs available.
   1. Chemotherapy is method of choice when there is suspected or confirmed spread of malignant cells.

2. Method used when the risk of recurrence systemically is high.
3. May be used as palliative measure to relieve pain or increase comfort.

B. Mechanism of action.
   1. Functions at cellular level by interrupting cell life—modifies or interferes with DNA synthesis.
   2. Chemotherapeutic agents eradicate cells, both normal and malignant, that are in the process of cell reproduction.

Drug Classification

A. Drugs classified by group into those that act on a certain phase of cell reproduction (cell cycle specific) or those that do not (cell cycle nonspecific).

B. Cell cycle specific agents: antimetabolites and mitotic inhibitors.
   1. Act on the cell during a particular phase of reproduction.
   2. Most effective in tumors where a large number of cells are dividing.
   3. Divided doses produce greater cytotoxic effects (not all cells will be in the same phase at the same time).
   4. Antimetabolites.
      a. Specific for the S-phase—replaces building blocks of DNA so cell can't divide.
      b. Examples of these drugs: Methotrexate, 6-mercaptopurine, 5-fluorouracil, Azacytidine, Cytarabine.
   5. Mitotic inhibitors.
      a. Specific for the M-phase—prevent cell division by destroying the mitotic spindle.
      b. Examples of these drugs: plant alkaloids— vincristine, vindesine, vinblastine, teniposide.

C. Cell cycle nonspecific drugs: alkylating agents, antitumor antibiotics, and nitrosoureas.
   1. Act on cells during any phase of reproduction— some drugs will attack cells in the resting phase (not actively dividing).
   2. Agents are dose-dependent—the more drug given, the more cells destroyed.
   3. These drugs are more toxic to normal tissue because they are less selective.
   4. Alkylating agents.
      a. These drugs prevent cell division by damaging the DNA "ladder" structure.
      b. Examples of these drugs: Cytoxan, Myleran, melphalan (L-PAM), Thiotepa, etc.
   5. Antitumor antibiotics.
      a. These drugs attack DNA (they act like alkylating drugs) by slipping between the DNA strands and prevent replication.
      b. Examples of these drugs: Adriamycin, Cosmegen, Dactinomycin.
   6. Nitrosoureas.
      a. Alkylating agents that are stronger and have a greater ability to attack cells in the resting phase of cell growth.
      b. These drugs can cross the blood-brain barrier.
      c. Examples of these drugs: streptozocin, methyl CCNU, BCNU.

D. Other miscellaneous agents (such as Procarbazine) are used in the chemotherapy group, but their exact mechanism of action is unknown.

E. Hormones (estrogens, androgens, progestins) are used in therapy to affect the hormonal environment.
   1. Affect the growth of hormone-dependent tumors.
   2. Steroids interfere with the synthesis of protein and alter cell metabolism (lymphomas and leukemias).
   3. Antihormones (Tamoxifen) block tumor growth by depriving the tumor of the necessary hormones.

F. Combination chemotherapy.
   1. Most often administered in combination which enhances the response rate.
   2. Cancer cells divide erratically on different schedules; thus drugs that are effective alone and have different mechanisms of action can combine to destroy even more cells.
   3. Drugs used in combination for synergistic activity.
   4. Guidelines for drug administration are carefully planned and referred to as protocols or regimens.
      a. Package inserts are based on single agent therapy, so it is important to adhere to the ordered protocol.
      b. Many protocols represent three or four drugs. (Example: the protocol for Hodgkin's lymphoma is based on four drugs, called MOPP.)
         (1) First day of drug administration is called DAY 1. Completing 28 days (in the Hodgkin's example) is the end of one cycle.

(2) Most chemotherapy is given for several cycles, sometimes as different combinations.

   c. Dosages of drugs are based on height and weight calculated as body surface area.

Planning/Goals of Treatment

A. The major goal is to cure the malignancy.
  1. Chemotherapy, as primary mode of treatment, may include curing certain malignancies such as acute lymphocytic leukemia, Hodgkin's disease, lymphosarcomas, Wilms' tumor.
  2. Cure may also occur in combination with other modes of treatment, radiation, or surgery.
B. Control may be the goal when cure is not realistic; the aim is to extend survival and improve the quality of life.
C. Palliation may be the goal when neither cure nor control may be achieved; this goal is directed toward client comfort.

Chemotherapeutic Administration

A. Chemotherapeutic agents are administered through a variety of routes.
  1. Oral route—used frequently. Safety precautions must be observed.
  2. Intramuscular and SubQ used infrequently as drugs are not vesicants.
  3. Intravenous is the most common route—provides for better absorption.
    a. Potential complications: infection, phlebitis.
    b. Prevention of complications: use smallest gauge needle possible; maintain aseptic technique; monitor IV site frequently, change IV fluid every 4 hours.
  4. Central venous catheter infusion—used for continuous or intermittent infusions.
    a. Potential complications: infection, catheter clotting, sepsis, malposition of needle.
    b. Prevention of complications: maintain aseptic technique and monitor site daily; flush catheter daily and between each use with heparin solution; assess client for signs of sepsis.
  5. Venous Access Devices (VADs)—used for prolonged infusions.
    a. Potential complications: infection and infiltration from malposition.

   b. Assess site frequently and assess for systemic infection.
  6. Intraarterial route—delivers agents directly to tumor in high concentrations while decreasing drug's systemic toxic effect.
    a. Potential complications: infection or bleeding at catheter site, catheter clotting, or pump malfunction.
    b. Change dressing site daily and assess for signs of infection; irrigate catheter with heparin solution and avoid kinks in tubing.
  7. Intraperitoneal—used for ovarian and colon cancer. High concentration of agents delivered to peritoneal cavity via a catheter, then drained.
  8. Other less frequently used routes are intrapleural, intrathecal, and a ventricular reservoir.
B. Factors for deciding dosage and timing of drugs.
  1. Dosage calculated on body surface area and kilograms of body weight.
  2. Time lapse between doses to allow recovery of normal cells.
  3. Side effects of each drug and when they are likely to occur.
  4. Liver and kidney function, as most antineoplastics are metabolized in one of these organs.
C. Common side effects.
  1. Damage to rapidly growing normal cells.
    a. Bone marrow (most serious damage).
      (1) Infection.
      (2) Abnormal bleeding.
    b. Hair follicles—alopecia.
    c. Mucous lining of gastrointestinal tract.
      (1) Nausea, vomiting, anorexia.
      (2) Fluid and electrolyte imbalances.
      (3) Dietary deficiency.
      (4) Stomatitis.
  2. Elevated uric acid and crystal and urate stone formation.
  3. Time of most severe depression of cells (termed nadir); different for each type of cell.
  4. Chemotherapeutics—have specific side effects in addition to these.

Chemotherapy Safety Guidelines

A. Antineoplastic drugs are potentially hazardous to personnel and may have teratogenic and/or carcinogenic effects.

B. Safety guidelines have been issued by the Occupational Safety and Health Administration (OSHA).
  1. Obtain special training for drug administration.
  2. Wear surgical latex gloves and a disposable, closed, long-sleeved gown.
  3. Use Luer-lok syringes.
  4. Label all prepared drugs appropriately.
  5. Double bag chemotherapy drugs once prepared, before transport.
  6. Have equipment ready to clean up any accidental spill.
  7. Dispose of all materials in marked containers labelled hazardous waste.
  8. Dispose of all needles and syringes intact.

Side Effects of Chemotherapy

A. Side effects occur primarily due to the mechanism of action of potent drugs on normal cells.
  1. Normal cells most affected are bone marrow cells, epithelial cells of the GI tract and hair follicles, and cells of the gonads.
  2. Since other normal cells are not actively reproducing (except with tissue injury and repair), they are not severely affected.
B. Skin and mucosa, protective linings of the body, are damaged.
  1. Mucositis (cells of the mucosa are affected)—may extend from oral cavity and stomach through GI tract.
    a. Assess for erythema, tenderness, and ulceration.
    b. Clients at high risk are those with dental caries, gum disease, smokers, and those who drink.
    c. Implementation includes good oral hygiene, mouthwashes, avoiding foods that are sharp, spicy, or acidic.
  2. Alopecia, or hair loss, caused by damage to rapidly dividing cells of the hair follicles.
    a. Hair loss begins 2–3 weeks after chemotherapy and continues through the cycles of chemotherapy; regrowth occurs following the course of therapy.
    b. Scalp hypothermia (ice cap) and scalp tourniquet reduces the amount of drug reaching the hair follicle and may prevent hair loss.
  3. Nausea, vomiting and anorexia are common in clients receiving chemotherapy.
    a. Support changes in food preferences, additional or less seasoning, small and more frequent meals.
    b. Offer high calorie and protein supplements.
    c. Antiemetic regimens (Reglan) may counteract these symptoms.
  4. Elimination disturbance occurs when the client does not eat well, is not exercising, or has mucositis.
    a. Diarrhea is related to toxicity of the drugs on the mucosal lining; diet bland and low residue.
    b. Implementation includes low residue foods, adequate fluid intake, and foods high in potassium.
    c. Stool softeners are ordered to minimize constipation.
C. Hematological disruptions: damage to normal cells in the bone marrow can be life-threatening.
  1. White blood cells and platelets have a shorter life span than red blood cells so they are more susceptible to damage.
  2. White blood cell suppression—leukopenia (less than 5,000/mm when normal white blood cell is 5,000–10,000/mm).
    a. Granulocytes are the most suppressed, which places client at risk for bacterial infection.
    b. Common sites of infection are the lung, urinary tract, skin, and blood.
    c. Implementation includes meticulous aseptic technique for IV therapy as well as handwashing; avoid exposure to infected persons.
    d. Teach signs and symptoms of infection to the cancer client with instructions to report symptoms to the doctor or nurse.
  3. Platelet suppression to below normal (less than $150,000–300,000/mm^3$) is called thrombocytopenia.
    a. A number less than $50,000/mm^3$ makes the client susceptible to bleeding gums, nose, easy bruising, heavier menstrual flow, etc.
    b. Teach client precautions: soft toothbrush, avoidance of douches and enemas, care with trimming nails, avoiding venipunctures when possible, and avoidance of any activity that might increase ICP.
  4. Red blood cell suppression—anemia is not usually a severe toxicity.

Psychosocial Impact of Chemotherapy

A. Assessment.
 1. Client's reaction of illness and chemotherapy.
 2. Prior experience with those receiving chemotherapy.
 3. Coping style under stress.
 4. Support network.
 5. Psychosocial changes resulting from cancer.
  a. Threats to the roles client has in life: career, marriage, parent, etc.
  b. Threat to life goals.
  c. Altered independence.
B. Implementation.
 1. Support client's coping style without attempting to change style.
 2. Provide accurate information, encourage questions, and expression of concerns.
 3. Allow time for client to communicate, express fears, concerns and adjustment to both disease and treatment.
 4. Refer client to appropriate health care providers and to help groups.

Pain in Cancer

Characteristics

A. Incidence.
 1. Various studies suggest that 50 percent of persons with cancer will not experience significant pain.
 2. Severe pain is experienced by about 60–80 percent of hospitalized clients.
 3. In early stages of cancer there is little pain—the pain that is felt is associated with treatment (surgery).
B. Causes of pain in cancer.
 1. Physiological causes.
  a. Bone destruction with infraction results from metastatic lesions secondary to primary carcinomas.
  b. Obstruction of an organ by tumor growth (intestinal obstruction).
  c. Compression of peripheral nerves produces sharp, continuous pain—pain follows nerve distribution.
  d. Infiltration or distention of tissue produces a localized, dull pain and increases in intensity as tumor grows.
  e. Inflammation, infection, and necrosis causes pain from pressure or dilatation and distention of tissue distal to an obstruction.
 2. Psychological causes.
  a. This form of pain depends on client's perceived threat of the condition or stress and reaction to it.
   (1) Fear or anxiety generated from the effects the disease may have on the person's life style or relationships.
   (2) Loss or threat of loss may produce a reactive depression with feelings of despair.
   (3) Frustration of drives or lack of need satisfaction may also contribute to psychological pain.
  b. Perception of threat or stress is influenced by client's personality characteristics: self-concept, independence-dependence, emotional stability, education, age, etc.
C. The nature of cancer pain falls into two general categories: chronic and intractable pain.

Assessment

A. Physical dimension of cancer pain is variable.
 1. The severity of pain may be assessed using a scale of 1 (pain free) to 3 (severe pain).
 2. Teach "pain tasks" to the client.
  a. Encourage client to identify and state what, where, and when pain occurs.
  b. This method will help determine which symptoms are most troublesome.
 3. Evaluate the meaning of the pain experienced by the client—understand pain as the client views it.
B. Scope of pain assessment must encompass several factors (Rowlingson).
 1. Severity and duration of pain.
 2. Nature of the disease process.
 3. Probable life expectancy.
 4. Temperament and psychological state.
 5. Occupational, domestic, and economic background of the client.
C. Assess vital signs as indicators of pain.
 1. Low to moderate pain and superficial in origin—the sympathetic nervous system is stimulated.
  a. Increased blood pressure and pulse.
  b. Increased respiratory rate and muscle tension.

2. Severe pain or visceral in origin—the parasympathetic nervous system is affected.
   a. Decreased blood pressure and pulse.
   b. Nausea, vomiting, and weakness.
3. Pain present for a month or longer (late-stage pain); there will probably be no change in vital signs.

D. Assess client's behavior as an indicator of pain.
   1. Alterations in body posture/gestures.
   2. Alterations in activities of daily living.

E. Assess verbalizations, both verbal and nonverbal, as indicators of pain.
   1. Ask systematic questions to determine degree of pain: location, radiation, onset, frequency, duration, quality.
   2. Determine situational factors that influence pain level: level of consciousness, meaning of pain, attitudes and feelings of others, presence of secondary gains, fatigue level, and stressful life events.

Implementation

A. Various neurological and neurosurgical interventions effectively manage pain experienced by cancer clients.
   1. Nerve blocks, either peripheral or intrathecal, can relieve pain.
   2. Procedures involve interruption of pain pathways some place along the path of transmission from the periphery to the brain.

B. Electrical stimulation may be used for pain relief.
   1. Transcutaneous methods (TENS): stimulation to the skin surface over the painful area.
   2. A peripheral nerve implant applies stimulation to peripheral nerves.
   3. Electrodes implanted in the dorsal column stimulate spinal column fibers.

C. A new technique for pain relief is electrical stimulation of the peri-ventricular gray matter in the brain.
   1. An electrode is implanted through a burr hole on the side opposite the most intense pain.
   2. Electrical pulses are then sent periodically into the brain.

D. Intraspinal morphine administration.
   1. An implantable infusion pump delivers a continual supply of opiate to the epidural or subarachnoid space.
   2. Useful for eliminating intractable pain below the mid- to low-thoracic level where spinal cord opiate receptors respond to morphine.

E. Hypnosis is currently viewed as one component of pain management.
   1. A hypnotic state can achieve significant analgesia.
   2. Self-control over pain and its associated anxieties can be assisted with hypnosis.

Cancer Nursing

A. Key stress periods for client with cancer are: time of diagnosis, period of hospitalization, and release from the hospital.
   1. Shock and fear are the major reactions.
   2. Severe depression is experienced by some clients.
   3. The emotional pain of the diagnosis initially outweighs the physical component of the cancer.

B. Adjustment to cancer depends on past life experiences.
   1. A client's previous attitude toward medical practices, hospitalization, and treatment methods influence adjustment.
   2. The manner in which a client has coped with previous stress or crises will determine, in part, how this stress is handled.

C. Phases of psychological adaptation to terminal illness include: denial, anger, bargaining, depression, and acceptance.
   1. These phases may be experienced differently, clients may experience them in a different order, or they may not experience all of the phases.
   2. It is important for the nurse to understand the characteristics of these phases and to recognize which phase the client is in.

D. The client will experience a range of feelings and defense mechanisms.
   1. Denial may occur initially with the diagnosis; this is a protective mechanism necessary until the diagnosis can be confronted.
      a. Allow the client to be in denial until he or she is ready to face reality.
      b. Provide opportunities for the client to confront her illness—be open to questions and clarification.

2. Fear and anxiety may manifest in physical symptoms: insomnia, nausea, vomiting, diarrhea, headaches, etc.
3. Anger and resentment, especially in the initial phases of the disease, may be a healthy way of expressing feelings.
   a. Encourage expression of anger—let the client know that you are able to listen to anger, resentment, and frustration.
   b. Encourage client to focus anger on external problem-solving and more adaptive coping patterns.
4. Depression may be considered normal for a period of time following surgery.
   a. Observe for the signs of depression.
   b. Because suicide is always a risk with depression, interventions should be aimed at safety for the client.

Psychosocial Aspects of Caring for the Cancer Client

A. Develop a collaborative relationship with the client.
   1. Identify and attempt to solve problems together.
   2. Engage with the client so that he or she will not feel they have to cope alone.
   3. Provide emotional support to help allay fears and anxieties.
B. Always be honest with the client.
   1. Truth is easier to cope with than uncertainty and the unknown.
   2. Honesty provides the foundation for a nurse-client relationship.
   3. Accurate information can be followed by an open discussion of the disease, the prognosis, the client's feelings, etc.
   4. Knowing the truth enables the client to begin to accept and work out the future without being immobilized by fears.
C. Assist the client to cope with pain.
   1. Stay with the client, especially when the pain is severe.
   2. Explore the nature of pain with the client.
   3. Respect the client's response to pain and believe what the client tells you.
D. Provide general comfort measures.
   1. Position for proper alignment.
   2. Use touch and massage for painful areas.
   3. Exercise extremities gently to maintain range of motion.
   4. Maintain patency of tubes and keep free of infection using meticulous handwashing and aseptic techniques.
   5. Preserve the client's energy by prioritizing activities.
   6. Assist the client to obtain adequate rest at night and during the day to reduce fatigue.
E. DO NOT undermedicate for cancer pain.
   1. Undertreatment with analgesics has been identified as a major problem (70 to 80 percent) for cancer patients—and nursing has a crucial responsibility to correct this problem.
   2. Two forms of undertreatment: physicians underprescribe and nurses routinely administer less than half the amount clients could receive.
   3. The danger of overuse of narcotics is a potential problem.
      a. This concern should not result in undertreatment.
      b. Only a very small percentage of clients are overmedicated.
F. Support family of the client as they move through the grieving process.
   1. Be honest with family members to establish a firm relationship.
   2. Encourage expression of feelings.
G. Introduce the hospice concept—provides care for the terminally ill client and family.
   1. Primary goal is to provide emotional support for the client and family.
   2. An accompanying goal is to provide for physical care.
   3. Relief of pain is just as important to a dying person as emotional support.

4

MEDICAL-SURGICAL NURSING*

Medical-Surgical Nursing requires the broadest and most extensive mastery of nursing knowledge and expertise, for it encompasses every system of the body and includes all disease processes. We believe that the student can more easily accomplish a review of nursing content from a system point of view. Therefore, we have organized this chapter first by systems and then by the Nursing Process. It is important that the student approach the study of each system remembering that the body is an integrated whole; what is happening in one system will affect and be affected by all other systems in the body. Each system's coverage includes basic principles of physiology, pathophysiology, various disease processes, their treatment, and nursing interventions. The material is organized and presented to enable the student to transfer basic principles to any manifestation of illness, while understanding the total interaction which takes place inside the body.

---

* **NCLEX-RN candidates:** Please refer to the Drug Chart on page 85. These are drugs you must be familiar with for NCLEX.

NEUROLOGICAL SYSTEM

The nervous system (together with the endocrine system) provides the control functions for the body. Unique in its incredible ability to handle thousands of bits of information and stimuli from the sensory organs, this system of nerves and nerve centers coordinates and regulates all of this data and determines the responses of the body.

ANATOMY AND PHYSIOLOGY OF THE NERVOUS SYSTEM

Central Nervous System—Brain and Spinal Cord

A. Brain.
  1. Cerebrum (two hemispheres).
     a. Function.
        (1) Highest level of functioning.
        (2) Governs all sensory and motor activity, thought, and learning.
        (3) Analyzes, associates, integrates, and stores information.
     b. Cerebral cortex (outer gray layer)—divided into four major lobes.
        (1) Frontal.
           (a) Precentral gyrus—motor function.
           (b) Broca's area—motor speech area.
           (c) Prefrontal—controls morals, values, emotions, and judgment.
        (2) Parietal.
           (a) Postcentral gyrus—integrates general sensation.
           (b) Interprets pain, touch, temperature, and pressure.
           (c) Governs discrimination.
        (3) Temporal.
           (a) Auditory center.
           (b) Wernicke's area—sensory speech center.
        (4) Occipital—visual area.
     c. Basal ganglia.
        (1) Collections of cell bodies in white matter.
        (2) Control motor movement.
        (3) Part of extrapyramidal tract.
  2. Diencephalon.
     a. Thalamus.
        (1) Screens and relays sensory impulses to cortex.
        (2) Lowest level of crude conscious awareness.
     b. Hypothalamus—regulates autonomic nervous system, stress response, sleep, appetite, body temperature, fluid balance, and emotions.
  3. Brainstem.
     a. Midbrain—motor coordination, conjugate eye movements.
     b. Pons.
        (1) Contains projection tracts between spinal cord, medulla, and brain.
        (2) Controls involuntary respiratory reflexes.
     c. Medulla oblongata.
        (1) Contains all afferent and efferent tracts.
        (2) Decussation of most upper motor neurons (pyramidal tracts).
        (3) Contains cardiac, respiratory, vomiting, and vasomotor centers.
  4. Cerebellum.
     a. Connected by afferent/efferent pathways to all other parts of CNS.
     b. Coordinates muscle movement, posture, equilibrium, and muscle tone.
B. Spinal cord.
  1. Structure.
     a. Conveys messages between brain and the rest of the body.
     b. Extends from foramen magnum to second lumbar vertebra.
     c. Inner column of H-shaped gray matter which contains two anterior and two posterior horns.
     d. Posterior horns—contain cell bodies which connect with afferent (sensory) nerve fibers from posterior root ganglia.
     e. Anterior horns—contain cell bodies giving rise to efferent (motor) nerve fibers.

f. Lateral horns—present in thoracic segments; origin of autonomic fibers of sympathetic nervous system.

g. White matter of cord contains nerve tracts.

  (1) Principal ascending tracts (sensory pathways).

    (a) Lateral spinothalamic—governs pain, temperature (contralateral).

    (b) Anterior spinothalamic—governs touch, pressure (contralateral).

    (c) Posterior column to medial lemniscus—governs proprioception, vibration, touch, pressure (epsilateral).

    (d) Spinocerebellar—governs bilateral proprioception to posterior and anterior portions of the cerebellum.

  (2) Principal descending tracts (motor pathways).

    (a) Pyramidal, upper motor neuron, or corticospinal—from motor cortex to anterior horn cell. Tract crosses in medulla.

    (b) Extrapyramidal tracts consist of corticorubrospinal, corticoreticulospinal, and vestibulospinal. These tracts facilitate or inhibit flexor/extensor activity.

2. Protection for CNS.

a. Skull—rigid chamber with opening at the base (foramen magnum).

b. Meninges.

  (1) Dura mater—tough, fibrous membrane—forms falx, tentorium.

  (2) Arachnoid membrane—delicate membrane that contains subarachnoid fluid.

  (3) Pia mater—vascular membrane.

  (4) Subarachnoid space—formed by the arachnoid membrane and the pia mater.

c. Ventricles.

  (1) Four ventricles.

  (2) Communication between subarachnoid space.

  (3) Produce and circulate cerebrospinal fluid.

d. Cerebral spinal fluid.

  (1) Secreted from choroid plexuses in lateral ventricles, third ventricle, and fourth ventricle.

  (2) Circulates within interconnecting ventricles and subarachnoid space.

  (3) Protective cushion; aids exchange of nutrients and wastes.

  (4) Normal pressure: 60–180 mm/H_2O.

  (5) Volume: 125–150 cc.

e. Blood-brain barrier.

  (1) CSF.

  (2) Brain parenchyma.

f. Blood supply—conductor of oxygen vitally needed by nervous system.

  (1) Internal carotids branch to form anterior and middle cerebral arteries.

  (2) Vertebral arteries arise from the subclavians and merge to form the basilar arteries which then subdivide into the two posterior cerebral arteries.

  (3) Circle of Willis—formed as the anterior communicating artery bridges the anterior cerebral arteries, and as the posterior communicating artery bridges each posterior and middle cerebral artery.

Neuron Structure and Function

A. Structure.

1. Cell body (gray matter).

2. Processes (nerve fibers).

  a. Axon conducts impulses from cell body.

  b. Dendrites receive stimuli from the body and transmit them to the axon.

3. Synapse—chemical transmission of impulses from one neuron to another.

B. Myelin sheath (white matter).

1. Surrounds axon.

2. Insulates; correlates with function and speed of conduction.

3. Produced by neurolemmal cells in peripheral nerve fibers (sheath of Schwann).

4. Produced by neuroglial cells in CNS fibers.

C. Classification by function.

1. Sensory (afferent)—conducts impulses from end organ to CNS.

2. Motor (efferent)—conducts impulses from CNS to muscles and glands.

3. Internuncial (connector)—conducts impulses from sensory to motor neurons.

4. Somatic—innervates body wall.

5. Visceral—innervates the viscera.

D. Reflex arc (basic unit of function).
  1. Receptor—receives stimulus.
  2. Afferent pathway—transmits impulses to spinal cord.
  3. CNS—integration takes place at synapse between sensory and motor neurons.
  4. Efferent pathway—motor neurons transmit impulses from CNS to effector.
  5. Effector—organ or muscle that responds to the stimulus.
E. Regeneration of destroyed nerve fibers.
  1. Peripheral nerve—can regenerate, possibly due to neurolemma.
  2. CNS—cannot regenerate; lacks neurolemma.

Peripheral Nervous System—Cranial and Spinal Nerves

A. Carries voluntary and involuntary impulses.
B. Lower motor neuron—motor cell in anterior horn and its peripheral processes (final common path).
C. Cranial nerves—12 pairs of parasympathetic nerves with their nuclei along the brainstem.
  1. Olfactory—sensory.
  2. Optic—conducts sensory information from the retina.
  3. Oculomotor—motor nerve that controls four of the six extraocular muscles. Raises eyelid and controls the constrictor pupillae and ciliary muscles of the eyeball.
  4. Trochlear—a motor nerve that controls the superior oblique eye muscle.
  5. Trigeminal nerve—a mixed nerve with three sensory branches and one motor branch. Corneal reflex is supplied by the opthalmic branch.
  6. Abducens—controls the lateral rectus muscle of the eye.
  7. Facial—a mixed nerve. The anterior tongue receives sensory supply. Motor supply to glands of nose, palate lacrimal, submaxillary, and sublingual. The motor branch supplies hyoid elevators and muscles of expression and closes eyelid.
  8. Acoustic—a sensory nerve with two divisions—hearing and semicircular canals.
  9. Glossopharyngeal—a mixed nerve. Motor innervates parotid gland and sensory innervates auditory tube and posterior portion of taste buds.
  10. Vagus—a mixed nerve with motor branches to the pharyngeal and laryngeal muscles and to the viscera of the thorax and abdomen. Sensory portion supplies the pinna of the ear, thoracic, and abdominal viscera.
  11. Accessory nerve—a motor nerve innervating the sternocleidomastoid and trapezius muscles.
  12. Hypoglossal—a motor nerve controlling tongue muscles.
D. Spinal nerves (31 pairs).
  1. All mixed nerve fibers formed by joining of anterior motor and posterior sensory roots.
  2. Anterior root—efferent nerve fibers to glands and voluntary and involuntary muscles.
  3. Posterior root—afferent nerve fibers from sensory receptors. Contains posterior ganglion—cell body of sensory neuron.

Autonomic Nervous System

A. Structure and function.
  1. The term autonomic means that this system operates independently of desires and intentions.
  2. Part of peripheral nervous system controlling smooth muscle, cardiac muscle, and glands.
  3. Two divisions make involuntary adjustments for integrated balance (homeostasis).
B. Diseases of sympathetic nerve trunks result in specific syndromes.
  1. Dilation of pupil.
  2. Bowel paralysis.
  3. Variations in pulse rate and rhythm.
C. Structure of sympathetic nervous system—thoracolumbar division.
  1. Long postganglionic (adrenergic) fibers.
  2. Fibers arise in brainstem and descend to gray matter in spinal cord from C_8 to L_2.
D. Structure of parasympathetic nervous system—craniosacral division.
  1. Short postganglionic (cholinergic) fibers.
  2. Cells lie in brainstem and sacral region of spinal cord.

System Assessment

A. Evaluate client's history regarding common signs and symptoms.
  1. Numbness, weakness.

2. Dizziness, fainting, loss of consciousness.
3. Headache, pain.
4. Speech disturbances.
5. Visual disturbances.
6. Disturbances in memory, thinking, personality.
7. Nausea, vomiting.

B. Assess client's level of consciousness.
1. Evaluate cerebral function (most sensitive and reliable index of consciousness).
2. Evaluate level of consciousness.
   a. Orientation to person, place, purpose, time.
   b. Response to verbal/tactile stimuli or simple commands.
   c. Response to painful stimuli: purposeful, nonpurposeful, decorticate, decerebrate, no response.
3. Assess behavior to determine level of consciousness: clouding, confusion, delirium, stupor, coma.

C. Evaluate pupillary signs.
1. Assess size: measure in millimeters.
2. Assess equality: equal, unequal, fluctuations.
3. Assess reactions to light: brisk, slow, fixed. Light reflex is most important sign differentiating structural from metabolic coma.
4. Evaluate unusual eye movements or deviations from midline.
   a. Unilateral pupil dilation: compression of third cranial nerve (controls pupillary constriction).
   b. Midposition, fixed pupils (often unequal): midbrain injury.
   c. Pinpoint, fixed pupils: pontine damage.

D. Evaluate motor function.
1. Assess face and upper and lower extremities for:
   a. Muscle tone, strength, equality.
   b. Voluntary movement.
   c. Involuntary movements.
   d. Reflexes: Babinski, corneal, gag.
2. Evaluate patterns of motor function.
   a. Pattern of motor dysfunction gives information about anatomic location of lesions, independent of level of consciousness.
   b. Appropriate—spontaneous movement to stimulus or command.
   c. Absence: hemiplegia, paraplegia, quadriplegia.
3. Inappropriate—nonpurposeful.

   a. Posturing in response to noxious stimuli.
      (1) Decorticate—nonfunctioning cortex, internal capsule (flexion, upper extremity).
      (2) Decerebrate—brainstem lesion (total extension).
   b. Involuntary.
      (1) Choreiform (jerky, quick).
      (2) Athetoid (twisting, slow).
      (3) Tremors.
      (4) Spasms.
      (5) Convulsions.

E. Assess reflexes.
1. Evaluate for presence of reflexes.
   a. Babinski: dorsiflexion ankle and great toe with fanning of other toes; indicates disruption of pyramidal tract.
   b. Corneal: loss of blink reflex indicates dysfunction of fifth cranial nerve (danger of corneal injuries).
   c. Gag: loss of gag reflex indicates dysfunction on the ninth and tenth cranial nerves (danger of aspiration).
2. Identify reflex response.
   a. Scale is 0 to 4.
   b. Absence of reflex is rated 0.
   c. Hyperactive reflex is rated 4.

F. Evaluate sensory function.
1. Assess general sensory function in all extremities: touch, pressure, pain.
2. If no motor response to command, may elicit response by sensory stimuli such as supraorbital pressure.
3. Use minimal amount of stimulus necessary to evoke a response.
4. Assess for bladder control.
   a. Spastic: automatic, hypertonic, reflex.
   b. Flaccid: autonomous, atonic, hypotonic, nonreflex.
5. Evaluate bowel control.
   a. Observe ability to evacuate stool.
   b. Assess consistency and number of stools.
   c. Identify need for bowel training program.

G. Evaluate vital signs.
1. Monitor for trends; changes are often unreliable and occur late with increasing intracranial pressure.
2. Observe blood pressure and pulse.

a. Increasing blood pressure with reflex slowing of pulse—compensatory stage with increasing intracranial pressure.

b. Fall in blood pressure with increasing or irregular pulse—decompensation.

3. Observe respiration.

a. Rate, depth, and rhythm more sensitive indication of intracranial pressure than blood pressure and pulse.

b. Cheyne-Stokes.

(1) Rhythmically waxes and wanes, alternating with periods of apnea.

(2) Cerebral hemisphere, basal ganglia, or metabolic.

c. Neurogenic hyperventilation.

(1) Sustained regular, rapid, and deep.

(2) Low midbrain, middle pons.

d. Apneustic.

(1) Irregular with pauses at end of inspiration and expiration.

(2) Mid or caudal pons.

e. Ataxic.

(1) Totally irregular, random rhythm and depth.

(2) Medulla.

f. Cluster.

(1) Clusters of breaths with irregularly spaced pauses.

(2) High medulla, low pons.

4. Check temperature (rectal).

a. Early rise may indicate damage to hypothalamus or brainstem.

b. Slow rise may indicate infection.

c. Elevated temperature increases brain's metabolic rate.

H. Observe for signs of meningeal irritation.

1. Brudzinski's sign: flexion of head causes flexion of both thighs at hips and knee flexion.

2. Kernig's sign: supine position, thigh and knee flexed to right angles. Extension of leg causes spasm of hamstring, resistance, and pain.

3. Nuchal rigidity.

4. Irritability.

5. Increased temperature.

I. Evaluate intracranial pressure.

1. Assess level of consciousness (most sensitive indication of increasing intracranial pressure)—changes from restlessness to confusion to declining level of consciousness and coma.

2. Check for headache—tension, displacement of brain.

3. Observe for vomiting—irritation vagal nuclei in floor of fourth ventricle.

4. Assess pupillary changes—unilateral dilation of pupil; slow reaction to light; fixed dilated pupil is ominous sign requiring immediate action.

5. Observe motor function—weakness, hemiplegia, positive Babinski, decorticate, decerebrate, seizure activity.

6. Measure vital signs—rise in blood pressure; widening pulse pressure; reflex slowing of pulse; abnormalities in respiration, especially periods of apnea; temperature elevation.

J. Evaluate autonomic nervous system.

1. Assess for sympathetic function.

a. Fight, flight, or freeze; diffuse response.

b. Increases heart rate, blood pressure.

c. Dilates pupils, bronchi.

d. Decreases peristalsis.

e. Increases perspiration.

f. Increases blood sugar.

2. Assess for parasympathetic function.

a. Repair, repose; discrete response.

b. Decreases heart rate, blood pressure.

c. Constricts pupils, bronchi.

d. Increases salivation and peristalsis.

e. Dilates blood vessels.

f. Bladder contraction.

K. Evaluate for hyperthermia.

1. Assess for shivering.

2. Assess respiratory function—ventilation and patent airway.

3. Evaluate cardiac function—pulse and rhythm.

4. Observe urinary function—color, specific gravity, and amount.

5. Check for nausea and vomiting.

L. Assess for pain.

1. Assess for nonverbal signs of pain, i.e., facial grimaces, retracting from painful stimuli.

2. Evaluate onset, location, intensity, duration, and aggravating factor.

3. Observe for precipitating factors, associated manifestations, and alleviating factors.

Diagnostic Procedures

Radiologic Procedures

A. Skull series.

1. Procedure: x-rays of head from different angles.
2. Purpose: to visualize configuration, density, and vascular markings.
3. Tomograms: layered vertical or horizontal x-ray exposures.

B. Ventriculography.
1. Procedure: injection of air directly into lateral ventricles followed by x-rays.
2. Purpose: to visualize ventricles, localize tumors. May be used if increased intracranial pressure contraindicates pneumoencephalography.
3. Potential complications: headache, nausea and vomiting, meningitis, increasing intracranial pressure.
4. Nursing implementation.
   a. Monitor vital signs.
   b. Check neurological status.
   c. Elevate head.
   d. Administer icebag and analgesics for headache.

C. Myelography.
1. Procedure: injection of dye or air into lumbar or cisternal subarachnoid space followed by x-rays of the spinal column.
2. Purpose: to visualize spinal subarachnoid space for distortions caused by lesions.
3. Potential complications.
   a. Same as for lumbar puncture.
   b. Cerebral meningeal irritation from dye.
4. Nursing care.
   a. Same as for lumbar puncture.
   b. If dye is used, elevate head and observe for meningeal irritation.
   c. If air is used, keep head lower than trunk.

D. Cerebral angiography.
1. Procedure: injection of radiopaque dye into carotid and/or vertebral arteries followed by serial x-rays.
2. Purpose: to visualize cerebral vessels and localize lesions such as aneurysms, occlusions, angiomas, tumors, or abscesses.
3. Potential complications.
   a. Anaphylactic reaction to dye.
   b. Local hemorrhage.
   c. Vasospasm.
   d. Adverse intracranial pressure.
4. Nursing implementation.
   a. Prior to procedure.
      (1) Check allergies.
      (2) Take baseline assessment.
      (3) Measure neck circumference.
   b. During procedure and postprocedure.
      (1) Have emergency equipment available.
      (2) Monitor neurological and vital signs for shock, level of consciousness, hemiparesis, hemiplegia, and aphasia.
      (3) Monitor swelling of neck and difficulty in swallowing or breathing.
      (4) Administer ice collar.

Magnetic Resonance Imaging (MRI)

A. Procedure: visualization of distribution of hydrogen molecules in the body in three dimensions.
B. Technique has revolutionized diagnostic medicine and is surpassing more conventional methods.
   1. Procedure is noninvasive.
   2. Does not use harmful ionizing radiation.
   3. Superior imaging of body's soft tissue.
C. Purpose.
   1. Differentiate types of tissues, including those in normal and abnormal states.
   2. Clinical applications include: brain, both tumors and vascular abnormalities; cardiac and respiratory conditions; cardiac anomalies; blood vessels; liver disease, renal abnormalities, gallbladder, and tumors.
D. Safety measures.
   1. Clients with pacemakers are excluded from MRI.
   2. Metal objects must be removed from clients.
   3. Clients with metal implants (hip prostheses, vascular clips, artificial valves, etc.) are prohibited from MRI imaging.
   4. Closely monitor clients with potential respiratory or cardiac collapse.
E. Nursing implementation.
   1. Maintain safety measures with MRI use.
   2. Explain procedure and machine to allay anxiety.
   3. Provide client and family teaching.
F. Brain scan.
   1. Procedure intravenous injection of radioactive isotope substance followed by anterior-posterior and lateral scanning. Concentration of substance is greatest in pathological areas.
   2. Purpose: to localize tumors with high degree of accuracy. Accuracy is increased if scanning is combined with either arteriography or encephalography.
   3. Keep npo 4–6 hours before exam.
G. Tomography.

1. Type of brain scan that relies on tissue density and shadows to reflect internal state of brain tissue.
2. EMI and/or CAT.

Electroencephalography (EEG)

A. Procedure: graphic recording of brain's electrical activity by electrodes placed on the scalp.
B. Purpose: to detect intracranial lesion and abnormal electrical activity (epilepsy).
C. Nursing implementation.
   1. Wash hair.
   2. Withhold sedatives or stimulants.
   3. Administer fluids as ordered.

Echoencephalogram

A. Procedure: recording of reflected ultrasonic waves from brain structures.
B. Purpose.
   1. To measure position and shifting of midline structures.
   2. To detect subdural hematoma or tumors.

Electromyography (EMG)

A. Procedure: recording of muscle action potential by surface or needle electrodes.
B. Purpose: to diagnose or localize neuromuscular disease.

Lumbar Puncture (LP)

A. Procedure: insertion of spinal needle through L_3–L_4 or L_4–L_5 interspace into lumbar subarachnoid space.
B. Purpose.
   1. To obtain cerebral spinal fluid (CSF).
   2. To measure intracranial pressure and spinal fluid dynamics.
   3. To instill air, dye, or medications.
C. Potential complications: headache, backache, and herniation with brainstem compression (especially if intracranial pressure is high).
D. Nursing implementation.
   1. Have client empty bowel and bladder.
   2. Assist with specimens and spinal fluid dynamics.
   3. Maintain strict asepsis.
   4. Monitor vital signs.
   5. Place client in horizontal position.
   6. Encourage fluids if not contraindicated.
   7. Inspect puncture site.
E. Spinal fluid dynamics—Queckenstedt-Stookey test.
   1. Normal: pressure increases with jugular compression and drops to normal 10 to 30 seconds after release of compression.
   2. Partial block: slow rise and return to normal.
   3. Complete block: no rise.

Cisternal Puncture

A. Procedure: needle puncture into cisterna magna just below the occipital bone.
B. Purpose: same as for lumbar puncture. May be used if intracranial pressure is high or for infants.
C. Potential complications: respiratory distress.
D. Nursing implementation.
   1. Same as for lumbar puncture.
   2. Observe for cyanosis, dyspnea, and apnea.

System Planning and Analysis

A. Alterations in neurological function are identified in early stages of dysfunction.
B. Neurological complications are prevented or identified before major neurological dysfunction occurs.
C. Motor function is maintained at optimal level.
D. Sensory dysfunction is identified as means to determine neurological damage.
E. Cranial nerve dysfunction is identified and appropriate interventions established to minimize physiological alterations.
F. Client is adequately prepared for diagnostic tests or surgical intervention.
G. Adequate respiratory function is maintained.
H. Body temperature is maintained within normal range.
I. Circulatory function is maintained within normal parameters.
J. Level of consciousness is monitored frequently.
K. Goals for rehabilitation are established.
L. Safe environment is established for clients with altered sensorium.
M. Source and level of pain are identified.

System Implementation

A. Observe for and treat seizure activity.

B. Monitor vital signs for signs of hyperthermia, increased intracranial pressure, and infection.

C. Observe motor and sensory function.

D. Observe pupillary signs for metabolic or structural complications.

E. Prevent muscle weakness and atrophy through range of motion exercises.

F. Promote bowel and bladder function.

G. Maintain nutritional status.

H. Prevent complications of immobility, i.e., skin breakdown.

I. Provide emotional support for client and family during hospitalization and upon discharge.

J. Monitor cardiac and respiratory function for early identification of potential complications.

K. Provide appropriate preoperative and postoperative nursing interventions.

L. Establish an individualized rehabilitative program.

M. Administer drug therapy and monitor side effects.

N. Institute nursing implementation to assist in decreasing intracranial pressure.

O. Establish appropriate measures for pain relief.

System Evaluation

A. Complications identified early and appropriate nursing interventions established.

B. Rehabilitation program improves client's motor and sensory function to optimum level.

C. Seizure activity is controlled through medication administration.

D. Intracranial pressure is decreased through nursing implementation and medical intervention.

E. Nutritional needs are met through appropriate interventions determined by client's condition.

F. Complications of immobility are prevented through skin care, range of motion, bowel and bladder training, and turning and positioning.

G. Emergency interventions are established to prevent major alterations in cerebral or spinal cord function.

H. Pain is controlled.

NEUROLOGIC DYSFUNCTION

The Unconscious Client

Definition: Unconsciousness is a state of depressed cerebral functioning with altered sensory and motor function.

Assessment

A. Evaluate client for possible causes: vascular disorders, intracranial mass, head trauma, cerebral toxins, metabolic disorders, acute infection.

1. Intracranial.
   a. Supratentorium mass lesion compressing or displacing brainstem.
   b. Infratentorium destructive lesions.
2. Extracranial.
   a. Metabolic encephalopathy (most common).
   b. Psychiatric conditions.

B. Assess comatose state using Glasgow coma scale.

1. Comatose state based on three areas associated with level of consciousness.
2. Scoring system.
   a. Based on a scale of 1 to 15 points.
   b. Any score below 8 indicates coma is present.
3. Eye opening is the most important indicator.
4. Coma scale.

a. Motor response.	Points
(1) Obeys	6
(2) Localizes	5
(3) Withdrawn	4
(4) Abnormal flexion	3
(5) Extensor response	2
(6) Nil	1
b. Verbal response.	Points
(1) Oriented	5
(2) Confused conversation	4
(3) Inappropriate words	3
(4) Incomprehensible sounds	2
(5) Nil	1
c. Eye opening.	Points
(1) Spontaneous	4
(2) To speech	3
(3) To pain	2
(4) Nil	1

C. Evaluate respiratory function and airway patency.

D. Assess for adequate circulation.

E. Assess fluid and electrolyte balance.

Implementation

A. Maintain open airway and adequate ventilation.

1. Check for airway obstruction.
   a. Can result in retention of carbon dioxide (with cerebral vasodilation, edema, and increased intracranial pressure).
   b. Hypoxia (with potential irreversible brain damage).

2. Complete continuous assessment.
   a. Color, chest expansion, deformities.
   b. Rate, depth, and rhythm of respirations.
   c. Air movement at nose/mouth or endotracheal tube.
   d. Breath sounds, adventitious sounds.
   e. Accumulation of secretions or blood in mouth.
   f. Signs of respiratory distress: hypoxemia, hypercapnia, or atelectasis.
3. Provide airway.
   a. Head tilt; modified jaw thrust if cervical injury suspected.
   b. Cuffed endotracheal or tracheostomy tube (maintain airway, avenue for suctioning and/or mechanical ventilation).
4. Provide assisted ventilation.
   a. If mechanical ventilator is used, ensure proper functioning.
   b. Watch pO_2 and pCO_2.
5. Position client.
   a. Semiprone (to prevent tongue from occluding airway and secretions from pooling in pharynx).
   b. Frequent change of position.
6. Provide pulmonary toilet.
   a. Deep breathing and coughing if not contraindicated.
   b. Suctioning of secretions as necessary.
7. Have emergency equipment available.

B. Maintain adequate circulation.
   1. Blood pressure.
      a. Hypertension—result of increased intracranial pressure.
      b. Hypotension—result of immobility.
   2. Pulse.
      a. Check quality and presence of all pulses.
      b. Check rate and rhythm of apical and/or radial pulse.
   3. Heart sounds.
      a. Arrhythmias due to hypoxia.
      b. Usually premature ventricular contractions.
   4. Skin.
      a. Color.
      b. Temperature.
   5. Edema.
      a. Dependent areas.
      b. Generalized.
   6. Signs of shock.

7. Positioning.
   a. Perform passive ROM to all extremities.
   b. Change position at least every two hours.
   c. Avoid Trendelenburg's position.
C. Monitor neurological status.
   1. Level of consciousness.
   2. Pupillary signs.
   3. Motor function.
   4. Sensory function.
D. Maintain nutrition, fluid and electrolyte balance.
   1. Keep client n.p.o. while unconscious (check for gag and swallowing reflex).
   2. Give intravenous fluids, hyperalimentation as required.
   3. Use caution with IV rates in presence of increased intracranial pressure.
   4. Administer tube feeding for long-term management. Refer to page 48.
   5. Maintain oral and nasal hygiene.
   6. Resume oral intake carefully as consciousness returns.
      a. Check gag reflex.
      b. Use ice chips or water as first liquid.
      c. Keep suction equipment ready.
E. Monitor homeostasis.
   1. Intake—n.p.o., oral, tube feedings, IV.
   2. Output—urinary, feces; check emesis, nasogastric tube.
   3. Daily weight.
   4. Electrolyte studies.
   5. Clinical signs of hydration.
F. Promote elimination.
   1. Urinary: retention catheter.
      a. Maintain daily hygiene of meatus.
      b. Ensure patency to prevent bladder distention, urinary stasis, infection, and urinary calculi.
      c. Evaluate amount, color, consistency of output; check specific gravity.
   2. Bowel: suppositories and enemas.
      a. Establish routine elimination patterns.
      b. Observe for complications.
      c. Check for paralytic ileus.
         (1) Abdominal distention.
         (2) Constipation and/or impaction.
         (3) Diarrhea.
G. Maintain integrity of the skin.
   1. High risk of decubitus ulcers due to:
      a. Loss of vasomotor tone.
      b. Impaired peripheral circulation.

c. Paralysis, immobility, and loss of muscle tone.

d. Hypoproteinemia.

2. Loss of sensation of pressure, pain or temperature—decreased awareness of developing decubitus ulcers or burns.

3. Skin care.

  a. Clean and dry skin; avoid powder because it may cake.

  b. Massage with lotion around and toward bony prominences once a day.

  c. Use alcohol to toughen skin.

  d. Alternate air mattress with sheepskin pad.

  e. Keep linen from wrinkling; avoid mechanical friction against linen.

H. Maintain personal hygiene.

1. Eye: loss of corneal reflex may contribute to corneal irritation, keratitis, blindness.

  a. Assess corneal reflex and signs of irritation.

  b. Irrigate eyes and instill artificial tears or patch.

2. Nose: trauma or infection in nose or nasopharynx may cause meningitis.

  a. Observe for drainage of CSF.

  b. Clean and lubricate nares; do not clean inside nostrils.

  c. Change nasogastric tube at intervals.

3. Mouth: mouth breathing contributes to drying and crusting excoriation of mucous membranes, which may contribute to aspiration and respiratory tract infections.

  a. Examine the mouth daily with a good light.

  b. Clean teeth, gums, mucous membranes, tongue, and uvula to prevent crusting and infection; lubricate lips.

  c. Inspect for retained food in the mouth of clients who have facial paralysis; follow with mouth care.

4. Ear: drainage of CSF from the ear indicates damage to the base of the brain and a danger of meningitis.

  a. Inspect ear for drainage of CSF.

  b. Loosely cover ear with sterile, dry dressing.

I. Maintain optimal positioning and movement.

1. Prevent further trauma.

  a. Maintain body alignment, support head and limbs when turning, logroll.

  b. Do not flex or twist spine or hyperextend neck if spinal cord injury suspected.

2. Provide adequate positioning.

  a. Disuse of muscle leads to contractures, osteoporosis, and compromised venous return.

  b. Maintain and support joints and limbs in most functional anatomic position.

  c. Avoid improper use of knee gatch or pillows under knee.

3. Avoid complete immobility.

  a. Perform ROM (against resistance if possible), weight bearing, tilt table.

  b. Encourage self-help.

J. Provide psychosocial support for client and family.

1. Assume that an unconscious client can hear; frequently reassure and explain procedures to client.

2. Encourage family interaction.

K. Institute safety precautions.

1. Use siderails at all times.

2. Remove dentures and dental bridges.

3. Remove contact lenses.

4. Avoid restraints.

5. Do not leave unattended when unstable for more than 15 to 30 minutes.

6. Tongue blade at bedside.

Increased Intracranial Pressure

Definition: An increase in intracranial bulk due to blood, CSF, or brain tissue leading to an increase in pressure.

Characteristics

A. Causes: trauma, hemorrhage, tumors, abscess, hydrocephalus, edema, or inflammation.

B. Increased pressure impedes cerebral circulation, absorption of CSF, and function of the nerve cells.

C. Increasing pressure is transmitted downward toward the brainstem with eventual tentorial herniation, brainstem compression, and death.

Assessment

A. Evaluate level of consciousness (most sensitive indication of increasing intracranial pressure)—changes from restlessness to confusion to declining level of consciousness and coma.

B. Check for headache—tension, displacement of brain.

C. Observe for vomiting—irritation of vagal nuclei in floor of fourth ventricle.

D. Observe pupillary changes—unilateral dilation of pupil; slow reaction to light; fixed dilated pupil is ominous sign requiring immediate action.

E. Assess motor function—weakness, hemiplegia, positive Babinski, decorticate, decerebrate, seizure activity.

F. Assess vital signs—rise in B/P; widening pulse pressure; reflex slowing of pulse; abnormalities in respiration, especially apnea; temperature elevation.

G. Assess for hyperthermia—possible complication.

Implementation

A. Acute phase: medical management.
   1. Elevate head of bed; avoid Trendelenburg's.
   2. Limit fluid intake (1200 cc/day).
   3. Administer medications: steroids, osmotic diuretics.
      a. Steroids (Decadron) decrease cerebral edema by their anti-inflammatory effect; decrease capillary permeability in inflammatory processes, thus decreasing leakage of fluid into tissue.
      b. Mannitol decreases cerebral edema; provides diuretic action by carrying out large volume of water through nephrons.
      c. Hypertonic IV solution administered because it is impermeable to blood-brain barrier; reduce edema by rapid movement of water out of ventricles into bloodstream.
   4. Administer mechanical ventilation.
   5. Prevent further complications.
      a. Monitor neurological dysfunction versus cardiovascular shock.
      b. Prevent hypoxia: avoid morphine.
      c. Monitor fluids: electrolyte and acid-base balance.

B. Chronic phase: surgical management.
   1. Ventriculo-peritoneal shunt systems (most common). Designed to shunt cerebrospinal fluid from the lateral ventricles into the peritoneum.
   2. Preoperative care.
      a. Follow care of client with increased intracranial pressure.
      b. Prepare client for craniotomy if necessary.
   3. Postoperative care.
      a. Monitor closely for signs and symptoms of increasing intracranial pressure due to shunt failure.
      b. Check for infection (a common and serious complication). If present, removal of the shunt system is indicated in addition to appropriate chemotherapy.

Hyperthermia

Definition: Temperature of 41° C (106° F); associated with increased cerebral metabolism, increasing risk of hypoxia.

Characteristics

A. Dysfunction of thermoregulatory center—trauma, tumor, cerebral edema, CVA, intracranial surgery.

B. Prolonged exposure to high environmental temperatures—heatstroke.

C. Caused by infection.

Assessment

A. Assess vital signs frequently, especially increased temperature.

B. Evaluate peripheral pulses for systemic blood flow.

C. Observe skin and mucous membranes for signs of dehydration.

D. Measure urine output to determine fluid balance.

E. Observe for signs of seizure activity with high temperature.

F. Assess heart sounds for arrhythmias.

G. Evaluate effects of hypothermia treatments.
   1. Reduces cerebral metabolism and demand for oxygen.
   2. Decreases cerebral and systemic blood flow.
   3. Reduces CSF pressure.
   4. Decreases endocrine, liver, and kidney function.
   5. Decreases pulse, blood pressure, and respiration; may affect cardiac pacemaker.

Implementation

A. Provide for patent airway if temperature is very high.

B. Provide safety measures for possible seizure activity.

C. Monitor fluid balance by observing skin condition, urine output, lung sounds, peripheral pulses.

D. Provide methods for inducing hypothermia.
   1. External—cool bath, fans, ice bags, hypothermic blanket (most common).
   2. Drugs.
      a. Chlorpromazine—reduces peripheral vasoconstriction, muscle tone, shivering; depresses thermoregulation in hypothalamus.
      b. Meperidine—relaxes smooth muscle, reduces shivering.

c. Promethazine—dilates coronary arteries, reduces laryngeal and bronchial irritation.

3. Extracorporeal—usually reserved for surgery.

E. Monitor effects of hypothermia.

  1. Prevent shivering.

    a. Shivering increases CSF pressure and oxygen consumption.

    b. Treatment: chlorpromazine.

  2. Prevent trauma to skin and tissue.

    a. Frostbite—crystallization of tissues with white or blue discoloration, hardening of tissue, burning, numbness.

    b. Fat necrosis—solidification of subcutaneous fat creating hard tissue masses.

    c. Initially give complete bath and oil the skin; during procedure, massage skin frequently with lotion or oil to maintain integrity of the skin.

  3. Monitor and prevent respiratory complications.

    a. Hypothermia may mask infection, cause respiratory arrest.

    b. Institute measures to maintain open airway and adequate ventilation.

  4. Monitor and prevent cardiac complications.

    a. Hypothermia can cause arrhythmias and cardiac arrest.

    b. Monitor cardiac status and have emergency equipment available.

  5. Monitor renal function.

    a. Insert Foley catheter.

    b. Monitor urinary output, BUN; may monitor specific gravity.

  6. Prevent vomiting and possible aspiration; client may have loss of gag reflex and reduced peristalsis.

  7. Monitor changes in neurological function during hypothermia.

PAIN MANAGEMENT

Characteristics

A. Classification of pain fibers.

  1. Class A—large myelinated (fast pain).

  2. Class B—smaller unmyelinated.

  3. Class C—unmyelinated (slow pain).

B. The experience of pain.

  1. Pain source—direct causative factor.

  2. Stimulation of pain receptor—mechanical, chemical, thermal, electrical, ischemic.

  3. Pain pathway.

    a. Sensory pathways through dorsal root, ending on second order neuron in posterior horn.

    b. Afferent fibers cross over to anterolateral pathway, ascend in lateral spinothalamic tract to thalamus.

    c. Fibers then travel to postcentral gyrus in parietal lobe.

C. Gate control theory.

  1. Pain impulses can be modulated by a transmission blocking action within CNS.

  2. Large diameter cutaneous pain fibers can be stimulated (rubbing, scratching) and may inhibit smaller diameter excitatory fibers and prevent transmission of that impulse.

  3. Cerebral cortical mechanisms that influence perception and interpretation may also inhibit transmission.

D. Pain perception—thalamus/awareness and parietal/integration.

E. Pain interpretation—cerebral cortex; delayed response influenced by previous experiences, culture, existing physical/psychological state.

F. Reactions—psychic and/or physiologic.

Assessment

A. Assess for type of pain.

  1. Superficial—localized, shorter duration, sharp sensation.

  2. Deep pain—long duration, diffuse, dull aching quality; associated autonomic responses, musculoskeletal tension, nausea.

    a. Visceral—internal organs.

    b. Somatic—neuromuscular, segmental distribution.

    c. Referred—area stimulated (deep) and area pain referred to (superficial) are innervated by nerve fibers arising from same segment of spinal cord.

    d. Secondary to skeletal muscle.

  3. Central pain—autonomic reflex pain syndrome.

    a. Causalgia—lesion peripheral nerve.

    b. Phantom—after amputation.

    c. Central—lesion in CNS, affecting pain pathway.

  4. Psychogenic—due to emotional factors without anatomic or physiological explanation.

B. Assess onset of pain.

C. Assess location, where it originates and travels.

D. Evaluate intensity and character of pain.

E. Check precipitating factors.
F. Assess associated factors.
   1. Nausea and/or vomiting.
   2. Bradycardia/tachycardia.
   3. Hypotension/hypertension.
   4. Profuse perspiration.
   5. Apprehension or anxiety.
G. Assess duration of pain.
H. Evaluate previous experience of pain.

Implementation

A. Assess pain before treating.
B. Give reassurance, reduce anxiety and fears.
C. Offer distraction.
D. Give comfort measures: positioning, rest, elevation, heat/cold applications; protect from painful stimuli.
E. Massage—but never massage calf due to danger of emboli.
F. Administer pain medication as needed: monitor therapeutic, toxic dose, and side effects.
G. Monitor alternative methods to control pain.
   1. Dorsal column stimulator: stimulation of electrodes at dorsal column of spinal cord by client-controlled device to inhibit pain.
   2. Analgesics: alter perception, threshold, and reaction to pain.
   3. Anesthesia: block pain pathway.
   4. Local nerve block.
   5. Neurosurgical procedures: interrupt sensory pathways; usually also affect pressure and temperature pathways.
      a. Neurectomy: interrupt cranial or peripheral nerves.
      b. Sympathectomy: interrupt afferent pathways (ganglia).

SEIZURE DISORDERS

Convulsions

Definition: The forceful involuntary contractions of voluntary muscles; may be one component of a seizure.

Characteristics

A. Causes: cerebral trauma, congenital defects, epilepsy, infection, tumor circulatory defect, anoxia, metabolic abnormalities, excessive hydration.
B. Classification.
   1. Tonic convulsion: sustained contraction of muscles.
   2. Clonic convulsion: alternating contraction/relaxation of opposing muscle group.
   3. Epileptiform: any convulsion with loss of consciousness.

Assessment

A. Identify if aura present.
B. Observe type of motor activity.
C. Observe pattern of seizure activity.
D. Identify length of seizure activity.
E. Evaluate loss of bowel or bladder control.
F. Evaluate loss of consciousness.
G. Observe for signs of respiratory distress.
H. Identify characteristics during the postictal state.

Implementation

A. Observe and record characteristics of seizure activity.
   1. Level of consciousness.
   2. Description of any aura.
   3. Description of body position and initial activity.
   4. Motor activity: initial body part involved, character of movements (tonic/clonic), progression of movement, duration, biting of the tongue.
   5. Respiration, color.
   6. Pupillary changes, eye movements.
   7. Incontinence, vomiting.
   8. Total duration, frequency, number of seizures, injuries.
   9. Postictal state.
      a. Loss of consciousness.
      b. Sleepiness.
      c. Impaired speech, motor or thinking.
      d. Headache.
      e. Neurological and vital signs.
B. Protect client from trauma.
   1. Ensure patent airway.
   2. Do not force any object between teeth if they are already clenched.
   3. Avoid use of any restraints, loosen restrictive clothing.
   4. Remove any objects from environment that may cause injury.
   5. Stay with client.
C. Provide nursing care after seizure.
   1. Keep turned to side to prevent aspiration.
   2. Reorient to environment when awakened.

Epilepsy

Definition: A combination of several disorders characterized by chronic seizure activity; a symptom of brain or CNS irritation. A seizure is an abnormal, sudden, excessive discharge of electrical activity within the brain.

Characteristics

A. Incidence in U.S. may be as low as 1 million or as high as 2.5 million—many clients hide their seizure disorder.

B. Major problems may be an electrical disturbance (dysrhythmia) in nerve cells in one section of the brain.

C. Seizures are associated with changes in behavior, mentation and motor or sensory activity.

D. Causes may be related to several factors.
   1. Genetic factors, trauma, brain tumor, circulatory or metabolic disorders, toxicity, or infection.
   2. May be symptoms of underlying brain pathology such as scar tissue, vascular disease, or meningitis.
   3. Heredity may play a part in absence, akinetic or myoclonic seizures.

E. Diagnostic tests include CT to determine underlying CNS changes, EEG for a distinctive pattern, MRI, blood studies, etc.

Assessment

A. Obtain seizure history through client report or observation: onset, pattern or sequence of progression, precipitating events, frequency, description.

B. Assess whether seizure is simple staring spell or prolonged convulsive movements.

C. Observe if there is excess or loss of muscle tone or movement.

D. Assess disturbance of behavior, mood, sensation, and/or perception.

E. Determine if autonomic functions of the body are disturbed.

F. Assess for prodromal signs or symptoms: mood changes, irritability, insomnia, etc.

G. Explore with client effect of epilepsy on life and life style (work limitations, social interaction, psychological adjustment).

H. Assess for Generalized Seizures: four types.
   1. Tonic-clonic seizures, traditionally known as "grand mal."
      a. May begin with an aura, then a tonic phase— stiffening or rigidity of muscles, particularly arms and legs, followed by loss of consciousness.
      b. Clonic phase follows—hyperventilation with rhythmic jerking of all extremities.
      c. Full recovery may take several hours.
   2. Absence seizures, formerly "petit mal."
      a. Brief, often just seconds, loss of consciousness; almost no loss or change in muscle tone.
      b. May occur 100 times/day. More common in children; may appear to be "day dreaming."
   3. Myoclonic seizure.
      a. Characterized by a brief, generalized jerking or stiffening of the extremities.
      b. May occur as single movement or in groups; seizure may throw person to the floor.
   4. Atonic or akinetic seizures, also called "drop attacks."
      a. Characterized by sudden, momentary loss of muscle tone.
      b. Usually causes person to fall to the ground.

I. Assess for partial seizures (focal seizures).
   1. Simple partial seizure.
      a. Localized (confined to a specific area) motor symptoms, accompanied by sensory symptoms.
      b. Client remains conscious throughout episode and may report an aura before seizure takes place.
   2. Complex partial (psychomotor) seizure.
      a. Area of brain most involved in temporal lobe (thus, this type of seizure is called psychomotor).
      b. Characterized by period of altered behavior and automatism (client is not aware of behavior); evidenced by such mannerisms as lip smacking, chewing, picking at clothes, etc.
      c. Client loses consciousness for a few seconds.

J. Idiopathic or unclassified seizures.
   1. This type of seizure accounts for half of all seizure activity.
   2. Occurs for no known reason and fits into no generalized or partial classification.

K. Assess for specific phases of seizure activity.
   1. Occurs without warning or following an *aura* (peculiar sensation that warns of an impending seizure—dizziness, visual or auditory sensation).
   2. Behavior at onset of seizure.

a. Change in facial expression—fixation of gaze, flickering eyelids, etc.

b. Sound or cry at time of seizure.

3. Movements of body.

a. Tonic phase—parts of body involved, length of time (usually 10–20 seconds).

b. Clonic phase—parts of body that jerk, sequence of jerking movements, how long activity lasts (usually about 30 seconds).

4. Behavior following seizure.

a. State of consciousness, orientation.

b. Motor ability, speech ability, activity.

Implementation

A. Prevent injury during seizure.

1. Remove objects that may cause harm.

2. Remain with client during seizure.

3. Do not force jaws open during seizure.

4. Do not restrict limbs or restrain.

5. Loosen restrictive clothing.

6. Turn head to side, if possible, to prevent aspiration and allow secretions to drain.

7. Check that airway is open. Do not initiate artificial ventilation during a tonic-clonic seizure.

B. Observe and document seizure pattern.

1. Note time, level of consciousness, and presence of aura before seizure.

2. Record type, character, progression of movements.

3. Note duration of seizure and client's condition throughout.

4. Observe and record postictal state.

C. Administer and monitor medications.

1. Seizure control may be achieved with one or a combination of drugs.

2. Dosage is adjusted to achieve seizure control with few side effects.

3. Medications must be given on time to maintain therapeutic blood levels.

4. Phenytoin (Dilantin).

a. Prevents seizures through depression of motor areas of the brain.

b. Side effects: GI disturbance, visual changes, rash, anemia, gingival hyperplasia.

c. Check CBC and calcium levels.

d. Give p.o. drug with milk or meals; supplemental vitamin D and folic acid.

5. Diazepam (Valium).

a. Given to stop motor activity associated with status epilepticus; for restlessness.

b. Side effects: if given IV, monitor for respiratory distress.

6. Phenobarbital (Luminal).

a. Reduces responsiveness of normal neurons to impulses arising in focal site.

b. Side effects: drowsiness, ataxia, nystagmus.

7. Carbamazepine (Tegretol).

a. Inhibits nerve impulses by limiting influx of sodium ions across cell membranes.

b. Give with meals; monitor for side effects—diplopia, blurred vision, ataxia, vomiting, leukopenia.

8. Clonazepam (Clonopin).

a. Decreases frequency, duration and spread of discharge in minor motor seizures (absence, akinetic, myoclonic seizures).

b. Side effects: lethargy, ataxia, vertigo thrombocytopenia—monitor CBC.

D. Promote physical and emotional health.

1. Establish regular routines for eating, sleeping and physical activity.

2. Avoid alcohol, stress and excessive fatigue.

3. Foster self-esteem and promote self-confidence.

4. Contact Epilepsy Foundation of America.

E. Status epilepticus—a seizure that lasts longer than 4 minutes or successive seizures without regaining consciousness.

1. A potential complication with all seizures—a neurological emergency with generalized tonic-clonic seizures.

2. Cause may be sudden withdrawal from medication, infection, head trauma, metabolic disorders, alcohol withdrawal.

3. Management includes maintaining airway, notifying physician, administering oxygen and IV medication: Valium, Dilantin, phenobarbital.

TRAUMA

Head Injury

Definition: A trauma to the skull resulting in varying degrees of injury to the brain by compression, tension, and/or shearing force.

Characteristics

A. Causes.

1. Auto accidents—acceleration/deceleration.

2. Falls, assaults, missiles, blunt objects.

B. Concussion—violent jarring of brain within skull; temporary loss of consciousness.

C. Contusion—bruising, injury of brain.
1. Acceleration—slower moving contents of cranium strike bony prominences or dura (coup).
2. Deceleration—moving head strikes fixed object and brain rebounds, striking opposite side of cranium (contrecoup).

D. Fracture—linear, depressed, compound, comminuted.

E. Hematoma.
1. Epidural—most serious; hematoma between dura and skull from tear in meningeal artery; forms rapidly.
2. Subdural—under dura due to tears in veins crossing subdural space; forms slowly.

F. Subarachnoid hemorrhage—bleeding directly into brain, ventricles or subarachnoid space.
1. Monitor symptoms suggestive of complications.
   a. Sudden onset: headache, nausea, vomiting.
   b. Change in LOC, nuchal rigidity.
   c. Change in vital signs.
2. Interventions.
   a. Keep BP within normal limits—administer drugs as ordered.
   b. Administer phenobarbital to control seizures; codeine for pain, corticosteroids for edema, fibrinolytic inhibitor (Amicar) to minimize risk of rebleed.
   c. Maintain bedrest, prevent exertion, keep room quiet and dark.
   d. Prevent straining, administer laxatives and stool softeners.
   e. Avoid stimulants like coffee, caffeine.

G. Intracerebral hemorrhage—usually multiple hemorrhages around contused area.

Assessment

A. Assess for level of consciousness, unconsciousness, or confusion.

B. Check for headache, nausea, vomiting.

C. Observe for pupillary changes—epsilateral dilated pupil.

D. Monitor changes in vital signs, reflecting increased intracranial pressure or shock.

E. Observe for vasomotor or sensory losses.

F. Assess for rhinorrhea, otorrhea, nuchal rigidity.

G. Identify any overt scalp or skull trauma.

Implementation

A. Primary nursing objective is to recognize, prevent, and treat complications.

B. Maintain adequate respiratory exchange—increased CO_2 levels increase cerebral edema.

C. Treat cerebral edema and increased intracranial pressure.
1. Awaken client as completely as possible for assessment.
2. See section on increased ICP.

D. Monitor temperature.

E. Control pain and restlessness.
1. Avoid morphine, a respiratory depressant that might increase ICP.
2. Use codeine or other mild, safe analgesic.

F. Monitor and treat seizure activity.

G. Observe for complications.
1. Shock—significant cause of death.
2. Cranial nerve paralysis.
3. Rhinorrhea (fracture ethmoid bone) and otorrhea (temporal).
   a. Check discharge—bloody spot surrounded by pale ring; positive testtape reaction for sugar.
   b. Do not attempt to clean nose or ears.
   c. Do not suction nose.
   d. Instruct client not to blow nose.
4. Ear—drainage of CSF from the ear indicates damage to the base of the brain and a danger of meningitis.
   a. Inspect ear for drainage of CSF.
   b. Loosely cover ear with sterile, dry dressing.

H. Prevent infection.
1. High risk of meningitis, abcess, osteomyelitis, particularly in presence of rhinorrhea, otorrhea.
2. Maintain strict asepsis.

I. Prevent complications of immobility.

J. Establish individualized rehabilitation program.

Spinal Cord Injury

Definition: Partial or complete disruption of nerve tracts and neurons resulting in paralysis, sensory loss, altered reflex activity, and autonomic nervous system dysfunction.

Characteristics

A. Trauma associated with cord damage is usually related to vertebra fracture resulting from severe hyperflexion, extension, or rotation.

B. Common traumas.

1. Automobile and motorcycle accidents.
2. Sports and industrial injuries.
3. Falls and crushing injuries, or stab wounds.
C. Other conditions associated with spinal cord pathology.
   1. Infections, tumors.
   2. Disruption of blood supply to cord—thrombus.
   3. Degenerative diseases.
   4. Congenital or acquired anomalies—spina bifida, myelomeningocele.
D. Improper handling and transport may result in extension of cord damage.
E. Vascular disruption, biochemical changes, and direct tissue damage cause pathology associated with trauma.
   1. Inflammatory process leads to edema and neuronal dysfunction.
   2. Ischemia and hypoxia due to vasoconstriction, edema, and hemorrhage.
   3. Hypoxia of gray matter stimulates release of catecholamines which increases hemorrhage and necrosis.

Assessment

A. Assess level of injury. The last cord segment in which normal motor, sensory, and reflex can be demonstrated is labeled level of injury, i.e., "C_5 level of injury" means neurofunction is intact for C_5 but not C_6.
B. Evaluate systems affected.
   1. Spinal shock—absence of reflexes slightly above and completely below level of lesion.
      a. Temporary condition: lasts days to months.
      b. Initial flaccid paralysis, absent reflexes, loss of sensation, loss of urinary and bowel retention, hypotension (especially positional).
   2. Degree of sensory, motor, and reflex loss depends upon severity of cord damage.
   3. Respiratory insufficiency or failures occur in injuries above C_4 due to lack of diaphragm innervation.
C. Identify classification of cord involvement.
   1. Functional deficiencies.
      a. Quadriplegia (tetraplegia)—all four extremities functionally involved—cervical injuries (C_1 through C_8).
      b. Paraplegia—both lower extremities functionally involved—thoracic-lumbar region (T_1 through L_4).
   2. Partial or complete cord damage.
      a. Complete cord transection.
         (1) All voluntary motor activity below injury is permanently lost.
         (2) All sensation dependent on ascending pathway of segment is lost.
         (3) Reflexes may return if blood supply to cord below injury is intact.
      b. Incomplete injuries.
         (1) Motor and sensory loss varies and is dependent on degree of incompleteness.
         (2) Extent of reflex dysfunction dependent on location of neurological deficit.
      c. Central cord syndrome—leg function returns, arm function does not, as damage has occurred to peripheral cord which innervates arms.
      d. Brown-Séquard's syndrome—one side of cord damaged resulting in paralysis on one side of body and loss of sensation on the other side.
   3. Upper and lower motor neuron damage.
      a. Upper motor neuron originates in cerebral cortex and terminates at anterior horn cell in cord.
         (1) Post-spinal shock reflexes return resulting in spastic paralysis. No reflex return if blood supply to cord is lost.
         (2) Spasms and reflexes used to retrain activities of daily living—bowel evacuation and bladder control.
      b. Lower motor neuron begins at anterior horn cell and becomes part of peripheral nerve to muscle, motor side of reflex arc.
         (1) Areflexia continues, flaccid paralysis.
         (2) Usually cauda equina injuries.
D. Assess for signs of autonomic dysreflexia.
   1. Absence of sweating below lesion.
   2. Paroxysmal hypertension.
   3. Fluctuations in temperature.
   4. Neurogenic bowel and bladder.
   5. Paralytic ileus.

Implementation

A. Complete a head-to-toe neurological examination to determine motor, sensory, and reflex loss due to spinal cord injury.
B. Provide emergency care—suspect spinal cord injury if neurological deficits present in extremities.
   1. Immobilize entire body, especially head and neck; do not flex head.
   2. Transport log fashion with sufficient help.

3. Maintain open airway and adequate ventilation—high cervical injuries can cause complete paralysis of muscles for breathing; observe for signs of respiratory failure.

C. Immobilize client, as ordered, to allow fracture healing and prevent further injury.
1. Stryker frame permits change of position between prone and supine.
   a. Maintain optimal body alignment.
   b. Place client in center of frame without flexing or twisting.
   c. Position arm boards, footboards, canvas.
   d. Turn; reassure client while turning.
   e. Free all tubings; secure bolts and straps.
2. Regular hospital beds used in many rehabilitation centers.
3. Halotraction with body cast allows early mobilization.
4. Soft and hard collars and back braces used about six weeks post-injury.
5. Maintain skeletal traction if part of treatment.
   a. Cervical tongs for hyperextension (Crutchfield, Gardner-Wells, Vinke).
      (1) Apply traction to vertebral column by attaching weights to pair of tongs.
      (2) Insert tongs into outer layer of parietal area of skull.
   b. Facilitates moving and turning of client while maintaining spine immobilization.
   c. Observe site of insertion for redness or drainage, alignment and position of traction, and pressure areas.

D. Complete frequent neurological assessment: note changes in muscle tone, motor movement, sensation, bladder and bowel function, presence or absence of sweating, temperature, and reflexes.

E. Monitor for autonomic nervous system disturbances.
1. Heart, lung, and bowel sounds for complications, such as embolus, ileus.
2. Temperature fluctuations—unable to adapt to environmental changes or infection-related.
   a. Excessive perspiration causes dehydration.
   b. Absence of perspiration leads to hyperthermia.

F. Prevent postural hypotension and syncope, which occur when head is elevated.
1. Apply ace bandage or teds.
2. Administer ephedrine p.o. one-half hour before client is to get up.

G. Manage autonomic hyperreflexia (or dysreflexia).
1. Signs and symptoms: extreme hypertension, flushing, bradycardia, headache (usually occipital), sweating, diplopia, convulsions.
2. Provide immediate treatment.
   a. Catheterize bladder or manually evacuate bowel.
   b. May administer parasympatholytic (Banthine) or ganglionic blocking agent (Hyperstat, Apresoline).
   c. If client is lying down and fracture status permits, immediately elevate the head of bed or elevate client to sitting position.
3. Control factors that precipitate episode to prevent recurrence.
   a. Set up regular bowel and bladder programs.
   b. Apply nupercainal ointment prior to rectal stimulation.
   c. Administer alpha-adrenergic blocking agents (phenoxybenzamine) b.i.d.

H. Prevent infections.
1. Administer prophylactic antibiotics while client is on catheterizations.
2. Evaluate elevated temperatures for urinary or respiratory infection.

I. Prevent circulatory complications.
1. Turn entire body every two hours. Give range-of-motion exercises to extremities.
2. Apply ace bandages and teds to legs.
3. Monitor for edema, thrombus, and emboli; provide prompt anticoagulant therapy if needed.
4. Do not overhydrate based on blood pressure (normal BP is 100/60 or below).

J. Maintain optimal positioning.
1. Logroll with firm support to head, neck, spine, and limbs; do not allow neck flexion.
2. Maintain good body alignment with 10 degree flexion of knees, heels off mattress or canvas, and feet in firm dorsiflexion.
3. During convalescence, provide cervical collar, tilt table, wheelchair, braces, parallel bars.

K. Promote optimal physical activity.
1. Provide physical therapy, exercises, range of motion.
2. Encourage independent activity.
3. Provide extensive program of rehabilitation and self-care.

L. Maintain integrity of the skin.
1. Turn client every two hours and check skin.

2. Do not administer IM medication below the level of the lesion due to impaired circulation and potential skin breakdown.
3. Provide elastic stockings to improve circulation in legs.
4. Later, instruct client how to look for and prevent injury; reinforce the necessity for self-care.
5. Provide prompt treatment of pressure areas.

M. Promote adequate nutrition, fluid, and electrolyte balance.
1. Provide diet adequate in protein, vitamins, calories, and bulk; limit milk.
2. Avoid citrus juices which alkalize the urine; give cranberry juice and vitamin C tabs to acidify urine.
3. Avoid gas-forming foods.
4. Monitor calcium, electrolyte, and hemoglobin.
5. Restrict fluids if client is on intermittent catheterization.

N. Establish optimal bladder function.
1. During spinal shock, bladder is atonic with urinary retention; danger of overdistention, stretching.
2. Possible reactions.
   a. Hypotonic, retention with overflow—sacral reflex center injury (lower motor neuron).
   b. Hypertonic, sudden reflex voiding—injury above sacral area (upper motor neuron).
3. Check for bladder distention, voiding, incontinence, and symptoms of infection.
4. Provide aseptic intermittent catheterizations—prophylactic antimicrobials (nitrofurantoin).
5. Prevent urinary tract infection, calculi.
   a. Monitor urinary residuals.
   b. Take periodic bladder and kidney function studies—IVP, cystogram.
6. Initiate bladder retraining.
   a. Hypertonic—sensation of full bladder, trigger areas, regulation of fluid intake.
   b. Hypotonic—manual expression of urine (Credé).
7. Administer medications to treat incontinence.
   a. Hypertonic—propantheline bromide, diazepam.
   b. Hypotonic—bethanechol chloride.

O. Establish optimal bowel function.
1. Incontinence and paralytic ileus occur with spinal shock; later, incontinence, constipation, impaction.
2. For severe distention, administer neostigmine methylsulfate and insert rectal tube, which decompresses intestinal tract.
3. Give enema only if necessary. Excessive amount of fluid distends bowel. Manual evacuation is preferred.
4. Initiate bowel retraining.
   a. Record bowel habits before and after injury.
   b. Provide well-balanced diet with bulky foods.
   c. Encourage fluid intake.
   d. Provide stool softeners, bulk producers, mild laxative.
   e. Encourage the development of muscle tone.
   f. Administer suppository (glycerin or Dulcolax) as indicated.
   g. Emphasize importance of a regular, consistent routine.

P. Provide psychological support to client and family.
1. Support client and family through grief process.
2. Promote sustained therapeutic relationships.
3. Provide diversionary activities, socialization.
4. Promote independence; teach client to problem-solve.
5. Give encouragement and reassurance but never false hope.
6. Encourage family involvement in care.
7. Provide sexual counseling if needed.
   a. Client should be aware of his or her sexual abilities postinjury.
   b. Role perception may need expansion.
8. During rehabilitation stage, provide employment counseling if needed.

Q. Establish individualized rehabilitation program for client.
1. Based on level of injury.
2. Determined by willingness of client to adapt to new body image.
3. Availability of family and community support services.

INFECTIOUS PROCESSES

Brain Abscess

Definition: Infectious process resulting in an encapsulated collection of pus usually found in the temporal lobe, frontal lobe, or cerebellum.

Assessment

A. Monitor for increased temperature unless abscess

walled off, in which case temperature can be sub-normal.
B. Check for headache, anorexia, malaise, vomiting.
C. Evaluate neurological deficits relative to area involved (focal seizures, blurred vision, etc.).
D. Monitor for signs of increased intracranial pressure.
E. Observe for weight loss.

Implementation

A. Observe neurological signs for alterations.
B. Decrease temperature.
   1. Sponge bath.
   2. Antipyretic drugs (Tylenol).
   3. Cooling blanket.
C. Administer appropriate antibiotics for causative agent.
D. Prepare client and family for surgical intervention.
E. Provide appropriate postoperative care.

Meningitis

Definition: An acute infection of the pia-arachnoid membrane.

Characteristics

A. Usually the result of another bacterial infection.
B. Organisms: meningococcus, staphylococcus, streptococcus, pneumococcus, Haemophilus influenzae, tubercle bacillus, Escherichia coli.
C. Inflammatory reaction with exudate in pia-arachnoid.
D. Results in a degeneration of nerve cells.
E. Congestion of adjacent brain tissue.

Assessment

A. Assess for painful stiff neck—nuchal rigidity, Kernig's and Brudzinski's signs, deep tendon knee reflexes.
B. Observe for severe headache, photophobia, vomiting.
C. Check for fever, chills, malaise.
D. Irritability, stupor, coma, possible seizures.

Implementation

A. Maintain open airway.
B. Treat the infective organism—antimicrobial therapy by intravenous route for two weeks.
C. Isolate for 48 hours after antibiotic therapy is initiated.
D. Treat increased intracranial pressure or seizures.

E. Control body temperature.
F. Provide adequate fluid and electrolyte balance.
G. Provide bedrest and a quiet environment; sedate if needed.
H. Prevent complications of immobility.
I. Relieve headache with acetaminophen.

Encephalitis

Definition: Severe inflammation of the brain caused by arboviruses or enteroviruses.

Assessment

A. Check for fever, headache, vomiting.
B. Evaluate for signs of meningeal irritation.
C. Evaluate neuronal damage, drowsiness, coma, paralysis, ataxia.

Implementation

A. Monitor vital signs frequently.
B. Monitor neurological signs for alterations in client's condition.
C. Administer anticonvulsant medications such as phenytoin.
D. Administer glucocorticoids to reduce cerebral edema.
E. Administer sedatives to relieve restlessness.
F. Manage fluid and electrolyte balance to prevent fluid overload and dehydration.
G. Position client to maintain patent airway and prevent contractures. Provide range-of-motion exercises.
H. Promote adequate nutrition through tube feedings, and parenteral hyperalimentation if necessary.
I. Provide hygenic care, i.e., skin care, oral care, and perineal care.
J. Provide safety measures if client confused.

ALTERED BLOOD SUPPLY TO BRAIN

Cerebral Vascular Accident (CVA)

Definition: A sudden focal neurological deficit due to cerebral vascular disease; the most common cause of brain disturbances.

Characteristics

A. Causes.
   1. Thrombosis.
   2. Embolism.

3. Hemorrhage (extradural, subdural, subarachnoid or intracerebral).

B. Risk factors.
1. Atherosclerosis.
2. Hypertension.
3. Anticoagulation therapy.
4. Cardiac valvular disease.
5. Synthetic valve and organ replacement.
6. Atrial arrhythmias.
7. Diabetes.

C. Interruption of blood supply to brain via carotid and vertebral-basilar arteries—causes cerebral anoxia.

D. Cerebral anoxia longer than ten minutes to a localized area of brain—causes cerebral infarction (irreversible changes).

E. Surrounding edema and congestion causes further dysfunction.

F. Lesion in cerebral hemisphere (motor cortex, internal capsule, basal ganglia)—results in manifestations on the contralateral side.

G. Permanent disability unknown until edema subsides. Order in which function may return: facial, swallowing, lower limbs, speech, arms.

Assessment

A. Evaluate transient ischemic attack (TIA), a precursor symptom or warning of impending CVA.
1. Rapid onset and short duration (30 minutes to 24 hours); by definition must be resolved within this time period. No permanent neurological deficit.
2. Most common symptoms: vision loss, diplopia, contralateral hemiparesis, aphasia, confusion, slurred speech and vertigo.

B. Carotid endarterectomy is surgical procedure for carotid stenosis—often done following TIA or presence of bruit indicating stenosis.
1. Procedure removes atherosclerotic plaque from arterial wall.
2. Monitor closely first 24 hours for cerebral iscemia or thrombosis or intolerance from carotid clamping.

C. Observe for generalized signs: headache; hypertension; changes in level of consciousness, convulsions; vomiting, nuchal rigidity, slow bounding pulse, Cheyne-Stokes respirations.

D. Observe for focal signs—upper motor lesion in motor cortex, and pyramidal tracts: hemiparesis, hemiplegia, central facial paralysis, language disorders, cranial dysfunction, conjugate deviation eyes toward lesion, flaccid hyporeflexia (later, spastic hyperreflexia).

E. Evaluate residual manifestations.
1. Lesion left hemisphere.
   a. Usually dominant, containing speech center; right hemiplegia; aphasia, expressive and/or receptive.
   b. Behavior is slow, cautious, disorganized.
2. Lesion right hemisphere.
   a. Left hemiplegia; spatial-perceptual deficits.
   b. Behavior is impulsive, quick; unaware of deficits; poor judge of abilities, limitations; neglect of paralyzed side.
3. General.
   a. Memory deficits; reduced memory span; emotional lability.
   b. Visual deficits such as homonomous hemianopia (loss of half of each visual field).
   c. Apraxia (can move but unable to use body part for specific purpose).

F. Evaluate client for rehabilitative program.

Implementation

A. Initial nursing objective is to support life and prevent complications.

B. Give oxygen as needed. Begin at 6 1/min. unless client has COPD.

C. Maintain patent airway and ventilation—elevate head of bed 20 degrees unless shock is present.

D. Monitor clinical status to prevent complications.
1. Neurological.
   a. Include assessment of recurrent CVA, increased intracranial pressure, bulbar involvement, hyperthermia.
   b. Continued coma—negative prognostic sign.
2. Cardiovascular—shock and arrhythmias, hypertension.
3. Lungs—pulmonary emboli.

E. Maintain optimal positioning.
1. During acute stages, quiet environment and minimal handling to prevent further bleeding.
2. Upper motor lesion—spastic paralysis, flexion deformities, external rotation of hip.
3. Positioning schedule—two hours on unaffected side; twenty minutes on affected side; thirty minutes prone, b.i.d.-t.i.d.
4. Complications common with hemiplegia—frozen shoulder, footdrop.

F. Maintain skin integrity: turn and provide skin care every two hours.

G. Maintain personal hygiene: encourage self-help.

H. Promote adequate nutrition, fluid, and electrolyte balance.
   1. Encourage self-feeding.
   2. Food should be placed in unparalyzed side of mouth.
   3. Tube feeding or gastrostomy feeding may be necessary.
I. Administer tube feeding.
J. Promote elimination.
   1. Bladder control may be regained within three to five days.
   2. Retention either may not be part of treatment regime.
   3. Offer urinal or bedpan every two hours day and night.
K. Provide emotional support.
   1. Behavior changes as consciousness is regained—loss of memory, emotional lability, confusion, language disorders.
   2. Reorient, reassure, and establish means of communication.
L. Promote rehabilitation to maximal functioning.
   1. Comprehensive program—begin during acute phase and follow through convalescence.
   2. Guidelines to assist client with left hemisphere lesion.
      a. Do not underestimate ability to learn.
      b. Assess ability to understand speech.
      c. Act out, pantomime communication; use client's terms to communicate; speak in normal tone of voice.
      d. Divide tasks into simple steps; give frequent feedback.
   3. Guidelines to assist client with right hemisphere lesion.
      a. Do not overestimate abilities.
      b. Use verbal cues as demonstrations; pantomimes may confuse.
      c. Use slow, minimal movements and avoid clutter around client.
      d. Divide tasks into simple steps; elicit return demonstration of skills.
      e. Promote awareness of body and environment on affected side.

Cerebral Aneurysm

Definition: A dilation of the walls of a weakened cerebral artery leading to rupture from arteriosclerosis or trauma.

Assessment
A. Observe eyes for diplopia, pain, blurred vision, or ptosis.
B. Evaluate for hemiparesis, nuchal rigidity.
C. Check for headache, tinnitus, nausea.
D. Observe for irritability, seizure activity.

Implementation
A. Establish and maintain a patent airway.
B. Administer oxygen at 6 l/min. unless client has COPD.
C. Place client on bedrest in semi-Fowler's or side lying position.
D. Turn and deep breathe client every two hours.
E. Suction only with specific order.
F. Provide darkened room without stimulation, i.e., limit visitors and lengthy discussions.
G. Avoid strenuous activity; provide range-of-motion exercises.
H. Provide diet low in stimulants such as caffeine. Restrict fluid intake to prevent increased intracranial pressure.
I. Monitor intake and output.
J. Monitor vital signs for hypertension or cardiac irregularities. Do not take rectal temperature due to vagal stimulation leading to cardiac arrest.
K. Observe for complications indicating rebleeding, clot formation, or increased size of aneurysm.

DEGENERATIVE DISORDERS

Multiple Sclerosis

Definition: A chronic, slowly progressive, noncontagious, degenerative disease of the CNS. Characterized by demyelinization of the neurons, this disease affects the brain and spinal cord.

Characteristics
A. Definite cause unknown; may be auto-immune, associated with a deficit in the T-lymphocytes.
B. Precipitating factors: pregnancy, fatigue, stress, infection, and trauma.
C. Incidence is greater in colder climate, equal in the sexes, and usually occurs between ages twenty to forty years.
D. Demyelinization of nerve fibers occurs within long conducting pathways of spinal cord and brain.

E. Lesions (plaques) are irregularly scattered—disseminated in pyramidal tract, posterior column, and ventricle of brain.

F. Destruction of myelin sheath creates patches of sclerotic tissue, degeneration of the nerve fiber, and disturbance in conduction of sensory and motor impulses.

G. Initially, the disease is characterized by periods of remission with exacerbation and variable manifestations, followed by irreversible dysfunction.

H. Clinical course may extend over 10 to 20 years.

I. Diagnostic tests; abnormal EEG, LP indicating increased gamma globulin but normal serum levels.

Assessment

A. Evaluate clinical manifestations—variable, depending on area of involvement: sensory fibers, motor fibers, brainstem, cerebellum, internal capsule.

B. Initial signs and symptoms: ataxia, diplopia, impaired speech.

C. Observe for weakness, paralysis, incoordination, intention tremor, spasticity, numbness, tingling, analgesia, anesthesia, loss of position sense.

D. Evaluate bladder/bowel retention or incontinence.

E. Observe for impaired vision (nystagmus), dysphagia.

F. Check client's emotional instability, impaired judgment.

G. Observe for Charcot's triad—nystagmus, intention tremor, scanning speech.

Implementation

A. Avoid precipitation of exacerbations.
1. Avoid fatigue, stress, infection, overheating, chilling.
2. Establish regular program of exercise and rest.
3. Provide a balanced diet, low in fat, rich in linoleic acid.

B. Administer and assess effects of medications.
1. Steroids hasten remission. Prednisone is used for short-term therapy.
2. Chlordiazepoxide for mood swings.
3. Baclofen or dantrolene for spasticity.
4. Bethanechol to relieve urinary retention, or oxybutynin to increase bladder capacity.

C. Promote optimal activity.
1. Moderation in activity with rest periods.
2. Physical and speech therapy.
3. Diversionary activities, hobbies.
4. During exacerbation, client is usually put on bed rest.

D. Promote safety.
1. Sensory loss—regulate bath water; caution with heating pads; inspect skin for lesions.
2. Motor loss—avoid waxed floors, throw rugs; provide rails and walker.
3. Diplopia—eye patch.

E. Promote regular elimination—bladder/bowel training programs.

F. Provide education and emotional support to client and family.
1. Encourage independence and realistic goals; assess personality and behavior changes; observe for signs of depression.
2. Provide instruction and assistive devices; provide information about services of the National Multiple Sclerosis Society.

G. Assess and prevent potential complications.
1. Most common: urinary tract infection, calculi, decubitus ulcers.
2. Common cause of death: respiratory tract infection, urinary tract infection.
3. Contractures, pain due to spasticity, metabolic or nutritional disorders, regurgitation, depression.

Myasthenia Gravis

Definition: A neuromuscular disease characterized by marked weakness and abnormal fatigue of voluntary muscles.

Characteristics

A. Cause unknown; question autoimmune reaction.

B. Clients with myasthenia have a high incidence of thymus abnormalities and frequently have systemic lupus erythematosus.

C. Basic pathology is a defect in transmission of nerve impulses at the myoneural junction, the junction of motor neuron with muscle.

D. Normally, acetylcholine is stored in synaptic vesicle of motor neurons to skeletal muscles. Defect may be due to:
1. Deficiency in acetylcholine/excess acetylcholinesterase.
2. Defective motor-end plate and/or nerve terminals.
3. Decreased sensitivity to acetylcholine.

E. Muscles supplied by bulbar nuclei (cranial nerves) are commonly involved.

F. Muscle involvement usually progresses from ocular to oropharyngeal, facial, proximal muscles, respiratory muscles.

G. Generally there is no muscle atrophy or degeneration; there may be periods of exacerbations and remissions.

H. Symptoms are related to progressive weakness and fatigue of muscles when used; muscles generally strongest in the morning.

Assessment

A. Observe eyes, which are affected first: ptosis, diplopia, and eye squint.

B. Assess for impaired speech; dysphagia; drooping facies; difficulty chewing, closing mouth, or smiling; breathing difficulty and hoarse voice.

C. Observe for respiratory paralysis and failure.

D. Assess for severe weakness during Tensilon test.

Implementation

A. Assist with disease diagnosis.
   1. Have Tensilon available for physician to inject.
   2. Assess results of Tensilon injections.
      a. Positive for myasthenia—improvement in muscle strength.
      b. Negative—no improvement or even deterioration.

B. Administer medications as ordered.
   1. Anticholinesterase drugs increase levels of acetylcholine at myoneural junction.
      a. Neostigmine, pyridostigmine, ambenonium—main difference is duration of effect.
      b. Edrophonium (Tensilon)—rapid, brief-acting anticholinesterase for testing purposes.
      c. Monitor side effects.
         (1) Related to effects of increased acetylcholine in parasympathetic nervous system: sweating, excessive salivation, nausea, diarrhea, abdominal cramps; possibly bradycardia or hypotension.
         (2) Excessive doses lead to cholinergic crisis—atropine given as cholinergic blocker.
      d. Nursing measures.
         (1) Give medication exactly on time, thirty minutes before meals.
         (2) Give medication with milk and crackers to reduce gastrointestinal upset.
         (3) Observe therapeutic or any toxic effects; monitor and record muscle strength and vital capacity.
   2. Steroids.
      a. Suppress immune response.
      b. Usually the last resort after anticholinesterase and thymectomy.

3. The following drugs must be avoided.
   a. Steptomycin, kanamycin, neomycin, gentamicin—block neuromuscular transmission.
   b. Ether, quinidine, morphine, curare, procainamide, innovar, sedatives—aggravate weakness of myasthenia.

C. Monitor client's condition for complications.
   1. Vital signs.
   2. Respirations: depth, rate, vital capacity, ability to deep breathe and cough.
   3. Swallowing: ability to eat and handle secretions.
   4. Muscle strength.
   5. Speech; provide method of communication if client unable to talk.
   6. Bowel and bladder function.
   7. Psychological status.

D. Promote optimal activity.
   1. Plan short periods of activity and long periods of rest.
   2. Time activity to coincide with maximal muscle strength.
   3. Encourage normal activities of daily living.
   4. Encourage diversionary activities.

E. Provide education and emotional support for client and family.
   1. Give reassurance and facts about the disease, medications and treatment regime, importance of adhering to medication schedule, difference between myasthenic/cholinergic crisis, and emergency care.
   2. Instruct client to avoid infection, stress, fatigue, and over-the-counter drugs.
   3. Instruct client to wear identification medal and carry emergency card.
   4. Provide information about services of Myasthenia Gravis Foundation.

F. Prevent myasthenic or cholinergic crisis.
   1. Myasthenic crisis.
      a. Acute exacerbation of disease may be due to rapid, unrecognized progression of disease; failure of medication; infection; or fatigue or stress.
      b. Myasthenic symptoms—weakness, dyspnea, dysphagia, restlessness, difficulty speaking.
   2. Cholinergic crisis.
      a. Cholinergic paralysis with sustained depolarization of motor-end plates is due to over-medication with anticholinesterase.

b. Symptoms similar to myasthenic state—restlessness, weakness, dysphagia, dyspnea.

c. Cholinergic symptoms—fasciculations, abdominal cramps, diarrhea, nausea, vomiting, salivation, sweating, increased bronchial secretion.

3. Tensilon test to differentiate crises, as symptoms are similar.

a. Give Tensilon; if strength improves, it is symptomatic of myasthenic crisis and the client needs more medication; if weakness is more severe, it is symptomatic of cholinergic crisis and overdose has occurred.

b. Be prepared for emergency with atropine, suction, and other emergency equipment for respiratory arrest.

4. Crisis with respiratory insufficiency—client cannot swallow secretions and may aspirate.

a. Maintain bed rest.

b. May require endotracheal or tracheostomy tube to assist with ventilation.

c. Monitor vital capacity, blood gases.

d. Give atropine and may hold anticholinesterase (cholinergic).

e. Begin anticholinesterase (myasthenic).

G. Provide appropriate nursing measures in the event of thymectomy surgery.

Parkinson's Disease

Definition: A degenerative disease resulting in dysfunction of the extrapyramidal system.

Characteristics

A. Possible causes: atherosclerosis, drug induced, postencephalitis, idiopathic.

B. Degeneration of basal ganglia due to depleted concentration of dopamine.

C. Depletion of dopamine correlated with degeneration of substantia nigra (midbrain structures which are closely related functionally to basal ganglia).

D. Loss of inhibitory modulation of dopamine to counterbalance cholinergic system and interruption of balance-coordinating extrapyramidal system.

E. Slowly progressive disease with high incidence of crippling disability; mental deterioration occurs very late.

Assessment

A. Assess stage of disease—five stages: unilateral, bilateral, impaired balance, fully developed severe disease, confinement to bed or wheelchair.

B. Identify presence of initial symptoms.

1. Slowing of all movements.
2. Aching shoulders and arms.
3. Monotonous and indistinct speech.
4. Writing becomes progressively smaller.

C. Evaluate major symptoms.

1. Tremor at rest, especially in hands and fingers (pill-rolling).

a. Increases when stressed or fatigued.

b. May decrease with purposeful activity or sleep.

2. Rigidity—blank facial expression (mask-like).

a. Drooling, difficulty swallowing or speaking.

b. Short, shuffling steps with stooped posture.

c. Propulsive gait.

d. Immobility of muscles in flexed position, creating jerky cogwheel motions.

e. Loss of coordinated and associated automatic movement and balance.

3. Bradykinesia—abnormal slowness and reduction in automatic movement; sluggishness of responses.

Implementation

A. Administer and monitor drugs.

1. Amantadine: used to treat clients with mild symptoms but no disability; side effects uncommon with usual dose.

2. Anticholinergic drugs: most effective is Ethopropazine; used to treat tremors and rigidity, and inhibit action of acetylcholine; side effects include dry mouth, dry skin, blurring vision, urinary retention, and tachycardia.

3. Levodopa (converted in body to dopamine).

a. Reduces akinesia, tremor, and rigidity.

b. Passes through blood-brain barrier.

c. Effectiveness may decline after 2–3 years.

d. Side effects.

(1) Anorexia, nausea, and vomiting (administer drug with meals or snack; avoid coffee, which seems to increase nausea).

(2) Postural hypotension, dizziness, tachycardia, and arrhythmias (monitor vital signs; caution client to sit up or stand

up slowly; have client wear support stockings).

   e. Contraindicated in clients with closed-angle glaucoma, psychotic illness, and peptic ulcer disease.

4. Sinemet—combination of carbidopa and levodopa; has fewer side effects than levodopa.

5. Antihistamines: reduce tremor and anxiety; side effect is drowsiness.

6. Antispasmodics (Artane, Kemadrin): improve rigidity but not tremor.

7. Bromocriptine (drug often used to replace levodopa when it loses effectiveness).

   a. Acts on dopamine receptors.

   b. Side effects: anorexia, nausea, vomiting, constipation, postural hypotension, cardiac arrhythmias, headache.

   c. Contraindicated in clients with mental illness, myocardial infarction, peptic ulcers, peripheral vascular disease.

B. Avoid the following drugs:

1. Phenothiazines, reserpine, pyridoxine, vitamin B_6: block desired action of levodopa.

2. Monamine oxidase inhibitors: precipitate hypertensive crisis.

3. Methyldopa: potentiate effects.

C. Maintain regular patterns of elimination.

1. Constipation is often a problem due to side effects of medications, reduced physical activity, muscle weakness, and excessive drooling.

2. Provide stool softeners, suppositories, mild cathartics.

D. Promote physical therapy and rehabilitation.

1. Provide preventive, corrective, and postural exercises.

2. Institute massage and stretching exercises, stressing extension of limbs.

3. Encourage daily ambulation—have client lift feet up when walking and avoid prolonged sitting.

4. Facilitate adaptation for activities of daily living and self-care; encourage rhythmic patterns to attain timing; foster independence; utilize special aids and devices.

5. Remove hazards that might cause falls.

E. Provide education and emotional support to client and family.

1. Remember, intellect is usually not impaired.

2. Assess changes in self-consciousness, body image, sexuality, moods.

3. Instruct client to avoid emotional stress and fatigue, which aggravate symptoms.

4. Instruct client to avoid foods high in vitamin B_6 and monamine oxidase.

F. Complete preoperative teaching for specific surgical intervention.

1. Stereotactic surgery to reduce tremor.

   a. Pallidotomy—lesion in globus pallidus.

   b. Thalamotomy—lesion in ventrolateral portion of thalamus.

2. Implantation of electrodes through burr holes into target area of brain; creation of lesion with high-frequency coagulation probe.

G. Provide appropriate nursing care following surgery.

CRANIAL AND PERIPHERAL NERVE DISORDERS

Trigeminal Neuralgia (Tic Douloureux)

Definition: A sensory disorder of the fifth cranial nerve, resulting in severe, recurrent paroxysms of sharp, facial pain along the distribution of the trigeminal nerve. Etiology and pathology are unknown; incidence is higher in older women.

Assessment

A. Assess for trigger points on the lips, gums, nose, or cheek.

B. Evaluate what stimulates symptom: cold breeze, washing, chewing, food/fluids of extreme temperatures.

C. Assess pain—limited to those areas innervated by the three branches of the fifth nerve.

MEDICAL IMPLICATIONS

A. Medical.

1. Massive doses of B_{12}.

2. Inhalation: 10–15 drops of trichloroethylene on cotton.

3. Anticonvulsants: Dilantin and Tegretol.

4. Alcohol injections to produce anesthesia of the nerve.

B. Surgical.

1. Peripheral—avulsion of supraorbital, infraorbital, or mandibular division.

2. Intracranial.

   a. Division of the sensory nerve root for permanent anesthesia.

b. Client may experience numbness, stiffness, or burning after surgery.

c. Microsurgery allows for selective sectioning of the fifth nerve.

d. Pain and temperature fibers are destroyed, and sensation of touch and corneal reflex are preserved.

Implementation

A. Observe and record characteristics of the attack.

B. Record method client uses to protect face.

C. Avoid extremes of heat or cold.

D. Provide small feedings of semi-liquid or soft food.

E. Administer medication and record effects.

F. Complete postoperative care.

1. Ophthalmic nerve—client needs protective eye care.

2. Maxillary and mandibular nerves.

a. Avoid hot food and liquids which might burn.

b. Instruct client to chew on unaffected side to prevent biting denervated portion.

c. Encourage client to visit dentist within six months.

d. Provide frequent oral hygiene to keep the mouth free of debris.

Bell's Palsy (Facial Paralysis)

Definition: A lower motor neuron lesion of the seventh cranial nerve, resulting in paralysis of one side of the face.

Characteristics

A. Etiology and pathology unknown.

B. May occur secondary to intracranial hemorrhage, tumor, meningitis, trauma.

C. Majority of clients recover in a few weeks without residual effects.

Assessment

A. Assess for flaccid muscles.

B. Check for shallow nasolabial fold.

C. Evaluate ability to raise eyebrows, frown, smile, close eyelids, or puff out cheeks.

D. Assess upward movement of eye when attempting to close eyelid.

E. Check for loss of taste in anterior tongue.

Implementation

A. Palliative measures comprise majority of interventions.

B. Monitor use of analgesics and steroids.

C. Provide face sling to prevent stretching of weakened muscles and loss of tone.

D. Promote active facial exercises to prevent loss of muscle tone and support of facial muscles.

E. Instruct to chew food on unaffected side.

F. Provide attractive, easy-to-eat foods to prevent anorexia and weight loss.

G. Provide special eye care to protect cornea and prevent keratitis.

H. Reassure and support.

Meniere's Disease

Definition: Dilatation of the endolymphatic system causing degeneration of the vestibular and cochlear hair cells.

Characteristics

A. Etiology is unknown.

B. Possible causes may include allergies, toxicity, localized ischemia, hemorrhage, viral infection, and edema.

C. Surgical division of vestibular portion of nerve or destruction of labyrinth may be necessary for severe cases.

Assessment

A. Assess for a chronic, recurrent process.

B. Assess for severe vertigo, nausea, vomiting, nystagmus, and loss of equilibrium.

C. Check impaired hearing and tinnitus.

D. Assess nutritional needs, which will depend on amount of nausea and vomiting.

Implementation

A. Maintain bedrest during acute attack.

1. Prevent injury during attack.

2. Provide side rails if necessary.

3. Keep room dark when photophobia present.

B. Provide drug therapy.

1. Vasodilators (nicotinic acid).

2. Diuretics, antihistamines (Benadryl).

3. Sedatives.

C. Monitor diet therapy.

1. Low sodium.

2. Lipoflavonoid vitamin supplement.

3. Restricted fluid intake.

D. Assist with ambulation if necessary.

Bulbar Palsy

Definition: A dysfunction of the ninth and tenth cranial nerves. The disease is secondary to tumors, infections, vascular, or degenerative diseases.

Assessment

A. Assess for glossopharyngeal paralysis: absent gag reflex; difficulty swallowing, increased salivation; anesthesia posterior palate and base of tongue.
B. Assess for vagal paralysis: difficulty with speech, breathing, and regurgitation.
C. Assess for possible aspiration.
D. Assess for breathing capability.
E. Check for difficulty in swallowing.
F. Evaluate state of depression and fear.

Implementation

A. Medical/surgical treatment is directed toward underlying cause.
B. Nursing care is directed toward prevention of complications.
C. Keep suction equipment at bedside.
D. Elevate head of bed.
E. Provide oral care.
F. Maintain open airway.
G. Keep emergency equipment available.
H. Avoid milk products and sticky carbohydrates.
I. Use small cup instead of straw for liquids.
J. Provide relationship therapy.
  1. Give client time to express fears and concerns.
  2. Provide consultation for depression if present.

Guillain-Barré Syndrome

Definition: An acute infectious neuronitis of cranial and peripheral nerves. Immune system overreacts to an infection destroying the myelin sheath.

Characteristics

A. Etiology is unknown.
B. Occurs at any age but increased incidence between thirty and fifty years of age.
C. Both sexes equally affected.
D. Presyndrome clients may report a mild upper respiratory infection or gastroenteritis.
E. Recovery is a slow process, taking 2 months to 2 years.
F. Diagnostic test results: CSF contains high protein, abnormal EEG.

Assessment

A. Assess for initial symptom of weakness of lower extremities.
B. Check gradual progressive weakness of upper extremities and facial muscles (24–72 hours); paresthesias may precede weakness.
C. Assess for respiratory failure that occurs in some clients.
D. Assess for cardiac arrhythmias, tachycardia.
E. Check sensory changes—usually minor, but in some cases severe impairment of sensory information occurs.

Implementation

A. No specific treatment available; supportive treatment includes monitoring for complications (respiratory, circulatory).
B. Carefully observe for respiratory paralysis and inability to handle secretions.
C. Provide chest physiotherapy and pulmonary toilet.
D. Maintain cardiovascular function.
  1. Monitor vital signs and cardiac rhythm.
  2. Vasopressors and volume replacement.
E. Prevent complications of immobility.
  1. Turn frequently.
  2. Provide skin care.
F. Provide appropriate diversion.
G. Reassure client, especially during paralysis period.
H. Previous treatment included corticosteroids; this is now considered controversial.

Amyotrophic Lateral Sclerosis (Lou Gehrig's Disease)

Definition: The most common motor neuron disease of muscular atrophy. It is a rapidly fatal, upper and lower motor neuron deficit affecting the limbs.

Characteristics

A. May result from several causes.
  1. Nutritional deficiency related to disturbance in enzyme metabolism.
  2. Vitamin E deficiency resulting in damage to cell membranes.
  3. Metabolic interference in nucleic acid production by nerve fibers.
  4. Autoimmune disorders.
B. Inherited as an autosomal dominant trait in 10 percent of cases.

C. Occurs after age 40; most common in men.

D. Is fatal within 3–10 years after onset.

E. Diagnostic tests: EMG and muscle biopsy; increased protein in CSF.

Assessment

A. Assess for atrophy and weakness of upper extremities.

B. Observe for difficulty swallowing and chewing.

C. Check respiratory excursion and breathing patterns.

D. Assess for impaired speech.

E. Assess for secondary depression.

Implementation

A. Assist with rehabilitation program to promote independence.

B. Monitor for complications.
   1. Prevent skin breakdown: reposition regularly, provide back care, and utilize pressure-relieving devices.
   2. Prevent aspiration of food or fluids: offer soft foods and keep patient in upright position during meals.
   3. Promote bowel and bladder function.

C. Provide emotional support.

SURGICAL INTERVENTION

General Preoperative Care

Assessment

A. Follow general assessment modalities for preoperative care.

B. Observe and record neurological symptoms relative to site of problem (clot, lesion, aneurysm, etc.); for example:
   1. Paralysis.
   2. Seizure foci.
   3. Pupillary response.

Implementation

A. Provide psychological support to client and family.

B. Prep and shave cranial hair (save hair).

C. Apply scrub solution to scalp, as ordered.

D. Avoid using enemas unless specifically ordered; the strain of defecation can lead to increased intracranial pressure.

E. Explain postoperative routine orders such as neurological checks and headaches.

F. Administer steroids or mecurial diuretics as ordered, to decrease cerebral edema.

G. Insert NG tube and/or Foley catheter, as ordered.

General Postoperative Care

Assessment

A. Follow general assessment modalities for postoperative clients.

B. Observe neurological signs.
   1. Evaluate level of consciousness.
      a. Orientation to time and place.
      b. Response to painful stimuli: pinch Achilles tendon or test with safety pin.
      c. Ability to follow verbal command.
   2. Evaluate pupil size and reactions to light.
      a. Are pupils equal, not constricted or dilated.
      b. Do pupils react to light.
      c. Do pupils react sluggishly or are they fixed.
   3. Evaluate strength and motion of extremities.
      a. Are handgrasps present and equal.
      b. Are handgrasps strong or weak.
      c. Can client move all extremities on command.
      d. Are movements purposeful or involuntary.
      e. Do the extremities have twitching, flaccid, or spastic movements (indicative of a neurological problem).

C. Observe vital signs.
   1. Keep client normothermic to decrease metabolic needs of the brain.
   2. Observe respirations for depth and rate to prevent respiratory acidosis from anoxia.
   3. Observe blood pressure and pulse for signs of shock or increased intracranial pressure.

D. Evaluate reflexes.
   1. Babinski—positive Babinski is elicited by stroking the lateral aspect of the sole of the foot, backward flexion of the great toe or spreading of other toes.
      a. Most important pathological reflex in neurology.
      b. If positive, indicative of pyramidal tract involvement (usually upper motor neuron lesion).
   2. Romberg—when client stands with feet close together, he or she falls off balance. If positive, may have cerebellar, proprioceptive, or vestibular difficulties.
   3. Kernig—client is lying down with thigh flexed at a right angle; extension of the leg upward

results in spasm of hamstring muscle, pain, and resistance to additional extension of leg at the knee (indicative of meningitis).

E. Observe for headache, double vision, nausea, or vomiting.

Implementation

A. Maintain patent airway.
  1. Oxygen deprivation and an increase of carbon dioxide may produce cerebral hypoxia and cause cerebral edema.
  2. Intubate if values indicate to be necessary:
    a. pO_2 below 80 mm Hg.
    b. pCO_2 above 50 mm Hg.
B. Suction if necessary, but not through nose without specific order.
C. Maintain adequate oxygenation and humidification.
D. Place client in semi-prone or semi-Fowler's position (or totally on side). Turn every two hours, side to side.
E. Maintain fluid and electrolytes.
  1. Do not give fluid by mouth to semiconscious or unconscious client.
  2. Weigh to determine fluid loss.
  3. Administer IV fluids slowly; overhydration leads to cerebral edema.
F. Record accurate intake and output.
G. Watch serial blood and urine samples; sodium regulation disturbances accompany head injuries.
H. Keep temperature down with cooling blanket if necessary. If temperature is down, the metabolic requirement of brain as well as oxygen requirements are less.
I. Take vital and neurological signs every fifteen to thirty minutes until stable.
J. Use seizure precautions. Administer anticonvulsants as ordered.
K. Provide hygienic care, including oral hygiene.
L. Observe dressing for unusual drainage (bleeding, cerebral spinal fluid).
M. Prevent straining with bowel movements.
N. Administer steroids and osmotic diuretics to decrease cerebral edema.
O. Observe for and treat postoperative complications.
  1. Increased intracranial pressure.
  2. Seizures.
  3. Hemorrhage.
  4. Wound infection.
  5. Brain abscess.
  6. Meningitis.

Precautions for Care of Neurosurgical Client

A. Do not lower head in Trendelenburg position or place in supine position.
B. Do not suction through nose without specific order.
C. Be careful when administering sedations and narcotics.
  1. Cannot evaluate neurological status.
  2. May cause respiratory embarrassment.
D. Do not give oral fluids unless client is fully awake.
E. Do not administer enemas or cathartics (may cause straining, therefore increasing intracranial pressure).
F. Do not place on operative side if large tumor or bone removed.

EYE AND EAR

Glaucoma

Definition: Abnormally increased intraocular pressure, which may produce serious visual defects.

Characteristics

A. Chronic open-angle glaucoma.
  1. Results from an overproduction or obstruction to the outflow of aqueous humor. Aqueous humor flows from the trabecular network, Schlemm's canal, or aqueous veins.
  2. Ninety percent of all glaucoma cases are of this type.
B. Chronic closed-angle glaucoma follows an untreated attack of acute closed-angle glaucoma.
C. Acute closed-angle (narrow-angle) glaucoma.
  1. Results from an obstruction to the outflow of aqueous humor.
  2. Causes of obstruction.
    a. A narrow angle between the anterior iris and the posterior corneal surface.
    b. Shallow anterior chambers.
    c. A thickened iris that causes angle closure upon pupil dilation.
    d. A bulging iris that presses on the trabecula to close the angle.
  3. Caused by trauma, drugs, or inflammation.

Assessment

A. Evaluate type of glaucoma.
  1. Chronic.
     a. Open angle—slow, progressive course.
     b. Closed-angle—gradual onset.
  2. Acute closed-angle—rapid onset.
B. Evaluate risk conditions: over forty years of age, diabetes, black client, hypertensive, familial history of glaucoma, and history of eye injury.
C. Identify results of Schiotz Tonometer Test (7 to 21 mm Hg is normal) and optic-disc cupping.
D. Assess chronic open-angle.
  1. Loss of peripheral vision and eventual loss of central vision.
  2. Mild aching in the eyes.
  3. Halos around lights.
E. Assess acute closed-angle glaucoma.
  1. Unilateral inflammation.
  2. Pain.
  3. Pressure over eye.
  4. Moderate pupil dilation, nonreactive to light.
  5. Cloudy cornea.
  6. Blurring and decreased visual acuity.
  7. Photophobia.
  8. Halos around light.
  9. Nausea and vomiting.
F. Assess chronic closed-angle glaucoma.
  1. Usually no symptoms.
  2. Halos around lights may occur.

Implementation

A. For chronic open-angle glaucoma.
  1. Decrease aqueous humor production through beta blockers, especially timolol maleate.
  2. Lower intraocular pressure with epinephrine or diuretics.
  3. Administer miotic eyedrops, such as pilocarpine, to facilitate the outflow of aqueous humor.
  4. When medication no longer controls intraocular pressure and peripheral vision is lost, prepare client for argon laser treatments.
     a. Trabeculoplasty—laser alters trabecular meshwork and facilitates aqueous humor drainage.
     b. Trabeculectomy—creates a new opening at limbus to allow drainage of aqueous humor.
B. For acute closed-angle glaucoma.
  1. Treat as a medical emergency problem.
  2. Administer drugs to lower intraocular pressure.

3. Prepare client for peripheral iridectomy.
   a. Allows aqueous humor to flow from posterior to anterior chamber.
   b. Administer ordered drugs: acetazolamide, mannitol, pilocarpine.
C. Provide postoperative care.
  1. Administer cycloplegic eyedrops to affected eye to relax the ciliary muscle and decrease inflammation.
  2. Encourage early ambulation.
  3. Observe unaffected eye for symptoms of acute closed-angle glaucoma if cycloplegic drops are given by mistake.

EYE SURGERY

Cataracts

Definition: Clouding or opacity of the lens that leads to blurring vision and eventual loss of sight.

Characteristics

A. Opacity is due to physical changes of the fibers or chemical changes in protein of the lens—most often caused by the slow degenerative changes of age.
B. Surgical procedure is usually based on individual needs; that is, how much the client can see out of the other eye.
  1. If any inflammation is present, surgery is not performed.
  2. Cataracts are removed under local anesthesia.
  3. Some simple cataracts are removed by use of alphachymotrypsin, which weakens the zonular fibers that hold the lens in position.
  4. Surgery is performed on one eye at a time.
C. Types of surgical extraction.
  1. Intracapsular—the lens is removed within its capsule through a small incision.
  2. Extracapsular—the lens is lifted out without removing the lens capsule.
  3. Phacoemulsification (ultrasonic)—the lens is broken up by ultrasonic vibrations and extracted via extracapsular route.
D. Intraocular lens implant at time of surgery is a common alternative to sight correction with glasses.

Implementation

A. Check that client understands preoperative instructions.
1. Client must be transported to and from hospital.
2. Client must have someone at home for assistance following surgery.
3. Client should shampoo hair before surgery.
4. Review instructions to decrease intraocular pressure (do not bend, cough, strain, or lift).

B. Administer prescribed preoperative medications.
1. Mydriatics (atropine sulfate, epinephrine HCl, cyclopentolate HCl)—note whether pupil dilates following drug instillation.
2. Antibiotics or topical anti-infective (Gentamicin)—prevention of infection.
3. Cycloplegics (Cyclogyl)—paralyzes ciliary muscles.
4. Narcotics (meperidine)—for pain relief.
5. Antiemetics (Compazine, Vistaril).

C. Provide postoperative care. Most procedures are done on outpatient basis.
1. Instruct client in postoperative drugs.
   a. Mydriatics (atropine sulfate)—2 to 6 weeks after surgery.
   b. Miotic agents (Pilocarpine HCl, carmylcholine) prescribed for certain types of lens implants.
   c. Steroids (prednisolone suspension) and antibiotic drops.
   d. Analgesics and antibiotics.
2. Instruct in ways to alleviate symptoms that could result in complications.
   a. Increased intraocular pressure may occur with nausea and vomiting; restlessness; coughing or sneezing; lifting more than 15 pounds; constipation.
   b. Observe for signs of infection: increasing redness, tearing, green drainage, or photophobia.
3. Instruct client to notify physician of sudden pain in operative eye—may be due to ruptured vessel or suture.
4. Apply dressing and shield at night to prevent injury to operative eye. Unoperative eye is usually left uncovered.
5. Instruct client to maintain low-Fowler's position the day of surgery and to turn only to unoperative side (as ordered).
6. Instruct client to avoid rapid movements and not to bend over—may be ambulatory first postoperative day.
7. Reinforce instructions on dressing changes and eye drops. (Client returns to physician's office first postoperative day for dressing to change).
8. Inform client that temporary glasses are prescribed 1–4 weeks postoperatively if lens is not implanted.

D. Assist client with specific adjustment problems.
1. Intraocular lens implant at time of surgery is very common.
   a. This lens provides means of focusing light on the retina—approximates human lens.
   b. If no implant, the eye cannot accommodate and glasses must be worn at all times.
   c. Mydriatic drops frequently used to prevent lens displacement.
2. Cataract glasses magnify—objects appear closer. Teach client to accommodate, judge distance, and climb stairs carefully.

Ophthalmic Drugs

A. Miotics: Pilocarpine HCl 1–4% solution; Carbamylcholine 1.5–3% solution.
1. Action is contraction of ciliary muscle which increases flow of aqueous humor.
2. Treatment for glaucoma and certain types of lens implants.
3. Side effects: headache, conjunctiva irritation, and inflammation.

B. Mydriatics: Atropine sulfate 0.25–2% solution; Epinephrine HCl 0.1% solution; Cyclopentolate HCl 0.5–1%.
1. Action is to block sphincter muscle response—dilates pupil.
2. Treatment for ocular surgery and used in eye examinations.
3. Side effects: headache, dizziness, dry mouth, flushing, and hyperemia.

C. Beta-blockers: Timolol maleate.
1. Action is to reduce intraocular pressure by decreasing formation of aqueous humor or may facilitate outflow of aqueous humor.
2. Treatment for glaucoma.
3. Side effects: eye irritation.

D. Carbonic Anhydrase Inhibitors: Acetazolamide, po or IV.
1. Action is to restrict action of the enzyme necessary to produce aqueous humor—mild diuretic action.
2. Treatment for glaucoma.

3. Side effects: CNS disturbance, GI irritation, acidosis, hypokalemia.

E. Hyperosmotic agents: glycerol (oral) or Mannitol (IV).
   1. Action is to increase blood osmolarity—reduce intraocular pressure.
   2. Treatment for cataract surgery as preoperative medication.
   3. Side effects: CNS—headache, confusion, blurred vision; GI irritability; nausea; dehydration.

Retinal Detachment

Characteristics

A. The retina is the part of the eye that perceives light; it coordinates and transmits impulses from its seeing nerve cells to the optic nerve.
B. There are two primitive retinal layers: the outer pigment epithelium and an inner sensory layer.
C. Retinal detachment occurs when:
   1. The two primitive layers of the retina separate, due to the accumulation of fluid between them.
   2. Both retinal layers elevate away from the choroid, due to a tumor.
D. As the detachment extends and becomes complete, blindness occurs.

Assessment

A. Assess if client sees opacities before the eyes.
B. Assess for flashes of light.
C. Ask client if he or she sees floating spots—blood and retinal cells that are freed at the time of the tear and that cast shadows on the retina as they drift about the eye.
D. Evaluate progressive constriction of vision in one area.
   1. The area of visual loss depends on the location of detachment.
   2. When the detachment is extensive and rapid, the client feels as if a curtain has been pulled over his or her eyes.

Implementation

A. Provide preoperative care.
   1. Keep client on bed rest.
   2. Cover both eyes with patches to prevent further detachment.
   3. Position client's head so the retinal hole is in the lowest part of the eye.
   4. Immediate surgery with drainage of fluid from subretinal space so that retina returns to normal position.
   5. Retinal breaks are sealed by various methods that produce inflammatory reactions (chorioretinitis).
      a. Cryosurgery—cold probe applied to sclera causes a chorioretinal scar. Most common procedure.
      b. Diathermy—causes retina to adhere to choroid.
      c. Laser—seals small retinal tears before detachment occurs.

B. Provide postoperative care.
   1. Maintain safe environment.
      a. Keep side rails up.
      b. Feed patient.
      c. Maintain bedrest for 1 or 2 days.
   2. Prevent complications.
      a. Observe for hemorrhage, which is a common complication. Notify physician immediately of any sudden, sharp eye pain.
      b. Cover both eyes.
      c. Position so area of detachment is in dependent position. (If air bubble is present, position on abdomen.)
      d. Prevent clinical manifestations which can cause hemorrhage.
         (1) Nausea and vomiting.
         (2) Restlessness.
      e. Encourage client to do deep breathing but to avoid coughing.
      f. Administer good skin care to prevent breakdown.
   3. Provide emotional support.
      a. Provide audible stimulation.
      b. Warn client as you enter the room and always speak before touching.
      c. Orient to surroundings.

C. Provide client instruction.
   1. Convalescent period.
      a. Wear patch at night to prevent rubbing of eyes.
      b. Wear dark glasses, avoid squinting.
      c. No reading for three weeks.
   2. Postconvalescent period.
      a. Avoid straining and constipation.
      b. Avoid lifting heavy objects for six to eight weeks.
      c. Avoid bending from the waist.

Removal of Foreign Body from Eye

A. Have client look upward.

B. Expose and evert lower lid to expose conjunctival sac.

C. Wet cotton applicator with sterile normal saline and gently twist swab over particle and remove it.

D. If particle cannot be found, have client look downward. Place cotton applicator horizontally on outer surface of upper lid.

E. Grasp eyelashes with fingers and pull upper lid outward and upward over cotton stick.

F. With twisting motion upward, loosen particle and remove.

G. If penetrating object—do not remove. Cover with cup, do not bend, and notify physician stat.

EAR SURGERY
Stapedectomy

Characteristics

A. Surgery performed when the client has otosclerosis.

B. Otosclerosis is a condition in which the normal bone of the inner ear is replaced by abnormal osseous tissue.
   1. The new growth of bone forms about the oval window and then about the stapes.
   2. It blocks the movements of the stapes so that it is unable to vibrate effectively in response to sound pressure.

C. Surgical procedure.
   1. An incision is made deep in the ear canal, close to the eardrum, so that the drum can be turned back and the middle ear exposed.
   2. The surgeon frees and removes the stapes and the attached footplate, leaving an opening in the oval window.
   3. The client can usually hear as soon as this procedure has been completed.
   4. The opening in the oval window is closed with a plug of fat or Gelfoam, which the body eventually replaces with mucous membrane cells.
   5. A steel wire or a Teflon piston is inserted to replace the stapes.
      a. It is attached to the incus at one end and to the graft or plug at the other end.
      b. The wire transmits sound to the inner ear.
   6. External canal is packed, covered with eye dressing over auricle.

Implementation

A. Position client in low-Fowler's, unoperated side or as ordered.

B. Do not turn the client.

C. Put side rails up.

D. Have client deep breathe every two hours until ambulatory, but do not allow client to cough.

E. Check for drainage; report excessive bleeding.

F. Prevent vomiting.

G. Give antibiotics as ordered.

H. Client may have vertigo when ambulatory; stay with the client and avoid quick movements.

I. Advise client not to smoke.

Irrigation of External Auditory Canal

A. Remove any discharge on outer ear.

B. Place emesis basin under ear.

C. Gently pull outer ear upward and backward for adult, or downward and backward for child.

D. Place tip of syringe or irrigating catheter at opening of ear.

E. Gently irrigate with solution at 95° to 105° F, directing flow toward the sides of the canal.

F. Dry external ear.

G. If irrigation does not dislodge wax, instillation of drops will need to be carried out.

CARDIOVASCULAR SYSTEM

The heart and the circulatory system, both systemic and pulmonary, comprise one of the most essential parts of the body; failure to function results in death of the organism. The heart is a hollow muscular organ which, by contracting rhythmically, effectively pumps the blood through the circulatory system to nourish all of the body tissues.

ANATOMY

Gross Structure of Heart

Layers

A. Pericardium.
1. Fibrous pericardium—fibrous sac.
2. Serous pericardium—allows for free cardiac motion.
B. Epicardium—covers surface of heart, extends onto great vessels, and becomes continuous with inner lining of pericardium.
C. Myocardium—muscular portion of heart.
D. Endocardium—thin, delicate layer of tissue that lines cardiac chambers and covers surface of heart valves.

Chambers of the Heart

Definition: The heart is a muscular organ divided by a septum into two halves—right or venous chamber and left or arterial chamber. The heart is actually a pump considered as two pumps working in sequence.

A. Right chamber.
1. Right atrium (receiving chamber) is a thin-walled, distensible, low-pressure collecting chamber for systemic venous system.
   a. Inlets: superior vena cava, inferior vena cava, coronary sinus, thebesian veins.
   b. Outlet: tricuspid valve.
2. Right ventricle (RV)—(ejecting chamber) is a thin-walled, low-pressure crescent-shaped pump for propelling blood into low resistance pulmonary circuit.
   a. Normal thickness: 0.5 cm.
   b. Type of contraction: bellows pumping action.
   c. Outlet: pulmonic valve into pulmonary artery.
B. Left chamber.
1. Left atrium (receiving chamber) is a thin-walled, medium-pressure collecting chamber for pulmonary venous system.
   a. Inlets: four pulmonary veins.
   b. Outlet: mitral valve.
2. Left ventricle (LV)—(ejecting chamber) is a thick-walled, high-pressure cone-shaped pump for propelling blood into high resistance systemic circuit.
   a. Normal thickness: 1.5 cm.
   b. Type of contraction: spiral squeezing-type pumping action.
   c. Outlet: aortic valve into aorta.

Valves

Definition: Valves are strong membranous openings that provide one-way flow of blood.

A. Atrioventricular valves prevent backflow of blood from the ventricles to the atria during systole.
1. Tricuspid—right heart valve.
   a. Three cusps or leaflets.
   b. Free edges anchored to papillary muscles in right ventricle by chordae tendineae which contract when the ventricular walls contract.
2. Mitral—left heart valve.
   a. Two cusps or leaflets.
   b. Free edges anchored to papillary muscles in left ventricle by chordae tendineae which contract when the ventricular walls contract.
B. Semilunar valves prevent backflow from the aorta and pulmonary arteries into the ventricles during diastole.
1. Pulmonic—three cusps or leaflets.
2. Aortic—three cusps or leaflets; orifices for coronary arteries arise from wall of aorta above two of the three cusps.

C. Valves function passively.
1. Close when backward pressure pushes blood backward.
2. Open when forward pressure forces blood in a forward direction.

Conduction System

Definition: Conduction system is composed of specialized tissue that allows rapid transmission of electrical impulses through the myocardium.

A. Sinoatrial (SA) node—main pacemaker of heart in which normal rhythmic self-excitatory impulse is generated.
1. 60 to 100 electrical impulses/min.
2. External control is through autonomic nervous system.
   a. Sympathetic—speeds rate.
   b. Parasympathetic—slows rate.
3. Nerves affect cardiac pumping in two ways.
   a. Change heart rate.
   b. Change strength of contraction of the heart.
4. Intrinsic automaticity—initiates electrical impulses automatically.
B. Internodal tracts—transmission of electrical impulses through atria from sinoatrial node to atrioventricular node.
C. Atrioventricular (AV) node—contains delay tissue to allow atrial contraction to eject blood into ventricle before ventricular contraction.
D. Bundle of His—conducts the electrical impulse from the atria into ventricles.
E. Left and right bundles to Purkinje's fibers—conduct impulses to all parts of the ventricles.

Coronary Blood Supply

Definition: Coronary blood flow is regulated by local blood flow regulation in the heart in response to needs of cardiac muscle for oxygen; thus, the rate of oxygen consumption is the major factor in determining coronary blood flow.

A. Arteries.
1. Right coronary artery supplies mainly the right ventricle but also part of the left ventricle. Coronary arteries fill on diastole.
2. Left coronary artery divides into two branches and supplies mainly the left ventricle.
   a. Left anterior descending artery.
   b. Circumflex artery.

B. Veins—generally parallel arterial system.
1. Coronary sinus veins empty into right atrium.
2. Thebesian veins empty into right atrium.

Gross Structure of Vasculature

Arteries

A. The function of the arteries is to transport blood under high pressure to the body tissues.
1. Arteries have strong vascular walls.
2. Blood flows rapidly to the tissues.
B. Precapillary sphincters.
1. Offer most resistance to blood flow located between arterioles and capillary bed.
2. Allow for local autoregulation of blood flow to meet individual tissue needs.
C. Arteriovenous shunts.
1. Bypass capillary bed and provide direct communication between arterioles and venules.
2. Normally are closed but in shock states are open.

Capillaries

Definition: Minute passageways with the function of exchanging fluid and nutrients between blood and interstitial spaces.

A. Capillary walls are thin and permeable to small substances.
B. Blood flow is slowest in capillaries.

Veins

Definition: Primary function is to act as conduits for transport of the blood from tissues back to the heart.

A. Venous system.
1. Pressure is low.
2. Walls are thin but muscular.
3. Walls are able to contract or expand, thereby storing a small or large amount of blood.
B. Factors influencing venous return.
1. Muscle contraction.
2. Gravity.
3. Competent valves.
4. Respiration.
   a. Inspiration increases venous return.
   b. Expiration decreases venous return.
5. Compliancy of right heart.

PHYSIOLOGY

Regulation of Cardiac Function

Contraction

Definition: The heart muscle utilizes chemical energy to do the work of contraction—a shortening or increase in tension.

A. The sarcomere is the unit of contraction and contains the proteins actin and myosin.
B. Sliding theory of contraction.
   1. Actin slides inward on myosin causing shortening of sarcomere, resulting in systole.
   2. When calcium is used up, actin and myosin slide apart, resulting in diastole.
C. Each cardiac cell is composed of many sarcomeres.

Cardiac Muscle Principles

A. Frank-Starling law: the greater the heart is filled during diastole, within physiological limits, the greater the quantity of blood pumped into the aorta and pulmonary artery.
   1. The heart can pump a large amount of blood or a small amount depending on the amount that flows into it from the veins.
   2. It automatically adapts to whatever the load may be (within physiological limits of the total amount heart can pump).
   3. Decreased blood volume reduces cardiac output since muscle length is too short to perform properly.
   4. Factors affecting cardiac output.
      a. Length of diastole.
      b. Force of contractility of cardiac muscle.
      c. Venous return.
      d. Peripheral vascular resistance (blood pressure).
      e. Ventricular compliancy (distensibility).
B. All-or-none principle: cardiac muscle either contracts or does not contract when stimulated.
C. Two phases of contractility.
   1. Isometric—increasing tension while maintaining length of muscle fiber.
   2. Isotonic—shortening muscle fiber while tension remains constant.

Mechanisms of Cardiac Reserve

A. Response of increased stretch to increased force of contraction.
B. Alteration of heart rate.
C. Hypertrophy to meet increased demands.
D. Blood flow redistribution via sympathetic nervous system response.

Properties of Cardiac Cells

A. Automaticity: ability to initiate an electrical impulse without external stimuli.
   1. SA node.
   2. Junctional tissue.
   3. Bundle branch—Purkinje system.
   4. Phases—depolarization and repolarization.
B. Conductivity: ability to transmit electrical impulse.
C. Contractility: ability of muscle to shorten with electrical stimulation.
D. Excitability (irritability): ability to be stimulated.
E. Refractoriness: ability to return cells to resting state.
   1. Absolute refractory period—no amount of electrical stimulation will cause contraction.
   2. Relative refractory period—strong enough electrical stimulation will cause contraction.

Pulse

Definition: The rhythmic dilation of an artery caused by the contraction of the heart.

A. Pulse deficit—difference between apical and radial, due to weakened or ineffective contraction of heart.
B. Pulse pressure—difference between systolic and diastolic pressure.
C. Factors influencing blood pressure.
   1. Force of heart contractions.
   2. Volume of blood; for example, hemorrhage will decrease blood pressure.
   3. Diameter and elasticity of blood vessels; for example, arteriosclerosis will increase blood pressure.
   4. Viscosity of blood; for example, polycythemia vera will increase blood pressure.

Autonomic Nervous System Control

Cardiac Muscle

A. Sympathetic nervous system (adrenergic)—innervates all cardiac muscle.
   1. Secretes epinephrine and norepinephrine.

2. Response to stress—excitatory.
   a. Increases SA node rate.
   b. Increases conductivity, especially AV node.
   c. Increases contractility of cardiac muscle.
   d. Increases cell irritability.
B. Parasympathetic nervous system (cholinergic)—innervates all but ventricular muscle.
   1. Mediated via vagus nerve.
   2. Secretes acetylcholine.
   3. Maintenance of homeostasis—"brake of heart."
      a. Decreases SA node rate.
      b. Decreases conductivity, especially AV node.
      c. Decreases atrial contractility.

Systemic Blood Vessels

A. Sympathetic nervous system.
   1. Effect is vasoconstriction of blood vessels through action mainly on precapillary sphincter (one exception: vasodilation of coronary arteries).
   2. To obtain dilatation: sympathetic system inhibited.
B. Parasympathetic nervous system.
   1. Usually predominates so blood vessels not vasoconstricted.
   2. Effect is vasodilation in certain areas such as cerebrum, salivary glands and lower colon.

Baroreceptor Reflex

A. Most important circulatory reflex is called baroreceptor reflex.
   1. Initiated by baroreceptors (also called pressoreceptors) located in walls of large systemic arteries.
   2. Rise in pressure results in baroreceptors transmitting signals to CNS to inhibit sympathetic action.
   3. Other signals, in turn, sent to circulation reduce pressure back toward normal.
   4. Result is decreased heart rate, vasodilation, and decreased blood pressure.
B. Effect of decreased blood pressure.
   1. Sympathetic stimulation overrides vagal response.
   2. Result is increased heart rate, vasoconstriction, and increased blood pressure.

Other Chemical Controls of Blood Pressure

A. Kidney.
   1. Adrenal cortex releases aldosterone, causing sodium and water to be reabsorbed. This increases blood volume and blood pressure.
   2. Juxtaglomerular apparatus releases renin, which causes vasoconstriction to increase blood pressure.
B. Antidiuretic hormone (vasopressin)—acts on kidney tubules to reabsorb water, thereby increasing blood volume and blood pressure.
C. Histamine release.
   1. Arterioles dilate.
   2. Venules constrict.
D. Capillary fluid shift mechanism; for example, hemorrhage and decreased blood pressure allow capillaries to reabsorb interstitial fluid.

System Assessment

A. Evaluate client's history.
   1. Pain—character, location, duration, intensity, precipitating or aggravating factors, and relieving factors.
      a. Ischemic type of pain: pain of angina or myocardial infarction.
      b. Pain from dissecting aorta: tearing or burning.
      c. Pericarditis pain: aggravated by deep breathing, supine position, turning from side to side.
   2. Dyspnea—shortness of breath, feeling of inability to get enough air.
      a. Exertional dyspnea (DOE): occurs while exercising.
      b. Orthopnea: occurs while in a reclining position.
      c. Paroxysmal nocturnal dyspnea (PND): interrupts client's sleep.
      d. Differentiations.
         (1) Tachypnea: increase in rate of breathing.
         (2) Hyperpnea: increase in depth and rate of breathing.
      e. Productive or nonproductive cough.
   3. Cyanosis—deficiency of oxygen in blood.
   4. Fatigue—result of diminution of cardiac output.
   5. Palpitations—client aware of heartbeat, often with rapid heart rates.

6. Syncope—transient loss of consciousness due to inadequate cerebral blood flow.
7. Hemoptysis—cough accompanied by bloody sputum.
8. Edema—collection of fluid in interstitial spaces.
9. Condition of extremities—color, temperature, skin nutrition, presence of petechiae, presence of dryness or clamminess.

B. Evaluate venous and arterial pulses through inspection and palpation.
   1. Veins.
      a. Neck veins—jugular venous pulsations.
         (1) Indirect measurement: height in cm of jugular venous distention from sternal notch when client is at a 45-degree angle.
         (2) Direct measurement through a central venous catheter placed in superior vena cava or right atrium.
      b. Arms and hand veins.
      c. Leg and feet veins.
   2. Arteries.
      a. Central (precordial).
      b. Peripheral pulses.
         (1) Presence or absence; character.
            (a) Small, weak: low stroke volume (for example, aortic stenosis); narrowed pulse pressure (for example, cardiac tamponade); increased systemic vascular resistance (for example, arteriosclerosis).
            (b) Large, bounding: water-hammer (for example, aortic insufficiency).
         (2) Pulsus alternans: alteration in height of pulse wave, usually in left ventricular failure.
         (3) Pulsus paradoxus: systolic blood pressure drop greater than 10 mm Hg during inspiration, as in cardiac tamponade.

C. Assess heart sounds through auscultation.
   1. Heart sounds—frequency, pitch, intensity, duration, timbre.
      a. S_1—closure of mitral and tricuspid valve.
      b. S_2—closure of aortic and pulmonic valve.
      c. S_3 and S_4—gallop sounds, usually indicative of heart failure.
         (1) S_3—rapid filling of ventricle in early diastole; may be heard normally; after S_2.

(2) S_4 coincides with atrial contraction due to poorly compliant ventricle; prior to S_1.
   2. Murmurs: turbulence of blood flow through narrowed lumen or incompetent valve; classified by their timing.
      a. Systolic.
         (1) Mitral and tricuspid insufficiency.
         (2) Aortic and pulmonic stenosis.
         (3) Patent foramen ovale.
         (4) Ventricular septal defect.
      b. Diastolic.
         (1) Mitral and tricuspid stenosis.
         (2) Aortic and pulmonic insufficiency.
   3. Pericardial friction rub—timed with heart rate.

D. Evaluate arterial pressure.
   1. Measurement of blood pressure—indirect via cuff.
      a. Both arms.
      b. Both legs initially.
   2. Presence of bruits (sound of abnormal murmur): turbulence of blood flow usually around obstruction.

E. Palpate and percuss thorax to determine chest wall abnormalities and position of heart.

F. Evaluate chest x-ray to determine abnormalities of lung fluids and cardiac silhouette.

G. Assess lung sounds for adventitious sounds.
   1. Rales: fine, medium, coarse.
   2. Rhonchi: sibilant, sonorous.

H. Assess client's readiness for a cardiac rehabilitation program.

Diagnostic Procedures

Electrocardiogram

Definition: An electrocardiogram (ECG or EKG) is a record of the electrical activity of the heart reflected by changes in electrical potential at skin surface.

A. Purpose: to determine types and extent of heart damage, cardiac irregularities, electrolyte imbalances.
   1. Nonpainful procedure but should be explained to client.
   2. Relaxation of client important to reduce electrical interference from muscle movement.

B. Twelve lead EKGs and vectorcardiography are essential for diagnosing cardiac abnormalities.

1. EKG provides a two-dimensional view of the heart along one of two planes, horizontal or frontal.
2. Vectorcardiography views heart's electrical activity from additional directions.

C. EKG interpretation.
1. Normal cardiac cycle.
   a. P wave—atrial depolarization.
   b. P-R interval—atrial depolarization.
   c. QRS wave—ventricular depolarization.
   d. ST segment—ventricular repolarization.
   e. T wave—ventricular repolarization and ventricular diastole.

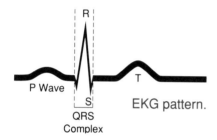

EKG pattern.

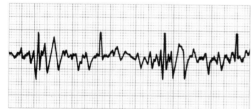

EKG pattern showing artifact

2. Interpretation of EKG.
   a. Determine heart rate by calculating atrial rate (P-P interval) and ventricular rate (R-R interval). Normal pulse 60 to 100.
   b. Determine regularity of rhythm (atrial and ventricular).
   c. Measure P-R interval to determine conduction time in atria and AV junction (0.12 to 0.20 seconds).
   d. Measure QRS duration to determine ventricular conduction (0.04 to 0.12 seconds).
   e. Measure Q-T interval (rate of 70 in one minute occurring 0.36 seconds apart).
   f. Check configuration and placement of P waves, QRS complex, ST segment, and T wave.
   g. Summarize findings to obtain interpretation.

3. Etiology of arrhythmias.
   a. Heart failure, electrolyte imbalance, acidosis or alkalosis, hypoxemia, drugs, hypotension, emotional stress.
   b. Precipitating or contributing diseases—infection, hypovolemia, anemia, thyroid disorders.

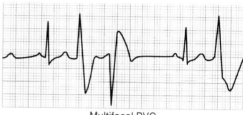

Multifocal PVC

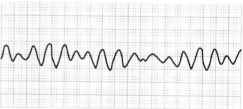

Ventricular tachycardia

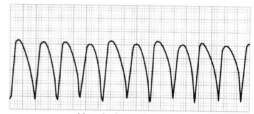

Ventricular fibrillation

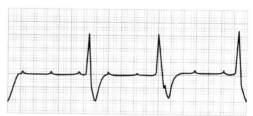

Third-degree heart block

His Bundle EKG

A. Intracardiac electrophysiologic test.
B. Directly measures heart's electrical activity from right side of client's heart.
C. Identify type of arrhythmia.
D. Identify location and extent of conduction block.
E. Evaluate the effectiveness of an artificial pacemaker.

Other Diagnostic Procedures

A. Routine chest films—silhouette of heart, chambers, and great vessels observed on x-ray.
B. Fluoroscopy—heart, lung, and vessel movements viewed on luminescent x-ray film screen in darkened room.
C. Angiography.
    1. Injection of radiopaque compounds into circulation at appropriate sites.
    2. Cineangiogram—dynamics of passage of contrast agent through vascular tree starting at injection site.
    3. Angiograms into chamber.
    4. Selective coronary arteriography.
D. Phonocardiogram—heart sounds translated into electrical energy by a microphone and recorded.
E. Echocardiography—records high-frequency sound vibrations; assists in evaluating structures of the heart, dimensions of the chambers, and thickness of septum and ventricular walls.
F. Jugular and carotid pulse wave tracings—record low-frequency, soundless vibrations from the vessels. These vibrations reflect the heart's pulsations during systole and diastole.
G. Treadmill test—increase in exercise provokes chest pain and EKG changes in presence of myocardial ischemia.
H. Holter monitor—tape-recorded ambulatory electrocardiogram. Monitors cardiac cycle for 24 hrs.

Nuclear Cardiology Tests

A. Technetium pyrophosphate scan.
    1. Special camera scans heart to identify areas of increased uptake of radioisotope.
    2. Radioisotope accumulates in damaged areas of the heart and will evidence a recent MI.
B. Thallium scan. A medication (^{201}TI) will be injected into the antecubital vein and scanning is done within 4 10 minutes.
    1. Necrotic or ischemic tissue will not reflect radioisotope as will tissue with normal blood supply and healthy cells.
    2. Detects myocardial scarring and perfusion, an acute or chronic MI, or evaluation of prior cardiac surgery.
C. Thallium scan with exercise.
    1. Test involves exercise; takes 1 hour and 15 minutes and 3 hours later, a 30-minute resting scan is performed.
    2. Imaging with exercise may demonstrate perfusion problems not apparent when client is at rest.
D. Gated cardiac blood pool scan.
    1. After an intravenous injection of a red blood cell tagging agent, the computer is synchronized with the EKG reading.
    2. This test evaluates left ventricular function.

System Planning and Analysis

A. Alterations in cardiac dysfunction are identified early and appropriate interventions instituted to prevent major complications.
B. Cardiac complications are treated immediately and effectively when they occur.
C. Client is adequately prepared for diagnostic tests.
D. Client is psychologically and physically prepared for surgical intervention.
E. Client is instructed in self-care such as medication, footcare, and exercise program.
F. Goals for rehabilitation are established.
G. Blood flow is increased to lower extremities through preventive measures.
H. Thrombophlebitis is prevented in clients with peripheral vascular disease and those on bed rest.
I. Adequate circulation is maintained for clients with aortic aneurysm.
J. Medications promote adequate cardiac output.
K. Cardiac arrest is identified and CPR established immediately.

System Implementation

A. Monitor apical pulse for alterations in cardiac rhythm.
B. Assess peripheral pulses to determine adequacy of circulation.
C. Monitor laboratory values for alterations in electrolytes, coagulation, and serum enzymes to prevent complications.
D. Provide diet appropriate for disease state.
E. Monitor vital signs for alterations, particularly in blood pressure and pulse.
F. Provide emotional support for clients and family when alterations in life-style are needed.
G. Administer and instruct client on drugs and their side effects.

H. Instruct client on preoperative and postoperative care modalities.
I. Monitor for complications following surgical intervention.
J. Plan an acceptable rehabilitation program with client and family.
K. Administer life saving measures when client's condition is compromised.

System Evaluation

A. Cardiac system functions within normal limits.
B. Cardiac surgery improves cardiac status.
C. Emergency interventions are established and cardiac status is improved.
D. Cardiac arrhythmias are detected early and definitive treatment started.
E. Diagnostic tests assist in diagnosis of cardiac dysfunction.
F. Cardiovascular symptoms are assessed and treated specifically.
G. Medications are administered and cardiovascular status improves.
H. Rehabilitation program is established and client reaches optimal level of functioning.

ACQUIRED HEART DISEASE

Coronary Artery Disease

Definition: Occurs as the result of accumulation of fatty materials (lipids, cholesterol being primary one), which narrows the lumen of coronary arteries. Clinical manifestations of disease reflect ischemia to myocardium, resulting from inadequate blood supply to meet metabolic demands.

Assessment

A. Assess for presence of risk factors.
 1. Diet—increased intake of cholesterol and saturated fats.
 2. Hypertension—aggravates atherosclerotic process.
 3. Cigarette smoking.
 4. Male sex.
 5. Age.
 6. Family history of CAD.
 7. Diabetes mellitus—accelerates atherosclerotic process.

 8. Lack of exercise; sedentary life style.
 9. Psychosocial tensions—may precipitate acute events; type A personality.
 10. Obesity—susceptibility to hypertension, diabetes mellitus, hyperlipidemia.
B. Evaluate chest pain.
 1. Angina, burning, squeezing, crushing tightness substernally or over prechordal area. Pain may radiate to neck, jaw, shoulder, arms.
 2. Associated with nausea, vomiting, increased perspiration, and cool extremities.
C. Assess heart sounds for presence of arrhythmias and/or murmurs.

Implementation

A. Monitor vital signs, particularly blood pressure and pulse.
B. Evaluate EKG findings.
C. Administer nitrates if chest pain present.
D. Evaluate chest pain—type, duration, relieved with medication.
E. Discuss risk factors and means to decrease or alter risk factors.
F. Monitor breath sounds and signs of peripheral edema to detect early complications.

Angina Pectoris

Definition: A severe chest pain due to the temporary inability of coronary arteries to meet oxygen needs of myocardium. Pathophysiology involves narrowing of coronary artery usually by vessel spasm, atherosclerotic or thrombic process.

Assessment

A. Assess for increased need for oxygen due to:
 1. Exertion and effort.
 2. Emotional upsets.
 3. Tachyarrhythmias.
 4. Over-eating.
 5. Extremes of temperature, especially cold.
 6. Smoking.
B. Identify presence of associated disease states: anemia, polycythemia, syphilitic heart disease, rheumatic heart disease, mitral and aortic stenosis, tachyarrhythmias, hypertension, hypotension, thyrotoxicosis, hypoglycemia.

C. Evaluate pain.
  1. Location: precordial, substernal.
  2. Character: compressing, choking, burning, squeezing, crushing heaviness.
  3. Radiation: left arm or right arm, jaw, neck, back.
  4. Duration: usually five to ten minutes, relieved by rest or nitroglycerin.
D. Observe for signs of dyspnea.
E. Assess EKG changes (may not be any at rest).
  1. ST segment depression or elevation during pain.
  2. T wave depressed or inverted.

Implementation

A. Current approach to therapy is to decrease oxygen demand of myocardium.
B. Understand medication usage for condition.
  1. Action of drugs.
    a. Dilate coronary arteries not atherosclerotic to increase blood flow to myocardium.
    b. Lessen cardiac work by decreasing venous return—decreases peripheral vascular resistance.
    c. Reduces cardiac response to exertion, stress.
    d. Inhibits platelet activity.
  2. Use—relief of pain from myocardial ischemia.
  3. Side effects—hypotension, headache, tachycardia.
  4. Administer IV nitroglycerin (Tridil) as ordered. (Potent, concentrated drug. Must be diluted in glass bottle of D_5W or sodium chloride 0.9%.)
    a. Given as a continuous infusion. Begin at 5 mcg/min.
    b. Increase by increments every 3–5 minutes, until the desired response occurs.
    c. IV infusion pump is used to deliver continuous flow rate.
    d. Closely monitor BP, PA, PCWP, HR, CO (cardiac output).
  5. Instruct in use of sublingual nitroglycerin (tablets or metered dose mouth spray).
    a. Effective only sublingually.
    b. Dosage (one to two tablets) may be repeated at five minute intervals.
    c. Physician should be called if no relief in 15 minutes.
    d. No limit to number taken in 24-hour period.
    e. Nonaddictive.
    f. May be used prophylactically before engaging in activity known to precipitate angina.
    g. Keep tablets in tightly closed dark glass bottle.
    h. Do not allow tablets to age—drug potency is 6 months.
    i. Wear Medi-Alert band and keep medication on person at all times.
  6. Instruct client in use of nitroglycerin ointment/transdermal patch.
    a. Apply directly to skin.
    b. Wash off remaining ointment before new application.
    c. Change skin placement with each application.
C. Provide client instruction.
  1. Learn to live in moderation—physical activity should be sufficient to maintain general physical state, but short of causing angina.
  2. Avoid stress and emotional upset.
  3. Reduce caloric intake if overweight.
  4. Refrain from smoking.
  5. Decrease use of stimulants (coffee, tea, cola).
  6. Instruct client in use of medication.
D. Other medications used.
  1. Long-acting nitrites (Isordil, Cardilate).
  2. Beta-blocker: propranolol (Inderal).
  3. Calcium blocking agents (Calan, Cardizem).

Myocardial Infarction

Definition: The process by which cardiac muscle is destroyed due to interruption of or insufficient blood supply for a prolonged period, resulting in sustained oxygen deprivation.

Characteristics

A. Causes.
  1. Atherosclerotic heart disease.
  2. Coronary artery embolism or vasospasm.
  3. Decreased blood volume with shock and/or hemorrhage.
  4. Direct trauma.
B. Infarction sites.
  1. Transmural—entire thickness of myocardium involved.

2. Subendocardial—damage has not penetrated through entire thickness of myocardial wall.
3. Inferior wall—right coronary artery lesion.
4. Anterior wall—left anterior descending.
5. Lateral—circumflex.
6. Posterior—right coronary artery.

C. Confirmation of diagnosis.
1. History (very important).
2. Serial 12 lead EKGs to observe for changes that reflect area of involvement.
   a. ST elevation (subendocardial): T wave inversion.
   b. Development of Q waves (transmural).
3. Serial chest x-rays.
4. Laboratory studies.
   a. Serum enzymes—released with death of tissue.
      (1) CPK-isoenzymes (CPK-MB)—most valuable measurement; level rises within six hours.
      (2) LDH, LDH_2-isoenzymes—level rises in 6–8 hours; persists longer.
      (3) SGOT+ — not specific to heart disease alone; serial tests helpful.
      (4) Alpha hydroxybutyric dehydrogenase.
   b. Increased white blood cells and sedimentation rate.
   c. Technetium 99 scan.
5. Radionuclide techniques.
   a. Thallium or technetium used.
   b. Identifies areas of diminished perfusion and weakened ventricular function.
   c. May be employed in conjunction with exercise testing.
6. Positron emission tomography (PET)
   a. New form of nuclear imaging.
   b. Performed with treadmill, bicycle, or IV dipyridamole-induced stress.
   c. Validate which drugs to be given or discontinued pre-scan.
7. Electrophysiologic testing.
   a. Intracardiac electrocardiography.
   b. Identifies mechanisms and optimal therapy for supra-ventricular arrhythmias and atrioventricular conduction disturbances.

Assessment

A. Evaluate pain—similar to angina but usually more intense and longer in duration (30 minutes or longer).

1. Location—left precordial, substernal.
2. Character—crushing, vise-like, tightness, burning.
3. Radiation—jaw, back, arms.

B. Identify anxiousness, feeling of doom, fatigue.
C. Observe for dyspnea or orthopnea.
D. Observe for nausea and vomiting.
E. Assess for diaphoresis.
F. Check for pallor or cyanosis, coolness of extremities.
G. Evaluate for arrhythmias.
H. Observe for signs of congestive heart failure.
I. Low grade temperature after first day.

Implementation

A. Treat death-producing arrhythmias immediately with lidocaine.
B. Administer IV or IM narcotic analgesics, as ordered, to relieve pain and anxiety.
C. Monitor cardiac rhythm continuously.
D. Monitor lidocaine drip.
E. Administer oxygen via cannula.
F. Provide bedrest and emotional support.
G. Monitor closely for signs of CHF (seen within first 24 hours).
H. Monitor IV nitroglycerin drip.
I. Monitor Swan-Ganz catheter and take PAWP and CO readings.
J. Provide physical rest and emotional support.
   1. Sedation, graduated activity.
   2. Use of commode and self-feed.
K. Maintain client on stool softeners and soft diet to prevent increased workload on heart and prevent Valsalva maneuver.
L. Provide low-fat, low-cholesterol, low-sodium diet.
M. Rehabilitate client to enable him to return to physical level according to cardiac capability.
   1. Plan exercise program.
   2. Provide psychological support.
   3. Avoid stressful environment.
   4. Consider possible change of life style.
   5. Start long-term drug therapy—might include antiarrhythmics, anticoagulants, and antihypertensives.
N. Encourage client to participate in organized cardiac rehabilitation program.
   1. Monitor exercise program based on METs.
   2. Stress reduction classes.
   3. Alterations in diet—low saturated fat, low cholesterol, no added salt, adequate fiber.

4. No smoking.
5. Instruction in CPR for family.
6. Cardiac anatomy discussion.

O. Monitor for complications.
   1. Arrhythmias, CHF, cardiogenic shock.
   2. Thrombophlebitis, papillary muscle dysfunction, pericarditis.
   3. Cardiogenic shock.
   4. Thrombophlebitis.
   5. Papillary muscle dysfunction.
   6. Pericarditis.
   7. Ventricular aneurysm or rupture (late complication) due to weakened area of myocardium as a result of myocardial infarction.

VALVULAR DISEASE

Mitral Stenosis

Definition: A progressive thickening of the valve cusps that results in the narrowing of lumen of mitral valve.

Assessment

A. Evaluate history for congenital heart disease or rheumatic heart disease.
B. Assess for signs of decreased cardiac output. Asymptomatic until valve area is less than 1.5 sq. cm and tachycardia or atrial fibrillation occurs.
C. Evaluate for symptoms and signs of left, and then right, ventricular failure.
D. Evaluate heart sounds for diastolic murmur, accentuated S_1 and opening snap.
E. Assess for complications.
   1. Atrial fibrillation.
   2. Subacute bacterial endocarditis.
   3. Thrombi formation.

Implementation

A. Treat heart failure and arrhythmias.
B. Decrease cardiac workload.
C. Prevent and/or treat infections.
D. Monitor administration of anticoagulants for treatment and/or prevention of thrombi in clients with atrial fibrillation.
E. Provide emotional support to client.
F. Prepare client for valvotomy if no calcification of valve or for surgical replacement of the mitral valve.

Mitral Insufficiency

Definition: Distortion of the valve that allows backward flow of blood from ventricle to atrium.

Assessment

A. Assess for presence of cardiac disease associated with mitral insufficiency.
   1. Rheumatic heart disease.
   2. Congenital disease.
   3. Bacterial endocarditis.
   4. Rupture of chordae tendineae.
   5. Rupture or dysfunction of papillary muscle.
   6. Dilatation of left ventricle.
B. Observe for evidence of left, then right, heart failure.
C. Evaluate for decreased intensity of S_1; pansystolic murmur; S_3.
D. Identify atrial fibrillation on monitor.
E. Evaluate for systemic emboli and hemoptysis—uncommon.

Implementation

Same as for mitral stenosis.

Aortic Stenosis

Definition: The narrowing of the aortic valve opening due to fibrosis and calcification. This results in inadequate ejection of blood from the left ventricle.

Assessment

A. Assess history for predisposing conditions.
   1. Rheumatic heart disease.
   2. Arteriosclerosis.
   3. Congenital defect.
B. Observe for dizziness and syncope.
C. Evaluate for angina.
D. Observe for symptoms of congestive heart failure.
E. Evaluate for systolic murmur; decreased S_2; gallop rhythm.
F. Measure EKG strip for presence of heart block (due to calcification in upper interventricular system).

Implementation

A. Follow nursing care protocols for clients with congestive heart failure.
B. Prepare client psychologically and physiologically for prosthetic valve replacement.

Aortic Insufficiency

Definition: Occurs when blood flows back into the venticle from the aorta. Usually results from aortic valve disease or aortic root disease.

Assessment

A. Assess for presence of the following conditions.
  1. Rheumatic heart disease.
  2. Congenital disease.
  3. Bacterial endocarditis.
  4. Syphilitic aortitis.
  5. Rheumatoid aortitis.
  6. Medial necrosis of aorta.
  7. Arteriosclerotic and hypertensive dilatation of aortic root.
  8. Dissecting aneurysm.
B. Observe for signs of left, then right, heart failure.
C. Evaluate for pounding arterial pulse (Corrigan-type arterial pulse).
D. Observe if diastolic blood pressure falls and systolic blood pressure remains normal or rises.
E. Evaluate for diastolic murmur.

Implementation

Same as for aortic stenosis.

Tricuspid Stenosis

Definition: The progressive narrowing of valve lumen.

Assessment

A. Assess for presence of the following conditions.
  1. Rheumatic heart disease with mitral valve involvement.
  2. Congenital disease.
  3. Bacterial endocarditis.
B. Observe for evidence of systemic venous congestion.
C. Evaluate for diastolic murmurs.

Implementation

A. Follow nursing protocols for clients with congestive heart failure.
B. Prepare client psychologically and physiologically for valvotomy or tricuspid valve replacement.

Tricuspid Insufficiency

Definition: Occurs when blood flows back into the atrium from the ventricle.

Assessment

A. Percuss and inspect chest to determine presence of cardiac hypertrophy.
B. Evaluate chest x-ray for heart dilatation and failure.
C. Assess for pansystolic murmur, S_3 accentuated during inspiration.
D. Observe for symptoms of right-sided heart failure.

Implementation

Same as for tricuspid stenosis.

COMPLICATIONS OF HEART DISEASE

Congestive Heart Failure

Definition: Results from insufficient cardiac output to meet the metabolic needs of the body.

Left Ventricular Failure

Definition: Congestion occurs mainly in the lungs due to inadequate ejection of the blood into the systemic circulation.

Characteristics

A. Causes.
  1. Arteriosclerotic heart disease.
  2. Acute myocardial infarction.
  3. Tachyarrhythmias.
  4. Myocarditis.
  5. High output states (e.g., anemia, pregnancy, hyperthyroidism).
  6. Valvular heart disease.
B. Pathological change.
  1. Decreased cardiac output to systemic circulation.
  2. Congestion in pulmonary circuit due to inability of left heart to accommodate pulmonary vein input (preload).
  3. Decrease in oxygen and carbon dioxide diffusion.

Assessment

A. Evaluate for presence of pulmonary symptoms.
   1. Dyspnea, orthopnea, PND, DOE.
   2. Moist cough.
   3. Wheezing.
   4. Rales, crackles.
   5. Cyanosis or pallor; cool extremities.
   6. Increased pulmonary artery and/or pulmonary wedge pressure.
B. Assess for anxiety, weakness, and fatigue.
C. Identify behavior changes.
D. Check for palpitations and diaphoresis.
E. Assess for gallop rhythm—presence of S_3.
F. Evaluate for tachycardia, arrhythmias and cardiomegaly.
G. Assess for reduced pulse pressure.

Implementation

A. Treat underlying cause.
B. Reduce pain and anxiety.
   1. Morphine sulfate.
   2. Physical and emotional rest; also decrease oxygen requirements.
C. Improve pulmonary ventilation and oxygenation.
   1. Oxygen—cannula usually better than mask since client already feels as though he or she cannot breathe. Administer at 2/ml for COPD clients.
   2. IPPB—also decreases venous return.
   3. Bronchodilator therapy.
   4. Mechanical ventilation (pulmonary edema).
D. Reduce preload (volume returning to heart).
   1. Administer nitrates—cause generalized vasodilation.
   2. Monitor diuretics; prevent fluid retention—restrict fluid and sodium.
   3. Rotating tourniquets (pulmonary edema).
   4. Fowler's position to facilitate breathing.
   5. Record intake and output; weight daily.
E. Reduce afterload (resistance against which heart must pump).
   1. Vasodilators.
   2. ACE inhibitors—control fluid retention.
F. Monitor drug administration when digitalizing client (improves myocardial contractility).
G. Treat arrhythmias.
H. Provide emotional support.
I. Teach client principles of care.
J. Prevent thrombophlebitis by applying antiembolic stockings.
K. Monitor for complications.
   1. Digitalis toxicity.
   2. Concurrent use of Quinidine or Ca^{++} channel blockers increase risk of toxicity.
   3. Electrolyte imbalance from diuretics, especially decreased potassium.
   4. Pulmonary emboli from bed rest, circulatory stasis.
   5. Oxygen toxicity especially with COPD clients.

Right Ventricular Failure

Definition: Congestion occurs when the blood is not pumped adequately from the systemic circulation into the lungs resulting in systemic congestion.

Assessment

A. Assess client for presence of conditions that could lead to right ventricular failure.
   1. Any disease resulting in left ventricular failure.
   2. Pulmonary embolism.
   3. Fluid overload.
   4. COPD.
      a. Pulmonary hypertension.
      b. Cor pulmonale.
   5. Cirrhosis—portal hypertension.
B. Evaluate symptoms primarily related to systemic congestion.
   1. Peripheral edema in dependent parts (necessitating good skin care and positioning).
      a. Feet and legs.
      b. Sacrum, back, buttocks.
   2. Ascites.
   3. Anorexia and nausea due to congestion in liver and gut.
   4. Weight gain.
   5. Oliguria during day and polyuria at night.
   6. Hepatomegaly, liver congestion.
C. Assess other symptoms.
   1. Jugular venous distention at 45 degrees.
   2. Arrhythmias.
   3. Increased central venous pressure.

Implementation

A. Treat underlying cause (usually pulmonary condition).

B. Reduce pain and anxiety.
  1. Morphine sulfate.
  2. Physical and emotional rest; also decrease oxygen requirements.
C. Improve pulmonary ventilation and oxygenation.
  1. Oxygen—cannula usually better than mask since client already feels as though he or she cannot breathe. Administer at 2 l/min for COPD clients.
  2. IPPB—also decreases venous return.
  3. Bronchodilator therapy.
  4. Mechanical ventilation for respiratory failure.
D. Reduce pulmonary and systemic congestion and blood volume.
  1. Diuretics.
  2. Moderate sodium restriction (1.5–2 gm)—also prevents fluid retention.
  3. Fowler's position.
E. Monitor drug administration when digitalizing client (improves myocardial contractility).
F. Prevent fluid retention.
  1. Record intake and output.
  2. Weigh daily.
G. Treat arrhythmias.
H. Provide support to client.
I. Teach client principles of care.
J. Monitor for complications of treatment.
  1. Digitalis toxicity.
  2. Electrolyte imbalance from diuretics, especially decreased potassium.
  3. Oxygen toxicity, especially with COPD clients.
  4. Myocardial failure.
  5. Cardiac dysrhythmias.
  6. Pulmonary infarction; emboli, pneumonia from bedrest—circulatory stasis.

Acute Pulmonary Edema

Definition: An excessive quantity of fluid in the pulmonary interstitial spaces or in the alveoli usually following severe left ventricular decompensation.

Characteristics

A. The most common cause is greatly elevated capillary pressure resulting from failure of left heart and damming of blood in lungs.
B. Alveoli filled with fluid and bronchioles congested.
C. Retention of fluid resulting from reduced renal perfusion.

Assessment

A. Assess for primary symptoms of moist rales and frothy sputum.
B. Observe for severe anxiety, feelings of impending doom.
C. Observe for marked dyspnea.
D. Listen for stertorous breathing.
E. Evaluate for marked cyanosis.
F. Observe for profuse diaphoresis—cold and clammy.
G. Evaluate for tachyarrhythmias.
H. Evaluate for gallop rhythm (S$_3$).
I. Inspect and percuss for cardiomegaly.
J. Evaluate for marked increase in pulmonary artery and/or pulmonary capillary wedge pressure.
K. Assess for increased CVP and neck vein distention in severe cases.

Implementation

A. Place in high-Fowler's position.
B. Administer oxygen at 6 liters/minute if client does not have COPD.
C. Administer drugs (diuretics, digitalis, morphine, nitroglycerin) to improve myocardial contractility and reduce pulmonary and systemic blood volume; aminophylline to relieve bronchospasm.
D. Instruct client in deep breathing coughing exercises.
E. Monitor fluid intake and output, weigh daily.
F. Monitor vital signs including PCWP.
G. Provide sedation with ordered medication. Observe respiratory rate and depth.
H. Monitor drug therapy used for preload or afterload (nitroglycerin, nitroprusside, hydralazine).
I. Place rotating tourniquets on client's extremities.
  1. Explain purpose to client.
    a. Reduce venous return to heart.
    b. Pool blood temporarily in extremities.
    c. Treatment for pulmonary edema.
  2. Complete procedure.
    a. Take blood pressure to determine midway between systolic and diastolic reading.
    b. Apply four pressure cuffs high up on all four extremities.
    c. Inflate three cuffs to pressure midway between systolic and diastolic pressure.
    d. Rotate the tourniquets every 15 minutes, using clockwise rotation.
    e. Release one tourniquet and then inflate the next tourniquet.

f. Observe for presence of arterial blood flow by checking peripheral pulses. Arterial pulses should be present, venous pulses absent.

g. Take frequent blood pressure readings to readjust cuff pressure.

h. Continue treatment for prescribed time, usually when diuretic has adequately functioned and signs of pulmonary edema lessened.

i. Discontinue tourniquets one at a time, continuing the cuff deflation in clockwise manner, and every 15 minutes.

Cardiogenic Shock

Definition: A severe form of pump failure resulting in severe pulmonary vascular congestion, and decreased cardiac output with compromised tissue perfusion.

Characteristics

A. Causes.
  1. Massive myocardial infarction with 40 to 60 percent muscle damage.
  2. Inadequate blood supply, compensatory mechanism, or changes in microcirculation leads to clinical manifestations.

B. Pathophysiology.
  1. Decreased contractility.
  2. Decreased arterial blood pressure, causing sympathetic nervous system stimulation, which produces vasoconstriction and opens AV shunts.
  3. Oxygen transport impairment causes increased anaerobic metabolism.
     a. Result is increased lactate.
     b. Increased lactate causes metabolic acidosis.
  4. Decreased cerebral perfusion.
  5. Decreased renal perfusion, resulting in renal failure.
  6. Myocardial ischemia leads to further pump failure.

Assessment

A. Observe for cold and clammy skin—vasoconstriction.

B. Check for tachycardia—(weak and feeble) sympathetic stimulation.

C. Evaluate if blood pressure is less than 80 mmHg systolic.

D. Observe for restlessness—cerebral anoxia due to decreased cardiac output.

E. Measure urinary output. May be less than 30 ml/hour due to poor renal perfusion.

F. Observe for pallor or cyanosis.

G. Evaluate for hypoxia.

H. Assess for acidemia.

I. Evaluate for signs of CHF due to inadequate ventricular emptying.

J. Differentiate from hypovolemic shock.
  1. Pulmonary capillary wedge pressure and CVP are increased in cardiogenic shock.
  2. Pulmonary capillary wedge pressure and CVP are normal or low in hypovolemic shock.

Implementation

A. Monitor drugs for improvement of left ventricular function.
  1. Dopamine (precursor of norepinephrine)—causes vasoconstriction peripherally but increases renal perfusion, generally BP and cardiac index rise.
  2. Norepinephrine if Dopamine ineffective (monitor for tachycardia, arrhythmias).

B. Monitor use of Nipride.
  1. Drug lowers peripheral vascular resistance.
  2. Decreases cardiac workload and increases cardiac output.

C. Maintain arterial blood pressure—vasopressors.
  1. Intraarterial blood pressure monitoring necessary to obtain accurate reading.
  2. Cuff pressures may be low (false reading) due to vasoconstriction and poor Korotkoff sounds.

D. Monitor Swan-Ganz catheter to assess heart failure.
  1. Balance and calibrate transducer.
  2. Connect catheter to a transducer and pressure monitor.
  3. Obtain measurements.
     a. Catheter positioned in pulmonary artery through percutaneous puncture.
        (1) PAP measures are: systolic (20–30 mmHg), diastolic (10–15 mmHg), and mean pressure (10–20 mmHg).
        (2) High PA pressures indicate (L) ventricular failure.

b. Pulmonary capillary wedge pressure (PCWP) is measured by inflating the distal balloon. PCWP pressures range from 4–12 mmHg. High PCWP pressures indicate (L) ventricular failure.

c. Cardiac output is measured by attaching the catheter to the computer monitor and injecting a bolus of IV fluid with a controlled temperature into the bloodstream.

4. Implement nursing interventions for Swan-Ganz catheter.

a. Apply sterile dressing over site.

b. Monitor client's vital signs and status.

c. Evaluate distal pulses in cannulated extremity (usually radial pulse).

d. Monitor PA pressures continuously and record with vital signs. Transducer should be at the level of the right atrium.

e. Obtain PCWP pressures as ordered.

f. Monitor for complications.

(1) Arrhythmias (especially PACs, PVCs).

(2) Catheter fling.

(3) Pulmonary infarction caused by wedging.

(4) Pulmonary emboli.

(5) Infection.

E. Maintain ventilation and oxygenation.

1. Airway.

2. Oxygen.

3. Artificial ventilation if necessary.

4. Arterial blood gases, to determine effect of therapy.

F. Establish fluid and electrolyte acid-base balance.

1. Replace fluid if hypovolemic.

2. Correct acidosis—for example, $NaHCO_3$.

3. Maintain urinary output—greater than 30 ml/hour.

G. Control pain and restlessness—IV analgesia most effective.

H. Treat arrhythmias—result of tissue hypoxia, acidosis, electrolyte imbalance, underlying disease, and drug therapy.

I. Decrease cardiac workload.

1. Physical and emotional rest.

2. Psychological support.

3. Comfortable position—flat with pillow, or semi-Fowler's position if client has difficulty breathing.

EMERGENCY INTERVENTIONS

Cardiopulmonary Resuscitation(CPR)

Suspect Unconsciousness

A. Call out for help.

B. Quickly approach victim.

C. Check responsiveness.

1. Shake shoulders.

2. Shout "Are you OK?"

D. Move to proper position.

1. Victim: flat on firm surface.

2. Rescuer: next to victim at approximately the same level.

Respiratory Management

A. Airway obstruction.

1. Food or other foreign body aspirant (if known cause of unconsciousness).

a. Tilt head—press backward on forehead and lift chin.

b. Attempt to ventilate will not be successful if obstructed.

c. If not successful, reposition head and reattempt to ventilate.

d. If not successful, presence of foreign body is assumed.

e. Turn client to one side and finger-probe for obstruction only if client is *not* breathing.

f. If this method proves unsuccessful institute Heimlich maneuver.

2. Heimlich maneuver—abdominal thrust.

a. Place client in sitting or standing position. Stand behind and place arms around waist of client.

b. Make a fist and place it halfway between xiphoid and umbilicus.

c. Place other hand on top of fist and perform a quick upward thrust.

d. Repeat this maneuver three more times before returning to first method of removing a foreign body.

e. Repeat entire procedure until open airway is obtained or advanced life support service is available.

3. Oral airway obstructants that are blood, emesis, mucus or water.

a. Turn head to side.

b. Suction (if available).

c. Finger swoops.

B. Open airway.

1. Adult.

a. Apply head-tilt method.

b. Apply jaw-thrust or chin-lift method (if neck injury even remotely possible).

2. Infant or toddler.

a. Tilt head back without hyperextension.

b. Use normal, horizontal alignment, flat surface.

C. Evaluate respiratory function.

1. Maintain open airway.

2. Observe for respiratory activity.

a. Put ear down near mouth.

b. Look for chest movement.

c. Feel for air flow with cheek.

d. Listen for exhalation.

D. Intervention.

1. Maintain open airway.

2. Form tight seal.

3. Adult management.

a. Replace victim's dentures (if any).

b. Pinch off nostrils.

c. Fit mouth-to-mouth seal.

4. Infant or toddler management.

a. Encircle nose and mouth.

b. Maintain tight seal.

c. Take fresh breath; do not allow complete deflation of lungs (stairstep volume).

d. Maintain position.

e. Assess volume: adult—800 cc minimum; infant—cheek full puffs.

5. Administer two full long breaths (1-1½ seconds).

a. Give breaths slowly to allow time for chest to expand.

b. Between breaths, release seal for exhalation.

Circulatory Management

A. Take major pulse.

1. Adult: carotid preferably (check for 5-10 seconds) and femoral as alternate.

2. Palpate one side, with two fingers, for five seconds.

B. If pulse absent begin CPR.

1. For adults.

a. Place hand on midline, lower half of sternum, two finger-widths above xiphoid.

b. Place heel of one hand on sternum, other hand superimposed.

c. Interlace fingers or extend off rib cage.

d. Rate 80 to 100 per minute, depth 1½ to 2 inches.

e. Count compressions: one-and, two-and, etc.

f. Release pressure between compressions for cardiac refilling.

g. Do not take hands off chest between compressions.

2. For children.

a. Place hand on midline sternum, midway between xiphoid process and cricothyroid notch.

b. Use heel of one hand only.

c. Rate 80 per minute, depth 1 to 1½ inches.

3. For infants.

a. Place fingers on midline sternum, midway between xiphoid process and cricothyroid notch.

b. Use two fingers only.

c. Rate 100 per minute, depth ½ to 1 inch.

d. Count compressions: one, two, three, four.

C. CPR protocol.

1. Shake and shout.

2. Open airway.

3. Look, listen, and feel for breathing.

4. Call code.

5. Ventilate patient with two slow breaths.

6. Check carotid pulse for 5 to 10 seconds.

7. Initiate CPR at 15 cardiac compressions to two ventilations at rate of 80-100 compressions per minute.

8. Check for carotid pulse after one minute. If absent, continue CPR.

Interpolation (Compressions: Ventilations)

A. Lone rescuer: (15:2 for adults, 5:1 for infants).

B. Two rescuers: 5:1 adults). Use 1½ second pause at each ventilation to allow adequate O_2 delivery.

C. Changing roles.

1. Compressor sets pace (one, one thousand, two, one thousand, three, one thousand, four, one thousand, breath).

2. Compressor observes for need and institutes change.

3. Compressor states, "Change, one-thousand; two, one-thousand."
4. Rescuer giving breaths gets into position to give compressions.
5. Rescuer giving compressions moves to victim's head after fifth compression, counts pulse for five seconds.
6. If no pulse, rescuer checking pulse states, "No pulse, start CPR," gives a breath, and CPR is begun again.

CPR Evaluation

A. In process.
1. Check major pulse after one minute of CPR.
   a. Equal to 4 sets of 15:2 by one rescuer.
   b. Equal to 12 sets of 5:1 by two rescuers.
2. Check major pulse every four to five minutes thereafter.
3. Pupil check every four to five minutes; optional if third trained person present (not always a conclusive indicator).
4. Observe for abdominal distention (all age groups).
   a. If evident, reposition airway and reduce force of ventilation.
   b. Maintain a volume sufficient to elevate ribs.
5. Ventilator must check carotid pulse frequently between breaths to evaluate perfusion.
6. Ventilator must observe each breath for effectiveness.
7. If respiratory arrest only, check major pulse after each minute (12 breaths) to ensure continuation of cardiac function.
B. After termination.
1. Diagnosis made (no pulse, no respirations) and intervention instituted within one minute after unconsciousness.
2. Assistance summoned and entry into Emergency Medical System done promptly and efficiently.
3. Proper CPR performed until acceptable termination.
4. No delay in CPR longer than five seconds (except extraordinary circumstances).
5. No delay in CPR longer than fifteen seconds for extraordinary circumstances (intubation, transportation down stairs).
6. Victim outcome.
   a. Condition.
   b. Potential for cardiac rehabilitation.
   c. Secondary complications (fractured ribs, ruptured spleen, lacerated liver, etc.).

Termination of CPR

A. Successful resuscitation.
1. Spontaneous return of adequate life support.
2. Assisted life support.
B. Transfer to emergency vehicle (other trained rescuers assume care).
C. Pronounced dead by physician.
D. Exhaustion of rescuer(s).

SURGICAL INTERVENTIONS FOR CARDIAC DISEASE

Cardiac Catheterization

Definition: Visualization of right and left sides of heart; visualization of coronary vessels (coronary angiography).

Assessment

A. Assess client's understanding of procedure.
B. Evaluate vital signs for baseline data.
C. Assess heart and lung sounds for baseline data.
D. Observe skin and mucous membranes for color.

Types of Catheterizations

A. Right heart.
1. Catheter is inserted through venous cutdown in antecubital vein or through femoral cutdown.
2. Catheter is threaded into right side of heart by way of superior vena cava.
   a. Measure oxygen saturation.
   b. Observe functioning of valves.
   c. Take pulmonary wedge pressure.
   d. Obtain chamber pressure.
B. Left heart—can be done by two methods.
1. Transarterial left catheter may be advanced retrograde across the aortic valve into left ventricle through the mitral valve into left atrium.
2. Brockenbrough transeptal catheter may be advanced through the femoral and external iliac veins and the inferior vena cava, to the right

atrium, and across into the left atrium.

    a. The needle inside the catheter penetrates the atrial septum to cross over from right to left atrium.

    b. Measurement is the same as for right heart catheterization.

    c. Selected coronary angiography may also be done.

3. Observe coronary blood flow.

4. Measure cardiac output and shunt flow.

Implementation

A. Obtain baseline data prior to test.

  1. History of allergy, especially shell fish.

  2. Assess characteristics of pulse, rate and rhythm.

  3. Identify respiratory pattern.

  4. Evaluate presence and characteristics of peripheral pulses.

  5. Obtain blood pressure.

B. Provide client teaching.

  1. Reinforce physician's explanation.

  2. Describe cath lab and equipment.

  3. Provide techniques to decrease anxiety and fear.

  4. Pretest medications.

C. Posttest: compare data with baseline data obtained prior to procedure.

  1. Notify physician if blood pressure is decreased by 10 percent from baseline.

  2. Take apical pulse to determine if arrhythmia is present.

  3. Record temperature and respirations to prevent infection and hemorrhage or cardiac tamponade.

D. Keep the leg straight with femoral insertion site.

E. Observe for signs of allergies to dye.

  1. Tachycardia.

  2. Erythema surrounding cutdown site.

  3. Nausea and vomiting.

  4. Shortness of breath.

F. Palpate pulses distal to catheter insertion site to observe for thrombophlebitis and vessel occlusion.

  1. Palpable pulses—bilateral and strong.

  2. Color—no cyanosis or blanching.

  3. Temperature of skin—warm.

G. Observe for signs of hemorrhage and shock.

H. Observe for complications.

  1. Respiratory complications—hypoventilation, hypoxia, pulmonary edema, and pneumonia.

2. Hemorrhage—apply pressure dressing and elevate extremity.

3. Thrombosis at cannulation site—notify physician if peripheral pulse is lost or if numbness, tingling, or coldness occurs.

4. Arrhythmias—if PVCs present, notify physician.

5. Cardiac tamponade—notify physician immediately.

Pacemaker Insertion

Definition: A temporary or permanent device to initiate and maintain heart rate when client's pacemaker is nonfunctioning.

Assessment

A. Assess client for conditions requiring pacemaker insertion.

  1. Conduction defect following open heart surgery.

  2. Heart block (usually third degree).

  3. Tachyarrhythmias.

  4. Stokes-Adams syndrome.

  5. Bradyarrhythmias.

B. Assess vital signs for baseline data.

C. Evaluate heart sounds to determine arrhythmias for baseline data.

D. Assess lung sounds for adventitious sounds.

E. Evaluate type of pacemaker inserted.

  1. External pacemaker—temporary, used in emergency situations.

    a. Pacing wire threaded through vein and attached to external power source.

    b. Used for heart block or bradycardia.

  2. Demand—functions only if client's own pacemaker fails to discharge, most common.

    a. The pacemaker is set at a fixed rate and will discharge only if client's own rate falls below it.

    b. Used mainly in Adams-Stokes or bradyarrhythmias or following cardiac surgery.

  3. Programmable pacemaker.

    a. Allows noninvasive adjustment of implanted pacemaker.

    b. Closely simulated normal cardiac electrical functioning.

F. Identify pacemaker placement.

  1. Epicardial — electrodes are implanted on outside of left ventricle, and they barely penetrate

myocardium. Battery pack is placed subcutaneously in a skin pocket.

2. Endocardial implantation—pacing electrode inserted through neck vein and placed near the apex of right ventricle.
   a. Permanent—battery is implanted beneath skin.
   b. Temporary—battery is located outside of skin.

Implementation

A. Observe for battery failure (pacemaker not firing as set).
   1. Faints easily.
   2. Hiccoughs.
   3. Rhythm change.
   4. Gradual decrease in pulse rate.
B. Observe for hematoma at site of insertion.
C. Observe for arrhythmias via cardiac monitoring.
   1. Competition from client's own pacemaker evidenced on rhythm strip.
   2. Absence of pacemaker artifact on rhythm strip.
   3. Premature ventricular contractions (PVCs) and ventricular tachycardia.
   4. Keep control box dry.
D. Monitor vital signs.
   1. Hemorrhage and shock.
   2. Cardiac tamponade.
   3. Infection.
E. Provide client teaching.
   1. Purpose for pacemaker.
   2. Medication dose and side effects.
   3. Method for utilizing and managing pacemaker.
   4. Monitoring pulse.
   5. Signs and symptoms of infection.
   6. No ROM on affected side for 3 days.
F. Counsel client to observe for pacemaker failure.
   1. Decreased urine output.
   2. Decreased blood pressure.
   3. Cyanosis.
   4. Shortness of breath.

Cardiac Surgery

Definition: Surgical procedures on the cardiac vessels or cardiac valves to prolong life for those who have heart disease.

Assessment

A. Assess type of open heart surgery to be done.

1. Coronary bypass surgery—healthy sections of a leg or chest blood vessel are grafted onto the blocked coronary artery.
2. Angioplasty—less invasive than bypass surgery and preferred when only one artery is involved.
   a. A catheter with a deflated balloon is threaded into artery at site of blockage.
   b. Balloon is inflated and widens artery by breaking up and compressing plaque against artery wall.
3. Commissurotomy of stenosed valve.
   a. Closed commissurotomy—finger inserted to dilate valvular opening.
   b. Open commissurotomy—dissection of scarred area by means of a scalpel.
4. Valve replacement: artificial, or prosthetic, valves; heterografts (porcine or bovine); homografts (human tissue or cadaver); autografts (client's own tissue).
B. Evaluate client's knowledge of operative procedure to prepare for preoperative teaching.
C. Assess vital signs, heart and lung sounds for baseline data.

Implementation

A. Observe for fluid and electrolyte imbalance.
   1. Obtain frequent lab specimens for hypokalemia and hyperkalemia.
   2. Measure CVP for hypovolemia and hypervolemia.
   3. Measure blood gases for acidosis and alkalosis.
   4. Measure hematocrit and hemoglobin for blood balance.
   5. Weigh daily.
B. Observe respiratory function.
   1. Place client on respirator for varying length of time postoperatively.
      a. Use endotracheal intubation with cuffed trach tube.
      b. Deflate cuff for five minutes each hour to prevent tracheal stricture.
   2. Suction at least every hour.
   3. Hyperinflate the lungs to prevent atelectasis (from anesthesia) every hour with respirator or ambu bag.
   4. Take frequent tidal volumes.
   5. Auscultate for abnormal lung sounds.
      a. Rales.
      b. Rhonchi.

C. Observe for cardiogenic shock.
1. Decreased blood pressure.
2. Tachycardia—thready pulse.
3. Absence of peripheral pulses.
4. Cardiac arrhythmias leading to arrest.
5. Decreased urine output.
6. Skin—cool, clammy, cyanotic.
7. Restlessness.
8. Central venous pressure above 15 cm water pressure (pulmonary edema).
9. Electrolyte imbalance.
D. Observe for signs of hemorrhage due to bleeders or coagulation disorders.
E. Place in semi-Fowler's position to facilitate cardiac and respiratory function.
F. Administer pain medication such as morphine sulfate IV.
G. Administer muscle relaxants such as Valium.
H. Monitor IV fluid and blood requirements by use of CVP, blood pressure readings, urine output.
1. Keep CVP between 5 to 15 cm water pressure or as directed by physician.
2. Keep urine above 30 cc/hour.
3. Hematocrit maintained at 35 to 40.
I. Maintain cardiac rhythm by use of antiarrhythmic drugs as necessary; Lidocaine prevents premature ventricular contractions.
1. Side effects include convulsions, respiratory arrest, and hypotension.
2. 50 to 100 mg IV bolus or 250 to 1000 mg in 500 cc D_5W. Do not administer more than 3 to 4 mg/minute.
J. Maintain blood pressure.
1. Sympathomimetics increase blood pressure.
   a. Adrenalin.
      (1) Increases cardiac output by increasing heart rate and myocardial contractility.
      (2) IV drip of 2 to 4 mg of Adrenalin in 500 cc D_5W titrated to keep blood pressure at desired level.
   b. Dopamine.
      (1) Stimulates heart by beta-adrenergic action.
      (2) Constricts resistance vessels by acting on alpha receptors.
      (3) Has a direct vasodilating effect on the kidneys and splenetic vascular bed.
   c. Isuprel.
      (1) Lowers peripheral resistance.
      (2) Causes increase in venous return leading to increase in cardiac output.
      (3) IV drip of 2 to 4 mg in 500 cc D_5W titrated to desired effect.
2. Antihypertensives (Arfonad).
   a. Quick-acting.
   b. Inhibits the transmission of nerve impulses through the sympathetic and parasympathetic ganglia.
   c. Produces peripheral vasodilatation.
   d. Administered via infusion pump in solution of 500 mg Arfonad to 500 cc D_5W. Begin at 0.08 to 0.1 mg/minute.
K. Maintain kidney function.
1. Keep urine output above 30 cc per hour with IV fluids or plasma expanders.
2. Administer diuretics to increase excretion of hemolyzed red cells caused by breakdown of the cell from cardiopulmonary bypass.
3. Maintain blood pressure above 90 systolic.
L. Maintain patent chest tubes.
1. Used to remove excessive fluid and air from chest cavity.
2. Connected to water-seal system.
3. Tubes should be milked frequently.
M. Maintain body temperature.
1. To raise body temperature.
   a. Thermal blankets, following hypothermic surgical procedure.
   b. Aqua K pads.
2. To decrease body temperature.
   a. Antipyretics to keep temperature below 100° F to prevent demands for increased cellular oxygen.
   b. Hypothermia blankets.
N. Assess level of consciousness.
1. Complications of coronary pulmonary bypass are air embolism or thrombus.
2. Depending on type of anesthesia used, client might awaken immediately upon return to recovery room or cardiac care unit, or remain unconscious up to several hours postoperatively.
   a. Neurological signs should be checked.
   b. All extremities should be checked for movement.
O. Administer anticoagulant therapy for valve replacements.
P. Monitor laboratory valves for anticoagulation.
1. Partial thromboplastin time or Lee-White clotting for heparin administration.

2. Prothrombin time for dicumarol therapy.

Q. Monitor for complications associated with valve replacement (in addition to common complications for any open heart surgery).
1. Conduction defects leading to arrhythmias.
2. Embolism resulting from the break-off of calcium deposits or from thrombus.
3. Hemorrhage.
4. Cardiac tamponade.
5. Supraventricular tachyarrhythmias.
6. Malfunction of prosthetic valve.

R. Monitor for complications associated with use of cardiopulmonary bypass.
1. Fluid and electrolyte imbalance.
2. Coagulation defects.
3. Pump fever—temperature rise after surgery without etiology.
4. Air embolism.
5. Thromboembolic disorders.
6. Renal failure due to clot formation or hypovolemia.
7. Postsurgery psychosis.
8. Postperfusion syndrome.

INFLAMMATORY HEART DISEASE

Bacterial Endocarditis

Definition: An infection of the lining of the heart caused by pathogenic microorganisms.

Characteristics

A. Acute—fulminating disease due to organisms engrafted on normal or diseased valve.
1. Occurs following open heart surgery or pulmonary infection.
2. Causative agents—group A nonhemolytic streptococcus, pneumococcus, and staphylococcus.

B. Subacute—slowly progressive disease from rheumatic or congenital lesions.
1. Occurs following dental, genitourinary, gynecological procedures.
2. Streptococcus most common organism.

Assessment

A. Observe for nonspecific causes—chills, diaphoresis, lassitude, anorexia, weight loss, arthralgia.

B. Check for fever and night sweats that recur for several weeks.

C. Assess for loud, regurgitant murmur or changing heart murmurs.

D. Identify history of recent infection, dental work, cystoscopy, IV drug addiction.

E. Assess for petechiae on skin or mucous membranes: tender, red nodules on fingers, palms, or toes.

F. Evaluate for systemic emboli.
1. Splenic infarction—pain, upper left quadrant, radiating to left shoulder.
2. Renal infarction—hematuria, pyuria, flank pain.
3. Cerebral infarction—hemiparesis or neurological deficits.
4. Pulmonary infarction—cough, pleuritic pain, dyspnea, hemoptysis.
5. Peripheral vascular—numbness and tingling in extremities.

G. Evaluate lab tests—increased WBC, ESR.

Implementation

A. Maintain intensive chemotherapy with antibiotic drugs for several weeks.

B. Follow general nursing measures.
1. Decrease cardiac workload—bedrest.
2. Ensure physical and emotional rest.

C. Encourage fluids.

D. Anticoagulant therapy contraindicated because of danger of cerebral hemorrhage.

E. Monitor for signs of CHF.

Pericarditis

Definition: Inflammation of the pericardium.

Assessment

A. Assess for possible cause of inflammation.
1. Transmural infarction—frequent cause.
2. Infection.
3. Hypersensitivity.
4. Trauma.
5. Neoplasms.

B. Evaluate type of pain—stabbing and knife-like; starts at sternum and radiates to neck and shoulder; aggravated by deep inspiration, supine position, and turning from side to side.

C. Observe for dyspnea, especially with deep inspiration.

D. Identify if pericardial friction rub is present.

E. Assess vital signs for indication of infection.

F. Evaluate lab tests—increased WBC, ESR, slightly elevated cardiac enzymes, and EKG changes (elevated ST segment).

Implementation

A. Maintain client on bed rest in semi-Fowler's position.

B. Administer and observe for side effects of salicylates and Indomethacin.

C. Monitor vital signs.

D. Monitor for pericordial friction rub on forced expiration with client in forward leaning position.

E. Relieve pain with analgesics.

F. Prepare client for pericardiocentesis if required.

G. Observe for complications following pericardiocentesis.
   1. Monitor vital signs and CVP for possible cardiac tamponade recurrence.
   2. Auscultate heart sounds to determine if decrease in intensity of heart sound is present.

H. Monitor for pericarditis complications.
   1. Pericardial effusion leading to tamponade.
   2. Constrictive pericarditis—prevents adequate diastolic filling of ventricles, leading to decreased cardiac output.

PERIPHERAL VASCULAR DISORDERS

Hypertension

Definition: Occurs when blood pressure is greater than 140 mm Hg systolically and 90 mm Hg diastolically.

Characteristics

A. Approximately 35 million people have disease in U.S.

B. Not linked to single etiology—heredity predisposes but environmental factors influence.

C. Twice as frequent in blacks. Higher incidence in white men than women before age 50; after age 50 this is reversed.

D. Risk factors.
   1. Age.
   2. Race.
   3. Obesity.
   4. Sex.
   5. Stress.

E. Type of hypertension.
   1. Primary or essential—no known etiology (accounts for 85–90 percent of clients).
   2. Secondary (accounts for 5–10 percent of clients).
      a. Renal disease.
      b. Endocrine disorders.
         (1) Pheochromocytoma.
         (2) Adrenal cortex lesions—aldosteronism, Cushing's syndrome.
      c. Coarctation of aorta.
      d. Toxemia of pregnancy.
      e. Acute autonomic dysreflexia.
      f. Increased intracranial pressure.

Assessment

A. Assess for risk factors by evaluating history.

B. Assess for common manifestations.
   1. Dizziness.
   2. Headache.
   3. Tinnitus.
   4. Flushed face.
   5. Epistaxis.

C. Identify if target organ involvement is present.
   1. Eyes—narrowing of arteries, papilledema (malignant hypertension), visual disturbances.
   2. Brain—mental and neurologic abnormalities, encephalopathy, CVA.
   3. Cardiovascular system—left ventricular hypertrophy and failure, angina, aggravation and acceleration of atherosclerotic process in coronary arteries and peripheral vessels.
   4. Kidneys—renal failure.

Implementation

A. Diet.
   1. Decrease sodium intake.
   2. Decrease calorie intake if overweight.

B. Drug therapy.
   1. Diuretics.
      a. Thiazides (Diuril, Esidrix, Enduron).
      b. Potassium sparing (Aldactone).
      c. Loop—potent diuretics (Lasix, Edecrin).
   2. Antihypertensives (Inderal, Aldomet, Catapres, Ismelin).

3. Vasodilators—Apresoline, Vasodilan.
4. Angiotension converting enzyme inhibitors.
C. Exercise—moderate; increase with reduced weight.
D. Assist client to utilize stress-reducing measures.
E. Educate client to decrease noncompliance.

Hypertensive Crisis

Definition: Hypertension that becomes acute and life-threatening. Diastolic pressure is usually over 120 mm Hg.

Assessment

A. Assess for severe symptoms.
1. Headache and confusion.
2. Drowsiness.
3. Vomiting.
4. Focal neurologic signs.
B. Monitor for potential complications.
1. Cerebral hemorrhage: symptoms same as for CVA.
2. Encephalopathy: headache, confusion, stupor, convulsions.
3. Heart failure (tachycardia, tachypnea, dyspnea, cyanosis).

Implementation

A. Monitor vital signs, ECG, and neurological signs closely.
1. Assess blood pressure q 5 min. with antihypertensive drug therapy.
2. Keep emergency drugs and resuscitative equipment readily available.
3. Monitor arterial pressure; rapid-acting antihypertensive agents require close monitoring of arterial pressure.
   a. Vasopressor if hypotension develops.
   b. Diuretics to maintain sodium diuresis.
B. Monitor parenteral therapy.
1. Administer all medication IV.
2. Assess for fluid overload.
C. Administer antihypertensive medications as prescribed.
1. Drugs frequently used are nitroprusside (Nipride), diazoxide (Hyperstat), and trimethaphan camsylate (Arfonad) because of their rapid-acting ability to work within a few minutes.
2. Drugs such as methyldopa (Aldomet) or hy-

dralazine hydrochloride (Apresoline) take longer to act and are used for long term therapy.
3. Potent diuretics such as furosemide (Lasix) and ethacrynic (Edecrin).
D. Monitor urinary output closely.
1. Indwelling urinary catheter may be indicated.
2. Oliguria or anuria should be reported immediately.
E. Maintain client on strict bedrest.
1. Elevate head of bed 45 degrees.
2. Place client in supine position if hypotension occurs suddenly due to medications.
3. Keep room quiet and free of unnecessary movement.
F. Support client and assist to remain calm.
1. Do not leave the client unattended.
2. Use anxiety-reducing measures—client may sense impending doom and be frightened.
G. Provide safety interventions.
1. Keep siderails up if client not fully alert.
2. Keep padded tongue blade at bedside for use according to hospital policy.
3. Place client on side if level of consciousness is diminished to prevent aspiration.
4. Keep suction equipment readily available.

Thromboangiitis Obliterans (Buerger's Disease)

Definition: The chronic inflammation of arteries and veins and secondarily of nerves. Process affects males under forty years of age.

Assessment

A. Observe for temperature and color changes (cyanosis); and for alterations in skin of lower extremities at rest and especially after exercise.
B. Evaluate type and severity of pain.
C. Evaluate presence of intermittent calf claudication.
D. Observe for decreased pulses.
E. Assess for cool, numb, tingling, or burning sensation of lower extremities.

Implementation

A. Encourage client to stop smoking.
B. Administer vasodilator drugs to increase blood supply to lower extremities.
C. Monitor peripheral pulses frequently.

D. Instruct client to prevent injury to feet and lower extremities to prevent complications.

E. Instruct client to maintain cleanliness of feet.

Raynaud's Disease and Phenomena

Raynaud's Disease: Primary vasospastic disorder of the small arteries caused by hypersensitivity to cold, release of serotonin, or congenital predisposition.

Raynaud's Phenomena: Intermittent episodes of small arteriole constriction in response to temperature or emotional changes.

Assessment

A. Raynaud's Disease.
 1. Intermittent arteriolar vasoconstriction evidenced by pain or coldness.
 2. Bilateral or symmetric numbness; tingling in hands.
B. Raynaud's Phenomena.
 1. Intermittent pallor, cyanosis, rubor, and changes in skin temperature in response to cold or strong emotion.
 2. Often related to underlying collagen or connective tissue disease.
 3. May be unilateral with severe changes.

Implementation

A. Encourage client to stop smoking.
B. Administer vasodilator drugs.
 1. Calcium channel blocker—nifedipine (Procardia). Causes coronary vasodilation by increasing myocardial oxygenation.
 2. Other drugs commonly used are Dibenzyline, Cyclospasmol, Tolazoline hydrochloride.
C. Encourage client to avoid precipitating factors such as cold temperature and emotional stress.
D. Wear warm clothing when in cold weather: boots, gloves, etc.
E. Surgical interventions: sympathectomy, femoropopliteal bypass grafting, amputation if severely impaired.

Deep Vein Thrombophlebitis

Definition: Formation of clot in a vein; occurs most often in left leg (due to right common iliac artery compressing left common iliac vein). Most prevalent sites: saphenous, posterior tibial, and peroneal veins.

Characteristics

A. Persons most vulnerable are from forty-five to sixty-five years of age.
B. Causes.
 1. Dehydration leads to increased cellular components in vessel.
 2. Decreased blood flow due to hypothermia and/or decreased metabolic rate during surgery.
 3. Injury to vessel during surgery.
C. Incidence most common following abdominal or circulatory surgery or fractures of leg or pelvis.
D. Use of oral estrogens.

Assessment

A. Assess for superficial vein thrombosis.
 1. Vein hard to the touch, edematous.
 2. Skin reddened, hot, tender.
 3. Induration along length of affected vein.
B. Assess for deep vein thrombosis.
 1. Leg swollen, tender, cyanosis.
 2. Increased temperature, pulse, white blood count, chills, malaise.
C. Palpate peripheral pulses for pressure. Use Doppler if necessary.
D. Evaluate for presence of Homan's sign.

Implementation

A. Maintain strict bed rest for seven to ten days.
B. Do not use knee gatch or pillows under knees.
C. Elevate lower extremities slightly, if ordered; raise entire foot of bed.
D. Administer thrombolytic and anticoagulant only after checking lab values. Observe for signs of bleeding.
E. Check for extension of clot.
 1. Breath sounds for possible emboli.
 2. Tenderness further up leg or in groin.
 3. Circulatory difficulties.
F. Position client to avoid venous stasis and turn every two hours.
G. Take vital signs at least every four hours.
H. Apply hot packs, if ordered, for two to three days.
I. Use range-of-motion exercises on unaffected limbs only.
J. Do not massage or exercise affected leg unless specified by physician.
K. Apply antiembolic stocking to unaffected leg.
L. Have client begin exercise gradually; first leg raises, then stand briefly every hour, then ambulate.

M. Medicate with salicylates and Butazolidin for pain control; watch for synergistic effect if anticoagulants are used.

N. Measure and compare leg circumference daily.

O. Provide client education.
1. Avoid standing in one position for any length of time (either walk or lie flat).
2. Avoid wearing constrictive clothing or garments.
3. Keep extremities at consistent, moderate temperature.
4. Wear support hose consistently.
5. Understand correct use of anticoagulants and the necessity for lab tests.
6. Do leg exercises when in bed.
7. Do not smoke.

Thrombolytic Agents

A. Action is to dissolve formed blood clots.

B. Stimulate conversion of plasminogen to plasmin (fibrinolysin).

C. Prescribed for acute pulmonary emboli, deep vein thrombosis, arterial thrombosis, and coronary thrombosis.

D. Agents.
1. Streptokinase; Urokinase.
2. Tissue plasminogen activator.

E. Major side effects.
1. Bleeding.
2. Ventricular dysrhythmias with coronary thrombosis.
3. Fever up to 100 degrees F.
4. Rash.

F. Contraindications for use.
1. Recent major surgery, GI bleed.
2. Uncontrolled hypertension.
3. Hepatic or renal disease.

G. Nursing management.
1. Obtain TT, APTT, PT, hematocrit and platelet count.
2. Infuse 250,000 IU over 30 minutes for loading dose.
3. Monitor infusion of 100,000 IU per hour (use controller or pump).
   a. 24 hours for pulmonary embolism.
   b. 24–72 hours for deep vein or arterial thrombosis.
4. Monitor closely for signs of bleeding.

Anticoagulant Therapy

A. Specific chemotherapeutic agents used to prevent intravascular thrombosis by decreasing blood coagulability.

B. Keep clotting time at one-and-a-half to two-and-a-half times normal.

C. Usual agents.
1. Heparin (IV sub q).
2. Coumadin (p.o.).

D. Pharmacological action.
1. Prevents fibrin deposits.
2. Prevents extension of a thrombus.
3. Prevents thromboembolic complications.

E. Major side effects of agents.
1. Hematuria.
2. Epistaxis.
3. Ecchymosis.
4. Bleeding gums.

F. Contraindications for use of drug.
1. Blood dyscrasia.
2. Liver and kidney disease.
3. Peptic ulcer.
4. Chronic ulceration colitis.
5. Active bleeding (except DIC).
6. Spinal cord or brain injuries.

G. Drugs and foods to avoid when on anticoagulant therapy.
1. Leafy green vegetables and foods high in vitamin K.
2. Salicylates.
3. Phenylbutazone.
4. Reserpine.
5. Steroids.
6. Barbiturates.

H. Safety precautions.
1. Observe for signs of bleeding (gums, hematoma, etc.).
2. Carry identification card.
3. Keep antagonist in close proximity.
4. Keep appointments for blood work.
5. Do not use straight edge razors or work with equipment that could cause injuries.

Heparin

A. Mode of administration: IV or sub q due to inactivation of drug when given orally.

B. Action.
1. Interferes with formation of thrombin from prothrombin.

2. Prevents thrombin from converting fibrinogen to fibrin.
3. Prevents agglutination and disintegration of platelets.
4. Dose lasts three to four hours if given IV.

C. Lab findings.
   1. Keep partial thromboplastin time (PTT) at 50 to 80 seconds (normal 39 to 53 seconds).
   2. Keep clotting time at 15 to 20 minutes (normal 9 to 12 minutes).

D. Antagonist.
   1. Protamine sulfate: 1 mg protamine sulfate for each 100 u of heparin in last dose.
   2. Effective within minutes.
   3. Anticoagulation therapy is reinstituted when needed.

E. Nursing management.
   1. Check PTT or clotting time before administration.
   2. Check patency of IV.
   3. Take following precautions when administering drug sub q into abdomen:
      a. Use small needle.
      b. Form pouch of skin no closer than 5 cm around umbilicus.
      c. Administer injection at 90-degree angle.
      d. Do not aspirate syringe and needle or massage skin around injection site to prevent ecchymosis.
      e. Keep protamine sulfate easily accessible.

Coumadin

A. Mode of administration: oral.
B. Action.
   1. Decreases prothrombin activity.
   2. Depresses hepatic synthesis of several clotting factors.
   3. Prevents utilization of vitamin K by liver.
   4. Takes 24 to 72 hours for action to develop and continues for 24 to 72 hours after last dose.
C. Lab findings.
   1. Keep prothrombin time at 18 to 30 seconds (normal is 12 to 14 seconds).
   2. 15 to 30 percent of normal activity.
D. Antagonist.
   1. Vitamin K—aquaMephyton IM or IV.
   2. Returns to hemostasis within six hours.
   3. Blocks action of Coumadin for one week.
E. Nursing management.

1. Check prothrombin time before giving.
2. Give at same time each day.
3. Teach client to avoid foods high in vitamin K (cabbage, cauliflower, spinach, and leafy vegetables).

Varicose Veins

Definition: A condition in which the veins are dilated because of incompetent valves.

Characteristics

A. Causes.
   1. Pregnancy.
   2. Standing for long periods of time.
   3. Poor venous return.
   4. Heredity.
B. Pathology.
   1. Veins are dilated and tortuous.
   2. Affects subcutaneous veins—saphenous veins.

Assessment

A. Assess for ache in legs; dull aching after standing.
B. Observe for edematous ankles.
C. Skin brown from blood that has escaped from overloaded veins.
D. Ulceration.

Implementation

A. Limit disease and prevent complications.
B. Maintain adequate blood supply to affected areas.
   1. Warmth.
   2. Cleanliness.
   3. Infection control.
   4. Avoidance of heat and cold extremes.
C. Educate client to see need for cessation of smoking.
D. Prevent constrictive clothing and positions; protect legs from pressure.
E. Prevent emotional stress.
F. Teach client to recognize extension of symptoms.
   1. Increase in pain in extremities.
   2. Changes in skin color.
   3. Ulceration.
   4. Change in temperature in extremities.
G. Have client recognize limitations caused by disease.
H. Encourage client to use antiembolic stockings.
I. Prepare client for vein stripping or sclerosing injections.

SURGICAL INTERVENTIONS FOR PERIPHERAL VASCULAR DISORDERS

Vein Stripping and Ligation

Definition: The ligation and removal of affected veins in the legs. Usually affects greater and lesser saphenous veins.

Assessment

A. Assess for completion of preoperative scrub.
B. Observe for physician's marks on veins.
C. Evaluate pulses for baseline data.
D. Assess client's knowledge of procedure and post-operative care.

Implementation

A. Have client scrub legs and lower abdomen once a day for three days prior to surgery.
B. Instruct on ambulation postoperatively.
C. Provide postoperative care.
D. Observe feet for edema, warmth, color (tight elastic bandages applied following surgery can impede circulation).
E. Evaluate peripheral pulses.
F. Elevate feet above level of heart.
G. Position flat in bed or have client walk. Do not allow client to dangle legs or sit in a chair for at least one week.
H. Ambulate early—five minutes every hour.
I. Following bandage removal, utilize elastic stockings.

Femoral Popliteal Bypass Graft

Definition: Prosthetic graft is anastomosed to the artery proximal and distal to the obstruction.

Assessment

A. Observe peripheral pulses for patency of graft.
  1. Check for presence of distal pulses.
  2. Check that extremities are warm and pink.
  3. Compare both extremities.
B. Check vital signs, particularly blood pressure.

Implementation

A. Mark areas on skin where pulses are palpated.
B. Monitor vasopressors for at least twelve hours.
C. Maintain blood pressure approximately 20 mm Hg above normal (keep suture line taut to prevent leakage).
D. Elevate foot of bed to prevent edema and promote arterial blood flow.
E. Do not allow flexion at hips (decreases blood flow).
F. Provide good skin care to prevent decubiti (poor vascularization).
G. Record accurate intake and output hourly for 24 hours.

Aortic Aneurysms

Definition: A localized abnormal dilatation of the vascular wall occurring most often in the ascending aorta and secondly in the aortic arch.

Characteristics

A. Caused by arteriosclerosis and syphilis.
B. Infections occur within vessel, trauma.
C. Highest incidence in older men.
D. High mortality if not surgically treated.
E. Major cause of death is spontaneous rupture.

Assessment

A. Evaluate symptoms to determine area involved.
  1. Thoracic aneurysm.
    a. Pain—sudden in onset with tearing or ripping sensation in thorax or anterior chest.
    b. Pain extends to neck, shoulders, lower back, or abdomen.
    c. Syncope.
    d. Pallor, perspiration.
    e. Dyspnea, increased pulse, cyanosis.
    f. Weakness, transient paralysis.
    g. Loss of pulses in affected extremities.
  2. Abdominal aneurysm.
    a. Pulsating mass in abdomen.
    b. Systolic bruit over aorta.
    c. Tenderness on deep palpation.
    d. Large aneurysm react as renal calculi, lumbar disc disease.
    e. Lumbar pain radiating to flank and groin indicates impending rupture.
B. Assess vital signs to obtain baseline data.
C. Evaluate peripheral pulses.
D. Assess intensity of pain.
E. Evaluate for dissecting aneurysms—simulates coronary occlusion.
  1. Originate in ascending aorta.
  2. Usually associated with severe hypertension.
  3. Pain described as tearing, referred pain.

Implementation

A. Maintain blood pressure with Arfonad or nitroprusside at below 140 systolic if aneurysm is dissecting.

B. Administer propranolol to decrease force of contraction.

C. Administer oxygen to prevent respiratory embarrassment.

D. Monitor fluid balance. Administer whole blood when needed.

E. Prepare client for immediate surgery if aneurysm is dissecting or for thoracic aneurysm. Abdominal aneurysm repair is not an emergency unless dissecting.

F. Provide postoperative nursing management.
   1. Follow same procedures as for open heart surgery if client has thoracic aneurysm.
   2. Observe circulatory status distal to graft site.
   3. Observe all peripheral pulses and temperature of extremities.
   4. Monitor renal function with accurate intake and output (cross clamp of aorta during surgery).
   5. Observe for emboli to brain or lung.
   6. Monitor neurological signs.
   7. Monitor for complications.
      a. Hypertensive preoperatively, but can easily become hypotensive due to excessive bleeding.
      b. Acute renal failure.
      c. Hemorrhage from graft site.
      d. Cerebral vascular accident.
      e. Paraplegia.
      f. Infection.

COMMONLY USED CARDIOVASCULAR DRUGS

Digitalis

A. Effects.
   1. Increases contractile force of heart (positive inotropism), which increases cardiac output in failing heart.
   2. Slows heart rate.
      a. Direct effect.
      b. Increases vagal tone and decreases sympathetic tone as heart failure lessens.
   3. Slows conduction through AV node.
   4. Increases automaticity which may cause many arrhythmias.

B. Uses.
   1. Congestive heart failure—increases contractility which in CHF reduces oxygen needs, increases cardiac efficiency, and reduces heart size.
   2. Supraventricular tachyarrhythmias—slows ventricular rate by slowing conduction of impulses through AV node.

C. Dosage—individualized to client and clinical situation (usually 0.25 mg q.d.).

D. Precautions.
   1. Hypokalemia predisposition.
   2. Renal failure predisposition to digitalis toxicity, especially with preparation of digoxin.
   3. Generally should not be given with AV block.

E. Major side effects.
   1. Cardiac.
      a. Arrhythmias, due to increased automaticity.
      b. Conduction disturbances—AV block.
   2. Gastrointestinal.
      a. Anorexia.
      b. Nausea and vomiting.
      c. Diarrhea.
   3. Others.
      a. Gynecomastia.
      b. Allergic reactions.

Calcium Blocking Agents

A. Effects.
   1. Inhibits the influx of calcium ions across cell membrane.
   2. Decreases heart rate as conduction is slowed through SA and AV nodes.
   3. Increases myocardial oxygenation by causing coronary vasodilation.
   4. Decreases peripheral vascular resistance by causing vasodilation of peripheral arteries.

B. Uses.
   1. Prescribed for angina.
   2. Utilized when beta blocker and nitrate therapy are not effective.

C. Agents and side effects.
   1. Cardizem (diltiazem hydrochloride)—nausea, edema, arrhythmia, headache.
   2. Procardia (nifedipine)—vertigo, nausea, peripheral edema, headache, and flushing.
   3. Calan, Isoptin (verapamil hydrochloride)—hy-

potension, peripheral edema, vertigo. (Verapamil is also being used to treat supraventricular arrhythmias.)

Coronary Vasodilators

A. Effects.
1. Dilates vascular smooth vessels.
2. Decreases peripheral arterial vascular resistance (afterload).
3. Decreases venous blood return to heart (preload).
4. Reduces myocardial oxygen consumption.
B. Uses—angina.
C. Side effects.
1. Flushed face.
2. Headache.
3. Vertigo and faintness.
4. Postural hypotension.
D. Agents.
1. Short acting.
   a. IV—Tridil, Nitrobid, Nitrostat.
   b. Sublingual—nitroglycerin.
   c. Topical—Nitrol.
   d. Oral—Nitrobid.
2. Long acting.
   a. Sublingual—Cardilate, Isordil.
   b. Oral—Peritrate, Sorbitrate.
   c. Topical disk—Nitrodisk, Nitro-Dur, Transderm.

Antiarrhythmic Drugs: Quinidine, Pronestyl, Lidocaine

A. Effects.
1. Increases recovery time of atrial and ventricular muscle.
2. Decreases myocardial excitability.
3. Increases conduction in cardiac muscle, Purkinje's fibers, and AV junction (exception: lidocaine).
4. Decreases contractility (exception: lidocaine).
5. Decreases automaticity.
B. Uses.
1. Quinidine—atrial fibrillation, atrial flutter, supraventricular and ventricular tachycardia, premature systoles.
2. Procainamide hydrochloride (Pronestyl)—premature ventricular systoles.
3. Norpace—premature ventricular contractions (uni-focal, multi-focal or coupling).

4. Xylocaine (lidocaine)—ventricular tachyarrhythmias.
C. Side effects.
1. Quinidine.
   a. Hypersensitivity, thrombocytopenia.
   b. Cinchonism—nausea, vomiting, diarrhea, tinnitus, vertigo, visual disturbances.
   c. Sudden death from ventricular fibrillation.
   d. Congestive heart failure due to negative inotropism.
   e. Conduction disturbances (not used in clients with conduction disturbances).
2. Pronestyl.
   a. Anorexia, nausea, vomiting, diarrhea.
   b. Systemic lupus erythematosus and agranulocytosis.
   c. Cardiac AV block (not used in clients with AV block).
   d. May be used in congestive heart failure due to less negative inotropic effect.
3. Norpace
   a. CNS—vertigo, syncope, fatigue.
   b. CV—hypotension, edema, weight gain, SOB.
   c. GI—nausea, vomiting, diarrhea.
   d. GU—urinary retention.
4. Lidocaine.
   a. CNS disturbances—drowsiness, paresthesias, slurred speech, blurred vision, seizures, coma.
   b. Cautious use in clients with liver disease or low cardiac output (metabolism of drug slowed).

Epinephrine (Adrenalin)

A. Effect: beta stimulation—increases heart rate and contractility.
B. Use: cardiac arrest most common.

Propranolol (Inderal)

A. Effect: blocks beta stimulation.
1. Decreases heart rate and contractility; that is, it decreases oxygen consumption.
2. Depresses automaticity of pacemakers and AV conduction.
3. Produces bronchoconstriction.
B. Uses.
1. To decrease ventricular rate from atrial flutter, fibrillation, and tachycardia.
2. To suppress ectopic arrhythmias, especially ventricular arrhythmias.

3. For angina.

C. Side effects—should not be used in AV block, bradycardia, congestive heart failure, or lung disease (bronchospasm).

Atropine

A. Effects: anticholinergic.
1. Increases rate of SA node.
2. Increases conduction through AV node.

B. Uses.
1. Symptomatic sinus bradycardia.
2. Partial AV block.

C. Side effects.
1. Inability to void, especially with prostate enlargement.
2. Dry mouth, skin, flushing, dilation of pupil.
3. Decrease in bronchial secretions.

Dopamine (Intropin)—Precursor of Norepinephrine

A. Effects.
1. Increases myocardial contractility.
2. Causes mild vasoconstriction.
3. Increases cardiac output and stroke volume.
4. Dilates renal vessels.

B. Uses.
1. Cardiogenic shock.
2. Chronic cardiac failure with congestive heart failure.

Dobutrex (Dobutamine Hydrochloride)

A. Effects.
1. Cardiac stimulation.
2. Increased cardiac output.
3. Reduces peripheral resistance.

B. Uses.
1. Organic heart disease.
2. Cardiac surgical procedures.

C. Side effects.
1. Arrhythmias, palpitations, increased heart rate.
2. Angina, chest pain.

Isoproterenol (Isuprel)

A. Effects: beta stimulation.
1. Increases heart rate, contractility, and oxygen consumption.
2. Decreases peripheral vascular resistance.

B. Uses.
1. Cardiogenic shock with high peripheral vascular resistance.

2. AV block—increases pacemaker automaticity and improves AV conduction.

C. Side effects.
1. Tachyarrhythmias, especially ventricular tachycardia.
2. Hypotension when hypovolemia is not corrected.
3. Headache, skin flushing, angina, dizziness, weakness.

Norepinephrine (Levophed)

A. Effects.
1. Alpha stimulation—peripheral vasoconstriction.
2. Beta stimulation mild.

B. Uses: cardiogenic shock with low peripheral resistance and normal cardiac output; requires careful monitoring of blood pressure.

C. Side effects.
1. Anxiety, headache.
2. Severe hypertension from overdosage.
3. Arrhythmias.
4. Infiltration into tissues, causing sloughing.

Antihypertensive Drugs

A. Purpose: reduce blood pressure to normal or near-normal without side effects.

B. Drugs.
1. Thiazides—when used in combination with other antihypertensive drugs, potentiate second drug.
2. Hydralazine (Apresoline).
   a. Effect: adrenergic blocker.
   b. Side effects: headache, tachycardia, and postural hypotension.
3. Methyldopa (Aldomet).
   a. Effect: decreases blood pressure.
   b. Side effect: postural hypotension.
4. Ganglionic blocking agents—pentolinium tartrate (Ansolysen), mecamylamine (Inversine).
   a. Effect: blocks parasympathetic and sympathetic ganglia.
   b. Side effect: postural hypotension.
5. Postganglionic blocking agents—guanethidine (Ismelin).
   a. Effect: blocks norepinephrine.
   b. Side effect: postural hypotension.
6. Diazoxide (Hyperstat).
   a. Effects: decreases peripheral vascular re-

sistance in all circulatory beds; affects arterial smooth muscles.
b. Use: hypertensive crisis only.
c. Administration: IV, rapidly.
d. Side effects: hypotension (rarely severe), GI disturbances, angina, atrial and ventricular arrhythmias, palpitations, headache, hyperglycemia, fluid retention due to reabsorption of sodium, propranolol potentiates action.

7. Sodium nitroprusside (Nipride).
a. Effect: acts on vascular smooth muscle causing peripheral vasodilation. Effect occurs in two minutes but it is transitory.
b. Administration: IV infusion.
c. Side effects: restlessness, agitation, muscle twitching, vomiting, or skin rash.

8. Captopril (Capoten).
a. The first of a new class of anti-hypertensive agents.
b. Effective for heart failure.
c. Works by suppressing the renin-angiotension-aldosterone system.
d. Serious adverse effects have been reported—must be used with discrimination under close medical supervision.
e. Warnings—proteinuria, agranulocytosis, hypotension.

Diuretics

A. Purpose: most diuretics block sodium reabsorption in proximal tubule of kidney and decrease ionic exchange of sodium in distal tubule, thereby eliminating water.
B. Drugs.
1. Thiazides.
a. Common preparations: chlorothiazide (Diuril), hydrochlorothiazide (Hydrodiuril), chlorthalidone (Hygroton).
b. Administration: oral and parenteral.
c. Advantages: potent by mouth; effective antihypertensives.

d. Disadvantages: electrolyte imbalances; loss of potassium.
   (1) Hyperuricemia and secondary aldosteronism.
   (2) Allergic reactions.
   (3) Hyperglycemia.
   (4) Hematologic complications.

2. Potassium-sparing agents.
a. Common preparations: spironolactone (Aldactone), triamterene (Dyrenium).
b. Administration: oral only.
c. Advantages. conserve potassium.
d. Disadvantages.
   (1) Usually not effective when used alone (best used with thiazides).
   (2) Electrolyte imbalance.
   (3) Gynecomastia and nitrogen retention.

3. Potent diuretics.
a. Common preparations: furosemide (Lasix), ethacrynic acid (Edecrin).
b. Administration: oral and parenteral.
c. Advantages: rapid, potent action useful in cases of severe pulmonary edema and refractory edema.
d. Disadvantages.
   (1) Allergic reactions.
   (2) Severe electrolyte imbalance (potassium and chloride loss).
   (3) Hypovolemia.
   (4) Hyperuricemia, secondary aldosteronism, hyperglycemia.

Afterload and Preload Drugs

A. Afterload—vasodilators (calcium channel blockers and apresoline).
1. Increase left ventricle stroke volume and cardiac output.
2. Decrease peripheral vascular resistance, pulmonary, and peripheral venous pressure.
B. Preload—vasodilators, diuretics, digitalis drugs.
1. Decreases venous blood return to heart.
2. Exerts force on ventricles to contract.

RESPIRATORY SYSTEM

The respiratory system is that body process which accomplishes pulmonary ventilation. The act of breathing involves an osmotic and chemical process by which the body takes in oxygen from the atmosphere and gives off end products, mainly carbon dioxide, formed by oxidation in the alveolar tissues.

ANATOMY OF RESPIRATORY SYSTEM

Upper Airway

A. Nasal passages.
  1. Filter the air.
  2. Warm the air.
  3. Humidify the air.
B. Nasopharynx.
  1. Tonsils.
  2. Eustachian tube: opens during swallowing to equalize pressure in the middle ear.
C. Oropharynx.
  1. Part of both the respiratory and digestive tract.
  2. Swallowing reflex initiated here.
  3. Epiglottis closes entry to trachea as foodstuff passes enroute to the stomach.

Lower Airway

A. Larynx.
  1. Protects the tracheobronchial tree from aspiration of foreign materials.
  2. Cough reflex initiated here, whether voluntary or involuntary.
  3. Houses the vocal cords, which are considered to be the dividing point between the upper and lower airways.
B. Trachea.
  1. Cylindrical structure.
  2. Extends from the cricoid cartilage into the thorax, branching into the right and left mainstem bronchi.

C. Right lung.
  1. Contains three distinct lobes: upper, middle, and lower.
  2. Lobes are divided by interlobar fissures.
D. Left lung.
  1. Contains two lobes—upper and lower.
  2. Lingula is part of the upper lobe but is sometimes referred to as the middle lobe of the left lung.
  3. Lobes are divided by one interlobar fissure.
E. Bronchi.
  1. Right mainstem bronchus (RMSB): shorter and wider than left bronchus; nearly vertical to trachea.
    a. Most frequent route for aspirated materials.
    b. Endotracheal tube might enter the RMSB if tube is passed too far.
  2. Left mainstem bronchus (LMSB): branches off the trachea at a 45-degree angle.
  3. The bronchi subdivide into bronchioles, terminal bronchioles, respiratory bronchioles, and alveoli.
F. Alveoli.
  1. Air cells in which gas exchange takes place: oxygen, carbon dioxide.
  2. House a substance known as surfactant, which keeps the alveoli expanded. Without surfactant the alveoli would collapse.
G. Pleura.
  1. The pleural fluid is a thin film of fluid, encasing each lung, which allows for a smooth, gliding motion between the lung and the chest wall.
  2. Even though this fluid is film-like, it would be difficult to pull it away from the chest wall (analogous to two glass slides with fluid between them; the slides move back and forth easily but are difficult to pull apart).

PRINCIPLES OF VENTILATION

Respiration

Definition: A process in which oxygen is transported from the atmosphere to the cells and carbon dioxide is carried from the cells to the atmosphere.

A. Respiration is divided into four phases.

1. Pulmonary ventilation.
2. Diffusion of oxygen and carbon dioxide between alveoli and blood.
3. Transportation of oxygen and carbon dioxide in blood to and from cells.
4. Regulation of ventilation.

B. Respiratory cycle.
   1. Inspiration (active process)—diaphragm descends and external intercostal muscles contract; alveolar pressure decreases, allowing air to flow into the lungs.
   2. Expiration (normally a passive process)—alveolar pressure increases, allowing air to flow from the lungs.

Respiratory Pressures

A. At inspiration the intra-alveolar pressure is more negative than the atmospheric pressure.
B. At expiration the intra-alveolar pressure is more positive, thereby pressing the air out of the lungs.
C. A negative pressure exists in the intrapleural space and aids in keeping the visceral pleura of the lungs against the parietal pleura of the chest wall. Lung space enlarges as the chest wall expands.
D. Recoil tendency of the lungs is due to the elastic fibers in the lungs and the surfactant.

Surfactant

A. Surface-active material that lines the alveoli and changes the surface tension, depending on the area over which it is spread.
B. Surfactant in the lungs allows the smaller alveoli to have lower surface tension than the larger alveoli.
   1. Results in equal pressures within both and prevents collapse.
   2. Production of surfactant depends on adequate blood supply.
C. Conditions that decrease surfactant.
   1. Hypoxia.
   2. Oxygen toxicity.
   3. Aspiration.
   4. Atelectasis.
   5. Pulmonary edema.
   6. Pulmonary embolus.
   7. Mucolytic agents.
   8. Hyaline membrane disease.

Compliance

A. Relationship between pressure and volume: elastic resistance. This is determined by dividing the tidal volume by peak airway pressure (V_t PAP). Total compliance equals chest wall compliance plus lung compliance.
B. Conditions that decrease chest wall compliance.
   1. Obesity—excess fatty tissue over chest wall and abdomen.
   2. Kyphoscoliosis—marked resistance to expansion of the chest wall.
   3. Scleroderma—expansion of the chest wall limited when the involved skin over the chest wall becomes stiff.
   4. Chest wall injury—as in crushing chest wall injuries.
   5. Diaphragmatic paralysis—as a result of surgical damage to the phrenic nerve, or disease process involving the diaphragm itself.
C. Conditions that decrease lung compliance.
   1. Atelectasis—collapse of the alveoli as a result of obstruction or hypoventilation.
   2. Pneumonia—inflammatory process involving the lung tissue.
   3. Pulmonary edema—accumulation of fluid in the alveoli.
   4. Pleural effusion—accumulation of pleural fluid in the pleural space compressing lung on the affected side.
   5. Pulmonary fibrosis—scar tissue replacing necrosed lung tissue as a result of infection.
   6. Pneumothorax—air present in the pleural cavity; lung is collapsed as volume of air increases.

Airway Resistance

A. Opposition or counterforce. Resistance depends on the diameter and length of a given tube (respiratory tract).
   1. Flow may be laminar (smooth) or turbulent.
   2. Resistance equals pressure divided by flow (Poiseuille's law).
B. Conditions that increase airway resistance.
   1. Secretions.
   2. Bronchial constriction.

Lung Volumes

A. Total lung capacity (TLC)—total volume of air that is present in the lungs after maximum inspiration.

B. Vital capacity (VC)—volume of air that can be expelled following a maximum inspiration.

C. Tidal volume (TV)—volume of air with each inspiration.

D. Inspiratory reserve volume (IRV)—volume of air that can be inspired above the tidal volume.

E. Inspiratory capacity (IC)—volume of air with maximum inspiration; comprises tidal volume and inspiratory reserve volume.

F. Expiratory reserve volume (ERV)—volume of air that can be expelled following a resting expiration.

G. Reserve volume (RV)—volume of air remaining in the lungs at the end of maximum expiration.

H. Functional reserve capacity (FRC)—volume of air remaining in the lungs at the end of resting expiration; comprises ERV and RV.

I. Forced expiratory volume$_1$ (FEV$_1$)—volume of air that is expelled within the first second of the vital capacity.

Alveolar Ventilation

Definition: The rate at which the alveolar air is renewed each minute by atmospheric air—the most important factor of the entire pulmonary ventilatory process.

A. Rate of alveolar ventilation.
   1. Alveolar ventilation is one of the major factors determining the concentrations of oxygen and carbon dioxide in the alveoli.
   2. Alveolar ventilation per minute is the total volume of new air entering the alveoli each minute equal to the respiratory rate times the amount of new air that enters the alveoli with each breath.

B. Dead space.
   1. Dead space air is the air that fills the respiratory passages with each breath.
   2. The volume of air that enters the alveoli with each breath is equal to the tidal volume minus the dead space volume.
   3. Anatomical dead space refers to volume of all spaces of the respiratory system besides the gas exchange areas (the alveoli and terminal ducts).
   4. Physiological dead space refers to alveolar dead space (occurring because of nonfunctioning or partially functioning alveoli) included in the total measurement of dead space.

   5. In the normal person anatomical and physiological dead space are equal because all alveoli are functional.

Oxygen and Carbon Dioxide Diffusion and Transportation of Respiratory Gases

Ventilation

A. The first phase in respiration is ventilation, which is the constant replenishment of air in the lungs.

B. Composition of alveolar air.
   1. Alveolar air is only partially replenished by atmospheric air each inspiratory phase.
      a. Approximately 350 cc of new air (tidal volume minus dead space) is exchanged with the functional residual capacity volume each respiratory cycle (FRC = 2300 cc).
      b. Sudden changes in gaseous concentrations are prevented when alveolar air is replaced slowly.
   2. Alveolar air contains more carbon dioxide and water vapor than atmospheric air.
   3. Alveolar oxygen concentration depends on the rate of oxygen absorbed into the blood and the ability of the lungs to take in carbon dioxide.
   4. Carbon dioxide content is likewise affected by the rate carbon dioxide is passed into the alveoli from the blood and the ability of the lungs to expire it.

Diffusion of Gases

A. The next phase is movement of oxygen from the alveolar air to the blood and movement of carbon dioxide in the opposite direction.

B. Movement of gases through the respiratory membrane depends on the following factors.
   1. Thickness of membrane.
   2. Permeability of membrane (diffusion coefficient).
   3. Surface area of the membrane.
   4. Differences in gas pressures in the alveolar and blood spaces.
   5. Rate of pulmonary circulation.

C. Blood low in carbon dioxide and high in oxygen leaves lungs.

D. Throughout the body there again is exchange of respiratory gases in the capillary beds.

1. Oxygen out of the blood and into the cells.
2. Carbon dioxide from cells into the blood.

Oxygen Transport in the Blood

A. About 3 percent of the oxygen is carried in a dissolved state in the water of plasma and cells.
B. About 97 percent is carried in chemical combination with hemoglobin in red blood cells.
   1. The percent of oxygen combined with each hemoglobin molecule depends on the partial pressure of oxygen (pO_2).
   2. The relationship is expressed as the oxygen-hemoglobin dissociation curve.
      a. It shows the progressive increase in the percent of the hemoglobin that is bound with oxygen as the pO_2 increases.
      b. When the pO_2 is high, oxygen binds with the hemoglobin, but when pO_2 is low (tissue capillaries), oxygen is released from hemoglobin.
      c. This is the basis for oxygen transport from the lungs to the tissues.
   3. Febrile states and acidosis permit less oxygen to bind with Hb, thereby limiting the amount of oxygen available for the tissues.
   4. The amount of oxygen that is available to the tissues depends on the oxygen content of the blood and the cardiac output.
C. Inadequate oxygen transport to the tissues—hypoxia.
   1. Hypoxic hypoxia: low arterial pO_2.
      a. Alveolar hypoventilation.
      b. Ventilation-perfusion inequalities.
      c. Diffusion defects.
      d. Fraction of inspired oxygen (FIO_2) is less than atmosphere, such as in high altitudes.
   2. Anemic hypoxia: decreased oxygen-carrying capacity to the blood.
      a. Anemia—less Hb; therefore, less oxygen is able to combine with it.
      b. Carbon monoxide poisoning—carbon monoxide combines with the Hb, preventing oxygen from combining with the Hb.
   3. Circulatory hypoxia: circulatory insufficiency.
      a. Shock—decreased cardiac output.
      b. Congestive heart failure.
      c. Arterial vascular disease—localized obstruction to arterial blood flow.
      d. Tissue need for oxygen surpasses supply available.
   4. Histotoxic hypoxia: prevents tissues from utilizing oxygen.

Carbon Dioxide Transport in the Blood

A. A small amount of carbon dioxide is dissolved in plasma and red blood cells in the form of bicarbonate.
B. Inside the red blood cells, carbon dioxide combines with water to form carbonic acid.
   1. It is catalyzed by the enzyme called *carbonic anhydrase.*
   2. The enzyme accelerates the rate to a fraction of a second.
C. In another fraction of a second carbonic acid dissociates to form hydrogen ions and bicarbonate in the red cells.
D. Carbon dioxide combines with the hemoglobin molecule.
   1. The hemoglobin molecule has given off its oxygen to the tissues, and carbon dioxide attaches itself.
   2. The venous system carries the combined carbon dioxide back to the lungs where it is expired.

Regulation of Respiration

A. Respiratory centers.
   1. Pons—two respiration areas: pneumotaxic and apneustic.
   2. Medulla oblongata—major brain area controlling rhythmicity of respiration.
   3. Spinal cord—facilitory role in maintaining respiratory center.
   4. Hering Breuer reflexes—stretch receptors located in lung tissue which assist in maintaining respiratory rhythm and prevent overstretch of the lung. Afferent fibers are carried in the vagus nerve.
B. Humoral regulation of respiration (chemical).
   1. Central chemoreceptors.
      a. Directly stimulated by an increase in hydrogen ion concentration (acidity) in the cerebral spinal fluid.
      b. An increase in arterial pCO_2 effects a rapid change in pH of the cerebral spinal fluid, increases the depth and rate of respiration, and decreases the pCO_2 level.

c. Changes in hydrogen ion and bicarbonate ion concentrations are not as quickly recognized as changes in the pCO_2 by the central chemoreceptors; therefore, responses to metabolic imbalances are slower.

d. Receptors are located in the medulla oblongata and adjacent structures.

2. Peripheral chemoreceptors.

a. Receptor cells are located in the carotid body at the bifurcation of the common carotid arteries and at the aortic arch.

b. Impulses from the aortic arch are transmitted to the brain via the vagus nerve.

c. Impulses from the carotid body are transmitted to the brain via the glossopharyngeal nerve.

d. The peripheral chemoreceptors primarily respond quickly to a decreased pO_2 (below 50 mm Hg) and to some extent to alteration of the pCO_2 and hydrogen ion concentration in the arterial blood.

System Assessment

A. Check for airway patency.
1. Clear out secretions.
2. Insert oral airway if necessary.
3. Position client on side if there is no cervical spine injury.
4. Place hand or cheek over nose and mouth of client to feel if client is ventilating.

B. Listen to lung sounds.
1. Absence of breath sounds: indicates lungs not expanding, due either to obstruction or deflation.
2. Rales (crackling sounds): indicate vibrations of fluid in lungs.
3. Rhonchi (coarse sounds): indicate partial obstruction of airway.
4. Decreased breath sounds: indicate poorly-ventilated lungs.
5. Detection of bronchial sounds that are deviated from normal position: indicates mediastinal shift due to collapse of lung.

C. Determine level of consciousness; decreased sensorium can indicate hypoxia.

D. Observe sputum or tracheal secretions; bloody sputum can indicate contusions of lung or injury to trachea and other anatomical structures.

E. Evaluate vital signs for temperature, respiratory rate, pulse, and changes in skin color.

F. Evaluate for tightness or fullness in chest.

G. Determine degree of pain client is experiencing.

H. Observe for PVCs if client is on monitor.

I. Assess for respiratory complications.
1. Assess for abnormal breathing patterns.
   a. Dyspnea—labored or difficult breathing.
   b. Hyperpnea—abnormal deep breathing.
   c. Hypopnea—reduced depth of breathing.
   d. Orthopnea—difficulty breathing in other than upright position.
   e. Tachypnea—rapid breathing.
   f. Stridor—noisy respirations as air is forced through a partially obstructed airway.
2. Evaluate cough.
   a. Normally a protective mechanism utilized to keep the tracheobronchial tree free of secretions.
   b. Common symptom of respiratory disease.
3. Assess bronchospasm.
   a. Bronchi narrow and secretions may be retained.
   b. Condition may lead to infection.
4. Observe for hemoptysis—expectoration of blood or blood-tinged sputum.
5. Assess for cyanosis—late sign of hypoxia, due to large amounts of reduced hemoglobin in the blood (PaO_2 of about 50 mm Hg).
6. Observe for hypoxia (anoxia)—a deficiency of oxygen in body tissues.
7. Evaluate for hypercapnia.
   a. Occurs when carbon dioxide is retained.
   b. High levels of oxygen depress and/or paralyze the medullary respiratory center.
   c. Peripheral chemoreceptors (sensitive to oxygen) become the stimuli for breathing.
8. Assess for presence of respiratory alkalosis or acidosis.

J. Assess for other system complications.
1. Evaluate for polycythemia—increase in RBCs as a compensatory response to hypoxemia.
2. Observe for clubbing of fingers. Pathogenesis is not well understood.
3. Evaluate for cor pulmonale—enlargement of the right ventricle as a result of pulmonary arterial hypertension following respiratory pathology.
4. Evaluate for chest pain.
5. Assess for atelectasis.

6. Check for abdominal distention.
7. Assess for hypertension.
8. Evaluate cardiac status: CHF, cerebral edema, arrhythmias.
9. Assess for trauma to thorax.
K. Assess oxygen concentration with noninvasive pulse oximetry.
   1. Sensor probe on earlobe, finger or toe registers light passing through vascular bed.
   2. Allows continual monitoring of arterial oxygen saturation.
L Assess for conditions associated with respiratory failure.
   1. Infectious diseases: tuberculosis, pneumonia.
   2. Obstruction of airway: pulmonary embolism, chronic bronchitis, bronchiectasis, emphysema, asthma, cardiac disorders leading to pulmonary congestion.
   3. Restrictive lung disease: pleural effusion, pneumothorax, atelectasis, pulmonary tumors, obesity.
   4. CNS depression: drugs, head injury, CNS infection.
   5. Chest wall trauma: flail chest, neuromuscular disease, congenital deformities.

Diagnostic Procedures

Radiologic Studies

A. Chest x-ray.
B. Lung scintigraphy: measures concentration of gamma rays from lung after intake of isotope.
C. Perfusion studies: outline pulmonary vascular structures after intake of radioactive isotopes IV.
D. Bronchography.
   1. An opaque substance is inserted into trachea, and an x-ray is taken of the tracheobronchial tree and lungs.
   2. Client is n.p.o. to prevent dangers of regurgitation and aspiration.

Bronchoscopy

A. A tube-like lighted scope to visualize the interior of the tracheobronchial tree.

B. Used as a therapeutic tool to remove foreign materials.
C. Procedure and nursing care.
   1. Place client supine with neck hyperextended.
   2. Postprocedure: check client's ability to control secretions.
   3. Observe for potential complications of laryngospasm, laryngeal edema, anesthesia complications, subcutaneous emphysema.
   4. Inform client to expect hoarseness and sore throat.

Biopsy of Respiratory Tissue

A. May be done by needle, via bronchoscope, or an open lung procedure biopsy.
B. Nursing care: observe for hemothorax and/or pneumothorax.

Thoracentesis

A. A needle puncture through the chest wall to remove air or fluid.
B. Used for diagnostic and/or therapeutic purposes.
C. Nursing care: observe for possible pneumothorax postprocedure.

Pulmonary Function Tests

A. Measure body's ability to mechanically ventilate and to effect gaseous exchange.
B. See Lung Volumes under Principles of Ventilation.

Tuberculin Skin Test

A. Mantoux intradermal test (more reliable).
   1. Tuberculin injected intradermal, intermediate PPD.
   2. Test read 48 to 72 hours postintradermal wheal production.
   3. Erythema not important.
   4. Area of induration more than 10 mm: indicates positive reaction (client has had contact with the tubercle bacillus).
   5. Reactions of 5 to 9 mm require retest.
B. Tine test.
   1. Not recommended for diagnosis.
   2. Test read on third day.
   3. Mantoux test if induration more than 2 mm.

Arterial Blood Studies

A. Arterial blood gases.
   1. Indicate respiratory function by measuring:
      a. Oxygen (pO_2).
      b. Carbon dioxide (pCO_2).
      c. pH.
      d. Oxygen saturation and bicarbonate (HCO_3).
   2. Determine state of acid-base balance.
   3. Reveal the adequacy of the lungs to provide oxygen and to remove carbon dioxide.
   4. Assess degree to which kidneys can maintain a normal pH.
B. Normal arterial values.
   1. Oxygen saturation: 93 to 98 percent.
   2. PaO_2: 95 mm Hg.
   3. Arterial pH: 7.35 to 7.45 (7.4).
   4. pCO_2: 35 to 45 mm Hg (40).
   5. HCO_3 content: 23 to 27 mEq (25).
   6. Base excess: -3 to $+3$ (0).

System Planning and Analysis

A. Breath sounds clearer to auscultation. Decreased rales and/or rhonchi. No adventitious sounds auscultated.
B. Shortness of breath reduced.
C. Coughing is more productive/effective.
D. Respiratory rate decreased; ventilation and air exchange increased.
E. Potential complications minimized.
F. Correction of hypoxic condition so that client is adequately oxygenated.
   1. Arterial pO_2 returns to normal range.
   2. Improved vital capacity and pulmonary ventilation.
   3. Increased tissue oxygenation (pink color).
G. Client's energy is conserved.
   1. Abdominal breathing is more automatic and respirations are more efficient and relaxed.
   2. Clients with chronic lung disease experience increased comfort and breathing efficiency.
H. Closed water-seal drainage is maintained, drainage is evacuated, and lung reexpanded.
I. If necessary, a route is established for mechanical ventilation.
J. An artificial airway is provided when upper airway is obstructed.
K. For clients with chronic obstructive lung disease, a route is established for long-term ventilatory assistance.
   1. Anatomic dead space is decreased.
   2. Pulmonary toilet with hyperinflation of lungs is accomplished.
   3. Effective treatment for atelectasis or other pulmonary complications is provided.

System Implementation

A. Maintain patent airway.
   1. Suction.
   2. Intubation.
      a. Oral airway.
      b. Endotracheal intubation.
B. Maintain adequate ventilation.
   1. If client needs help breathing, a ventilator may be used.
      a. Ventilator simulates breathing action usually provided by diaphragm and thoracic cage.
      b. Type of ventilator depends on specific needs of client.
   2. Ventilators are classified by function based on cycles and delivery.
C. Administer oxygen therapy using specific oxygen equipment according to the percentage of oxygen required by client.
D. Monitor blood gases to determine how well client's oxygen needs are being met.
E. Maintain fluid and electrolyte balance.
   1. When blood and fluid loss is replaced, watch carefully for fluid overload, which can lead to pulmonary edema.
   2. Record intake and output.
F. Maintain acid-base balance; make frequent blood gas determination as acid-base imbalances occur readily with compromised respirations or with mechanical ventilation.
G. Provide for relief of pain.
   1. Analgesics should be used with caution as they depress respirations. (Demerol is the drug of choice.)
   2. Atropine, morphine sulfate, and barbiturates should be avoided.
   3. Nerve block may be used.
H. Administer electrocardiogram to establish if there is associated cardiac damage.

I. Provide for chest physiotherapy.
J. Maintain hydration status.
   1. Necessary to liquefy secretions or prevent formation of thick, tenacious secretions.
   2. Monitor oral intake of fluids, IV administration of fluids, or humidification to tracheobronchial tree.
K. Administer appropriate drug therapy for respiratory condition.

System Evaluation

A. Respiratory status is maintained.
B. Vital capacity and pulmonary ventilation are improved, and tissue oxygenation is increased.
C. Client's energy is conserved.
D. Secretions are loosened, and lungs are fully expanded.
E. Client is able to breathe deeply, and shortness of breath is reduced.
F. Breath sounds are clear to auscultation with no apparent adventitious sounds.
G. Client is able to cough without assistance, and coughing is productive.
H. Arterial pO_2 returns to normal range, and correction of hypoxic condition occurs.
I. Client experiences increased comfort, and anxiety level is decreased.

INFECTIOUS DISEASES

Pulmonary Tuberculosis

Definition: Airborne, infectious, communicable disease thought to be caused by *Mycobacterium tuberculosis*. May affect any part of the body, but is most common in the lungs. Disease may be acute or chronic.

Characteristics

A. Tubercle bacilli is rod-shaped and gram-positive, acid fast.
B. Diagnostic findings.
   1. Early AM sputum for stain and culture: positive acid-fast bacillus.
   2. Fiberoptic bronchoscopy and chest x-ray (to determine presence and extent of TB).
   3. Increased WBC and ESR.
   4. Mantoux skin test: positive.
      a. Purified protein derivative (PPD) tuberculin antigen.
      b. PPD tuberculin injected intradermally to form wheal 6–10 mm.
      c. Test read 48–72 hours: significant induration is 10 mm diameter or more. Results mean client has had contact—does not signify active disease is present. Insignificant reaction is induration less that 10 mm.
C. Most people infected do not develop clinical illness because the immune system brings infection under control.
D. Persons at risk: persons with HIV, the elderly, certain minority groups, persons in close contact with infectious TB, or who have live dormant bacilli from an initial infection acquired years before.
E. Pathophysiology.
   1. Inhaled droplets containing the bacteria infect the alveoli that become the focus of infection.
   2. After entrance of tubercle bacilli, the body attempts to wall off the organism by phagocytosis and lymphocytosis.
   3. Macrophages surround the bacilli and form tubercles.
   4. Tubercles go through the process of caseation—a necrotic process. (Cells become an amorphous cheese-like mass and may be encapsulated to form a nodule.)
   5. Caseous nodule erodes and sputum is released leaving an air-filled cavity.
   6. Initial lesion may disseminate by extension, via bloodstream or lymph system, and through bronchi.

Assessment

A. Evaluate pulmonary symptoms.
   1. Cough (at cavitation stage).
   2. Sputum production—initially dry, then purulent.
   3. Dyspnea.
   4. Hemoptysis.
   5. Pleuritic pain (with pleural involvement).
   6. Rales.
B. Evaluate systemic symptoms.
   1. Fatigue, malaise.
   2. Night sweats, low-grade fever in afternoon.
   3. Weight loss.
   4. Anorexia.
   5. Irritability, lassitude.
   6. Tachycardia.
C. Complete physical examination.
D. Complete social and medical history.
E. Examine sputum—takes 3–8 weeks for results.
F. Check tuberculin test.

Implementation

A. Maintain respiratory precautions.
  1. Client not considered infectious 2–4 weeks after initiation of chemotherapy.
  2. Teach client methods to prevent spread of droplets when coughing.
B. Monitor administration of medications.
  1. A combination of drugs used to destroy variable microbial organisms.
  2. Current regimen is 2 months of isoniazid (INH), rifampin (RIF), and pyrazinamide (PYZ) followed by 4 months of isoniazid and rifampin. Streptomycin and Ethambutol are also recommended for initial treatment.
     a. Six months of drug therapy is usually sufficient for killing the bacilli. Treatment may continue for 1 year; at least 9 months for HIV positive.
     b. Sputum smears obtained every 2–4 weeks until negative (sputum cultures become negative in 3–5 months).
  3. Second-line drugs used for resistant clients: capreomycin, kanamycin, para-aminosalicylic acid, and cycloserine.
  4. Drugs more effective when administered in single daily dose.
  5. Drug resistance is a problem, especially in Asians.
  6. Corticosteroids may be used together with antituberculosis agents in severe cases to reduce symptoms.
C. Chemoprophylaxis.
  1. Isoniazid and vitamin B_6 therapy for 6 months to 1 year given to those infected with tubercle bacillus without the disease or to those at high risk for development of the disease.
  2. Evaluate for potential complications of INH therapy: liver dysfunction and liver damage.
     a. Check for fatigue, loss of appetite, joint pain, dark urine, fever, right upper quadrant tenderness, nausea, and vomiting.
     b. Encourage client to report for frequent prescribed liver function studies.
D. Work with client to maintain compliance—the major problem in eliminating TB.
  1. Strict compliance to drug regimen.
  2. Monthly follow-up visits for sputum smear until conversion.
E. Instruct client in ways to prevent spread of disease.
  1. Cover nose and mouth with a few layers of disposable tissue when sneezing or coughing.
  2. Expectorate into a disposable sputum container.
  3. Maintain adequate air ventilation.
F. Decontaminate infected air by nonrecirculated air or ultraviolet rays.
G. Provide well-balanced diet: high carbohydrate, high protein, high vitamin B_6.
H. Provide frequent oral hygiene.

Pneumonia

Definition: An acute inflammatory process of the alveolar spaces resulting in a lung consolidation as the alveoli fill with exudate.

Assessment

A. Evaluate for type of pneumonia.
  1. Bacterial pneumonias.
     a. Lobar.
        (1) Pneumococcus is the most common organism.
        (2) Communicable disease.
        (3) Young males most affected.
        (4) Clinical manifestations.
           (a) Rapid onset, severe chills, high temperature (103° to 106°F, reduced by crisis).
           (b) Constant dry, hacking cough.
           (c) Pleuritic pain.
           (d) Anxiety.
           (e) Dyspnea.
           (f) Sputum—watery to rust-colored.
     b. Bronchopneumonia.
        (1) Strep and staph common organisms.
        (2) Aspiration frequently of this type (food, chemical, smoke, oil).
        (3) Secondary to other conditions such as age, debilitation, stasis.
        (4) Common in very young and very old.
        (5) Clinical manifestations.
           (a) Temperature—101° to 103° F (reduced by lysis).
           (b) Cough productive—yellow or green sputum.
  2. Atypical pneumonia.
     a. Known etiology—rickettsial: Q fever, Rocky Mountain spotted fever, psittacosis.
     b. Nonspecific etiology—known as "walking pneumonia."
        (1) Found in common living conditions.
        (2) Most common in young adults.

(3) Temperature not usually above 99° F (reduced by lysis).
(4) Clinical manifestations.
   (a) Malaise.
   (b) Fatigue.
   (c) Chills.
   (d) Cough—usually nonproductive ("goose honk").
   (e) Sputum—clear or white (if productive).
B. Assess for exacerbation of chronic obstructive pulmonary disease as respiratory infections precipitate this condition.
C. Observe for an increase in the amount of sputum.
  1. Change in the character of sputum (particularly color—yellow to green).
  2. Onset of malaise or febrility may indicate infection.

Implementation

A. Maintain bed rest until temperature is normal.
B. Limit visitors.
C. Force fluids to 3000 cc or more to provide hydration.
D. Observe and record type and amount of sputum.
E. Administer antibiotics as ordered.
  1. Given for a period of 10 to 14 days.
  2. Antibiotics most commonly used are ampicillin and tetracycline.
F. Provide physiotherapy as ordered.
G. Obtain throat, sputum, and blood cultures for specific organisms.
H. Administer oxygen at 6 l/minute unless COPD.
I. Administer antipyretic drugs.

Hypoxic Condition

Definition: Oxygen deficiency—the primary indication for initiation of oxygen therapy.

Assessment

A. Check to see if client has a patent airway.
B. Assess client's vital signs.
C. Observe existence of PVCs if client is on monitor.
D. Observe client for any of the following signs. If these signs are evident, you may need to administer oxygen.
  1. Tachycardia.
  2. Gasping and/or irregular respirations (dyspnea).
  3. Restlessness.
  4. Flaring nostrils.
  5. Cyanosis.
  6. Substernal or intercostal retractions.
  7. Increased blood pressure followed by decreased blood pressure.
  8. Abnormal ABGs.
E. Evaluate for stages of hypoxia.
  1. Early symptoms.
    a. Restlessness.
    b. Headache, visual disturbances.
    c. Slight confusion.
    d. Hyperventilation.
    e. Tachycardia.
    f. Hypertension.
    g. Dyspnea.
  2. Late symptoms.
    a. Hypotension.
    b. Bradycardia.
    c. Metabolic acidosis (production of lactic acid).
  3. Chronic oxygen lack.
    a. Polycythemia.
    b. Clubbing of fingers and toes.
    c. Thrombosis.
F. Assess for side effects of oxygen therapy.
  1. Atelectasis.
    a. Nitrogen is washed out of the lungs when a high FIO_2 is delivered to client.
    b. In alveoli free of nitrogen, oxygen diffuses out of the alveoli into the blood faster than ventilation brings oxygen into the alveoli.
    c. This results in a collapse (atelectasis) of the affected alveoli.
  2. Pulmonary oxygen toxicity.
    a. High FIO_2 delivered over a long period of time (48 hours) results in destruction of the pulmonary capillaries and lung tissue.
    b. The clinical picture resembles that of pulmonary edema.
  3. Retrolental fibroplasia.
    a. Blindness resulting from high FIO_2 delivered to premature infants.
    b. This condition is seen in prolonged FIO_2 of 100 percent when high levels of oxygen not needed.
  4. Carbon dioxide narcosis.
    a. Carbon dioxide narcosis can develop if hypoxic drive is removed by administering

FIO$_2$ to return the arterial pO$_2$ to normal range.

  b. Symptoms of carbon dioxide narcosis.
    (1) Comatose.
    (2) Flushed, pink skin.
    (3) Flaccid (sometimes twitching) extremities.
    (4) Shallow breathing.
G. Evaluate client for clinical manifestations of COPD.
  1. Ventilatory drive is hypoxemic.
  2. Oxygen administration requires critical observation. Start at 2 l/minute.

Implementation

A. Monitor lung sounds for adequate ventilation.
B. Monitor client for signs of oxygen toxicity.
C. Provide skin care for areas surrounding oxygen equipment.
D. Administer oxygen at appropriate flow with specified equipment.
  1. Nasal prongs and cannula.
    a. Easily tolerated by clients.
    b. The FIO$_2$ will vary depending on the flow.
      (1) FIO$_2$: 24–28%.   Flow: 1–2 l.
      (2) FIO$_2$: 30–35%.   Flow: 3–4 l.
      (3) FIO$_2$: 38–44%.   Flow: 5–6 l.
  2. Mask without reservoir bag.
    a. Requires fairly high flows to prevent rebreathing of carbon dioxide.
    b. Accurate FIO$_2$ difficult to estimate.
      (1) FIO$_2$: 35–45%.   Flow: 8–12 l.
      (2) FIO$_2$: 45–55%.   Flow: 8–12 l.
      (3) FIO$_2$: 55–65%.   Flow: 8–12 l.
  3. Mask with reservoir bag.
    a. Higher FIO$_2$ is delivered because of the reservoir.
    b. At flows less than 6 l/minute, risk of rebreathing carbon dioxide increases.
      (1) FIO$_2$: 50–60%   Flow: 6 l.
      (2) FIO$_2$: 60–70%.   Flow: 7 l.
      (3) FIO$_2$: 70–100%.   Flow: 8–10 l.
  4. Venturi mask.
    a. Delivers fixed or predicted FIO$_2$.
    b. Utilized effectively in clients with COPD when accurate FIO$_2$ is necessary for proper treatment.
      (1) FIO$_2$: 24%.   Flow: 2–4 l.
      (2) FIO$_2$: 28%.   Flow: 4–6 l.
      (3) FIO$_2$: 35%.   Flow: 6–8 l.

  5. Face tent.
    a. Well-tolerated by clients but sometimes difficult to keep in place.
    b. Convenient for providing humidification with compressed air in conjunction with nasal prongs.
    c. FIO$_2$: 35–50%.   Flow: 8–10 l.
  6. Oxygen hood.
    a. Hood fits over child's head.
    b. Provides warm, humidified oxygen at high concentrations.
    c. FIO$_2$: 40–85%.   Flow: 5–12 l.
  7. Intratracheal oxygen device for long-term therapy.

CHRONIC OBSTRUCTIVE PULMONARY DISEASE (COPD)

Definition: A functional category applied to respiratory disorders that obstruct the pathway of normal alveolar ventilation either by spasm of the airways, mucus secretions, or changes in airway and/or alveoli.

Chronic Bronchitis

Definition: A long-term inflammation of the mucous membrane of the bronchial tubes with recurrent cough and sputum production.

Characteristics

A. Cigarette smoking is probably the biggest culprit, inhibiting the ciliary activity of the bronchi, and resulting in increased stimulation of the mucous glands to secrete mucus.
B. Immunological factors and familial predisposition may also be implicated for those individuals who do not smoke.

Assessment

A. Assess for bronchoconstriction.
B. Evaluate malaise.
C. Check for exertional dyspnea.
D. Assess for hemoptysis.
E. Evaluate cough—may not be productive but may be purulent.
F. Assess for hypoxia.
G. Evaluate lung fields for the following:
  1. Atelectasis.
  2. Percussion—hyperresonant.

3. Tactile fremitus decreased.
4. Prolonged expiratory phase.
5. Expansion decreased.
6. Trachea midline.
7. Wheezes, rales.

Implementation

A. Administer antibiotics when infection occurs.
B. Administer bronchodilators to relieve broncho-spasm and facilitate mucus expectoration.
C. Force fluids to 3000 cc daily.
D. Provide chest physiotherapy.
E. Monitor oxygen therapy.

Bronchiectasis

Definition: Thought to develop following airway obstruction or atelectasis as a result of disease, such as tuberculosis, or infection, such as pneumonia.

Assessment

A. Evaluate for frequent, severe paroxysms of coughing.
B. Assess for hemoptysis.
C. Check for fetid breath.
D. Assess for thick, profuse sputum.
E. Observe for breathlessness, fatigue.
F. Assess for profuse night sweats.
G. Assess for weight loss, anorexia.
H. Evaluate lung fields and chest for the following:
   1. Trachea deviates to the affected side.
   2. Decreased expansion.
   3. Percussion—dull.
   4. Vocal fremitus and breath sounds absent if bronchus occluded.
   5. Vocal fremitus increased; bronchovesicular/bronchial breath sounds if bronchus open.
   6. Rales, rhonchi.

Implementation

A. Administer antibiotics as ordered. Usually given for 7 to 10 days.
B. Provide chest physiotherapy.
C. Administer bronchodilators to assist in removal of secretions.
D. Monitor oxygen therapy if hypoxia occurs.
E. Prepare client for surgery if severe hemoptysis occurs.

F. Encourage client to rest by providing quiet environment.
G. Provide high-protein diet with increased fluid intake.
H. Provide frequent mouth care.

Emphysema

Definition: The permanent overdistention of the alveoli with resulting destruction of the alveolar walls. (Emphysema is a Greek word meaning "overinflated.")

Assessment

A. Alpha, antitrypsin deficiency causes condition to develop at a younger age.
B. Observe for dyspnea—chief complaint.
C. Assess sputum production.
D. Observe for weight loss.
E. Assess for hypoxia, hypercapnia.
F. Observe for barrel chest.
G. Observe if expansion decreased.
H. Assess for flat diaphragm.
I. Observe if accessory muscles of respiration are used.
J. Assess for decreased tactile fremitus.
K. Percuss for hyperresonance.
L. Auscultate for distant breath sounds.
M. Assess for prolonged expiratory phase.
N. Assess for wheezes, forced expiratory rhonchi.
O. Assess for complications.
   1. Pulmonary hypertension.
   2. Right-sided heart failure.
   3. Spontaneous pneumothorax.

Implementation

A. Monitor for signs of impending hypoxia.
B. Monitor for alterations in lung sounds.
C. Instruct on pursed lip breathing exercises.
D. Administer low concentration oxygen. Usually 2 l/min.
E. Monitor for signs of carbon dioxide narcosis.
F. Provide hydration.
   1. Necessary to liquefy secretions present, or to prevent formation of thick, tenacious secretions in clients with pulmonary disease.
   2. Modalities.
      a. Oral intake of fluids.
      b. IV administration of fluids.

c. Humidification to tracheobronchial tree via face tent or aerosol mask, using compressed air.

3. Humidification and aerosol therapy.
   a. Humidity.
      (1) Water content of a gas at a given temperature.
      (2) Humidification can be delivered through humidifier or nebulizer.
   b. Aerosol.
      (1) Suspension of water particles in a gas medium.
      (2) Nebulizers deliver aerosols.
   c. Clinical implications.
      (1) Relief of bronchospasm and mucosal edema.
      (2) Mobilization of secretions.
      (3) Administration of medications such as bronchodilators, mucolytics, detergents, and selected antibiotics.
      (4) Humidification of the tracheobronchial tree.

Positions for Chest Physiotherapy
- To affect RUL and LUL, place client in upright position.
- To affect RML, position client on left side with head slanted down, right shoulder one-quarter turn onto pillow. Cup anteriorly over left nipple.
- To affect lingula LL, position client on right side with head slanted down, left shoulder one-quarter turn onto pillow. Cup anteriorly over left nipple.
- To affect RLL and LLL, place client in Trendelenburg's position, alternating sides, or prone.

G. Provide for chest physiotherapy.
   1. Postural drainage.
      a. Positions are utilized to promote gravitational drainage and mobilization of secretions of affected lung segments.
      b. This allows the client to expectorate them.
      c. They may also be aspirated through a sterile suctioning procedure.
   2. Cupping and vibration.
      a. Valuable and necessary adjunct to postural drainage.
      b. Vibration of the chest is performed only during the expiratory phase of respiration.
   3. Deep breathing and coughing.
      a. Should be encouraged often.

b. Clients with COPD should be taught the mechanics of an effective cough.
   (1) Contract intercostal muscles.
   (2) Contract diaphragm.
   (3) Fill lungs with air.

4. Breathing exercises or exercise regimen—an integral part in the management of clients with pulmonary disease.
   a. Diaphragmatic breathing.
      (1) Breathe in via nose.
      (2) Exhale through slightly pursed lips.
      (3) Contract abdominal muscles while exhaling.
      (4) Chest should not move, but abdomen should do the moving. (Abdomen contracts at expiration.)
      (5) Exercises can be learned with client flat on back and then done in other positions.
   b. Accelerated diaphragmatic breathing.
   c. Chest expansion—apical, lateral (unilateral, bilateral), basal.
   d. Controlled breathing with daily activities and graded exercises to improve general physical fitness.
   e. Relaxation and stretching.
   f. General relaxation.

5. Intermittent positive pressure breathing (IPPB).
   a. Purposes.
      (1) Improve oxygenation to the lungs.
      (2) Improve alveolar ventilation.
      (3) Deliver aerosolized bronchodilators.
      (4) Decrease the work of breathing.
      (5) Mobilize secretions.
      (6) Improve or prevent atelectasis.
      (7) Treat pulmonary edema.
   b. IPPB treatments should be administered by a respiratory therapist or trained nursing personnel.
   c. Client should not be left unattended during the IPPB treatments.
   d. Postural drainage, cupping and vibration, and coughing and deep breathing should follow each treatment.

H. Monitor carefully for complications of right-sided heart failure (cor pulmonale) and left-sided failure.

Chronic Asthma

Definition: A condition manifested by difficult breathing and characterized by generalized broncho-constriction, excess mucus secretion, and mucosal edema.

Assessment

A. Assess for type of asthma.
  1. Extrinsic—early onset in life and often associated with history of allergy.
  2. Intrinsic—usually adult onset and often associated with environmental factors.
B. Evaluate for precipitating factors.
  1. Etiology unknown.
  2. Emotion.
  3. Infection.
  4. Seasonal changes.
  5. Pets.
  6. Smoking.
  7. Family history.
  8. Occupational exposure to dusts or chemical irritants.
  9. Drugs.
C. Evaluate for respiratory problems.
  1. Respiratory distress.
  2. Air hunger.
  3. Tachypnea.
  4. Prolonged expiratory phase.
  5. Cough may be nonproductive or very purulent.
  6. Tachycardia.
  7. Hypoxia, cyanosis, hypercapnia.
  8. Assess physical signs.
    a. Retraction of intercostal and sternal muscles.
    b. Percussion—hyperresonant.
    c. Distant breath sounds.
    d. Rhonchi, wheezes, rales.

Implementation

A. Provide supportive respiratory care.
B. Administer drug therapy.
  1. Bronchodilators.
    a. Epinephrine and derivatives.
    b. Aminophylline and derivatives.
    c. Cromolyn (Intal).
    d. Isoetharine (Bronkosol).
  2. Corticosteroids.

C. Sedatives and narcotics should be used with caution.
D. Administer oxygen via nasal cannula.
E. Force fluids to 3000 cc daily.
F. Monitor IPPB treatments.

CHRONIC RESTRICTIVE DISORDERS

Pleural Effusion

Definition: A collection of non-purulent fluid in the pleural space. Many pathological processes can irritate the pleurae and cause effusion, but in older clients cancer is a common cause.

Assessment

A. Assess for dyspnea.
B. Check fatigue level.
C. Assess for elevated temperature.
D. Assess for dry cough.
E. Assess for pleural pain.
F. Assess physical signs.
  1. Absence of movement on side of effusion.
  2. Percussion—dull.
  3. Decreased breath sounds.
  4. Pleural friction rub occurs in dry pleurisy, but as effusion develops, the friction rub disappears.
  5. Collapse of lung—when fluid increases in amount.
  6. Mediastinal structures shift position.
  7. Cardiac tamponade.

Implementation

A. Assist with thoracentesis, which is used to aid in diagnosis and to relieve pressure by draining excess fluid.
  1. Explain procedure to client.
  2. Instruct client to tell you any compromising symptoms such as difficulty in breathing or discomfort.
  3. Give client reassurance during procedure.
B. Monitor vital signs.
C. Following removal of fluid, observe for bradycardia, hypotension, pain, or pulmonary edema.
D. Monitor administration of drugs if ordered for empyema.

E. Administer oxygen as ordered.

F. Teach deep-breathing exercises to increase lung expansion.

G. Monitor chest tubes and drainage.

Pneumothorax

Definition: A collection of air in the pleural cavity. As the air collects in the pleural space, the lung is collapsed and respiratory distress ensues. The condition occurs as a result of chest wall penetration by surgery or injury or when disease process interrupts the internal structures of the lung.

Characteristics

A. Tension pneumothorax is a medical emergency.
1. The mediastinum shifts away from the side of the pneumothorax compressing the unaffected lung.
2. A large-bore needle is introduced into the pleural cavity to release the pressure.
3. A tube thoracostomy is then performed.

B. A small pneumothorax may reabsorb on its own.
1. If the pneumothorax is large or increasing in size, closed tube thoracostomy is performed.
2. Water-seal is utilized to reexpand the lung.

C. Hemothorax (blood in the thoracic cavity).
1. Hemothorax occurs with pneumothorax, especially if trauma is the causative factor.
2. Treatment: evacuate the blood through chest tube insertion.

Assessment

A. Assess for sharp, sudden chest pain.

B. Check anxiety, vertigo.

C. Assess for hypotension.

D. Assess for gasping respirations, dyspnea.

E. Look for pallor.

F. Evaluate cough.

G. Check tachycardia.

H. Evaluate elevated temperature, diaphoresis.

I. Assess for hypoxia, hypercapnia.

J. Assess for physical signs.
1. Paradoxical or diminished movement on the affected side.
2. Percussion—hyperresonant.
3. Absent breath sounds.
4. Tactile fremitus decreased.

Implementation

A. Monitor vital signs frequently for impending shock.

B. Auscultate lungs frequently.

C. Monitor for respiratory distress.

D. Assist client to semi- or high-Fowler's position.

E. Reassure client who will be anxious.

Cancer of the Lung

Definition: Pulmonary tumors are either primary or metastatic and interrupt the normal physiological functioning of the lung.

Characteristics

A. Classification of lung cancer is designated by anatomic location or by histological pattern.
1. Anatomic classification.
   a. Central lesions involve the tracheobronchial tube up to the distal bronchi.
   b. Peripheral lesions extend from the distal bronchi and includes the broncioles.
2. Four histologic types.
   a. Squamous cell (epidermoid).
      (1) Most frequent lung lesions.
      (2) Affects more men than women.
      (3) Associated with cigarette smoking.
      (4) Lesion usually starts in bronchial area and extends.
      (5) Metastasis not usually a rapid process.
   b. Adenocarcinoma.
      (1) Usually develops in peripheral tissue (smaller bronchi).
      (2) Metastasizes by blood route.
      (3) May be associated with focal lung scars.
      (4) Affects more women than men.
   c. Bronchiole-alveolar cell.
      (1) Rare multimodular lesion.
      (2) Affects bronchiolar or alveolar linings.
   d. Undifferentiated carcinoma.
      (1) Metastisizes early.
      (2) Affects younger age group.
      (3) Affects more men than women.

B. Detection—pulmonary lesions are not usually detected by physical exam, and symptoms do not occur until process is extensive. Chest x-ray is very helpful in diagnosis.

Assessment

A. Assess for pulmonary symptoms.

1. Persistent cough.
2. Dyspnea.
3. Bloody sputum.
4. Long-term pulmonary infection.
5. Atelectasis.
6. Bronchiectasis.
7. Chest pain.
8. Chills, fever.

B. Assess for systemic symptoms.
   1. Weakness.
   2. Weight loss.
   3. Anemia.
   4. Anorexia.
   5. Metabolic syndromes.
      a. Hypercalcemia.
      b. Inappropriate ADH.
      c. Cushing's syndrome.
      d. Gynecomastia.
   6. Neuromuscular changes.
      a. Peripheral neuropathy.
      b. Corticocerebellar degeneration.
   7. Connective tissue abnormalities.
      a. Clubbing.
      b. Arthralgias.
   8. Dermatologic abnormalities.
   9. Vascular changes.

Implementation

A. Comprehensive supportive care of client in the preoperative and postoperative state. (See section on care of the operative client.)
B. Give appropriate information to client to allay anxiety and clarify expectations.
C. Instruct client in postoperative procedures to minimize complications.
D. Give psychological support.

THORACIC TRAUMA

Trauma Assessment

A. Check for airway patency.
   1. Clear out secretions.
   2. Insert oral airway if necessary.
   3. Position client on side if there is no cervical spine injury.
   4. Place hand or cheek over nose and mouth of client to feel if client is breathing.

B. Inspect thoracic cage for injury.
   1. Inspect for contusions, abrasions, and symmetry of chest movement.
   2. If open wound of chest, seal off immediately with a pressure dressing to prevent air from entering thoracic cavity.
   3. Watch for symmetrical movement of chest. Asymmetrical movement indicates:
      a. Flail chest.
      b. Tension pneumothorax.
      c. Hemothorax.
      d. Fractured ribs.
   4. Observe color; cyanosis indicates decreased oxygenation.
   5. Observe type of breathing; stertorous breathing usually indicates obstructed respiration.

C. Auscultate lung sounds.
   1. Absence of breath sounds: indicates lungs not expanding, due either to obstruction or deflation.
   2. Rales (crackling sounds): indicate vibrations of fluid in lungs.
   3. Rhonchi (coarse sounds): indicate partial obstruction of airway.
   4. Decreased breath sounds: indicate poorly-ventilated lungs.
   5. Detection of bronchial sounds which are deviated from normal position: indicates mediastinal shift due to collapse of lung.

D. Determine level of consciousness; decreased sensorium can indicate hypoxia.
E. Observe sputum or tracheal secretions; bloody sputum can indicate contusions of lung or injury to trachea and other anatomical structures.

Trauma Implementation

A. Take history from client to aid in total evaluation of client's condition.
B. Administer electrocardiogram to establish if there is associated cardiac damage.
C. Maintain patent airway.
   1. Suction.
   2. Intubation.
      a. Oral airway.
      b. Endotracheal intubation.
D. Maintain adequate ventilation.
E. Maintain fluid and electrolyte balance.

1. When blood and fluid loss is replaced, watch carefully for fluid overload, which can lead to pulmonary edema.
2. Record intake and output.

F. Maintain acid-base balance; make frequent blood gas determinations as acid-base imbalances occur readily with compromised respirations or with mechanical ventilation.

G. Provide for relief of pain.
   1. Analgesics should be used with caution as they depress respirations. (Demerol is the drug of choice.)
   2. Atropine, morphine sulfate, and barbiturates should be avoided.
   3. Nerve block may be used.

TYPES OF TRAUMATIC INJURIES

Open Wounds of the Chest

Assessment

A. Evaluate if air from the atmosphere entered the pleural cavity causing collapse of lung.

B. Assess for air entering and leaving the wound during inspiration and expiration.

C. Evaluate if intrapleural negative pressure is lost, thereby embarrassing respirations, leading to hypoxia. Death can occur if not corrected promptly.

Implementation

A. Apply vaseline gauze to wound with pressure dressing.

B. Place client on assisted ventilation if necessary.

C. Prepare for insertion of chest tubes.

D. Place client in high-Fowler's position (unless contraindicated) to assist in adequate ventilation.

Hemothorax or Pneumothorax

Definition: Hemothorax refers to blood in pleural space. Pneumothorax refers to air in pleural space. As air or fluid accumulates in pleural space, positive pressure is built up, collapsing the lung.

Assessment

A. Evaluate pain.

B. Auscultate for decreased breath sounds.

C. Observe for tracheal shift to unaffected side.

D. Observe for dyspnea and respiratory embarrassment.

Implementation

A. Assist with the insertion of a number 18 needle into the second intercostal space, midclavicular line, followed by aspiration of the fluid or air by means of a thoracentesis.

B. Assist with insertion of chest tubes and connection to closed-chest drainage.

C. Continuously observe vital signs for complications such as shock and cardiac failure.

Fractured Ribs

Assessment

A. Evaluate pain and tenderness over fracture area.

B. Observe for bruising at injury site.

C. Evaluate respiratory embarrassment occurring from splinters puncturing lung and causing pneumothorax.

D. Observe client for splinting of chest causing shallow respirations. Splinting causes a reduction in lung compliance as well as respiratory acidosis.

Implementation

A. Administer mild analgesic, such as small doses of Demerol, for pain relief. (*Caution:* Narcotics can depress respiration and the cough reflex.)

B. Encourage deep breathing and coughing to prevent respiratory complications such as atelectasis and pneumonia.

C. Observe for signs of hemorrhage and shock.

D. Assist with intercostal nerve block if necessary to decrease pain.

Flail Chest

Definition: Multiple rib fractures that result in an unstable chest wall.

Assessment

A. Evaluate for pain.

B. Observe for dyspnea leading to cyanosis.

C. Assess if detached portion of flail chest is moving in opposition to other areas of chest cage and lung.

1. On inspiration, the affected chest area is depressed; on expiration, it is bulging outward.
2. This causes poor expansion of lungs, which results in carbon dioxide retention and respiratory acidosis.

D. Evaluate ability to cough effectively. Inability leads to accumulation of fluids and respiratory complications such as pneumonia and atelectasis.

E. Assess for signs of cardiac failure due to impaired filling of right side of heart. This condition results from high venous pressure caused by paradoxical breathing.

F. Observe for rapid, shallow, and noisy respirations.

Implementation

A. Prepare for tracheotomy with a cuffed trach tube.

B. Place client on volume-set respirator (MA-I), which delivers the same amount of tidal volume with each breath and is not dependent on client's respirations.

C. Suction frequently to prevent respiratory complications.

D. Prevent pain by administering nerve block or Demerol as ordered.

E. Observe for signs of shock and hemorrhage.

F. For client on ventilator, use nasogastric tube to prevent abdominal distention and emesis, which can lead to aspiration.

G. For client not on mechanical ventilator:
1. Encourage turning, coughing, and hyperventilating every hour.
2. Administer oxygen.
3. Maintain IPPB therapy.
4. Suction as needed.

Cardiac Tamponade

Definition: Acute accumulation of blood or fluid in the pericardial sac. Can occur from blunt or penetrating chest wounds (interferes with diastolic filling).

Assessment

A. Assess for increased CVP.

B. Assess for decreased blood pressure.

C. Assess for narrowed pulse pressure.

D. Evaluate paradoxical pulse (pulse disappears on inspiration and is weak on expiration because of changed intrathoracic pressure).
1. Paradoxical pulse is an exaggeration of the normal fall in arterial BP on inspiration.

2. Defined as a fall in systolic arterial BP to 10–20 mm Hg or more on inspiration.
3. Occurs with PE, pericardial constriction or tamponade and restrictive cardiomyopathy.

E. Observe for distended neck veins (jugular vein cannot empty properly).

F. Auscultate for distant heart sounds.

G. Observe for agitation.

H. Observe for cyanosis.

Implementation

A. Assist with needle insertion. Large needle (16–18 gauge) is inserted by physician into pericardium, and blood is withdrawn.

B. Maintain cardiac monitoring to observe for arrhythmias due to myocardial irritability.

C. Have cardiac defibrillator and emergency drugs available to treat cardiac arrhythmias.

D. Monitor vital signs and watch for shock.

TREATMENT FOR TRAUMATIC INJURY

Chest Tubes

Assessment

A. Evaluate client's safety while tubes inserted.

B. Assess patency of chest tubes.

C. Observe for mediastinal shift.

D. Auscultate breath sounds for air flow.

E. Observe for bilateral chest expansion.

F. Evaluate chest drainage.

Implementation

A. Assist physician in placement of tubes.
1. Tubes placed in pleural cavity following thoracic surgery.
2. Provides for removal of air and serosanguineous fluid from pleural space.

B. Attach to water-seal suction—maintains closed system.
1. Tape all connectors.
2. Ensure that all stoppers in bottles are tight fitting.

C. Apply suction.
1. Keep bottles below level of bed.
2. Keep suction level where ordered (be sure that bubbling is not excessive in the pressure-regulating bottle).
3. Maintain water level in bottle.

D. Maintain patency.

1. Milk chest tubes every 30 to 60 minutes.
   a. Milk away from client toward the drainage receptable (Pleur-evac or bottles).
   b. Pinch tubing close to the chest with one hand as the other hand milks the tube. Continue going down tube in this method until coming to the drainage receptacle.
2. Milking may be ordered—stripping should be avoided.

E. Maintain safety-clamp for less than a minute.
   1. Keep rubber-tipped hemostats at bedside to clamp tube. (If air leak develops in tube, lung may collapse.) Clamping is controversial—check hospital policy.
   2. Check that all connectors are taped.

F. Clamp chest tube only for following reasons.
   1. To locate source of air leak when bubbling occurs in water-seal chamber. Begin clamping close to chest—when clamp is between air leak and water-seal, bubbling will stop—leak is above it.
   2. To prevent air from entering pleural space; clamp while replacing drainage unit due to breakage or full collection chamber.
   3. To verify that client is ready to have chest tubes removed.
   4. Do not clamp to get client out of bed of if tubing comes apart (place end in sterile water as temporary seal).
      a. Clean tube ends and reconnect.
      b. Have client exhale to rid pleural space of air.

Water-Seal Chest Drainage

Characteristics

A. Three types—one-, two-, or three-bottle drainage.
B. General principles.
   1. Used after some intrathoracic procedures.
   2. Chest tubes placed intrapleurally.
   3. Breathing mechanism operates on principle of negative pressure (pressure in chest cavity is lower than pressure of atmosphere, causing air to rush into chest cavity when injury such as stab wound occurs).
   4. When chest has been opened, vacuum must be applied to chest to reestablish negative pressure.
   5. Closed water-seal drainage is method of reestablishing negative pressure.
      a. Water acts as a seal and keeps the air from being drawn back into pleural space.

b. Open drainage system would allow air to be sucked back into chest cavity and collapse lung.
6. Closed drainage is established by placing catheter into pleural space and allowing it to drain under water.
   a. The end of the drainage tube is always kept under water.
   b. Air will not be drawn up through catheter into pleural space when tube is under water.

Assessment

A. Assess client's respiratory rate, rhythm, and breath sounds for signs of respiratory distress.
B. Check that all connections on tubing are airtight and suction control is connected.
C. Examine system to see if it is set up and functioning properly.
D. Identify any malfunctions in system, i.e., air leaks, negative pressure, or obstructions.

Implementation

A. Maintain one-bottle suction system.

One-Bottle Suction System

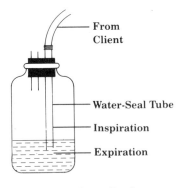

From Client

Water-Seal Tube

Inspiration

Expiration

Water Seal and Drainage Bottle

1. There is only one bottle; it functions as a collection bottle for drainage as well as a pressure regulator.
2. As the drainage increases in amount, the water-seal tube (immersed in the drainage) is pulled up slightly to decrease the amount of force that is required to permit the fluid to be drained from the pleural space.

3. The depth to which the water-seal tube is immersed below the fluid in the bottle determines the pressure exerted by the water.

4. Drainage is measured in the same way as two-bottle or three-bottle suction.

B. Maintain two-bottle suction system.

Two-Bottle Suction System

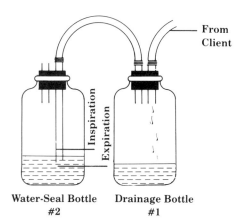

Water-Seal Bottle
#2

Drainage Bottle
#1

1. Two-bottle suction.
   a. Same as three-bottle suction except that the bottle connected to mechanical suction is not included.
   b. Drainage bottle (bottle number one) is connected from client and is between the client and the water-seal bottle (or bottle number two).
      (1) Short tube goes from client into drainage bottle (not to extend below drainage level).
      (2) Mark drainage level on outside of bottle.
      (3) Short tube with rubber tubing goes from the drainage bottle to water-seal bottle.
      (4) This tube extends below water level in the water-seal bottle.

2. Bottle number two.
   a. The long tube extends below water level (from bottle number one).
   b. A second short tube provides an air vent.
   c. Water in this bottle goes up the tube when client inhales and down the tube when client exhales.
   d. Water in this bottle should not bubble constantly.

C. Maintain three-bottle suction system.

Three-Bottle Suction System

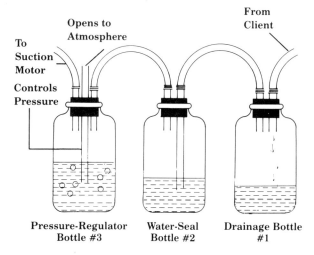

Pressure-Regulator
Bottle #3

Water-Seal
Bottle #2

Drainage Bottle
#1

1. Third bottle is connected to suction motor—called mechanical suction.

2. Bottle number three regulates the amount of negative pressure in the system.

3. Three tubes.
   a. Short tube, above water level, comes from water-seal bottle.
   b. Short tube connected to suction motor.
   c. Third tube, below water level in bottle, opens to the atmosphere outside of the bottle.
   d. The depth to which third tube is submerged in the water determines the suction pressure within the drainage system.

4. When drainage system pressure becomes too low, outside air is sucked into the system. Results in constant bubbling in the pressure regulator bottle.

5. Whenever the motor is off, drainage system must be open to the atmosphere.
   a. Intrapleural air can escape from the system.
   b. Detach the third bottle tubing from the suction motor to provide the air vent.

Mechanical Ventilation

Assessment

A. Assess respiratory status for need to use mechanical ventilation.

B. Identify type of mechanical ventilation needed.
   1. Negative pressure ventilator.
      a. Helpful in problems of a neuromuscular nature.

b. Not effective in the treatment of increased airway resistance.

c. Types—full body, chest, and chest-abdomen.

2. Positive pressure ventilator.

a. Uses positive pressure (pressure greater than atmospheric) to inflate lungs.

b. Types.

(1) Pressure cycle.

(a) Pressure ranges from 10 to 30 cm of water pressure.

(b) Air is actively forced into lungs.

(c) Expiration is passive.

(2) Volume cycle.

(a) Uses physiological limits.

(b) Predetermined total volume is delivered irrespective of airway pressure.

(c) Positive end expiratory pressure (PEEP) utilized to maintain positive pressure between expiration and beginning of inspiration.

C. Assess for complications of positive pressure therapy.

1. Respiratory alkalosis.

2. Gastric distention and paralytic ileus.

3. Gastrointestinal bleeding.

4. Diffuse atelectasis.

5. Infection.

6. Circulatory collapse.

7. Pneumothorax progressive alveolar capillary block.

8. Sudden ventricular fibrillation.

Implementation

A. Monitor ventilator for complications.

B. Suction client or check for kinks in tubing when pressure alarm sounds.

C. Monitor blood gas values frequently.

D. Maintain fluid therapy.

1. IV route.

2. Oral route if client able to swallow.

E. Monitor intake and output.

Thoracic Surgical Procedures

Assessment

A. Identify type of procedure done.

1. Exploratory thoracotomy: incision of the thoracic wall, performed to locate bleeding, injuries, tumors.

2. Thoracoplasty: removal of ribs or portions of ribs to reduce the size of the thoracic space.

3. Pneumonectomy: removal of entire lung.

4. Lobectomy: removal of a lobe of the lung (three lobes on right side, two on the left).

5. Segmented resection: removal of one or more segments of the lung (right lung has ten segments and left lung has eight).

6. Wedge resection: removal of a small, localized area of disease near the surface of the lung.

B. Evaluate time of client care required.

Implementation

A. Provide postoperative nursing management.

1. Closed chest drainage is employed in all but pneumonectomy. In pneumonectomy, it is desirable that the fluid accumulate in empty thoracic space. Eventually the thoracic space fills with serous exudate, which consolidates to prevent extensive mediastinal shifts.

2. Maintain patent chest tube drainage by chest tube milking—milk away from client toward drainage bottle.

3. Maintain respiratory function.

a. Have client turn, cough, and deep breathe.

b. Suction if necessary.

c. Provide oxygen therapy.

d. Provide IPPB therapy.

e. Ventilate mechanically if necessary.

4. Ambulate early to encourage adequate ventilation and prevent postoperative complications. (Ambulate clients with pneumonectomies in two or three days to facilitate cardiopulmonary adjustment.)

5. Provide range-of-motion exercises to all extremities to promote adequate circulation.

6. Monitor central venous pressure with vital signs—watch for indications of impaired venous return to heart.

7. Position client correctly.

a. Use semi-Fowler's position when vital signs are stable to facilitate lung expansion.

b. Turn every one to two hours.

c. Pneumonectomy

(1) No chest tubes inserted. Fluid left in space to consolidate.

(2) Position on operative side.

(3) Some physicians will allow positioning on either side after twenty-four hours.

  d. Segmental resection or wedge resection: position on back or unoperative side (aids in expanding remaining pulmonary tissue).

  e. Lobectomy: turn to either side (can expand lung tissue on both sides).

8. Maintain fluid intake as tolerated. Watch for overload in pneumonectomy clients.

9. Provide arm and shoulder postoperative exercises—prevent adhesion formation.

  a. Put affected arm through both active and passive range of motion every four hours.

  b. Start exercises within four hours after client has returned to room following surgery.

B. Monitor for postoperative complications.

1. Respiratory complications.

  a. Causes of inadequate ventilation.

    (1) Airway obstruction due to secretion accumulation.

    (2) Atelectasis due to underexpansion of lungs and anesthetic agents during surgery.

    (3) Hypoventilation and carbon dioxide buildup due to incisional splinting because of pain.

    (4) Depression of CNS from overuse of medications.

  b. Tension pneumothorax.

    (1) Caused by air leak through pleural incision lines.

    (2) Can cause mediastinal shift.

  c. Pulmonary embolism.

  d. Bronchopulmonary fistula.

    (1) Air escapes into pleural space and is forced into subcutaneous tissue around incision, causing subcutaneous emphysema.

    (2) Caused by inadequate closure of bronchus when resection is done.

    (3) Another cause is alveolar or bronchiolar tears in surface of lung (particularly following pneumonectomy).

  e. Atelectasis and/or pneumonia: caused by airway obstruction or as result of anesthesia.

  f. Respiratory arrest can occur.

2. Circulatory complications.

  a. Hypovolemia: due to fluid or blood loss.

  b. Arrhythmias: due to underlying myocardial disease.

  c. Cardiac arrest: can occur from either of these conditions.

  d. Pulmonary edema: can occur due to fluid overload of circulatory system.

Tracheostomy

Assessment

A. Determine need for tracheostomy as compared to less intrusive methods of providing patent airway.

B. Assess client's level of consciousness to determine client's ability to understand explanation and instructions.

C. Observe client's respiratory status: shortness of breath, severe dyspnea, tachypnea, or tachycardia.

D. Auscultate for presence and forced expiration of rhonchi, rales, or wheezes.

E. Observe for dried or moist secretions surrounding cannula or on tracheal dressing.

F. Observe for excessive expectoration of secretions.

G. Assess result of routine tracheal care to determine if routine care is adequate for this client.

H. Observe client's ability to sustain respiratory function by ability to breath through normal airway.

I. Assess respiratory status: breath sounds, respiratory rate, use of accessory muscles for breathing while tracheal tube is plugged.

J. Assess for labored breathing, flaring of nares, retractions, and color of nail beds.

Implementation

A. Provide tracheal suction as ordered or p.r.n.

1. Always apply oral or nasal suction first so that when cuff is deflated, secretions will not fall into lung from area above cuff.

2. Catheter must be changed before doing tracheal suctioning.

B. Provide humidity by using trach mist mask, if client is not on ventilator.

C. Monitor for hemorrhage around tracheostomy site.

D. Change dressings (nonraveling type) and cleanse surrounding area with hydrogen peroxide at least every four hours.

E. Provide care for cuffed tracheostomy tube.

1. Hyperventilate client before and after cuff is deflated with ambu bag.
2. Deflate tracheal cuff.
   a. Suction airway before deflating cuff.
   b. Attach 10 cc syringe to distal end of inflatable cuff, making sure seal is tight.
   c. Slowly withdraw 5 cc of air. Amount of air withdrawn is determined by type of cuff used and whether air leak is utilized.
   d. Keep syringe attached to end of cuff.
   e. Suction if cough reflex stimulated.
   f. Assess respirations, if labored reinflate cuff.
   g. If high volume/low pressure cuff is used, cuff is not routinely deflated. (In fact, deflating cuff does not help tracheal lining. The pooled secretions above the tracheal cuff are the problem.)
3. Inflate cuff.
   a. Suction airway before inflating cuff.
   b. If syringe is not already attached, attach 10 cc syringe to distal end of inflatable cuff, making sure seal is tight.
   c. Inflate prescribed amount of air to create leak-free system. Cuff is inflated correctly when you cannot hear the client's voice or any air movement from nose or mouth.
   d. Remove syringe and apply rubber-tipped forceps to maintain air in cuff.
   e. If high volume/low pressure cuff is used, cuff is not routinely deflated.

F. Administer inner cannula tracheal cleaning.
1. Suction before cleaning tracheal tube.
2. Unlock the inner cannula by turning the lock to the right about 90 degrees and secure the outer cannula of the neck plate with your left index finger and thumb.
3. Gently pull the inner cannula slightly upward and out towards you.
4. Wash cannula thoroughly with cool, sterile water, saline, or hydrogen peroxide to remove secretions. (Tapwater may be used if hospital policy allows.) Soak the cannula in a hydrogen-peroxide filled sterile bowl to further remove dried secretions.
5. Rinse cannula thoroughly with sterile water or saline, and dry tube thoroughly with absorbent paper.
6. Replace the inner cannula carefully by grasping the outer flange of the cannula with your left hand as you insert the cannula. Lock the inner cannula by turning the lock to the left so that it is in an upright position.
7. Cleanse around the incision site with applicator sticks soaked in normal saline and/or hydrogen peroxide (one-half strength). Apply antibiotic ointment around incision site if ordered.
8. Apply trach dressing around insertion site, and change trach ties if needed.
9. If trach ties are to be changed, ask another person to hold the tracheal tube in place while you change the ties. This procedure prevents accidental extubation if the client coughs.

G. Provide instillation of normal saline.
1. Attach sterile catheter to suction machine tubing.
2. Draw up normal saline (usually 3 to 5 cc) in syringe.
3. Remove needle from syringe.
4. Turn on oxygen supply to resuscitation bag.
5. Turn on suction equipment.
6. Remove needle before injecting saline into tube.
7. Instill prescribed amount of normal saline into tracheostomy or endotracheal tube with un-gloved hand.
8. Give client 3 to 5 breaths with resuscitation bag if client can tolerate this procedure.
9. Put on sterile glove and begin deep suctioning. Client may be hyperventilated with resuscitator bag after suctioning.

H. Provide tracheostomy plugging.
1. Suction nasopharynx.
2. Change suction catheters, and suction trachea.
3. Deflate tracheal cuff; suction again if necessary.
4. Place tracheal plug in either the inner cannula or outer cannula with inner cannula removed.
5. Observe client for respiratory distress.

Suctioning

Assessment

A. Determine need for suctioning.
B. Observe vital signs for increases in pulse and respiration and for changes in skin color.
C. Auscultate sounds to evaluate lung field.
D. Determine level of consciousness to assess hypoxia.

Implementation

A. Provide nasotracheal suction.
1. Gather equipment.

a. Sterile suction catheter, usually No. 14 or No. 16 French.

b. Sterile saline.

c. Suction machine.

d. Sterile gloves.

2. Complete suctioning procedure.

a. Preoxygenate before suctioning.

b. Lubricate catheter with normal saline.

c. Insert catheter into nose for 15 to 20 cm.

d. Do not apply suction while introducing catheter.

e. When advanced as far as possible, begin suctioning by withdrawing catheter slowly, rotating it with pressure applied. (Usually a whistle tip catheter or Y connector tube is used to apply pressure.)

f. Withdraw catheter slightly if cough reflex is stimulated.

g. Remember that hypoxia can occur if suctioning is done incorrectly.

(1) Excess of 10 seconds suctioning—oxygen decreased in respiratory tree.

(2) Causes chemoreceptors to respond by increasing ventilation rate.

h. Postoxygenate after suctioning.

B. Provide tracheostomy suctioning.

1. Gather equipment.

a. Same equipment as for nasotracheal.

b. Sterile syringe (5 cc) and sterile saline for instillation into trach tube.

2. Complete suctioning procedure.

a. Be sure that suction catheter is not more than half the diameter of tracheostomy tube.

b. Preoxygenate before suctioning.

c. Lubricate with sterile saline, then insert catheter through tracheostomy tube for 20 to 30 cm with suction turned off.

d. Do not suction for more than 10 seconds.

e. Rotate catheter while withdrawing it.

f. Do not repeat procedure for at least three minutes unless necessary to withdaw more secretions to permit adequate ventilation.

g. If secretions are very tenacious, 3 to 5 cc of sterile saline may be inserted through tube and allowed to remain for a few seconds before suctioning.

h. To remove secretions from right bronchus, turn client's head to left; to remove secretions from left bronchus, turning client's head to right may help.

Pulmonary Medications

Sympathomimetic Bronchodilators

A. Epinephrine (Adrenaline).

1. Beta and alpha stimulant; relaxes bronchial smooth muscle.

2. Routes: subq, IV, MDI (metered dose inhalant).

3. Used to treat asthma and for anaphylaxis.

4. May cause arrhythmias, increased BP, urinary retention, increased blood sugar, headache.

B. Ephedrine sulfate.

1. Relaxes smooth muscle of the tracheobronchial tree.

2. Route: p.o.

3. Used for mild bronchospasm.

4. Similar side effects as epinephrine.

C. Isoproterenol (Isuprel).

1. Pure beta agonist; relaxes smooth muscle of tracheobronchial tree; relieves bronchospasms.

2. Routes: IV, MDI.

3. May cause marked tachycardia, arrhythmias, angina, palpitations.

D. Albuterol (Proventil, Ventolin).

1. Very selective $beta_2$ agonist.

2. Routes: p.o., MDI.

3. Minimal cardiovascular side effects.

E. Isoetharine (Bronkosol, Bronkometer).

1. More $beta_2$ specific than Isuprel; relaxes smooth muscle of the tracheobronchial tree; less potent.

2. Route: Nebulized solution or MDI.

3. Side effects similar to Isuprel, but appear less frequently; may cause tachycardia.

4. Tolerance to bronchodilating effect may develop with too frequent use of medication.

F. Metaproterenol (Alupent).

1. Relieves bronchospasm.

2. Routes: p.o., MDI.

3. Side effects same as isoetharine.

G. Terbutaline (Bricanyl, Brethine).

1. Beta-adrenergic-receptor agonist; bronchodilator; relieves bronchospasms associated with COPD, asthma.

2. Routes: subq, p.o., Brethaire by MDI.

3. May cause nervousness, palpitations; nausea if taken on an empty stomach.

Anticholinergic Bronchodilators

A. Ipratropium bromide (Atrovent).

1. Bronchodilating effect primarily local and site specific; more potent than sympathomimetics in COPD.
2. Route: MDI.
3. Minimal side effects.

Methylxanthine Bronchodilators

A. Aminophylline.
  1. Relaxes smooth muscle of the tracheobronchial tree; bronchodilator.
  2. Routes: p.o., IV, rectal suppository.
  3. Therapeutic serum level 8–20 mcg/ml.
  4. May cause tachycardia, hypotension, arrhythmias, GI distress, tremors, anxiety, headache.
  5. Toxic levels cause arrhythmias, seizures.
B. Theophylline.
  1. Relaxes smooth muscle of the bronchi and pulmonary vessels.
  2. Routes: p.o., rectally.
  3. Therapeutic serum level 10–20 mcg/ml.
  4. Side effects similar to Aminophylline.
C. Oxtriphylline (Choledyl).
  1. Similar to other bronchodilators.
  2. Route: p.o.
  3. Less GI irritation than Aminophylline.

Antimediators/Antiinflammatory Agents

A. Cromolyn Sodium
  1. Used for younger clients with asthma.
  2. Route: MDI.

3. Prevents bronchospasm when used before exercise or exposure to cold air.
B. Corticosteroids.
  1. Used in conjunction with brochodilators for treatment of bronchospasms. Aerosol use prevents systemic side effects of steroids.
  2. Routes:
    a. Prednisone p.o.
    b. Methylprednisolone, hydrocortisone IV.
    c. Beclomethasone diproprionate (Beclovent, Vanceril) MDI.
    d. Thiamcinolone (Azmacort) MDI.
  3. Instruct client to rinse mouth after use to prevent oral candidiasis.
  4. Side effects include increased appetite, euphoria and psychosis.

Mucokinetic Agents

A. Acetylcysteine (Mucomyst)
  1. Used to loosen secretions; reduces viscosity.
  2. Routes: inhaled or instilled.
  3. May cause bronchospasm, nausea.
  4. Instruct client to rinse mouth after use.
B. Quaiafenesin
  1. Commonly used expectorant.
  2. Route: p.o.
C. Iodide preparations (SSKI, Organidin).
  1. Expectorant liquefies tenacious bronchial secretions.
  2. Route p.o.; bitter taste, give with juice or milk.
  3. Do not administer if allergic to iodine or hyperthyroid.

GASTROINTESTINAL SYSTEM

The alimentary tract's primary function is to provide the body with a continual supply of nutrients, fluids, and electrolytes for tissue nourishment. This system has three components: a tract for ingestion and movement of food and fluids; secretion of digestive juices for breaking down the nutrients; and absorption mechanisms for the utilization of foods, water, and electrolytes for continued growth and repair of body tissues.

ANATOMY AND PHYSIOLOGY

Main Organs

Description: The main organs of the gastrointestinal system include the mouth, pharynx, esophagus, stomach, small intestine, and large intestine.

Functions

A. Normally, it is the only source of intake for the body.
B. Provides the body with fluids, nutrients, and electrolytes.
C. Provides means of disposal for waste residues.

Activities

A. Secretion of enzymes and electrolytes to break down the raw materials ingested.
B. Movement of ingested products through the system.
C. Complete digestion of ingested nutrients.
D. Absorption of the end products of digestion into the blood.

Coats Composing the Walls

A. Mucous lining.

1. Rugae and microscopic gastric and hydrochloric acid glands in the stomach.
2. Villi, intestinal gland Peyer's patches, and lymph nodes.
3. Intestinal glands.
B. Submucous coat of connective tissue, in which the main blood vessels are located.
C. Muscular coat.
1. Digestive organs have circular and longitudinal muscle fibers.
2. The stomach has oblique fibers in addition to the circular and longitudinal fibers.
D. Fibroserous coat, the outer coat.
1. In the stomach, the omentum hangs from the lower edge of the stomach, over the intestines.
2. In the intestines, it forms the visceral peritoneum.

The Mouth, Pharynx, and Esophagus

A. The buccal cavity includes:
1. Cheeks.
2. Hard and soft palates.
3. Muscles.
4. Maxillary bones.
B. The pharynx.
1. Tubelike structure that extends from the base of the skull to the esophagus.
2. Compound of muscle lined with mucous membrane, composed of the nasopharynx, the oropharynx, and the laryngopharynx.
3. Functions include serving as a pathway for the respiratory and digestive tracts, and playing an important role in phonation.
C. The esophagus begins at the lower end of the pharynx and is a collapsible muscular tube about ten inches long.
1. It leads to the abdominal portion of the digestive tract.
2. The main portion is lined with many simple mucous glands; complex mucous glands are located at the esophagastric juncture.

The Stomach

A. Elongated pouch lying in the epigastric and left hypochondriac portions of the abdominal cavity.
B. Divisions are the fundus, the body, and the pylorus (the constricted lower portion).
C. Curvatures are the lesser curvature and the greater curvature.

D. Sphincters.
  1. Cardiac sphincter—at the opening of the esophagus into the stomach.
  2. Pyloric sphincter—guards the opening of the pylorus into the duodenum.
E. Coats.
  1. The mucous coat allows for distention and contains microscopic glands: gastric, hydrochloric acid, and mucous.
  2. The muscle coat contains three layers.
    a. Circular—forms the two sphincters.
    b. Longitudinal.
    c. Oblique.
  3. The fibroserous coat forms the visceral peritoneum; the omentum hangs in a double fold over the intestines.
F. Glands.
  1. Mucous—secrete mucus.
  2. Goblet cells—secrete viscid mucus.
  3. Gastric glands.
    a. Parietal—secrete hydrochloric acid.
    b. Chief cells—secrete pepsin, lipase, amylase, and rennin.
G. Function: mechanical and chemical digestion.
  1. Mechanical.
    a. Churning provides for forward and backward movement.
    b. Peristalsis moves material through the stomach and, at intervals with relaxation of the pyloric sphincter, squirts chyme into the duodenum.
  2. Chemical.
    a. Hydrochloric acid provides the proper medium for action of pepsin and aids in the coagulation of milk in adults.
    b. Pepsin splits protein into proteoses and peptones.
    c. Lipase is a fat-splitting enzyme with limited action.
    d. Rennin coagulates or curdles the protein of milk.
    e. Intrinsic factor—acts on certain components of food to form the antianemic factor.

The Small Intestine

A. Approximately twenty-one feet.
B. Divisions.
  1. The duodenum includes the Brunner's glands (the duodenal mucous digestive glands) and the openings for the bile and pancreatic ducts.
  2. The jejunum is approximately eight feet long and the ileum is approximately twelve feet long. Both have deep circular folds that increase their absorptive surfaces.
    a. The mucous lining has numerous villi, each of which has an arteriole, venule, and lymph vessel that serve as structures for the absorption of digested food.
    b. The small intestine terminates by opening into the cecum (the opening is guarded by the ileocecal valve).
C. Intestinal digestion.
  1. Intestinal juice has an alkaline reaction and contains a large number of enzymes.
  2. Enzymes.
    a. Peptidase splits fragments of proteins into free amino acids.
    b. Amylase digests starch to maltose.
    c. Maltase reduces maltose to monosaccharide glucose.
    d. Lactase splits lactose into galactose and glucose.
    e. Sucrase reduces sucrose to fructose and glucose.
    f. Nucleoses split nucleic acids into nucleotides.
    g. Enterokinase activates trypsinogen to trypsin.

The Large Intestine

A. Approximately five feet long, with a relatively smooth mucous membrane surface. The only secretion is mucus.
B. Muscle coats pucker the wall of the colon into a series of pouches (haustra) and contain the internal and the external anal sphincters.
C. Divisions.
  1. The cecum (the first part of the large intestine) is guarded by the ileocecal valve, which prevents regurgitation of the cecal contents into the ileum.
  2. Colon.
    a. Ascending—that portion of the colon extending from the ileocecal valve to the right hepatic flexure.
    b. Transverse—the largest, most mobile section extending from the right hepatic flexure to the left splenic flexure.

c. Descending—the narrowest portion of the large intestine, extending from the left splenic flexure to the brim of the pelvis.

d. Sigmoid—S-shaped portion of the colon, beginning at the brim of the pelvis and extending to the rectum.

D. Functions.

1. Absorption and elimination of wastes.

2. Formation of vitamins: K, B_{12}, riboflavin, and thiamin.

3. Mechanical digestion: churning, peristalsis, and defecation.

4. Absorption of water from fecal mass.

Accessory Organs

Description: The accessory organs of the gastrointestinal system include the teeth, tongue, salivary glands, pancreas, liver, gallbladder, and appendix.

Tongue

A. A skeletal muscle covered with a mucous membrane that aids in chewing, swallowing, and speaking.

B. Papillae on the surface of the tongue contain taste buds.

C. The frenulum is a fold of mucous membrane that helps to anchor the tongue to the floor of the mouth.

Salivary Glands

A. Three pairs—the submaxillary, the sublingual, and the buccal glands.

B. Secretion.

1. Saliva is secreted by the glands when sensory nerve endings are stimulated mechanically, thermally, or chemically.

2. pH ranges: 6.0–7.9. Between 1000 and 1500 ml are secreted in a 24-hour period in adults.

3. Contains amylase, an enzyme that hydrolyzes starch.

Teeth

A. Deciduous teeth (20 in the set) and permanent teeth (32 in the set).

B. The functions are mastication and mixing saliva with food.

Liver

A. Location and size.

1. Located in the right hypochondrium and part of the epigastrium.

2. It is the largest gland in the body, weighing three to four pounds.

3. It is protected by the lower ribs and is in contact with the undersurface of the dome of the diaphragm.

B. Lobes—right lobes (include the right lobe proper, the caudate, and the quadrate) and left lobe.

1. Lobes are divided into lobules by blood vessels and fibrous partitions.

2. The lobule is the basic structure of the liver and contains hepatic cells and capillaries.

C. Ducts include the hepatic duct from the liver, the cystic duct from the gallbladder, and the common bile duct (the union of the hepatic and cystic ducts).

Functions of the Liver

A. Metabolism of carbohydrates.

1. Converts glucose to glycogen and stores glycogen.

2. Converts glycogen to glucose.

3. Glycogenolysis—the supply of carbohydrate released into bloodstream.

B. Metabolism of fats.

1. Oxidation of fatty acids and formation of acetoacetic acid.

2. Formation of lipoproteins, cholesterol, and phospholipids.

3. Conversion of carbohydrates and protein to fat.

C. Metabolism of proteins.

1. Deamination of amino acids.

2. Formation of urea.

3. Formation of plasma proteins.

4. Interconversions among amino acid and other compounds.

D. Vascular functions for storage and filtration of blood.

1. Blood (200 to 400 ml) can be stored by the liver.

2. Vitamins (A, D, and B_{12}) and iron are stored in the liver.

3. Detoxifies harmful substances in the blood.

4. Breaks down worn-out blood cells.

5. Filters blood as it comes through the portal system.

E. Secretory functions.

1. Constant secretion (500 to 1000 ml in 24 hours) of bile, which is stored in the gallbladder.
2. Bile is a yellow-brown viscous fluid, alkaline in reaction, and consists of bile salts, bile pigments, cholesterol, and inorganic salts.
3. Bile emulsifies fats.
4. Red blood cell destruction releases hemoglobin which changes to bilirubin; bilirubin unites with plasma proteins and is removed by the liver and excreted in the bile.
5. The bile pigment bilirubin is converted by bacterial action into urobilin and to urobilinogen (appears in urine and gives feces brown color).

F. Hepatic reticuloendothelial functions.
1. Inner surface of the liver sinusoids contains Kupffer cells.
2. Kupffer cells are phagocytic and are capable of removing bacteria in the portal venous blood.

G. Sex hormone and aldosterone metabolism.

The Gallbladder

A. Small sac of smooth muscle located in a depression at the edge of the visceral surface of the liver, which functions as a reservoir for bile.
B. Ducts.
1. Cystic duct—the duct of the gallbladder joins the hepatic duct, which descends from the liver, to form the common bile duct.
2. The common bile duct is joined by the duct of the pancreas (Wirsung's duct) as it enters the duodenum.
3. The sphincter of Oddi guards the common entrance.
C. Secretion—the presence of fatty materials in the duodenum stimulates the liberation of cholecystokinin which causes contraction of the gallbladder and relaxation of the sphincter of Oddi.

The Pancreas

A. A soft, pink-white organ, 15 cm long and 2.5 cm wide, which adheres to the middle portion of the duodenum.
B. Divided into lobes and lobules.
1. Exocrine portion secretes digestive enzymes, which are carried to the duodenum by Wirsung's duct.
2. Endocrine secretion is produced by the islets of Langerhans; insulin is secreted into the bloodstream and plays an important role in carbohydrate metabolism.

C. Pancreatic juices contain enzymes for digesting proteins, carbohydrates, and fats.
1. Enzymes are secreted as inactive precursors which do not become active until secreted into the intestine (otherwise they would digest the gland).
2. Actions.
a. Trypsinogen to trypsin to act on proteins producing peptones, peptides, and amino acids.
b. Pancreatic amylase acts on carbohydrates, producing disaccharides.
c. Pancreatic lipase acts on fats, producing glycerol and fatty acids.

D. Two regulatory mechanisms of pancreatic secretion.
1. Nervous regulation—distention of the intestine.
2. Hormonal regulation.
a. Chyme in the intestinal mucosa causes the release of secretin (which stimulates the pancreas to secrete large quantities of fluid) and pancreozymin.
b. Pancreozymin passes by way of the blood to the pancreas and causes secretion of large quantities of digestive enzymes.

System Assessment

A. Evaluate client's history regarding reported signs and symptoms.
B. Assess over-all condition of client including vital signs and level of consciousness.
C. Evaluate condition of mouth, teeth, gums, and tongue.
1. Foul odor to breath may indicate diseased teeth, gums, or poor assimilation along gastrointestinal tract.
2. Coated tongue may indicate chemical imbalance in system.
D. Check for presence of gag reflex.
E. Assess general contour of abdomen with client lying flat. Look for concave or protuberant abdomen.
F. Assess for bowel sounds: decreased, increased, or hypoactive.
G. Check bowel habits and/or alterations in bowel elimination.

H. Palpate abdominal muscles for tenderness or rigidity; evaluate all quadrants of abdomen.
I. Assess bowel motility.
   1. Hypermotility may be result of irritation of autonomic nervous system or inflammatory process.
   2. Hypomotility may be result of blockage, intestinal muscle weakness, or chemical agents.
J. Check for amount of flatulence client reports, which indicates malfunction of system or dietary indiscretion.
K. Assess stool specimen.
   1. Check for presence of blood.
   2. Check for presence of mucus.
   3. Evaluate consistency, color, and odor of stool.
L. Assess fluid intake per day.
M. Evaluate dietary program, i.e. type of foods, amount, etc.
N. Evaluate laboratory tests.
O. Note presence or absence of hemorrhoids.
P. Assess degree of sphincter control through client reports of ability to control and regulate bowel movements.
Q. Assess for presence of pain along gastrointestinal tract and in accessory organs.
   1. Assess nonverbal signs, such as flinching, grimacing, etc.
   2. Evaluate onset, location, intensity, duration, and aggravating factors.
R. Palpate for rebound tenderness of spleen.
S. Check skin color for yellow tinge, pallor, or heavy flushing.
T. Assess for signs of shock following trauma to abdomen.
U. Evaluate tone of voice for hoarseness.
V. Assess client's knowledge of diagnostic tests or surgical interventions.

Diagnostic Procedures

Roentgenography of the Gastrointestinal Tract

A. The gastrointestinal tract cannot be visualized unless a contrast medium is ingested or instilled into it.
B. Barium sulfate—a white, chalky radiopaque substance that can be flavored—is normally used as a contrast medium.
C. For an upper gastrointestinal tract study, the client ingests an aqueous suspension of barium.

The progression of barium is followed by the fluoroscope.
D. Roentgenography of the upper tract reveals:
   1. Structure and function of the esophagus.
   2. Size and shape of the right atrium.
   3. Esophageal varices.
   4. Thickness of gastric wall.
   5. Motility of the stomach.
   6. Ulcerations, tumor formations, and anatomic abnormalities of the stomach.
   7. Pyloric valve patency.
   8. Emptying time of the stomach.
   9. Structural abnormalities of the small intestine.
E. X-rays are taken for permanent records.
F. Preparation of client for an upper GI roentgenograph.
   1. Maintain n.p.o. after midnight, prior to the test.
   2. Withhold medication.
   3. Explain procedure.
G. The lower GI roentgenograph involves rectal instillation of barium, which is viewed with the fluoroscope. Then permanent x-rays are taken.
H. The lower GI roentgenograph reveals the following information:
   1. Abnormalities in the structure of the colon.
   2. Contour and motility of the cecum and appendix.
I. Preparation of client for a lower GI roentgenograph.
   1. Empty intestinal tract by giving an enema, laxatives, or suppositories as ordered.
   2. Maintain n.p.o. after midnight, prior to the examination.
   3. Explain procedure to client.

Endoscopy

A. Visualization of the inside of a body cavity by means of a lighted tube.
B. Flexible scopes are used for these examinations; the scopes may be equipped with a camera.
C. Purposes.
   1. Direct visualization of mucosa to detect pathologic lesions.
   2. Obtaining biopsy specimens.
   3. Securing washings for cytologic examination.
D. Organs capable of being scoped: esophagus, stomach, duodenum, rectum, sigmoid colon, transverse colon, and right colon.

E. Nursing implementation.
   1. Explain procedure to client.
   2. Have client fast, prior to the examination.
   3. Prepare the lower bowel with laxatives, enemas, or suppositories as ordered.
   4. Prior to gastroscopy, a local anesthetic may be used in the posterior pharynx. Withhold fluids and food after the procedure until the gag reflex has returned.
   5. Support client during the procedure. The muscles of the GI tract tend to go into spasm with the passage of the scope, causing pain.
   6. Following the endoscopy, observe for hemorrhage, swelling, or dysfunction of the involved area.

Analysis of Secretions

A. Contents of the GI tract may be examined for the presence or absence of digestive juices, bacteria, parasites, and malignant cells.
B. Stomach contents may be aspirated and analyzed for volume and free and total acid.
C. *Gastric analysis,* performed by means of a nasogastric tube.
   1. Maintain n.p.o. six to eight hours prior to the test.
   2. Pass nasogastric tube; verify its presence in the stomach; tape to client's nose.
   3. Collect fasting specimens.
   4. Administer agents, such as alcohol, caffeine, histamine (0.2 mg subcutaneous), as ordered, to stimulate the flow of gastric acid.
      a. Watch for side effects of histamine, including flushing, headache, and hypotension.
      b. Do not give drug to clients with a history of asthma or other allergic conditions.
   5. Collect specimens as ordered, usually at 10 to 20 minute intervals.
   6. Label specimens and send to laboratory.
   7. Withdraw nasogastric tube; offer oral hygiene; make client comfortable.
   8. Gastric acid is high in the presence of duodenal ulcers, and is low in pernicious anemia.
D. *Tubeless gastric analysis.*
   1. Enables the determination of acidity or its absence.
   2. Have client fast for six to eight hours prior to the examination.
   3. Administer gastric stimulant, followed by Azuresin or Diagnex Blue, as ordered.
   4. Acid in the stomach displaces the dye, which is then released, absorbed by the bowel mucosa, and excreted in the urine.
   5. The bladder is emptied; the specimen saved. One hour after taking dye resin, client is instructed to void again. Urine is analyzed, and an estimation is made of the amount of free acid in the stomach.
E. Gastric washings for acid-fast bacilli.
   1. Have client fast six to eight hours prior to the procedure.
   2. Insert nasogastric tube and secure gastric washings.
   3. Send specimens to the laboratory to determine the presence of acid-fast bacilli.
   4. Wash your hands carefully and protect yourself from direct contact with specimens.
   5. This procedure is performed on suspected cases of active pulmonary tuberculosis when it is difficult to secure sputum for analysis.
F. Analysis of stools.
   1. Stool specimens are examined for amount, consistency, color, shape, blood, fecal urobilinogen, fat, nitrogen, parasites, food residue, and other substances.
   2. Stool cultures are also done for bacteria and viruses.
   3. Some foods and medicines can affect stool color: spinach, green; cocoa, dark red; senna, yellow; iron, black; upper GI bleeding, tarry black; lower GI bleeding, bright red.
   4. Stool abnormalities.
      a. Steatorrhea: bulky, greasy and foamy, foul odor.
      b. Biliary obstruction: light gray or clay-colored.
      c. Ulcerative colitis: loose stools, with copious amounts of mucus or pus.
      d. Constipation or obstruction: small, hard masses.
   5. Specimen collection.
      a. Specimens for detection of parasites should be sent to the laboratory while the stool is still warm and fresh.
      b. Examinations for blood are performed on small samples. A tongue blade may be used to place a small amount of stool in a disposable waxed container.

c. Stools for chemical analysis are usually examined for the total quantity expelled, so the complete stool is sent to the laboratory.

Biopsy and Cytology

A. Specimens for microscopic examination are secured by endoscopy examination, cell scrapings, and needle aspiration.
B. Specimens are examined, and the laboratory then determines their origin, structure, functions, and the presence of malignant cells.

Radionuclide Uptake

A. Radionuclides are used in diagnosis by measuring the localization of the substance, such as radioiodine in the thyroid, and the excretion of the material.
B. Various substances are studied, such as vitamin B_{12}, iron and fat, and major organs can be scanned.
C. Substances are tagged with radioactive isotopes to assess the degree of absorption.

Blood Examinations

A. Hematologic studies and electrolyte determinations reveal information about the general status of the client.
B. Results of these examinations in conjunction with other assessment procedures and clinical symptoms help to localize the disorder.

System Planning and Analysis

A. Alterations in bowel function are identified in the early stages of dysfunction.
B. Vital signs are stabilized.
C. Relief of abdominal distention occurs with increased client comfort.
D. Bowel sounds are present indicating no obstruction.
E. Bowel habits stabilize and no severe alterations occur.
F. Amount of flatulence lessens and client is more comfortable.
G. Stool specimens indicate absence of blood, pus, parasites, or other abnormalities.
H. Fluid and dietary intake are appropriate.
I. Pain and tenderness diminish, and client is comfortable.
J. Skin color reverts to normal.

K. Signs of shock and bleeding are absent.
L. Client is able to perform own colostomy or ileostomy care.
M. Client has adequate understanding of diagnostic procedures or surgical interventions.

System Implementation

A. Monitor vital signs.
B. Check for signs of dehydration.
   1. Dry mucous membranes.
   2. Poor skin turgor.
   3. Decreased urination.
   4. Increased pulse.
C. Monitor fluid intake or IV administration if ordered.
D. Monitor dietary intake or n.p.o. status as ordered.
E. Check and record stool pattern, consistency, color, odor, presence of blood or pus, etc.
F. Evaluate laboratory results of stool culture.
G. Observe skin tone, color, and changes.
H. Administer enema if ordered.
I. Promote bowel regulation through client teaching of dietary information.
J. Perform and teach colostomy or ileostomy care to client.
K. Place or assist physician in placing Miller-Abbott tube for relief of distention if ordered.
L. Instruct client on diagnostic tests.
M. Instruct client in preoperative and postoperative care.

System Evaluation

A. Gastrointestinal system functions normally.
   1. Abdominal distention is relieved.
   2. Flatulence is decreased.
   3. Bowel sounds are present.
   4. Alterations in elimination are corrected.
   5. Pain is not present.
B. Bowel habits stabilize and neither constipation nor diarrhea is present.
C. Stool specimens denote no abnormalities.
D. Fluid and dietary intake is modified to maintain hydration and dietary status.
E. Vital signs are stable.
F. No signs of shock are present.
G. Skin color is normal.

H. Client performs and understands principles of own colostomy or ileostomy care.

I. Client has appropriate knowledge of diagnostic tests and surgical interventions and is able to participate appropriately in tasks.

GENERAL DISORDERS

Definition: General symptoms of the gastrointestinal tract that may occur singly or concurrently and may be due to a wide variety of causes.

Anorexia

Definition: Loss of appetite.

Assessment

A. Assess for physiological basis for anorexia.
   1. Most illnesses, especially active stages of infections and disorders of the digestive organs, cause anorexia.
   2. Physical discomfort.
   3. Constipation.
   4. Fluid and electrolyte imbalances.
   5. Oral sepsis.
   6. Intestinal obstruction.
B. Assess for psychological source of anorexia.
   1. Fear and anxiety.
   2. Depression.
   3. Anorexia nervosa.
C. Assess for mechanical problems resulting in anorexia.
   1. Improperly fitting dentures.
   2. Excessive amounts of food.

Implementation

A. Be aware of client's eating habits, food likes and dislikes, and cultural and religious beliefs regarding food.
B. Permit choices of food when possible.
C. Show interest, but do not force client to eat.
D. Provide a pleasant environment.
E. Serve small, attractive portions of food.

Nausea and Vomiting

Definitions: Nausea is a feeling of revulsion for food, accompanied by salivation, sweating, and tachycardia. Vomiting is the contraction of the expiratory muscles of the chest, spasm of the diaphragm with contraction of the abdominal muscles, and subsequent relaxation of the stomach, allowing the gastric contents to be forced out through the mouth.

Characteristics

A. Accompanying symptoms: decreased blood pressure, increased salivation, sweating, weakness, faintness, paleness, vertigo, headache, and tachycardia.
B. Vomiting centers.
   1. Chemoreceptor emetic trigger zone.
   2. Vomiting center in the medulla.
C. Stimulation of vomiting centers.
   1. Impulses arising in the gastrointestinal tract.
   2. Impulses from cerebral centers.
   3. Chemicals via the bloodstream to the centers.
   4. Increased intracranial pressure.

Assessment

A. Assess for cerebromedullary causes.
   1. Stress, fear, and depression.
   2. Neuroses and psychoses.
   3. Shock.
   4. Pain.
   5. Hypoxemia.
   6. Increased intracranial pressure.
   7. Anesthesia.
B. Assess for toxic causes.
   1. Drugs ingested.
      a. Direct action on the brain.
      b. Irritant effects on the stomach or the small bowel.
   2. Food poisoning—ask foods recently ingested.
   3. Acute febrile disease—evaluate temperature.
C. Evaluate possible visceral causes.
   1. Allergy.
   2. Intestinal obstruction—evaluate bowel sounds.
   3. Constipation.
   4. Diseases of the stomach.
   5. Acute inflammatory disease of the abdominal and pelvic organs.
   6. Pregnancy.
   7. Cardiovascular diseases.
   8. Visceral disease.

9. Motion sickness.

D. Check for severe hypovitaminosis, especially B vitamins.

E. Assess for eating patterns: fasting or starvation.

F. Check for endocrine disorders, such as hypothyroidism and Addison's disease.

G. Observe character and quantity of emesis.

H. Evaluate hydration status and fluid and electrolyte balance.

I. Check daily weights.

J. Assess for complications: alkalosis, convulsions or tetany, atelectasis, or pneumonitis.

Implementation

A. Administer drugs: antiemetics, antihistamines, phenothiazines.

B. Monitor parenteral fluid and electrolyte replacements.

C. Perform gastric decompression.

D. Closely monitor prolonged vomiting as hemorrhage could result.

E. Monitor hydration status as dehydration will result in electrolyte imbalance leading to alkalosis.

F. Monitor for aspiration of vomitus, which may cause asphyxia, atelectasis, or pneumonitis.

G. Protect the client from unpleasant sights, sounds, and smells.

H. Promptly remove used emesis basin and equipment.

I. Promptly change soiled linens and dressings.

J. Ventilate room and use unscented air fresheners.

Constipation and Diarrhea

Definitions: Diarrhea is a condition characterized by loose, watery stools resulting from hypermotility of the bowel (not determined by frequency). Constipation is the undue delay in the evacuation of feces, with passage of hard and dry fecal material.

Assessment

A. Assess all other systems of the body to determine causal factors.

B. Assess for constipation.
1. Lack of regularity.
2. Psychogenic causes.
3. Drugs such as narcotics.
4. Inadequate fluid and bulk intake.
5. Mechanical obstruction.

C. Assess for diarrhea.
1. Fecal impaction.
2. Ulcerative colitis.
3. Intestinal infections.
4. Drugs such as antibiotics.
5. Neuroses.

D. Evaluate hydration status.

E. Assess for presence of metabolic acidosis.

F. Assess for fecal impaction—pain.

G. Observe the condition of the stool, such as color, odor, shape, consistency, amount, and any unusual features, such as mucus, blood, or pus.

Implementation

A. Administer drugs.
1. Laxatives may be used temporarily to relieve constipation, but regular use will cause loss of bowel tone.
2. Antidiarrheals, such as absorbents, astringents, and antispasmodics, may relieve symptoms.

B. Provide fluid and electrolyte replacement therapy to correct imbalances.

C. Prevent skin excoriation with emollients, powder, and cleanliness.

D. Change soiled linens and dressings.

E. Ventilate room.

DISORDERS OF THE UPPER GASTROINTESTINAL TRACT

Oral Infections

Definitions: Stomatitis is an inflammation of the mouth; glossitis, an inflammation of the tongue; and gingivitis, an inflammation of the gums.

Characteristics

A. Causes may be mechanical, chemical, or infection.

B. Types
1. Herpes simplex—a group of vesicles on an erythematous base.
   a. Usually located at the mucocutaneous junction of the lips and face.
   b. Caused by a virus that may be activated by sunlight, heat, fever, digestive disturbances, and menses.

c. Antimicrobial treatment is not effective unless there is secondary bacterial infection.

d. Treated symptomatically.

2. Vincent's angina (trench mouth)—purplish-red gums covered by pseudomembrane.

   a. Caused by fusiform bacteria and spirochetes.

   b. Symptoms include: fever, anorexia, enlarged cervical glands, and foul breath.

   c. May be acute, subacute, or chronic.

Assessment

A. Assess for anorexia.

B. Evaluate excessive salivation.

C. Check for foul breath.

D. Evaluate condition of gums and tongue.

E. Assess for jagged teeth or mouth breathing.

F. Check for foods or drinks that result in allergies.

G. Assess for presence of infection.

Implementation

A. Remove cause.

B. Provide frequent, soothing oral hygiene.

C. Administer topical medications or systemic antibiotics.

D. Provide a soft, bland diet.

E. Administer pain medications as needed.

Disorder of the Salivary Glands

Definition: Salivary gland infection is an inflammation (parotitis or surgical mumps) usually caused by *Staphylococcus aureus*.

Assessment

A. Assess for pain.

B. Check temperature.

C. Assess for enlargement of glands.

D. Assess for dysphagia.

Implementation

A. Administer preventive measures.

   1. Keep the glands active; calculus or calculi (stones) form when the gland is inactive.

   2. Provide adequate fluids.

   3. Give oral hygiene.

B. Provide warm packs.

C. Administer antibiotics.

D. Monitor hydration.

E. Care for incision.

F. Observe for drainage.

Malignant Tumors of the Mouth

Definition: Cancer of the mouth is a malignant tumor (squamous cell carcinomas) and usually affects the lips, the lateral border of the tongue, or the floor of the mouth.

Assessment

A. Assess for lesions that tend to be painless and hard and ulcerate easily.

B. Assess for poor oral hygiene.

C. Check for chronic irritation.

D. Evaluate for chemical and thermal trauma (tobacco, alcohol, and hot, spicy foods).

E. Assess for metastasis by local extension.

   1. Cause symptoms by occupying space and exerting pressure.

   2. Usually fibromas, lipomas, or neurofibromas.

Implementation

A. Provide postsurgical interventions.

B. Monitor for complications.

Radical Neck Dissection

Definition: Removal of cancerous lymph nodes in the neck.

Assessment

A. Assess for patent airway.

   1. Observe for airway obstruction (wheezing, stridor, retraction).

   2. Observe for respiratory distress, stertorous, labored breathing, increased respirations, and cyanosis.

B. Observe for edema that could constrict trachea.

C. Watch for difficulty in swallowing if allowed oral fluids. Difficulty may indicate nerve damage. If radical procedure, client will probably be fed through either nasogastric tube, gastrostomy, or IV therapy.

D. Observe dressings for hemorrhage, which could lead to respiratory embarrassment.

E. Assess vital signs for indications of bleeding and infection.

F. Assess for infection: increase in temperature, foul odor to dressings.

G. Observe for carotid rupture or chylous fistula— milky drainage.

H. Assess catheter drainage and suture lines.

I. Evaluate wound healing.

J. Observe for lower facial paralysis indicating facial nerve injury.

K. Assess mental state for depression, damage to self-image, feelings of loss, etc.

Implementation

A. Maintain adequate respiratory function.
   1. Place in high-Fowler's position.
   2. Monitor for respiratory distress.

B. Suction to prevent aspiration and pneumonia.

C. Administer oxygen as needed.

D. Encourage intake of fluids, which is necessary to thin secretions.

E. Provide care for laryngectomy (frequently performed with radical neck dissection).
   1. Use mist mask.
   2. Clean tube as you would tracheostomy tube.

F. Change dressings frequently to prevent infection.
   1. Drains are frequently placed in surgical site; Hemovac is the drain most commonly used.
   2. Observe for unusual drainage (amount, type, as well as odor).

G. Give oral hygiene every two to four hours.

H. Develop means to communicate as client will not be able to talk postoperatively if laryngectomy was also performed.
   1. Provide method of writing for the first few days.
   2. Explain to client that hoarseness is usual for the first few weeks.
   3. Provide bell or readily accessible means of communication for client who will be anxious following surgery.

I. Provide privacy for client.

J. Develop nurse-client relationship, for client may be depressed, may suffer feelings of loss, and may need to verbalize concerns about self-image.

K. Teach or follow through with rehabilitation exercises for head and shoulder.
   1. Rotate neck, tilt head to both sides, and drop chin to chest.
   2. Swing arm on operated side in arc to extend range of motion.

L. Provide general postoperative care.

Laryngectomy

Definition: Removal of larynx due to malignant tumors.

Characteristics

A. Total laryngectomy and radical neck dissection procedure of choice for cancer under following circumstances:
   1. If tumor does not extend more than 5 mm up base of tongue or below upper edge of cricoarytenoid muscle.
   2. If there is no evidence of distant metastasis.

B. Epiglottis, thyroid cartilage, hyoid bone, cricoid cartilage, and part of trachea are removed.

C. Stump of trachea is brought out to neck and sutured to skin. The pharyngeal portion is closed, and breathing through nose is eliminated.

D. Accompanied by radical neck dissection if neck tissue and lymph nodes are involved.

Assessment

A. Assess drainage from wound suction for amount, color, and odor.

B. Assess for carotid artery hemorrhage.

C. Evaluate lung fluids for atelectasis and pneumonia.

Implementation

A. Suction frequently with sterile technique until area has healed; then use clean technique.

B. Place pressure on neck wound for hemorrhage around site.

C. Instruct client regarding means for communication, as he or she will not be able to speak immediately postoperatively.

D. Speech rehabilitation is utilized after surgical area has healed.

Inflammation of the Esophagus

Definition: Esophagitis may be caused by local or systemic infection, or by chemical irritation from reflux of gastric juices into the lower esophagus.

Assessment

A. Assess for heartburn.

B. Assess for intolerance of spices, alcohol, and caffeine.

C. Check for dysphagia.

Implementation

A. Administer oral antacids.

B. Provide a bland diet.

C. Elevate head of bed.

Esophageal Varices

Definition: Tortuous dilated veins in the submucosa of the lower esophagus, possibly extending into the fundus of the stomach or upward into the esophagus; caused by portal hypertension and often associated with cirrhosis of the liver.

Assessment

A. Assess for bleeding.

B. Check for hypotension.

C. Evaluate neck vein for distention.

D. Assess for nutritional status.

E. Evaluate indications that lead to suspected varices.
   1. Hematemesis.
   2. Hematochezia.
   3. History of alcoholism.

F. Observe for strain of coughing or vomiting which could result in esophageal rupture.

Implementation

A. Carefully observe vital signs, watching for hemorrhage and shock.

B. Maintain prescribed pressure levels in esophagogastric balloons.

C. Provide frequent oral hygiene and aspiration of the mouth and throat since the client cannot swallow saliva with the balloons in place.

D. Prevent esophageal erosion by deflating the balloons (only with physician's order).

E. Safety measure: keep scissors at bedside. If tube dislodges and causes obstruction, cut tube to deflate balloons.

F. Prevent nasal breakdown.
   1. Keep nostrils lubricated and clean.
   2. Provide foam rubber padding to reduce pressure.

G. Observe for sudden respiratory crisis, which may occur with aspiration or upward displacement of the balloons.

H. Maintain fluid and nutritional balance.

I. Observe for complications of active bleeding varices.
   1. Hypovolemia.
   2. Hepatic encephalopathy due to increased ammonia production as blood protein is metabolized.
   3. Metabolic imbalances due to acid-base and electrolyte disturbances.

J. Comfort family and client.
   1. Explain procedures and utilize nursing comfort measures.
   2. Use sedatives and narcotics judiciously because the liver is usually impaired in its ability to detoxify.

MEDICAL IMPLICATIONS

A. Lowering portal pressure by Pitressin administration.
   1. Intravenous infusion.
      a. 20 to 50 units in 100 to 200 cc D_5W over 20 minutes.
      b. Side effects.
         (1) Abdominal colic.
         (2) Bowel evacuation.
         (3) Facial pallor.
         (4) Arterial hypertension and reduced hepatic blood flow.
   2. Intra-arterial infusion.
      a. 0.05 to 0.1 unit per minute via the superior mesenteric artery.
      b. The rate of infusion may be increased up to a limit of 0.4 unit per minute.
      c. Side effects at the catheter insertion site.
         (1) Bleeding.
         (2) Thrombosis.
         (3) Embolism.
         (4) Infection.
      d. Major complication: bowel necrosis from altered perfusion.

B. Sengstaken-Blakemore tube for pressure application against varices.
   1. Tube has three openings.
      a. One opening to gastric balloon (inflated with 200 cc of air).
      b. Second opening to esophageal balloon.

   c. Third opening for aspiration of gastric contents.
   2. Traction with a ¾ to 1½ pound weight used to prevent downward movement.
   3. Iced saline irrigations may be used to vaso-constrict the small collaterals.
C. Restoration of clotting factors.
   1. Vitamin K replacement.
   2. Platelet replacement (destroyed by damaged spleen).
   3. Fresh-frozen plasma.
D. Surgical repairs.
   1. Direct ligation of varices.
   2. Portasystemic shunts.
      a. Portacaval.
         (1) End to side.
         (2) Side to side.
      b. Splenorenal.
         (1) End to side.
         (2) Side to side.
      c. Mesocaval.
         (1) End to side.
         (2) Use of synthetic graft.

Esophageal Hernia (Hiatus Hernia)

Definition: In esophageal hernia, a portion of the stomach herniates through the diaphragm and into the thorax.

Characteristics

A. Congenital weakness.
B. Trauma.
C. Relaxation of muscles.
D. Increased intra-abdominal pressure.
E. Manifestations range from none to acutely severe manifestations.

Assessment

A. Assess for heartburn and pain.
B. Assess for dysphagia.
C. Check vomiting pattern.
D. Assess for complications.
   1. Ulceration.
   2. Hemorrhage.
   3. Regurgitation and aspiration of gastric contents.
   4. Incarceration of stomach in the chest, with possible necrosis, peritonitis, and mediastinitis.

Implementation

A. Provide small, frequent meals, avoiding highly seasoned foods.
B. Maintain upright position during and after meals.
C. Give antacids after meals and at bedtime.
D. Elevate head of bed to avoid regurgitation.
E. Avoid anticholinergic drugs which delay emptying of the stomach.
F. Prevent constricting clothing about the waist and sharp, forward bending.
G. Monitor medical treatment.
   1. Reduction of stomach distention.
   2. Reduction of stomach acidity.
   3. Reduction of increased levels of intra-abdominal pressure.
H. Give postoperative care for surgical reduction of hernia, via a thoracic or abdominal approach.

Esophageal Neoplasms

Characteristics

A. Benign lesions.
   1. Leiomyoma most common type.
   2. Asymptomatic.
B. Malignant lesions.
   1. Usually occur in lower two-thirds of esophagus.
   2. Mainly affect men over fifty.
   3. Smoking and alcohol are risk factors.
      a. Poor prognosis (less than five years' survival) due to early lymphatic spread and late development of symptoms.
      b. Dysphagia most common symptom.
      c. Diagnosis made by barium swallow, esophagoscopy, biopsy.
C. Treatment
   1. Surgical excision.
   2. Radiation therapy (fistulas may be a complication).

Assessment

A. Assess for extent of lesions.
B. Evaluate vital signs.
C. Observe for poor dietary status.
D. Observe for complications of ulceration and hemorrhage, fistula formation, and pneumothorax in end-stage disease.

Implementation

A. Maintain fluid and electrolyte balance.
B. Manage nutrition needs (hyperalimentation therapy may be used).
C. Administer gastrostomy tube feedings, if needed.
D. Monitor client's ability to handle secretions.
E. Provide emotional support.

GASTRIC DISORDERS

Dyspepsia Indigestion

Definition: Indigestion is caused by diseases of the gastrointestinal system, eating too rapidly, emotional problems, inadequate chewing, eating improperly cooked foods, systemic diseases, food allergies, and altered gastric secretion or motility.

Assessment

A. Assess for heartburn.
B. Assess for flatulence.
C. Observe for nausea.
D. Observe for eructations.
E. Identify feeling of fullness.

Implementation

A. Based on the cause of the disorder.
B. Antacids and bland diets.
C. Antispasmodics and tranquilizers.
D. Altered eating habits.

Anorexia Nervosa

Definition: Underlying emotional disorders cause psychogenic aversion to food, with resulting emaciation. It usually occurs in females during the late teens or early twenties.

Assessment

A. Assess weight—loss of one-fourth to one-half or more of the body weight occurs with this disorder.
B. Check for amenorrhea.
C. Observe vomiting when food is forced.
D. Assess for hypotension.
E. Evaluate for anemia.
F. Assess for hypoproteinemia.

Implementation

A. Give supportive care.
B. Administer tube feedings.
C. Monitor psychiatric treatment.
   1. Set firm limits.
   2. Monitor eating patterns.

Acute Gastritis

Definition: An inflammation of the stomach.

Characteristics

A. Ingestion of infectious, corrosive, or erosive substance (such as alcohol, aspirin, and food poisoning).
B. Acute systemic infections.
C. Radiotherapy or chemotherapy.

Assessment

A. Assess for pain.
B. Evaluate nausea and vomiting pattern.
C. Check for malaise.
D. Observe for hemorrhage.
E. Assess for anorexia.
F. Check for headache.

Implementation

A. Remove cause and treat symptomatically.
B. Monitor drugs that include antacids and phenothiazines.

Chronic Gastritis

Definition: A nondescript upper abdominal distress with vague symptoms which indicate that other causes should be explored.

Characteristics

A. Atrophic: decreased number of gastric cells, and shrinking of mucosa and muscular layers.
B. Hypertrophic: modular, thickened, irregular mucosa.
C. Superficial: edematous, reddened mucosa with erosions.
D. Symptoms vary greatly; majority of persons do not have symptoms.

Assessment

A. Assess for dyspepsia, anorexia, and eructations.
B. Check for foul taste in mouth.
C. Assess for nausea and vomiting.
D. Assess for pain and mild epigastric tenderness.
E. Observe for complications.
 1. Hemorrhage.
 2. Scarring of mucosa.
 3. Ulcer formation.
 4. Malnutrition.

Implementation

The same as for peptic ulcer.

Peptic Ulcer Disease

Definition: An ulceration in the mucosal wall of the stomach, pylorus, or duodenum, occurring in portions that are accessible to gastric secretions. Erosion may extend through the muscle to the peritoneum.

Characteristics

A. Pathophysiology
 1. Any condition that upsets the balance between digestion and protection.
  a. Digestive balance: hydrochloric acid and pepsin secretion.
  b. Protective balance: hormone mucin.
  c. Bacterial invasion of mucosa.
 2. The gastroduodenal mucosa is unable to withstand action of gastric acid and pepsin.
 3. This is due either to an increase in concentration or activity of acid and pepsin, and/or a decrease in normal resistance of mucosa.
 4. Predisposing factors.
  a. Emotional stress.
  b. Excessive smoking.
  c. Ingestion of steroids and ASA.
  d. Irregular eating patterns; eating hurriedly.
B. Diagnostic evaluation.
 1. Medical history and symptoms.
 2. Upper GI series—most definitive.
 3. Gastroscopy—fiberoptic panendoscopy.
 4. Gastric analysis—helpful in atypical cases.
 5. Laboratory examination of blood and stools.

Assessment

A. Assess pain.
 1. Location and intensity.
 2. Duration.
 3. Aggravating factors.
B. Check if pain is relieved by food.
C. Assess dietary patterns, types of foods, etc.
D. Evaluate vital signs.
E. Assess degree of stress and identify stressors.
F. Evaluate laboratory results.
G. Check stool for blood.
H. Observe for hemorrhage.
 1. Dark, granular (coffee ground) emesis is a result of acid digestion of blood in the stomach.
 2. Tarry, black stools result when blood is completely digested.
 3. Hematemesis (vomiting of bright-red blood).
 4. Bright-red blood from rectum. Occurs when bleeding originates from high in the gastrointestinal tract and there is concurrent rapid gastrointestinal motility.

Implementation

A. Administer and monitor medications.
 1. Histamine H_2 receptor antagonists: front-line therapy.
  a. Cimetidine (Tagamet), ranitidine (Zantac), famotidine (Pepcid), and nizatidine (Axid), p.o. or IV.
  b. Action: blocking action reduces production of gastric acid and allows ulcers to heal.
  c. Drugs over 90% effective when taken p.o. for 8 weeks.
  d. Minimal side effects: headache and skin rash.
 2. New drugs with limited FDA approval due to serious side effects (diarrhea and abdominal pain).
  a. Omeprazole (Prilosec), gastric acid pump inhibitor indicated for short-term treatment of duodenal ulcers.
  b. Misoprostol (Cytotec), a synthetic prostaglandin, particularly useful for persons using long-term NSAIDS. Protects stomach lining from erosive action of gastric acid. (This drug may induce abortions.)
 3. Antacids.
  a. Action: reduces gastric acidity; given for pain.
  b. Taken one hour after meals, effects last longer.
  c. Side effects: diarrhea and constipation.
  d. Types of nonabsorbable antacids.
   (1) Calcium carbonate is most effective but may cause hypercalcemia, hypercalciuria and constipation.

(2) Magnesium oxide is more potent than either magnesium trisilicate or magnesium carbonate.

(3) Aluminium hydroxide—high sodium content and constipation are disadvantages.

(4) Sodium bicarbonate is absorbed and should be avoided to prevent systemic alkalosis.

4. Sucralfate (Carafate).

  a. Action: stimulates release of prostaglandins; stimulates mucosal barrier.

  b. Duration is 5 hours; administer one hour before or after meals and at bedtime on an empty stomach.

  c. Prescribed when drug interactions or side effects negate use of H_2 antagonists.

  d. Side effects: constipation, nausea and vomiting.

5. Antibiotics (Amoxil).

  a. Used for treating ulcers caused by *Helicobacter Pylori* infection.

  b. Combined with bismuth preparations and H_2 antagonists.

6. Anticholingeric drugs.

  a. Used only for clients with severe pain in the early morning.

  b. Drug action increases risk of gastric outlet syndrome.

7. Assist client to understand medication regimen: medications, dosages, times administered, and desired effects.

B. Provide dietary control of symptoms.

1. Ensure three nutritious meals.

2. Avoid black pepper, foods that cause distress, e.g., highly seasoned, rough, greasy, gas-forming, or fried.

3. Avoid prolonged use of milk and cream as they actually stimulate acid production.

4. Avoid alcohol as it releases gastrin, stimulates the parietal cells, and may damage the mucosa.

5. Avoid tea, coffee, and cola because caffeine stimulates gastric secretion.

6. Do not provide any snacks, even at bedtime (stimulates acid secretion).

7. Provide iron and ascorbic acid to promote healing.

C. Reduce stressful situations.

1. Allow client to care for important business obligations.

2. Eliminate visitors or duties that increase stress.

3. Teach autogenic methods of stress reduction, relaxation, tension-releasing activities.

D. Promote rest.

1. Adequate sleep is strongly advised.

2. Business and social responsibilities should be curtailed during acute phase.

3. Hospitalization may be required if therapy is not effective in one week's time.

4. Sedatives and tranquilizers may be helpful for the anxious, tense client.

E. Provide client and family teaching regarding:

1. Diet.

2. Activity levels and rest.

3. Correct use of medications.

4. Potential complications and how to deal with them.

5. Avoid smoking—decreases healing rate.

F. Observe for complications.

1. Hemorrhage, ranging from slight blood loss (revealed by occult blood in stool) to massive blood loss, which may lead to shock.

  a. Promote bed rest.

  b. Observe vital signs.

  c. Observe consistency, color, and volume of vomitus and stools.

  d. Provide nasogastric suction to empty the stomach of clots and blood and to watch the rate of bleeding.

  e. Monitor blood, plasma, or IV fluids to support blood volume.

  f. Administer narcotics and/or tranquilizers to reduce restlessness and to relieve pain.

  g. Gavage with ice water to increase vasoconstriction.

2. Perforation: occurs almost exclusively in males twenty-five to forty years of age.

  a. Monitor acute onset of severe, persistent pain that increases in intensity and can be referred to the shoulder.

  b. Examine for tender, board-like rigidity of the abdomen.

3. Pyloric obstruction caused by scarring, edema, or inflammation at the pylorus.

  a. Monitor for the following signs: nausea and vomiting, pain, weight loss, and constipation.

  b. Be aware that persistent vomiting can lead to alkalosis.

Table 1. COMPARISON OF DUODENAL AND GASTRIC ULCER

	Chronic Duodenal Ulcer	Chronic Gastric Ulcer
Age	Usually twenty-five to fifty	Usually fifty and over
Sex	Male:female—4:1	Male:female—2:1
Blood group	Most frequently type O	Blood group A
Social class	Executives, competitive leaders	Lower socio-economic class
Incidence	80%	20%
General nourishment	Well nourished	Malnourished
Acid production in stomach	Hypersecretion	Normal to hyposecretion
Location	Within 3 cm. of pylorus	Lesser curvature
Pain	45–60 minutes after meals and at night. Usually absent before breakfast—worsens as day progresses. Ingestion of food, antacids or vomiting relieves pain.	On an empty stomach or shortly after the meal. Rarely is there pain at night. Relieved by food, antacids or vomiting.
Vomiting	Uncommon	Common
Hemorrhage	Melena more common than hematemesis	Hematemesis more common than melena
Malignancy possibility	None	Usually less than 10%

SURGICAL INTERVENTION FOR GASTROINTESTINAL DISEASES

Gastric Cancer

Definition: Carcinoma of the stomach is a common cancer of the digestive tract.

Characteristics

A. Responsible for twenty thousand deaths annually in the United States.
B. Has decreased in incidence during the last twenty years, but is a significant cause of death because of low cure rate.
C. Occurs twice as often in males as in females, and more often in Blacks than in other races.
D. Found frequently in conjunction with pernicious anemia and atrophic gastritis.
E. Worldwide incidence varies.
F. Early carcinoma causes no symptoms.

Assessment

A. Assess for weight loss and anorexia.
B. Check for feeling of vague fullness and sensation of pressure.
C. Assess for anemia from blood loss.
D. Examine stools for occult blood.
E. Assess vomiting if pylorus becomes obstructed.
F. Observe for late symptoms: ascites, palpable mass, and pain from metastasis.
G. Evaluate for metastasis.
   1. Occurs by direct extension into surrounding tissue.
   2. Spreads through lymphatic and hematogenous systems.

Implementation

A. Provide postoperative care for surgical resection.
   1. Surgical mortality is 5 to 12 percent.
   2. Five-year survival rate is 5 to 15 percent.
B. Monitor chemotherapy—response has not been consistent; may shorten lifespan if toxic effects occur.
C. Provide nursing implementation (same as for peptic ulcer disease).

SURGICAL IMPLICATIONS

A. Vagotomy and gastroenterostomy or pyloroplasty.
   1. Vagus nerve is cut.
   2. Drainage of stomach.
      a. Drainage operation necessary because vagotomy is often followed by gastric retention.
      b. Vagus nerve provides the motor impulses to the gastric musculature, whose division is often followed by gastric atony.
   3. The pyloroplasty or gastroenterostomy also reduces the stimulation of gastric acid by reducing the formation of gastrin produced in the antral area of the stomach.
B. Vagotomy and antrectomy.
   1. Decrease production of acid to a point where ulcers will not recur.
   2. Remove acid-stimulating mechanism of stomach (that is, divide vagus nerve and remove antral portion of stomach).
C. Partial gastrectomy and possible vagotomy.
   1. Billroth I—partial gastrectomy with remaining segment of stomach anastomosed to duodenum.
   2. Billroth II—remaining segment of stomach is anastomosed to jejunum. (Usual for duodenal ulcer.)

Postoperative Period

Assessment

A. Observe color, amount, and consistency of nasogastric drainage.
B. Evaluate patency of nasogastric tube.
C. Evaluate type and severity of pain.
D. Evaluate client's ability to deep breathe and cough.
E. Assess intravenous site for possible complications.
F. Listen for bowel sounds.
G. Assess all systems for possible complications.

Implementation

A. After anesthesia recovery, place in modified Fowler's for comfort and easy stomach drainage.
B. Prevent pulmonary complications—medicate before turning, coughing, or hyperventilating.
C. Institute nasogastric suction; drainage contains some blood first twelve hours.
   1. Physician inserts tube.
   2. Keep patent by irrigating with sodium chloride.
D. See that client is n.p.o. (no peristalsis).
E. Give intravenous fluids with potassium chloride.
F. After nasogastric tube is out, give small sips of clear water. (Do not use straw.)
   1. Do not give cold fluids (cause distress); give warm, weak tea.
   2. Offer bland foods to where client eats six small meals a day and drinks 120 cc fluid between meals.
G. Promote ambulation on first postoperative day unless contraindicated by physician.
H. Check drainage tubes if inserted. (Serosanguineous drainage is normal.)
I. Observe for postoperative complications.
   1. Shock (from hypovolemia).
   2. Vomiting—usually due to blood left in stomach. (Nasogastric tube prevents vomiting.)
   3. Hemorrhage.
   4. Pulmonary complications.
   5. Large fluid and electrolyte losses.
   6. Dumping syndrome—due to rapid emptying of gastric contents into small intestine, which has been anastomosed to the gastric stump.
      a. Mechanical result of surgery in which a small gastric remnant remains after surgery.
      b. From this there is a large opening from the gastric stump into the jejunum.
      c. Foods that are high in carbohydrates and electrolytes must be diluted in the jejunum before absorption can take place.
      d. The ingestion of fluid at mealtime is another factor in the rapid emptying of the stomach into the jejunum.
      e. Symptoms are caused by rapid distention of jejunal loop anastomosed to stomach.
         (1) There is a withdrawal of water from the circulating blood volume into the jejunum to dilute the high concentration of electrolytes and sugars.
         (2) A rapid movement of extracellular fluids into the bowel occurs and converts the hypertonic material to an isotonic mixture.
         (3) This rapid shift decreases the circulatory blood volume, like a hypovolemic shock.

f. Foods high in sugars and salt produce the symptoms.
   (1) Palpitation.
   (2) Perspiration.
   (3) Faintness.
   (4) Weakness that lasts from a few minutes to as long as thirty minutes and causes the client to lie down.
g. Prevention of dumping syndrome.
   (1) Avoid sugar and salt; maintain a high-protein, high-fat, low-carbohydrate diet.
   (2) Avoid drinking fluids with meals, thereby delaying gastric emptying.
   (3) Lie down after meals.
   (4) Physicians can prevent symptoms by forming smaller stomas and larger gastric stump.
   (5) Syndrome usually subsides in six months.
7. Diarrhea—complication of vagotomy (use Kaopectate).
8. Vitamin B_{12} deficiency.
   a. Production of "intrinsic factor" is halted. (The gastric secretion is required for the absorption of vitamin B_{12} from the gastrointestinal tract.)
   b. Unless supplied by parenteral injection throughout life, client suffers vitamin B_{12} deficiency.

INTESTINAL DISORDERS

Regional Enteritis (Regional Ileitis, Crohn's Disease)

Definition: An inflammatory disease of the small intestine that is chronic and relapsing. It results in thickening, scarring, and granulomas of intestinal tissues, which cause narrow lumen, fistulas, ulcerations, and abscesses. The etiology is unknown, but may be related to altered immunologic reactivity.

Characteristics
A. Occurs at all ages.
B. Usually observed in second and third decade of life.
C. High incidence of familial occurrence.
D. High incidence in Jewish population; low in Blacks.

Assessment
A. Assess for cramp-like pain after meals.
B. Evaluate for weight loss.

C. Check for malnutrition.
D. Assess for secondary anemia.
E. Check for chronic diarrhea.
F. Evaluate temperature.
G. Assess for acute perforation, generalized peritonitis, and massive melena, which are sometimes present at onset.

Implementation
A. Provide appropriate diet: low-residue, bland, with iron and vitamin supplements.
B. Administer medications.
   1. Antibiotics (nonabsorbable sulfonamides) to control infection.
   2. Antiinflammatory drugs to reduce swollen membranes.
   3. Antidiarrheal agents to control diarrhea.
   4. Sedatives and narcotics to reduce apprehension and pain.
C. Provide postoperative care for surgical intervention (ileostomy).

Intestinal Malignant Tumors

Characteristics
A. Adenocarcinoma of the duodenum is the most common lesion of small intestines.
   1. In the United States, less than one percent of gastrointestinal tract cancers arise in the small bowel.
   2. Occurs in younger age group; twice as common in men.
B. Malignant tumors of large intestine are second most frequent cause of death from cancer.
   1. Men and women equally affected.
   2. CA colon more common in women; CA rectum more common in men.
   3. Metastasis is by direct extension, usually to stomach from transverse colon, bladder, and bowel.

Assessment
A. Assess for abnormal stools, malabsorption, or intestinal bleeding.
B. Assess for weight loss.
C. Check for anorexia.
D. Check for vomiting.
E. Evaluate crampy pain.
F. Assess for intestinal obstruction or biliary obstruction.

Implementation

A. Provide postoperative care for surgical intervention.
   1. Large intestine tumors may result in a colostomy.
   2. Instruct client in colostomy procedure and care.
   3. Refer client to ostomy club.
B. Monitor cytotoxic drug therapy following surgery.
C. Provide psychological support.
D. Maintain low-residue or liquid diet.
E. Administer antibiotics if ordered.

Appendicitis

Definition: Appendicitis is an inflammation of the appendix due to infection.

Assessment

A. Assess for generalized, severe upper abdominal pain that localizes in the right lower quadrant.
B. Check for anorexia.
C. Evaluate slightly increased temperature.
D. Assess for nausea and vomiting.

Implementation

A. Place in semi-Fowler's position to relieve abdominal strain.
B. Give nothing by mouth until bowel sounds present.
C. Insert nasogastric tube as required.
D. Ensure adequate bowel evacuation with enema, if necessary.
E. Insert rectal tube for flatus.
F. Follow routine postoperative nursing care for any abdominal surgery.

Intestinal Obstructions

Definition: An impairment of the forward flow of intestinal contents by partial or complete stoppage.

Characteristics

A. Mechanical type of obstruction.
   1. Adhesions—fibrous bands of scar tissue, following abdominal surgery, may become looped over a portion of the bowel.
   2. Hernias—incarcerated or strangulated.
   3. Volvulus—twisting of the bowel.
   4. Intussusception—telescoping of the bowel upon itself.
   5. Tumors.
   6. Hematoma.
   7. Fecal impaction.
   8. Intraluminal obstruction.
B. Neurogenic type of obstruction.
   1. Paralytic, adynamic ileus.
   2. Ineffective peristalsis due to toxic or traumatic disturbance of the autonomic nervous system.
C. Vascular type of obstruction.
   1. Occlusion of the arterial blood supply to the bowel.
   2. Mesenteric thrombosis.
   3. Abdominal angina.
D. Pathophysiology.
   1. Fluids and air collect proximal to the obstruction.
      a. Peristalsis increases as the bowel attempts to force material through.
      b. Peristalsis ends and the bowel becomes blocked.
   2. Pressure increases in the bowel and decreases the absorptive ability.
   3. Circulating blood volume is reduced and shock may develop.
   4. Location of the obstruction determines the symptoms and progression of the clinical course.

Assessment

A. Assess for small bowel obstruction by evaluating following symptoms.
   1. Cramp-like pain in midabdomen.
   2. Nausea and early severe vomiting.
   3. Reverse peristalsis.
   4. Dehydration.
   5. Abdominal distention.
   6. Shock and death.
B. Assess for large bowel obstruction by evaluating following symptoms.
   1. Progression of symptoms is slower than with small bowel obstruction.
   2. Constipation.
   3. Abdominal distention.
   4. Cramp-like pain in lower abdomen.
   5. Fecal vomiting if ileocecal valve incompetent.

C. Assess for paralytic ileus by evaluating following symptoms.
  1. Dull, diffused pain.
  2. Gaseous distention.
  3. Constipation.
  4. Vomiting after eating.
D. Observe and report the nature, duration, and character of pain.
E. Assess the presence and progression of distention and the absence of flatus and stool.
F. Observe for signs and symptoms of fluid and electrolyte imbalance.

Implementation

A. Assist in placement of Miller-Abbott or Cantor tube for intestinal decompression to remove gas and fluid.
B. Monitor parenteral fluids to replace fluids and electrolytes.
  1. Sodium, potassium, and chloride.
  2. Dextrose and water.
C. Administer antibiotics to prevent secondary infections (especially peritonitis).
D. Measure and record vital signs, intake and output, and emesis.
E. Save stool for testing.
F. Prepare client for surgery, if indicated.

Herniorrhaphy

Definition: A hernia is a protrusion of the intestine through an opening in the abdominal wall.

Characterisitics

A. Femoral—below groin.
B. Umbilical—around umbilicus, due to failure of orifice to close.
C. Incisional—due to weakness in incisional area from infection or poor healing.
D. Inguinal—weakness in abdominal wall where round ligament is located in female and where spermatic cord emerges in male.

Assessment

A. Assess for possible wound healing at incision site.
B. Assess for edematous scrotum for inguinal hernia.
C. Check for constipation.
D. Assess for abdominal distention.

Implementation

A. Treatment.
  1. Reducing hernia—place an appliance over hernia area to prevent abdominal contents from entering hernia area and strangulating.
  2. Surgical intervention.
B. Postoperative Care.
  1. Maintain routine postoperative care.
  2. Ambulate day of surgery or next morning.
  3. Provide ice pack or scrotal support if inguinal hernia in male.
  4. Prevent urine retention.
  5. Report any abdominal distention.

Diverticulosis and Diverticulitis

Definitions: Diverticulum is the outpouching of the intestinal mucosa, which may occur at any point in the gastrointestinal tract but more commonly in the sigmoid colon. It is caused by congenital weakness and increased pressure in the lumen. Diverticulosis is the presence of multiple diverticula. Diverticulitis is the inflammation of diverticula.

Characteristics

A. No symptoms unless complications develop.
B. Large bowel diverticula are more apt to develop complications.
C. Complications are perforation, hemorrhage, inflammation, fistulas, and abscess.

Assessment

A. Assess for cramp-like pain.
B. Check for flatulence.
C. Assess for nausea.
D. Evaluate patterns of irregularity, irritability, and spasticity of the intestine.
E. Assess for fever.
F. Examine for dysuria associated with bladder involvement.

Implementation

A. Provide care during acute phase.
  1. Intravenous fluids with electrolytes.
  2. Bed rest.
  3. Nothing by mouth.
  4. Nasogastric decompression.

5. Drugs: antibiotics, analgesics, antispasmodics, and bulk former (Metamucil).
B. Monitor appropriate diet.
   1. Current studies indicate a high-residue diet using bran fiber for diverticulosis.
   2. Low residue regimen for severe inflammatory phase of diverticulitis.
   3. Provide vitamin and iron supplements.
C. Instruct client and family in pathology and rationale for treatment.
D. Administer anticholinergics: Donnatal, Pro-Banthine.
E. Provide sedatives and tranquilizers for anxiety.
F. Monitor stool normalization: bowel lubricant nightly, bulk preparation daily, evacuant suppository, vegetable oil, unprocessed bran in fruit juice daily.

Ulcerative Colitis

Definition: A chronic ulcerative and inflammatory disease of the colon and rectum, which commonly begins in the rectum and sigmoid colon and spreads upward. The disease is characterized by periods of exacerbations and remissions.

Characteristics

A. Cause unknown, but theories include autoimmune factor, allergic reaction, specific vulnerability of colon, emotional instability, and bacterial infection.
B. Most common in young adulthood and middle life. More prevalent among Jews; less common in blacks than whites.

Assessment

A. Assess for gradual onset.
   1. Malaise.
   2. Early—vague abdominal discomfort.
   3. Later—crampy abdominal pain.
   4. Bowel evacuation—pus, mucus, and blood.
   5. Stools scanty and hard.
   6. Painful straining with defecation.
B. Assess for abrupt onset.
   1. Severe diarrhea (15 to 20 watery stools a day that may contain blood and mucus).
   2. Fever.
   3. Anorexia.
   4. Weight loss.
   5. Abdominal tenderness.
   6. Rectal and anal spasticity.
   7. Consistency of stools vary with areas of colon involved.
C. Assess for complications.
   1. Dehydration.
   2. Magnesium and calcium imbalances.
   3. Anemia and malnutrition—malabsorption and iron and vitamin K deficiency.
   4. Perforation, peritonitis, and hemorrhage.
   5. Abscesses and strictures.
   6. Carcinomatous degeneration (if more than 10 years' duration).
   7. Hemorrhoids and anal fissures.
   8. Bleeding tendency.
D. Evaluate results of client's history and diagnostic tests.
   1. Medical history.
   2. Clinical manifestations.
   3. Lower GI series.
   4. Stool and blood examinations.
   5. Sigmoidoscopy.

Implementation

A. Major objective—prevent acute episodes and/or manage complications.
B. Maintain nutritional status.
   1. High-protein, high-calorie diet, high fiber.
   2. Avoid gas-forming foods and milk products.
   3. All foods should be cooked to reduce cramping and diarrhea.
   4. Vitamin and iron supplements.
   5. Eating may increase diarrhea and anorexia.
C. Replace fluid and electrolytes.
   1. 3 to 4 liters/day.
   2. Added potassium chloride.
D. Correct psychological disturbances.
   1. Allow client to ventilate feelings; accept client as he or she is.
   2. Help client live with chronic disease (a change in lifestyle may be necessary).
   3. Avoid emotional probing during periods of acute illness.
   4. Provide client and family with instructions about pathology of the disease and rationale for treatment.
E. Administer drugs as ordered.
   1. Steroid therapy for inflammation, toxicity, and emotional symptoms.

a. Induces remissions.

b. Given IV in acute episode.

c. Given rectally for long term.

2. Anti-infectives.

a. Routine sulfonamides to reduce severity of attack.

b. Antibiotic therapy for secondary bowel inflammation and systemic infections.

3. Immunosuppressives.

4. Tranquilizers: e.g., phenobarbital to relieve anxiety and decrease peristalsis.

5. Anticholinergics.

a. Relieve abdominal cramps.

b. Assist in controlling diarrhea.

6. In acute stages cathartics contraindicated.

F. Maintain bed rest during acute phase.

Table 2. SURGICAL CORRECTIONS FOR THE COLON

Colostomy

A. Causes.

1. Cancer of colon—permanent colostomy.

2. Traumatic or congenital disruption of intestinal tract (permanent or temporary).

3. Diverticulitis (double barrel)—can be put back after inflammatory process healed.

B. Procedure—portion of colon brought through abdominal wall.

C. Preoperative care.

1. Provide high calorie, low residue diet for several days.

2. Administer intestinal antiseptics with sulfa and neomycin (p.o.) to decrease bacterial content of colon and to soften and decrease bulk of contents of colon.

3. Cleanse bowel by administering laxatives and enemas.

4. Provide adequate fluids and electrolytes.

D. Postoperative care.

1. Depends on which part of colon involved; contents are liquid to formed.

2. Client has no voluntary control of bowel evacuation.

3. Ascending colostomy is hard to train for evacuation.

4. Evacuate bowel every 24 to 48 hours.

a. Irrigate with 200–500 cc at first.

b. Empty when one-third to one-half full.

5. Control with diet and/or irrigation.

6. Maintain skin care around stoma; use skin barrier.

7. Assure proper fit and placement of appliance—one-eighth inch from stoma.

8. Increase fluid intake.

9. Instruct client in colostomy self-care.

10. Suppositories may be given via colostomy.

Ileostomy

A. Causes.

1. Ulcerative colitis.

2. Crohn's disease (regional ileitis).

B. Procedure.

1. Total colectomy and ileostomy (anything less gives only temporary relief).

2. Portion of ileum brought through abdominal wall.

C. Preoperative care.

1. Provide intensified fluid, blood, and protein replacement.

2. Administer chemotherapy and antibiotics.

3. If on steroids, maintain therapy after surgery and then gradually decrease.

4. Provide low residue diet in small, frequent feedings.

5. Administer neomycin enemas.

D. Postoperative care.

1. Contents always liquid (from small intestine).

2. More chance of excoriation of skin around stoma.

3. Provide increased fluids because of excessive fluid loss through stoma.

4. Provide a low residue, high caloric diet until client is accustomed to new arrangement for bowel evcauation.

5. Do not give suppositories via ileostomy.

Continent ileostomy

A. Internal reservoir created by short segment of small intestines.

B. Nipple valve is formed from terminal ileum.

C. As reservoir fills, fecal pressure closes valve.

D. Client catheterizes stoma two to four times a day.

E. Appliance may be needed if leaking occurs.

Hemorrhoids

Definition: Dilated varicose veins of the anal canal that may be internal or external.

Characteristic

A. Types.
1. Internal hemorrhoids occur above the internal sphincter and are covered by mucous membrane.
2. External hemorrhoids occur outside the external sphincter and are covered by anal skin.
3. Thrombosed hemorrhoids are infected and clotted.
B. Causes.
1. Portal hypertension.
2. Straining from constipation.
3. Irritation and diarrhea.
4. Increased venous pressure from congestive heart failure.
5. Increased abdominal pressure as from pregnancy.

Assessment

A. Assess for itching.
B. Assess for pain.
C. Check bleeding.
D. Assess for complications: hemorrhage, strangulation, thrombosis, and prolapse.

Implementation

A. Treat constipation with diet, stool softeners, and laxatives.
B. Maintain diet low in roughage and high in fiber.
C. Provide suppositories, ointments, and systemic analgesics.
D. Administer hot sitz baths.
E. Internal hemorrhoids ligated with rubber bands— tissue necroses and drops off.

Anorectal Surgery

Characteristics

A. Hemorrhoids or varicose veins of anal canal.
1. External—outside rectal sphincter.
2. Internal—above internal sphincter.
B. Pilonidal cyst—cyst located on lower sacrum with hair protruding from sinus opening.

C. Anal fissure—crack in the anal canal.
D. Anal fistula—abnormal opening near the anus and continuing into the anal canal.

Implementation

A. Give routine postoperative care.
B. Keep perineal and rectal area clean by providing sitz baths (after first day) or irrigations.
C. Apply spray analgesics when needed to ease pain.
D. Medicate for pain but avoid codeine preparations as they are constipating.
E. Place in prone position or side-lying position for at least four hours postop to prevent hemorrhage.
F. Prevent urinary retention.
1. Keep accurate intake and output.
2. Observe for frequent, small voidings.
G. Clients usually have packing inserted with pressure dressing applied.
1. Reinforce dressing as needed to apply pressure.
2. Keep area clean.
H. Apply ice packs immediately postoperatively.
1. Prevents edema formation.
2. Provides vasoconstriction.
I. When client able to ambulate, encourage small steps; increase activity gradually.
J. When client sitting in chair, use flotation pads, not rubber rings; limit sitting to short periods of time.
K. Force fluids to aid in keeping bowel movements soft.
L. Administer stool softeners and laxatives every day.
M. On second day, before first bowel movement, enemas are sometimes ordered.
1. Medicate for pain.
2. Administer an enema with a pliable, soft, well-lubricated tube.
3. Place in sitz bath after expelling enema (will relieve excessive pain by relaxing anal area).

DISORDERS OF LIVER, BILIARY, AND PANCREATIC FUNCTION

Diagnostic Evaluation Studies

Physical Examination

A. Palpation of the abdomen to determine tenderness, size, and shape of liver and spleen.

B. Visual inspection for ascites, venous networks, and jaundice.

Radiologic Techniques

A. Cholecystogram—to visualize the gallbladder for detection of gall stones, and to determine the ability of the gallbladder to fill, concentrate, contract, and empty normally.
   1. Organic radiopaque dye may be given by mouth ten to twelve hours before x-ray, or intravenously ten minutes before x-ray.
   2. Dyes taken orally (e.g., Telepaque, Priodax, Oragrafin) are given one at a time at three to five minute intervals with at least 240 cc of water. A low-fat evening meal precedes the dye ingestion. Clients are n.p.o. until after examination. An enema is given before test.
B. Cholangiography—dye (e.g., Urokon Sodium) is injected directly into the biliary tree.
   1. May be injected into the common duct drain during surgery or postoperatively.
   2. Gallbladder disease is indicated by poor or absent visualization of the gallbladder.
   3. Stones will appear as shadows within the opaque medium.
C. Scanning of the liver—iodine 131 or other like substances are administered intravenously; then a scintillation detector is passed over the area.
   1. Lesions appear as filling defects.
   2. The isotopes are concentrated in functioning tissue.
D. Other procedures with contrast media: celiac angiography, hepatoportography, splenoportography, and pancreatic angiography.
   1. With all these procedures, organic iodine dye is injected into the vessel, flowing to and outlining the desired area.
   2. Reveals the patency of the vessels and the lesions that distort the vasculature.

Liver Biopsy

A. Sampling of liver tissues by needle aspiration to determine tissue changes and to facilitate diagnosis.
B. Nursing implementation prior to procedure.
   1. Verify test results of prothrombin times and blood typing; High PT may indicate deficiency in prothrombin, fibinogen, or factors V, VII, or X.
   2. Obtain baseline vital signs and written permission.
   3. Keep n.p.o. and provide sedation as ordered.
   4. Assemble equipment, position client, and assist with procedure.
   5. Support client; let client verbalize fears.
C. Nursing implementation following procedure.
   1. Position client on right side over biopsy site to prevent hemorrhage.
   2. Measure and record vital signs.
   3. Watch for shock.
   4. Observe for complications: hemorrhage, puncture of the bile duct, peritonitis, and pneumothorax.

Laboratory Tests

A. Biliary excretion.
   1. Serum bilirubin—abnormal in biliary and liver disease causing jaundice.
      a. Direct (conjugated)—normal: 0.2 mg/100 ml, soluble in H_2O.
      b. Indirect (unconjugated)—normal: 0.8 mg/100 ml, insoluble in H_2O.
      c. Total serum bilirubin—normal: 1.0 mg/100 ml.
   2. Urine bilirubin—normally none is found.
   3. Urine urobilinogen—0 to 4 mg/24 hours.
   4. Fecal urobilinogen—40 to 280 mg/24 hours.
   5. Serum cholesterol—150 to 250 mg/100 ml.
B. Protein studies.
   1. Total protein—6 to 8 g/100 ml.
   2. Serum albumin—3.5 to 5.0 mg/100 ml.
   3. Serum globulin—1.5 to 3.0 mg/100 ml.
   4. Prothrombin time—11 to 16 sec.
   5. Cephalin—0 to 1+.
   6. In liver damage, fewer plasma proteins are synthesized; thus, albumin synthesis is reduced.
      a. Serum globulins produced by the plasma cells are increased.
      b. PT is reduced in liver cell damage.
C. Fat metabolism—serum lipase 1.5 units.
D. Carbohydrate metabolism—glucose tolerance levels should return to normal in one to two hours.
E. Liver detoxification.
   1. Bromsulphalein excretion (BSP) should be less than 5 percent dye retention after one hour.
   2. Dye is injected intravenously and removed by the liver cells, conjugated, and excreted.
   3. Blood specimen is obtained at 30-minute and one-hour intervals after injection.

4. Increased retention occurs in hepatic disorders.

F. Enzyme production—elevations reflect organ damage.
   1. SGOT: 10 to 40 units/ml.
   2. SGPT: 5 to 35 units/ml.
   3. LDH: 120 to 340 units/ml.

G. Alkaline phosphatase (2 to 5 units) elevated in obstructive jaundice and in liver metastasis.

H. Blood ammonia (30–70 μ/100 ml)—ammonia level rises in liver failure since liver converts ammonia to urea. Metabolic alkalosis increases the toxicity of NH_3.

Jaundice

Definition: A symptom of a disease that results in yellow pigmentation of the skin due to accumulation of bilirubin pigment. Jaundice is usually first observed in the sclera of the eye.

Characteristics

A. Hemolytic.
   1. Results from rapid rate of red blood cell destruction which releases excessive amounts of unconjugated bilirubin.
   2. Caused by hemolytic transfusion reactions, erythroblastosis fetalis, and other hemolytic disorders.

B. Hepatocellular.
   1. Results from inability of the diseased liver cells to clear the normal amount of bilirubin from the blood.
   2. Caused by viral liver cell necrosis or cirrhosis of the liver.

C. Obstructive.
   1. Caused by intrahepatic obstruction due to inflammation, tumors, or cholestatic agents.
   2. Bile is dammed into the liver substance and reabsorbed into the blood.
   3. Deep orange, foamy urine; white or clay-colored stools; and severe itching (pruritus).

Assessment

A. Evaluate laboratory findings indicating hemolytic jaundice.
   1. Increased indirect (unconjugated) serum bilirubin.
   2. Absence of bilirubin in urine.
   3. Increased urobilinogen levels.

B. Evaluate laboratory findings indicating hepatocellular jaundice.
   1. Increased bilirubin.
   2. Increased SGOT.
   3. Increased SGPT.
   4. Increased alkaline phosphatase.
   5. Urobilinogen in urine.
   6. Increased PT.
   7. Decreased albumin.

C. Evaluate laboratory findings indicating obstructive jaundice.
   1. Increased bilirubin.
   2. Increased alkaline phosphatase.
   3. Decreased stool urobilinogen.

Implementation

A. Control pruritus.
   1. Starch or baking soda baths.
   2. Soothing lotions, such as calamine.
   3. Antihistamines, tranquilizers, and sedatives.
   4. Cholestyramine—binds bile salt.

B. Provide emotional support.
   1. Allow client to ventilate feelings of altered body image.
   2. Notify family and visitors of client appearance.

C. Provide dietary plan for anorexia and liver involvement.

Viral Hepatitis

Definition: An inflammation of the liver; the most common infection of the liver, often becoming a major health problem in crowded living conditions.

Characteristics

A. Hepatitis A (infectious hepatitis).
   1. Transmission.
      a. Oral-anal route.
      b. Blood transfusion with infected serum or plasma.
      c. Contaminated equipment, such as syringes and needles.
      d. Contaminated milk, water, and food (uncooked clams and oysters).
      e. Respiratory route is possible, but not yet established.
      f. Antibodies persist in serum.

2. Prevention.
   a. Good handwashing.
   b. Good personal hygiene.
   c. Control and screening of food handlers.
   d. Passive immunization.
      (1) ISG to exposed individuals.
      (2) ISG for prophylaxis for travelers to developing countries.
3. Incubation period: 20 to 50 days (short incubation period).
4. Incidence.
   a. More common in fall and winter months.
   b. Usually found in children and young adults.
   c. Client is infectious three weeks prior to and one week after developing jaundice.
5. Clinical recovery: three to sixteen weeks.
B. Hepatitis B (serum hepatitis, SH virus).
1. Transmission.
   a. Oral or parenteral route with infusion, ingestion, or inhalation of the blood of an infected person.
   b. Contaminated equipment, such as needles, syringes, and dental instruments.
   c. Oral or sexual contact.
   d. Infected people can become carriers.
   e. Caused by filtrable virus—Australian antigen.
   f. High risk individuals include homosexuals, IV drug abusers, medical workers.
2. Prevention.
   a. Screen blood donors for HB_3AG.
   b. Use disposable needles and syringes.
   c. Registration of all carriers.
   d. Passive immunization: ISG for exposure and HBIG for finger stick, contact with mucous membrane secretions.
   e. Active immunization: Hepatavax B Vaccine and formalin treated Hepatitis B Vaccine—purified antigen given in three doses (1 month, then 6 months).
C. Type C, formerly non-A, non-B.
1. Transmission.
   a. Transmitted primarily by contact with contaminated blood.
   b. Incidence noted following injectin of prophylactic gamma globulin.
   c. Increased incidence in population using drugs.
2. Usual incubation period 7–8 weeks.
3. May not show clinical jaundice.

Assessment

A. Perform general assessment; keep in mind that client is not immediately sick after being infected; onset depends on incubation period and degree of infection.
B. Assess preicteric phase.
1. Signs are generally systemic.
   a. Lethargy and malaise.
   b. Anorexia, nausea and vomiting.
   c. Headache.
   d. Abdominal tenderness and pain.
   e. Diarrhea or constipation.
   f. Low-grade temperature.
2. Above symptoms may precede jaundice or it may never appear.
C. In anicteric hepatitis client has symptoms of disease and altered lab tests, but no jaundice.
D. Assess icteric phase.
1. Dark urine and clay colored stools generally occur a few days prior to jaundice.
2. Jaundice is first observable in the eyes.
3. Pruritus—usually transient and mild.
4. Enlarged liver with tenderness.
5. Nausea may continue with dyspepsia and flatulence.
E. Assess posticteric phase.
1. Jaundice disappears.
2. The absence of clay-colored stools is an indication of resolution.
3. Fatigue and malaise continue.
4. Enlarged liver continues for several weeks.

Implementation

A. Type A.
1. Wash your hands carefully and take precautions during stool and needle procedures.
2. Use disposable equipment or sterilized reusable equipment.
3. Provide diet.
   a. High-calorie, well balanced diet; modified servings according to client response.
   b. Protein decreased if signs of coma.
   c. Ten percent glucose IV if not taking oral foods.
   d. Vitamin K supplements if prothrombin time is abnormally long.
   e. Promote adequate fluid intake.
4. Instruct client and family.
   a. Stress the importance of follow-up care.

b. Stress the restricted use of alcohol.

c. Stress that client never offer to be a blood donor.

d. Encourage gamma globulin for close contacts.

e. Advise correction if any unsanitary condition exists in the home.

5. Bedrest during acute phase with bathroom privileges; reasonable activity level during subsequent phases.

B. Type B.

1. Maintain bedrest until symptoms have decreased.

   a. Activities restricted while liver is enlarged.

   b. Activities discouraged until serum bilirubin is normal.

2. Provide well-balanced diet supplemented with vitamins.

3. Administer antacids for gastric acidity and soporifics for rest and relaxation.

4. Instruct client and family in pathology of the disease and rationale for treatment.

5. Counsel client to abstain from sexual activity during communicable period.

Cirrhosis

Definition: Cirrhosis is a progressive disease of the liver characterized by diffuse damage to the cells with fibrosis and nodular regeneration.

Characteristics

A. Types.

1. Laennec's portal cirrhosis (alcoholic/nutritional).

   a. Most common in the United States.

   b. Scar tissue surrounds the portal areas.

   c. Characterized by destruction of hepatic tissue, increased fibrous tissue, and disorganized regeneration.

2. Postnecrotic cirrhosis—a sequela to viral hepatitis in which there are broad bands of scar tissue.

3. Biliary cirrhosis.

   a. Pericholangitic scarring as a result of chronic biliary obstruction and infection.

   b. Least encountered of the three types.

B. Causes.

1. Repeated destruction of hepatic cells, replacement with scar tissue, and regeneration of liver cells.

2. Insidious onset with progression over a period of years.

3. Occurs twice as often in males; primarily affects forty- to sixty-year-old age group.

C. Clinical progression.

1. Early in the disease process, the liver becomes enlarged due to fat accumulation in the cells; accompanying this are gastrointestinal problems and fever.

2. Subsequent symptoms are usually anorexia, weight loss, fatigue and jaundice. (Jaundice is not always present in the active stage.)

3. Continued structural changes in liver result in obstruction of portal circulation. Collateral circulation increases to compensate for increased portal pressure.

   a. Obstruction of portal circulation results in portal hypertension which, in turn, leads to esophageal varices and changes in bowel functioning with chronic dyspepsia.

   b. Liver function deteriorates; leads to peripheral edema and ascites, accompanied by hormone imbalance, weakness, depression and potential bleeding.

4. As the liver is unable to synthesize protein, plasma albumin is reduced; leads to edema and contributes to ascites.

   a. Ascites, accumulation of serous fluid in the peritoneal cavity, increases as pressure in the liver increases.

   b. In addition, estrogen-androgen imbalance causes increased sodium and water to be retained.

5. Hepatic coma results from the incomplete metabolism of nitrogenous compounds, particularly ammonia, by the incompetent liver. When the liver cannot detoxify this product, it remains in the systemic circulation and hepatic encephalopathy ensues.

Assessment

A. Evaluate client's history of failing health, weakness, gastrointestinal distress, fatigue, weight loss, and low resistance to infections.

B. Assess for emaciation and ascites due to malnutrition, portal hypertension, and hypoalbuminemia.

C. Check for hematemesis.

D. Assess for lower leg edema from ascites obstructing venous return from legs.

E. Palpate liver.

F. Assess for prominent abdominal wall veins from collateral vessel bypass.

G. Assess for esophageal varices and hemorrhoids from portal hypertension.

H. Evaluate skin manifestations: spider angiomas, telangiectasia, vitamin deficiency, and alterations.

I. Evaluate laboratory tests.
1. Impaired hepatocellular function; elevated bilirubin, SGOT, SGPT, and LDH; reduced BSP; reduced albumin; and elevated PT.
2. Increased WBC, decreased RBC, coagulation abnormalities, increased gamma globulin, and proteinuria.

J. Assess for precoma state: tremor, delirium, and dysarthria.

Implementation

A. Assist in maximizing liver function.
1. Diet: ample protein to build tissue; carbohydrates to sustain weight and to provide energy.
2. Salt restriction in edema.
3. Multivitamin supplement (especially B).
4. Diuretics—spironolactones.

B. Eliminate hepatotoxin intake (aldosterone antagonist).
1. Completely restrict use of alcohol.
2. Lower the dosage of drugs metabolized by the liver.
3. Avoid sedatives and opiates.
4. Avoid all known hepatotoxic drugs (Thorazine, halothane).

C. Prevent infection by adequate rest, diet, and environmental control.

D. Administer plasma proteins as ordered.

E. Maintain adequate rest during acute phase.

F. Monitor intake and output due to fluid restriction.

G. Provide good skin care and control pruritus.

H. Evaluate client's response to diet therapy.

I. Measure, record, and compare vital signs.
1. Character of pain.
2. Progression of edema.
3. Character of emesis and stools.

J. Evaluate level of consciousness, personality changes, and signs of increasing stupor.

K. Instruct client and family in disease process and

rationale for treatment.

L. Prevent and control complications: ascites, bleeding esophageal varices, hepatic encephalopathy, and anemia.

M. Provide postoperative care if LeVeen peritoneovenous shunt is placed due to intractable ascites or circulatory failure.

COMPLICATIONS

Portal Hypertension

Definition: The result of altered liver structure that impedes normal hepatic blood flow and increases portal pressure.

Characteristics

A. Obstruction of portal circulation causes portal hypertension and congestion of the spleen, pancreas, and gastrointestinal tract.

B. As the body compensates for increased pressure in the hepatic system, collateral circulation increases.

Assessment

A. Assess for evidence of increased collateral circulation: hemorrhoids, veins observable on abdomen, esophageal varices that bleed easily.

B. Assess for presence of edema, especially in peripheral areas.

C. Check for weight gain and abdominal distention from ascites.

D. Assess for respiratory complications due to severe ascites.

E. Assess for abdominal pain (may be indication of infection or bleeding).

Implementation

A. Provide general nursing care for cirrhosis.

B. Provide specific care for management of edema.
1. Skin care to prevent breakdown.
   a. Use lanolin based products to soften skin.
   b. Guard against cutting or scratching skin.
2. Dietary control: decreased sodium intake, diuretics with potassium supplements, vitamin supplements of B complex, C, folate, and K.
3. Monitor intake and output; weigh daily.

C. Provide care for ascites.

1. Prevent complications associated with ascites i.e., respiratory impairment, infection.
2. Restrict fluids and sodium intake.
3. Position client in high-Fowler's to maximize respiratory capability.
4. Weigh daily and measure abdominal girth to estimate status of fluid accumulation.
5. Assist with paracentesis (will be avoided as long as possible due to the danger of precipitating shock, hypovolemia, or hepatic coma).
   a. Removal of fluid will relieve pressure on the diaphragm, stomach, or umbilical hernia.
   b. Because of high protein concentration in the ascitic fluid, IV infusion of salt-poor albumin may be administered over 24 hours.

Esophageal Varices

Refer to page 202.

Hepatic Coma
(Hepatic Encephalopathy)

Definition: Results from brain cell alterations caused by build-up of ammonia levels.

Characteristics

A. Increased blood ammonia levels.
  1. Normally, ammonia is formed in the intestines from the breakdown of protein and is converted by the liver to urea.
  2. In liver failure, ammonia is not converted into urea, and blood ammonia concentrations increase.
B. Any process that increases protein in the intestine, such as gastrointestinal hemorrhage and high-protein intake, will cause elevated blood ammonia.
C. Other factors involved in high ammonia levels.
  1. Electrolyte and acid-base imbalances. Alkalosis increases toxicity of NH_3.
  2. Constipation.
  3. Infectious diseases.
  4. Central nervous system depressants.
  5. Shunting of blood into systemic circulation without passing through the hepatic sinusoids.

Assessment

A. Assess for mental aberrations.

  1. Impaired memory, attention, concentration, and rate of response.
  2. Personality changes: untidiness, confusion, and inappropriate behavior.
B. Assess for depressed level of consciousness and flapping tremor (liver flap) upon dorsiflexion of hand.
C. Evaluate disorientation and eventual coma.

Implementation

A. Temporarily eliminate protein from the diet.
B. Give client bile salts to assist with the absorption of vitamin A.
C. Give folic acid and iron to prevent anemia.
D. Administer antibiotics to destroy intestinal bacteria and to reduce the amount of ammonia.
E. Administer Lactulose—acidifies colon contents resulting in retention of ammonium ion and decreased ammonia absorption.
F. Give enemas and/or cathartics to empty bowel and to prevent further ammonia formation.
G. Give salt-poor albumin to maintain osmotic pressure.
H. Use cation exchange resins to remove toxic substances from the bowel.
I. Correct fluid and electrolyte imbalances.
J. Weigh daily.
K. Measure and record intake and output.
L. Observe, measure, and record neurologic status daily.
  1. Test ability to perform mental tasks.
  2. Keep samples of handwriting.
M. Avoid depressants, which must be detoxified by the liver. Use agents, such as phenobarbital, that are excreted through the kidneys.
N. Prevent complications—decubitus, thrombophlebitis, or pneumonia.
O. With coma, utilize same nursing skills as with the unconscious client.

Cholecystitis and Cholelithiasis

Definition: Cholecystitis, either acute or chronic, is an inflammation of the gallbladder; cholelithiasis refers to stones in the gallbladder, formed of cholesterol (the most common) or pigment; choledocholithiasis refers to stones in the common bile duct.

Characteristics

A. Estimated 25 million in U.S. have gallstones.

B. Four times more common in women. Commonly occurs age 40 to 50.

C. Risk factors: cholesterol gallstones—obesity, estrogen, rapid weight loss, genetic predisposition, cholesterol-lowering drugs, and bile acid malabsorption; pigment gallstones—chronic liver disease, obstruction, or biliary infection.

Assessment

A. Laboratory values.
1. Serum amylase elevated—may indicate pancreatic involvement of stones in common bile duct; alkaline phosphatase, bilirubin increased.
2. White blood cell count elevated—indicates inflammation.

B. Differentiate between cholecystitis and cholelithiasis.

C. Assess for cholecystitis.
1. Epigastric distress—eructation after eating.
2. Pain—localized in right upper quadrant because of somatic sensory nerves.
   a. Murphy's sign: client cannot take a deep inspiration when assessor's fingers are pressed below hepatic margin.
   b. Pain begins two to four hours after eating fried or fatty foods and persists more than 4–6 hours.
4. Nausea, vomiting, and anorexia.
5. Low-grade fever.
6. Jaundice due to hepatocellular damage.
7. Weight loss.

D. Assess for cholelithiasis.
1. Pain—excruciating, upper right quadrant—radiates to right shoulder (biliary colic).
2. Pain is sudden, intense, paroxysmal—occurs with contraction of gallbladder.
3. Nausea and vomiting.
4. Jaundice due to obstruction and/or hepatocellular damage.

E. Observe for biliary obstruction.
1. Jaundice—yellow sclera.
2. Urine—dark orange and foamy.
3. Feces—clay colored.
4. Pruritus.

Implementation

A. Provide relief from vomiting.
1. Position nasogastric tube and attach to low suction. Tube reduces distention and eliminates gastric juices that stimulate cholecystokinin.
2. Provide good oral and nasal care; assure patency and flow of gastric secretions.

B. Maintain fluid and electrolyte balance.
1. Monitor intravenous fluids; record I & 0.
2. Observe serum electrolyte levels; watch for signs of imbalance.

C. Monitor drug therapy.
1. Administer broad spectrum antibiotics (Keflin) in presence of positive culture.
2. Chenodeoxycholic acid—bile acid dissolves cholesterol calculi (90 percent of stones).
3. Nitroglycerin or papaverine to reduce spasms of duct.
4. Synthetic narcotics (Demerol, methadone) to relieve pain. Morphine sulfate may cause spasm of sphincter of Oddi and increase pain.
5. Questran/Benadryl to relieve pruritus.

D. Provide low-fat diet; avoid alcohol and gas-forming foods.

E. Maintain bed rest.

Surgical Management

A. Cholecystectomy: removal of gallbladder after ligation of the cystic duct and vessels.
1. Common bile duct may be explored.
2. A penrose drain usually inserted for drainage following procedure.

B. Choledochostomy: opening into the common bile duct for removal of stones.
1. T-tube inserted into duct and connected to drainage bottle.
2. Purpose is to decompress biliary tree and allow for postoperative cholangiogram.

C. Cholesterol stones removed through dissolution therapy. For high risk clients—oral medications to decrease size or dissolve stones: chenodeoxycholic acid or ursodeoxycholic acid or combination of both.

D. Endoscopic cholecystectomy: removal of gallbladder through small puncture hole in abdomen.
1. Laser dissects gallbladder.
2. Discharged day of surgery—normal activities resumed in 2–3 days.

E. Extracorporeal shock wave lithotripsy: shock waves that disintegrate stones in the biliary system.
1. Ultrasound is used for stone localization before the lithotriptor sends waves through a water bag upon which the client is lying.
2. Analgesics and sedatives are given to reduce pain during procedure.

3. Oral dissolution medication follows to dissolve stone fragments.

Implementation

A. Position client in low- to semi-Fowler's to facilitate bile drainage.
B. Maintain skin integrity following surgery.
  1. Change position frequently; relieve pressure points.
  2. Protect skin around incision site from bile seepage.
    a. Change dressings frequently.
    b. Use protective skin paste or drainage pouches to prevent bile drainage from skin contact.
C. Prevent respiratory complications (the most common postoperative complication).
  1. Turn, cough and deep breathe every two hours.
  2. Use IPPB or Tri-flo every two hours.
  3. Auscultate for abnormal breath sounds.
  4. Observe for signs of respiratory distress.
  5. Ambulate and activate as early as allowed.
D. If nasogastric tube was inserted to relieve distention and increase peristalsis, irrigate tube every four hours and p.r.n.
E. If T-tube inserted:
  1. Place client in semi-Fowler's position to facilitate drainage.
  2. Measure amount and record character and color of drainage.
  3. Clamp tube before eating.
  4. Protect skin around incision and cleanse surrounding area.
F. Prevent wound infections; clients tend to be obese—healing is often delayed.
G. Prevent thrombophlebitis.
  1. Encourage range of motion.
  2. Ambulate early.
  3. Provide antiembolic stockings.
H. Provide diet: low fat, high carbohydrate and high protein.
  1. Instruct client to maintain diet for at least 2 or 3 months postoperatively.
  2. May require continued use of vitamin K as dietary supplement.
I. Prepare client for T-tube removal.
  1. As T-tube is clamped, observe for:
    a. Abdominal discomfort and distention.
    b. Chills and fever; nausea.
  2. Unclamp tube if any nausea or vomiting.

Acute Pancreatitis

Definition: An inflammation of the pancreas with associated escape of pancreatic enzymes into surrounding tissue.

A. Etiology.
  1. The most common precipitating factor in U.S. is alcoholic indulgence.
  2. Biliary tract disease with blocking of ampulla of Vater by gallstones.
  3. A result of prednisone or thiazide therapy.
  4. Complication of a viral or bacterial disease.
B. Pathology.
  1. Cholecystitis with reflux of bile components into the pancreatic duct.
  2. Spasm and edema of ampulla of Vater following inflammation of the duodenum.

Assessment

A. Assess for acute interstitial pancreatitis.
  1. Constant epigastric abdominal pain radiating to the back and flank. More intense in supine position.
  2. Nausea, vomiting, abdominal distention, and paralytic ileus.
  3. Low-grade temperature.
  4. Severe perspiration; anxiety
  5. Jaundice.
B. Laboratory values.
  1. Elevation of white count—20,000 to 50,000.
  2. Elevated serum lipase and amylase (5–40 times); glucose, bilirubin, and alkaline phosphatase.
  3. Urine amylase elevated.
  4. Abnormal low serum levels in calcium, sodium and magnesium—due to dehydration, binding of calcium in areas of fat necrosis.
C. Assess for acute hemorrhagic pancreatitis.
  1. Pancreatic enzymes erode major blood vessels causing hemorrhage into the pancreas and retroperitoneal tissues.
  2. Enzymatic digestion of the pancreas.
  3. Severe abdominal, back and flank pain.
  4. Ascites.
  5. Shock.

Implementation

A. Alleviate pain.
  1. Give meperidine (Demerol) as ordered (pain and anxiety increase pancreatic secretions).

2. Avoid opiates which may cause spasm of biliary-pancreatic ducts.
3. Give antispasmodic medication—atropine.
B. Reduce pancreatic stimulus.
1. Client is n.p.o. to eliminate chief stimulus to enzyme release.
2. Nasogastric tube to low suction to remove gastric secretions.
3. Drugs to reduce pancreatic secretion.
a. Anticholinergics (e.g., Pro-Banthine).
b. Sodium bicarbonate to reverse metabolic acidosis.
c. Diamox to prevent carbonic anhydrase from catalyzing secretion of bicarbonate into pancreatic juice.
d. Regular insulin to treat hyperglycemia.
4. Diet to avoid pancreatic secretion; low fat; no alcohol or caffeine; parenteral feedings if n.p.o.
C. Take vital signs every 15 to 30 minutes during acute phase.
D. Prevent or treat infection (and possible sepsis) with broad spectrum antibiotics.
E. Replace and maintain fluids and electrolytes.
1. Treat hypocalcemia with calcium gluconate IV. (Signs—nausea, vomiting; tetany; abdominal pain; positive Chvostek's sign.)
2. Treat hypokalemia—potassium is a major component in pancreatic juice. (Signs—muscle weakness; hyporeflexia; hypotension; apathy or irritability.)
3. Blood and plasma administration may be necessary to maintain circulatory volume.
F. Reduce body metabolism.
1. Oxygen for labored breathing.
2. Bed rest.
3. Cool, quiet environment.
G. Provide client and family instruction.
1. Discuss pathology of disease.
2. Give rationale for treatment.
3. Instruct client to avoid alcohol, coffee, heavy meals, and spicy foods.

Chronic Pancreatitis

Definition: Chronic fibrosis of the pancreatic gland with obstruction of ducts and destruction of secreting cells, following repeated attacks of acute pancreatitis.

Etiology

A. Alcohol abuse most common cause.
B. Other causes: hyperparathyroidism, malnutrition and trauma.

Assessment

A. Assess for pain—persistent epigastric and left upper quadrant pain radiating to upper left lumbar region.
B. Check for anorexia, nausea, vomiting, constipation, and flatulence.
C. Evaluate disturbances of protein and fat digestion.
1. Malnutrition.
2. Weight loss from decreased intake due to fear of pain.
3. Abdominal distention with flatus and paralytic ileus.
4. Foul fatty stools (steatorrhea).
D. Laboratory values.
1. Elevated serum amylase and lipase (indicates decreased pancreatic enzyme excretion).
2. Increased glucose and lipids.
3. Decreased calcium, potassium.
E. Assess for hyperglycemia with symptoms of diabetes.
F. Evaluate fecal fat in stool specimens; x-ray often shows pancreatolithiasis and mild ileus, indicating fibrous tissue and calcification.

Implementation

A. Provide low protein, low fat, high carbohydrate diet. Suggest bland and low gas-forming foods in small, frequent feedings.
B. Administer drug therapy.
1. Antacids (Maalox) to neutralize acid secretions.
2. Histamine antagonists (rantidine-Zantac and cimetidine-Tagamet) to decrease hydrochloric acid production so pancreatic enzymes are not activated.
3. Anticholinergics (atropine, Pro-Banthine) to decrease vagal stimulation, GI motility, and inhibit pancreatic enzymes.
4. Administer pancreatic replacements, such as pancreatin (Viokase) and pancrelipase (Cotazym) with meals or snacks to aid digestion. Dose depends on degree of malabsorption or maldigestion.
5. No narcotics.
C. Report diabetic symptoms—insulin or oral hypoglycemic agents will be administered; monitor blood glucose levels to control hyperglycemia and prevent insulin shock.
D. Monitor for potential complications: pseudocyst, ascites or pleural effusion, GI hemorrhage, biliary tract obstruction. Surgical treatment is done for specific complications and to relieve constant pain.

GENITOURINARY SYSTEM

The urinary system—the kidneys and their drainage channels—is essential for the maintenance of life. This system is responsible for excreting the end products of metabolism as well as regulating water and electrolyte concentrations of body fluids. The genitalia refers to the organs of reproduction.

ANATOMY AND PHYSIOLOGY

Kidney Structure

A. Paired organs located to the right and left of midline lateral to lower thoracic vertebrae.
B. Kidneys perform two major functions.
   1. Excrete most of the end products of body metabolism.
   2. Control the concentrations of most of the constituents of body fluids.
C. Composed of structural units, each of which functions the same as the total kidney and is capable of forming urine by itself.
D. The functional renal unit is called the nephron. Each nephron is composed of:
   1. A glomerulus (a network of many capillaries) that filters fluid out of the blood. It is encased by Bowman's capsule.
   2. Tubules (proximal, Henle's loop, distal) in which fluid is converted to urine as it goes to the pelvis of the kidneys.
E. Fluid from Bowman's capsule moves through the proximal tubule located in the cortex.
F. Fluid then flows through Henle's loop located in medulla of kidney.
G. Fluid flows from loop to the collecting tubule.
H. After flowing through many convolutions, the fluid goes into a collecting sac called the pelvis of the kidney.
I. From the pelvis, fluid flows through the ureter and empties into the bladder.

Kidney Function

A. Urine production.
   1. As the fluid filtrate flows through the proximal tubules, 80 percent of the water and solutes are reabsorbed into tubular capillaries.
   2. The water and solutes that are not reabsorbed become urine.
   3. The amount of fluid and solutes excreted is determined through selective reabsorption.
B. Nephron function.
   1. The basic function is to rid the body of unwanted substances, the end products of metabolism (fluid and electrolytes).
   2. The nephron filters much of the plasma through the glomerular membrane into the tubules.
   3. The tubules filter the wanted elements of the blood (e.g., water and electrolytes) from the unwanted elements and reabsorb them into the plasma through the peritubular capillaries.
   4. Reabsorption and secretion take place by both active and passive transport.
C. Tubular reabsorption and secretion.
   1. Three substances filtered at glomerulus.
      a. Electrolytes: Na^+, K^+, Ca^{++}, Mg^{++}, HCO_3^-, Cl^-, and HPO_4^{--}.
      b. Nonelectrolytes: glucose, amino acids, urea, uric acid, creatinine.
      c. Water.
   2. Proximal tubule reabsorption.
      a. 80 percent of filtrate reabsorbed actively through obligatory reabsorption.
      b. H_2O, Na^+, and Cl^- continue through loop of Henle where Cl^- is actively transported out of ascending loop followed passively by Na^+.
D. Glomerular filtration.
   1. Glomerular membrane is semipermeable (proteins and glucose do not cross the membrane).
   2. Amount of filtration is determined by hydrostatic pressure.
   3. A decrease in blood pressure leads to a decrease in GFR and therefore a decrease in urine output.
   4. Approximately 1000 to 2000 ml blood flows through kidney each minute to produce 60 cc urine output per hour.
E. Concentrating and diluting mechanisms.

1. Countercurrent flow of blood and tubular fluid increase concentration of NaCl and therefore H_2O reabsorption.
2. ADH (antidiuretic hormone) controls H_2O reabsorption at distal tubule.
   a. Concentrated urine leads to increased ADH secretion.
   b. Dilute urine leads to decreased ADH secretion.
3. Distal tubule and collecting duct.
   a. Secretion and reabsorption completed.
   b. Distal tubule—final regulation of H_2O and acid-base balance.
   c. Uric acid and K^+ secreted into distal tubules and excreted in urine.
4. Hormonal regulation.
   a. H_2O reabsorption depends on ADH.
   b. Na^+ and K^+ reabsorption influenced by aldosterone.
      (1) Increased aldosterone causes increased Na^+ reabsorption and increased K^+ secretion.
      (2) Decreased aldosterone exhibits opposite effect.
   c. Ca^{++} and HPO_4^{--} reabsorption regulated by parathyroid hormone.
      (1) Increased parathyroid hormone leads to increased Ca^{++} reabsorption and increased HPO_4^{--} excretion.
      (2) Decreased parathyroid hormone exhibits opposite effect.
5. Water balance maintained through homeostasis—all functions of kidney must be maintained.

F. Blood pressure regulation.
   1. Regulation occurs through release of renin from juxtaglomerular cells in response to low blood volume or ischemia.
   2. Renin stimulates conversion of angiotensinogen to angiotensin I in liver.
   3. Angiotensin I changed to angiotensin II in pulmonary capillary bed.
   4. Angiotensin II increases blood pressure by vasoconstriction of peripheral arterioles and secretion of aldosterone.
   5. Increased aldosterone stimulates Na^+ reabsorption.
   6. Increased Na^+ reabsorption causes increased H_2O retention and plasma volume, which leads to increased blood pressure.

Characteristics of Urine

A. Components of urine include organic and inorganic materials in urine solution.
B. Cloudy urine is of little significance and is usually the result of urates or phosphates which precipitate out.
C. Red blood cells in the urine or hematuria is significant and indicates the presence of some disease or disorder in the body.
   1. Acute nephritis or exacerbation of chronic nephritis.
   2. Neoplasms, vascular accidents, or infections.
   3. Renal stones.
   4. Renal tuberculosis.
   5. Trauma to the urinary tract.
   6. A manifestation of thrombocytopenia.
   7. May be the result of problems along the genitourinary tract, such as the ureter, the bladder, or the prostate gland.
D. The source of blood cells in urine must be determined.
   1. Blood during the initial period of voiding may be from the anterior urethra or prostate.
   2. Blood mixed with the total volume of urine may be from kidneys, ureters, or bladder.

RENAL REGULATION OF FLUID AND ELECTROLYTES

Composition of the Body

Body Fluids

Definition: Total body water represents the largest constituent (45 to 80 percent) of the total body weight, depending on the amount of fat present.

A. Intracellular—represents 40 percent of total body water fluid; contained inside the cell; includes the red blood cells.
B. Extracellular—represents 20 percent of total body water; includes remaining fluid not contained within the cell.
   1. Intravascular (plasma)—liquid in which the blood cells are suspended (5 percent).
   2. Interstitial—liquid surrounding tissue cells (15 percent).
   3. Percent varies with age and amount of fat.

a. Newborn—83 percent of baby's weight is water.

b. Thin person has more water.

Electrolytes

Definition: Electrolytes are compounds that dissolve in a solution to form ions; each particle then carries either a positive or negative electrical charge.

A. Types.
 1. Cations—positive charge (Na^+, K^+, Ca^{++}, Mg^{++}).
 2. Anions—negative charge (Cl^-, HCO_3^-, HPO_4^{--}, SO_4^{--}).
 3. Equal number of cations and anions (154 each).
B. Concentration in solution is expressed in mEq/l. Total number of cations (mEq) plus total number of anions (mEq) will be the same in both the intracellular fluid and extracellular fluid, thereby rendering the body's fluid composition electrically neutral.
C. Compartment composition.
 1. Extracellular—large quantities of sodium, chloride, and bicarbonate ions.
 2. Intracellular—large quantities of potassium, phosphate, and proteins.

Dynamics of Intercompartmental Fluid Transfer

Transport of Fluids and Electrolytes

A. Diffusion—movement of solutes (substances that are dissolved in a solution) or gases from an area of higher concentration to an area of lower concentration; a passive transport system.
B. Filtration—passage of fluids through a semipermeable membrane as a result of a difference in hydrostatic pressures (pressure exerted by a fluid within a closed system).
C. Osmosis—passage of water or solvent through a semipermeable membrane from an area of lesser concentration to an area of greater concentration of solute; a passive transport system.
D. Facilitated diffusion—transport of molecules that are too large or insoluble across the membrane by means of a carrier molecule, creating a complex which is soluble in the membrane.
E. Active transport—transport (requiring energy—ATP) of substances across a membrane from an

area of low concentration to an area of high concentration.
F. Oncotic pressure—osmotic pressure that results from dispersed colloid particles (the largest being proteins) in the blood capillaries; the pressure draws water back into the vascular system, thereby maintaining blood volume.
G. Lymphatics—vessels responsible for returning the large molecules that have escaped from the blood capillaries (including protein molecules) to the bloodstream, returning them from the interstitial fluid and the gastrointestinal tract.

Balance of Body Fluid

A. Intake.
 1. Ingestion of foodstuff and water.
 2. Oxidation of foodstuff.
B. Output.
 1. Skin and lungs.
 a. Water is lost through vaporization from the skin surface and through expired air from the lungs.
 b. The amount lost increases as metabolism increases.
 2. Gastrointestinal tract.
 a. Routes include saliva, gastric secretions, bile, pancreatic juices, and intestinal mucosa.
 b. A volume in excess of seven liters is transferred from the extracellular fluid (ECF) into the gastrointestinal tract, only to be reabsorbed, excepting some 200 ml which is passed with feces.
 3. Kidneys.
 a. Carry the heaviest load.
 b. Through glomerular filtration and tubular reabsorption, the kidneys maintain homeostasis.
 c. Three hormones influence the kidneys in fluid balance.
 (1) Antidiuretic.
 (2) Aldosterone.
 (3) Thyroid.

Fluid Imbalances

Assessment

A. Assess for dehydration (extracellular fluid volume deficit).

1. Evaluate possible causes.
   a. Vomiting, diarrhea.
   b. Increased urine output.
   c. Diuretics.
   d. Excessive loss through respiration.
   e. Insufficient IV replacement.
2. Assess skin.
   a. Loss of skin turgor (after being pinched and lightly pulled upward, skin returns to normal very slowly).
   b. Dry warm skin.
3. Assess febrile state (usually means there is fluid loss through perspiration).
4. Observe cracked lips, dry mucous membranes.
5. Assess decreased urinary output (normal output is 30 cc/hour).
6. Concentrated urine—dark amber color and odorous.
7. Weight loss.
8. Low central venous pressure.
9. Increased respiration.

B. Assess for circulatory overload (extracellular volume excess).
   1. Evaluate possible causes.
      a. Excessive IV fluids.
      b. Inadequate kidney function.
   2. Assess for headache.
   3. Observe flushed skin.
   4. Assess tachycardia.
   5. Assess for venous distention, particularly neck veins.
   6. Evaluate increased blood pressure and CVP.
   7. Assess tachypnea (increased respiratory rate), coughing, dyspnea (shortness of breath), cyanosis, and pulmonary edema.

Implementation

A. Take central venous pressure to determine fluid balance if CVP catheter is in place. The CVP reflects the competency of the heart (particularly the right side) to handle the volume of blood returning to it.
   1. CVP indicates the comparison of the pumping capacity of the heart and the volume of the circulating blood.
   2. Normal CVP reading: 5 to 10 cm H_2O.
   3. Increased CVP (above 15 cm H_2O) can be indicative of congestive heart failure or circulatory overload.
   4. Decreased CVP (below 5 cm H_2O) is indicative of hypovolemia (decreased fluid volume) whether from blood loss or other fluid losses.

B. Monitor client's condition every two hours.
   1. Check condition of skin.
      a. Dry, warm, cracked lips.
      b. Elasticity.
   2. Check body temperature—fever suggests loss of body fluids.
   3. Check for venous distention.
   4. Ask client about unusual related symptoms, if possible, such as headache, shortness of breath.
   5. Check urine output at least every eight hours for maintenance IV therapy, or as often as every hour for replacement fluid administration.
   6. Check for symptoms of electrolyte disturbances at least every four hours.

Electrolyte Imbalances

Potassium Imbalance

A. Normal serum level is 3.5 to 5.5 mEq/l.
B. Potassium deficiency and excess is a common problem in fluid and electrolyte imbalance.
C. Major cell cation.
D. General nursing management related to potassium imbalances.
   1. Observe ECG tracings for change in T wave, S-T segment, or QRS complex.
   2. Measure intake and output accurately.
   3. Draw frequent blood specimens for potassium level.
   4. Observe for signs of metabolic acidosis and alkalosis.

Hypokalemia

Definition: Hypokalemia is a very low concentration of potassium ions in extracellular fluid.

A. Signs and symptoms of hypokalemia.
   1. Muscle weakness, muscle pain, hyporeflexia, fatigue.
   2. Hypotension, shallow respiration.
   3. Arrhythmias—PVCs particularly.
   4. Anorexia advancing to nausea, vomiting.
   5. Apathy, drowsiness leading to coma.

6. ECG changes include peaked P wave, flat T wave, depressed S-T segment, and elevated U waves.
7. Paralytic ileus.

B. Causes of hypokalemia.
1. Renal loss most common (usually caused by use of diuretics).
2. Insufficient potassium intake.
3. Loss from gastrointestinal tract via NG tube placement without replacement electrolyte solution, or from vomiting or diarrhea.

C. Nursing management of hypokalemia.
1. Maintain IVs with KCl added.
2. Replace K$^+$ when excess loss occurs (NG tubes, diarrhea, etc.).
3. Replace no more than 20 mEq of KCl in one hour; observe ECG monitor if possible.
4. Dilute KCl in 30 to 50 cc IV fluid via volutrol.
5. Observe for adequate urine output.

Hyperkalemia

Definition: Hyperkalemia is an excess of potassium in extracellular fluid.

A. Signs and symptoms of hyperkalemia.
1. Weakness, muscle cramp, flaccid paralysis.
2. Hyperreflexia proceeding to paralysis.
3. Bradycardia, arrhythmias.
4. Ventricular fibrillation.
5. ECG changes depict elevated or tented T wave, widened QRS complex, prolonged P-R interval, and flattened P wave with depressed S-T segment.
6. Oliguria.
7. Diarrhea, nausea.

B. Causes of hyperkalemia.
1. Usually renal disease (cannot excrete potassium).
2. Burns (due to cellular destruction releasing potassium from cells into extracellular space).
3. Crushing injuries (due to cellular breakage releasing potassium from cells).
4. Adrenal insufficiency.
5. Respiratory or metabolic acidosis.

C. Nursing management of hyperkalemia.
1. Administer diuretics if kidney function adequate.
2. Administer hypertonic IV glucose with insulin.
3. Provide exchange resins through NG or enema (Kayexalate).
4. Provide calcium IV to stimulate heart if depressed action.
5. Administer sodium bicarbonate if client is acidotic.

Sodium Imbalance

A. Normal serum level is 135 to 145 mEq/l.
B. Sodium deficiency and excess are common problems in fluid and electrolyte imbalance.
C. General nursing management.
1. Observe skin condition.
2. Measure intake and output.
3. Auscultate lung sounds.
4. Observe urine for specific gravity and color.

Hyponatremia

Definition: Hyponatremia is caused by a very low concentration of sodium in extracellular fluid.

A. Signs and symptoms of hyponatremia.
1. Signs and symptoms are the same as those for extracellular fluid deficiency.
   a. Weakness.
   b. Restlessness.
   c. Delirium.
   d. Hyperpnea.
   e. Oliguria.
   f. Increased temperature.
   g. Flushed skin.
   h. Abdominal cramps.
   i. Convulsions.
   j. Nausea, anorexia.
2. If sodium is lost but fluid is not, the following signs and symptoms will be present (similar to those of water excess).
   a. Mental confusion.
   b. Headache.
   c. Muscle twitching and weakness.
   d. Coma.
   e. Convulsions.
   f. Oliguria.

B. Causes of hyponatremia.
1. Excessive perspiration.
2. Use of diuretics.
3. Gastrointestinal losses—severe diarrhea, vomiting, pancreatic and biliary fistulas.
4. Lack of sodium in diet.
5. Burns, fibrocystic disease.
6. Excessive IV administration without NaCl.
7. Diabetic acidosis.
8. Adrenal insufficiency.

C. Nursing management of hyponatremia.
   a. Administer IV fluids with sodium.
   b. Maintain accurate intake and output.

Hypernatremia

Definition: Hypernatremia is caused by a very high concentration of sodium in extracellular fluid.

A. Signs and symptoms of hypernatremia.
   1. Signs and symptoms are same as for extracellular fluid excesses.
      a. Pitting edema.
      b. Excessive weight gain.
      c. Increased blood pressure.
      d. Dyspnea.
   2. If hypernatremia is due to dehydration, in which there is a loss of fluid thereby increasing the number of ions, the signs and symptoms include:
      a. Concentrated urine and oliguria.
      b. Dry mucous membranes.
      c. Thirst.
      d. Flushed skin.
      e. Increased temperature.
      f. Tachycardia, hypertension.
B. Causes of hypernatremia.
   1. Severe diarrhea.
   2. Decreased water intake.
   3. Febrile states.
   4. Ingestion of sodium chloride.
   5. Excessive loss of water through rapid and deep respiration.
   6. Renal failure.
C. Nursing management of hypernatremia.
   1. Record intake and output.
   2. Restrict sodium in diet.
   3. Weigh daily.
   4. Observe vital signs.
   5. Administer fluids orally or IV.

Hypocalcemia

Definition: Hypocalcemia results from a deficit of calcium in the extracellular fluid.

A. Signs and symptoms of hypocalcemia.
   1. Abdominal cramps, muscle cramps.
   2. Tetany, carpopedal spasms.
   3. Circumoral tingling, especially in fingers.
   4. Convulsions.
B. Causes of hypocalcemia.

1. Acute pancreatitis.
2. Chronic renal insufficiency.
3. Burns.
4. Removal of parathyroid glands.
5. If transfused with over 2000 cc of blood requires calcium supplement.
6. Malabsorption syndrome.
C. Nursing management of hypocalcemia.
   1. Calcium gluconate IV.
   2. Serum albumin if condition due to low serum albumin concentration.
   3. Monitor for hypocalcemia.
      a. Trousseau test positive.
      b. Chvostek test positive.

Hypercalcemia

Definition: Hypercalcemia results from an excess of calcium in the extracellular fluid.

A. Signs and symptoms of hypercalcemia.
   1. Anorexia, nausea.
   2. Lethargy, weight loss, polydipsia, polyuria.
   3. Flank pain, bone pain, decreased muscle tone.
B. Causes of hypercalcemia.
   1. Excessive intake of vitamin D (milk).
   2. Hyperparathyroidism, neoplasm of parathyroids.
   3. Thyrotoxicosis.
   4. Immobilization.
   5. Paget's disease.
C. Nursing management of hypercalcemia.
   1. Treat the underlying cause of the high serum calcium level.
   2. Immediate reversal—sodium salts IV and diuretics (Lasix).

Hypomagnesemia

Definition: Deficit of magnesium due to chronic alcoholism, starvation, malabsorption, or vigorous diuresis.

A. Signs and symptoms of hypomagnesemia.
   1. Neuromuscular irritability.
      a. Jerks, twitches.
      b. Hyperactive reflexes.
      c. Convulsions.
      d. Tetany.
   2. Cardiovascular changes.
      a. Tachycardia.
      b. Hypotension.

B. Causes of hypomagnesemia.
1. Low intake.
2. Abnormal loss—diarrhea.
3. Chronic nephritis.
4. Diuretic phase of renal failure.
C. Nursing management of hypomagnesemia.
1. Magnesium sulfate.
   a. Administer IV or IM slowly.
   b. Observe for adequate urine output.
2. Antidote: calcium gluconate.

Hypermagnesemia

Definition: An excess of magnesium as a result of renal insufficiency or inability to excrete magnesium absorbed from food.

A. Causes of hypermagnesemia.
1. Renal insufficiency.
2. Overdose.
3. Severe dehydration.
4. Overuse of antacids with magnesium (Gelusil).
B. Signs and symptoms of hypermagnesemia.
1. Hypotension.
2. Curare-like paralysis.
3. Sedation.
4. Decreased respiration function.
5. Cardiac arrhythmias.
6. Warm sensation in body.
C. Nursing management of hypermagnesemia.
1. Administer calcium gluconate IV slowly.
2. Give in peripheral veins (not CVP line).

ACID-BASE REGULATION

Principles of Acid-Base Balance

A. Acid-base balance is the ratio of acids and bases in the body necessary in order to maintain a chemical balance conducive to life.
B. Acid-base ratio is 20 base to 1 acid.
C. Acid-base balance is measured by arterial blood samples and recorded as blood pH. Range is 7.35 to 7.45.
D. Acids are hydrogen ion donors. They release hydrogen ions to neutralize or decrease the strength of the base.
E. Bases are hydrogen ion acceptors. They accept hydrogen ions to convert strong acids to weak acids

(for example, hydrochloric acid is converted to carbonic acid).

Regulatory Mechanisms

A. The body controls the pH balance by use of:
1. Chemical buffers.
2. Lungs.
3. Cells.
4. Kidneys.
B. The chemical buffer system works fastest, but other regulatory mechanisms provide more reliable protection against acid-base imbalance.
1. A buffer is a substance that reacts to keep pH within normal limits. It functions only when excessive base or acid is present.
2. Chemical buffers are paired (for example, weakly ionized acid or base is balanced with a fully ionized salt).
   a. Pairing prevents excessive changes in normal acid-base balance.
   b. The buffers release or absorb hydrogen ions when needed.
3. The buffer systems in the extracellular fluid react quickly with acids and bases to minimize changes in pH.
   a. Once they react, they are used up.
   b. If further stress occurs, the body is less able to cope.
4. There are three primary buffer systems.
   a. Bicarbonate—maintains blood pH at 7.4 with ratio of 20 parts bicarbonate to 1 part carbonic acid.
   b. Plasma proteins—vary the amounts of hydrogen ions in the chemical structure of the protein (along with liver). They can both attract and release hydrogen ions.
   c. Hemoglobin—maintains the balance by the chloride shift. Chloride shifts in and out of red blood cells according to the level of oxygen in the blood plasma. Each chloride ion that leaves the cell is replaced by a bicarbonate ion.
C. Lungs.
1. Next to react are the lungs.
2. It takes 10 to 30 minutes for lungs to inactivate hydrogen molecules by converting them to water molecules.

3. The carbonic acid that was formed by neutralizing bicarbonate is taken to lungs.

   a. There it is reduced to carbon dioxide and water and exhaled.

   b. Therefore, when there is excessive acid in the body, the respiratory rate increases in order to blow off the excessive carbon dioxide and water.

4. When there is too much bicarbonate or base in the body, respirations become deeper and slower.

   a. This process builds up the level of carbonic acid.

   b. The result is the strength of the excessive bicarbonate is neutralized.

5. Lungs can only inactivate the hydrogen ions carried by carbonic acid. The other ions must be excreted by the kidneys.

D. Cells.

   1. They absorb or release extra hydrogen ions.

   2. They react in two to four hours.

E. Kidneys.

   1. Kidney most efficient regulatory mechanism.

   2. Begins to function within hours to days.

   3. Blood pH is maintained by balance of 20 parts of bicarbonate to 1 part carbonic acid.

   4. Four processes are involved in acid-base regulation.

      a. Dissociation of H^+ from H_2CO_3 (H^+ and HCO_3).

      b. Reabsorption of Na^+ from urine filtrate. (Na^+ and H^+ change places.)

      c. Formation and conservation of $NaHCO_3$ (Na^+ and HCO_3^-).

      d. NH_3 from metabolic process (Krebs cycle) enters kidney's tubular cell and adds a H^+ ion and then exchanges as ammonium with Na^+ (Na^+ and NH_4).

   5. Hydrogen and potassium compete with each other in exchange for Na^+ in the tubular urine.

      a. In acidosis the H^+ ion concentration is increased and K^+ ion must wait to be excreted as hydrogen has preference.

      b. In alkalosis the H^+ ion is low and K^+ is excreted in larger amounts.

ACID-BASE IMBALANCES

Metabolic Acidosis

Definition: Metabolic acidosis occurs when there is a deficit of bases or an accumulation of fixed acids.

A. Changes in pH and serum carbon dioxide.

   1. The pH will become acidotic as a result of insufficient base.

      a. Therefore, it falls below 7.35.

      b. There are either more hydrogen ions or less bicarbonate ions present in the blood.

   2. The serum CO_2 level will be below 22 mEq/l (normal range of CO_2 is 26 to 28 mEq/l).

      a. Serum CO_2 measures the amount of circulating bicarbonate.

      b. Serum CO_2 will be decreased due to the depletion of the bicarbonate ion in the neutralization process of the extra acids.

      c. In lab reports, the CO_2 may be reported as: HCO_3, CO_2 content, or CO_2 combining power, depending on the laboratory.

      d. Laboratory values will vary depending on the methods used for analysis.

      e. Normal ranges:

         (1) HCO_3: 22 to 26 mEq/l.

         (2) CO_2 content: 26 to 28 mEq/l.

         (3) CO_2 combining power: 58 volume percent.

B. Compensatory mechanisms.

   1. When compensating for metabolic acidosis, the one clinical manifestation usually observed is the "blowing off" of excessive acids. This can be noted by a respiratory rate increase.

   2. The lungs are the fastest mechanism used to compensate for metabolic acidosis.

      a. If the lungs are involved, as in respiratory acidosis, they cannot function as a compensatory mechanism.

      b. Therefore, the kidneys must take over and the process is much slower.

C. Laboratory values.

   1. The partial pressure of the blood gas carbon dioxide (pCO_2) will decrease below 35 mm of pressure when the client is compensating. (Normal values: 35 to 45 mm pressure.)

   2. The partial pressure of oxygen (pO_2) is usually increased due to increased respiratory rate. (Normal values pO_2: 80 to100 mm Hg.)

3. The serum potassium level is increased with acidosis, due primarily to the cause of the acidosis.

    a. For example, clients can go into metabolic acidosis from severe diarrhea.

    b. When this condition is present, the potassium moves out of the cell and into the extravascular space due to the dehydration process.

4. Sodium and chloride levels may be decreased. Again, this is usually due to excessive loss through urine or gastrointestinal disorders.

5. Laboratory values when a client is in metabolic acidosis and in the compensatory state.

    a. Metabolic acidosis.

        (1) pH: 7.30.

        (2) HCO_3: 16 mEq/l.

        (3) pCO_2: 38 mm.

        (4) pO_2: 95 mm.

        (5) Cl: 120 mEq/l.

        (6) K: 5.5 mEq/l.

    b. Compensated metabolic acidosis.

        (1) pH: 7.40.

        (2) HCO_3: 16 mEq/l.

        (3) pCO_2: 20 mm.

D. Causes of metabolic acidosis (seen particularly in the surgical client).

1. Diabetes—diabetic ketoacidosis.

    a. When insufficient insulin is produced or administered to metabolize carbohydrates, increased fat metabolism will result, thus producing excess accumulations of ketones and other acids.

    b. This is the most common problem associated with metabolic acidosis in the surgical client.

2. Renal insufficiency—kidneys retain the products of protein metabolism, thereby decreasing the bicarbonate that is available to maintain an acid-base balance.

3. Diarrhea—excessive amounts of base are lost from the intestines and pancreas, resulting in acidosis.

E. Clinical manifestations.

1. Headache.

2. Drowsiness.

3. Nausea, vomiting, diarrhea.

4. Stupor, coma.

5. Twitching, convulsions.

6. Kussmaul's respiration (increased respiratory rate).

7. Fruity breath (as evidenced in diabetic ketoacidosis as a result of improper fat metabolism).

F. Nursing management.

1. Administer sodium bicarbonate intravenously to alkalize the client and return client to normal acid-base balance as quickly as possible.

    a. Usual dosage: 1 to 3 ampules of 50 mEq bicarbonate/ampule.

    b. This is usually the immediate treatment rendered for metabolic acidosis.

2. Administer sodium lactate solution to increase the base level.

    a. Sodium lactate is converted to bicarbonate by the liver.

    b. Lactated Ringer's IV solution may be used.

3. Administer insulin in ketoacidosis. Insulin will move glucose out of the blood serum and into the cell, thereby decreasing ketosis. Insulin decreases ketones by decreasing the release of fatty acids from fat cells.

4. Monitor laboratory values closely while managing metabolic acidosis.

5. Watch for signs of hyperkalemia and dehydration in the client (oliguria, vital sign changes, etc.).

6. Record intake and output.

Metabolic Alkalosis

Definition: Metabolic alkalosis is a malfunction of metabolism, causing an increase in blood base or a reduction of available acids in the serum.

A. Changes in pH and serum carbon dioxide.

1. The pH will become more alkaline; therefore, it will be above 7.45.

2. The CO_2 will also increase above 35 mEq/l. Note that this measures the amount of circulating bicarbonate or the base portion of the plasma. (A good way to remember these acid-base values is to recall that as the pH increases, so does the CO_2. The reverse is true for acidosis.)

3. The pCO_2 will not change unless the lungs attempt to compensate.

4. Serum potassium and chloride levels will decrease, due to the basic cause of the alkalosis,

whether it be excessive vomiting or the use of diuretics.

B. Compensatory mechanisms.
1. The lungs will attempt to hold on to the carbonic acid in an effort to neutralize the base state; therefore, the rate of respiration will decrease.
2. When the lungs are compensating for the alkalotic state, the pCO_2 will increase above 45 mEq/l.

C. Laboratory values when client is in metabolic alkalosis and compensatory states.
1. Metabolic alkalosis.
   a. pH: 7.50.
   b. HCO_3: 38 mEq/l.
   c. pCO_2: 38 mm pressure.
   d. pO_2: 95 mm pressure.
   e. K: 3.0 mEq/l.
   f. Cl: 88 mEq/l.
2. Compensated metabolic alkalosis.
   a. pH: 7.40.
   b. HCO_3: 38 mEq/l.
   c. pCO_2: 50 mm pressure.
   d. pO_2: 95 mm pressure.

D. Causes of metabolic alkalosis.
1. Ingestion of excessive soda bicarbonate (used by individuals for acid indigestion).
2. Excessive vomiting which results in the loss of hydrochloric acid and potassium.
3. Placement of NG tubes that causes a depletion of both hydrochloric acid and potassium.
4. Use of potent diuretics, particularly by cardiac clients. They tend to lose not only potassium but also hydrogen and chloride ions, causing an increase in the bicarbonate level of the serum.

E. Clinical manifestations.
1. Nausea, vomiting, diarrhea.
2. Irritability, agitation, coma, convulsions.
3. Restlessness and twitching of extremities.
4. ECG changes indicate tachycardia, with the T wave running into the P wave.

F. Nursing management.
1. Maintain diet of foods high in potassium and chloride (bananas, apricots, dried peaches, Brazil nuts, dried figs, oranges).
2. Administer IV solution of added electrolytes.
   a. Estimate the potassium loss from gastric fluid at 5 to 10 mEq for each liter lost.
   b. In many institutions, the gastric fluid loss is replaced cc for cc every two to four hours.
   c. In other institutions, the approximate electrolyte loss is calculated and this amount is added to the 24-hour IV solution.
3. Give Diamox to promote kidney excretion of bicarbonate.
4. Administer potassium chloride maintenance doses to clients on long-term diuretics.
5. Give ammonium chloride to increase the amount of available hydrogen ions, thereby increasing the availability of acids in the blood.
6. Check laboratory values frequently to watch for electrolyte imbalance.
7. Watch client for physical signs indicative of hypokalemia or metabolic alkalosis.
8. Keep accurate records of intake and output and vital signs.

Respiratory Acidosis

Definition: Respiratory acidosis refers to increased carbonic acid concentration (accumulated CO_2 which has combined with water) caused by retention of carbon dioxide through hypoventilation. Differs from metabolic acidosis in that it is caused by defective functioning of the lungs.

A. Changes in pH, pCO_2, and pO_2.
1. With an increased acidic state, the pH will fall below 7.35.
2. The pCO_2 will be increased above 50 mm Hg.
3. The pO_2 will be normal (80 to 100 mm Hg) or it can be decreased as hypoxia increases.
4. The HCO_3 will be normal if respiratory acidosis is uncompensated.

B. Compensatory mechanisms.
1. Because the basic problem in respiratory acidosis is a defect in the lungs, the kidneys must be the major compensatory mechanism.
   a. The kidneys work much slower than the lungs.
   b. Therefore, it will take from hours to days for the compensation to take place.
2. The kidneys will retain bicarbonate and return it to the extracellular fluid compartment.
3. The bicarbonate level will be elevated with partial or complete compensation.

C. Laboratory values when client is in respiratory acidosis and compensated acidosis.

1. Respiratory acidosis.
   a. pH: 7.32.
   b. pCO_2: 52 mm Hg.
   c. pO_2: 90 mm Hg.
   d. HCO_3: 24 mEq/l.
2. Compensated acidosis.
   a. pH: 7.35.
   b. pCO_2: 50 mm Hg.
   c. pO_2: 90 mm Hg.
   d. HCO_3: 36 mEq/l.

D. Causes of respiratory acidosis.
   1. Sedatives.
   2. Over-sedation with narcotics in postoperative period.
   3. A chronic pulmonary disorder such as emphysema, asthma, bronchitis, or pneumonia leading to:
      a. Inability of the lungs to expand and contract adequately.
      b. Difficulty in the expiratory phase of respiration, leading to retention of carbon dioxide.
   4. Poor gaseous exchange during surgery.

E. Clinical manifestations.
   1. Dyspnea after exertion.
   2. Hyperventilation when at rest.
   3. Cyanosis.
   4. Sensorium changes (drowsiness leading to coma).
   5. Carbon dioxide narcosis.
      a. When body has adjusted to higher carbon dioxide levels, the respiratory center loses its sensitivity to elevated carbon dioxide.
      b. Medulla fails to respond to high levels of carbon dioxide.
      c. Client is forced to depend on anoxia for respiratory stimulus.
      d. If a high level of oxygen is administered, client will cease breathing.

F. Nursing management.
   1. Turn, cough, and deep breathe client at least every two to four hours postoperatively. Use oropharyngeal suction if necessary.
   2. When pulmonary complications present a threat, do postural drainage, percussion, and vibration, followed by suctioning.
   3. Keep client well hydrated to facilitate removal of secretions. If client is dehydrated, secretions become thick and more difficult to expectorate.

4. Watch vital signs carefully, particularly rate and depth of respirations.
5. Teach pursed-lip breathing to chronic respiratory clients.
6. If oxygen is administered, watch carefully for signs of carbon dioxide narcosis.
7. Place client on mechanical ventilation if necessary.
8. Administer aerosol medications through IPPB.
   a. Bronchodilators (aminophylline)—relieve bronchospasms.
   b. Detergents (tergemist)—liquefy tenacious mucus.
   c. Antibiotics specific to causative agent.
9. Administer drug therapy.
   a. Sodium bicarbonate IV (0.25 g/kg body weight).
   b. Sodium lactate IV.
   c. Ringer's lactate IV to replace electrolyte loss.

Respiratory Alkalosis

Definition: Respiratory alkalosis occurs when an excessive amount of carbon dioxide is exhaled, usually caused by hyperventilation. The loss of carbon dioxide results in a decrease in H^+ concentration along with a decrease in pCO_2 and an increase in the ratio of bicarbonate to carbonic acid. The result is an increase in the pH level.

A. Changes in pH, pCO_2, and pO_2.
   1. With an increased alkalotic state, the pH will increase above 7.45, indicating there is a decreased amount of carbonic acid in the serum.
   2. The pCO_2 will be normal-to-low, as this measures the acid portion of the acid-base system (30 to 45 mm Hg).
   3. The pO_2 should be unchanged.
   4. The bicarbonate level (HCO_3 or CO_2 content) should be normal unless the client is compensating.

B. Compensatory mechanisms.
   1. Since the basic problem is related to the respiratory system, the kidneys will compensate by excreting more bicarbonate ions and retaining hydrogen ions.
   2. This process will return the acid-base balance to a normal ratio.

C. Laboratory values when client is in respiratory alkalosis and compensated alkalosis.
  1. Respiratory alkalosis.
    a. pH: 7.51.
    b. pCO_2: 32 mm pressure.
    c. pO_2: 95 mm Hg.
    d. HCO_3: 24 mEq/l.
  2. Compensated alkalosis.
    a. pH: 7.45.
    b. pCO_2: 30 mm pressure.
    c. pO_2: 95 mm Hg.
    d. HCO_3: 18 mEq/l.
D. Causes of respiratory alkalosis.
  1. Hysteria: client hyperventilates and exhales excessive amounts of carbon dioxide.
  2. Hypoxia: stimulates client to breathe more vigorously.
  3. Following head injuries or intracranial surgery.
  4. Increased temperature.
  5. Salicylate poisoning.
    a. Stimulation of respiration causes alkalosis through hyperventilation.
    b. Acidosis may occur from excessive salicylates in the blood.
E. Clinical manifestations—increased neuromuscular irritability.
  1. Hyperreflexia.
  2. Muscular twitching.
  3. Convulsions.
  4. Gasping for breath.
F. Nursing management.
  1. Eliminate cause of hyperventilation.
  2. Remain with client and be supportive to reduce anxiety.
  3. Use rebreathing bag to return client's carbon dioxide to self (paper bag works just as well).

System Assessment

A. Evaluate urinalysis findings to determine presence of infection, bleeding, or signs of renal failure.
B. Assess pain for location, intensity and precipitating factors.
  1. Ureteral pain is related to obstruction and is usually an acute manifestation.
    a. Site of obstruction may be found by tracing the location of radiation of pain.
    b. Pain may be severe and usually radiates down ureter into scrotum or vulva and to the inner thigh.
  2. Bladder pain is due to infection and overdistention of the bladder in urinary retention.
  3. Testicular pain is caused by inflammation or trauma, and is acute and severe.
  4. Pain in the lower back and leg may be caused by prostate cancer with metastasis to pelvic bones.
  5. Pain caused by renal disease.
    a. Dull ache in flank, radiating to lower abdomen and upper thigh.
    b. Pain may be absent if there is no sudden distention of kidney capsules.
C. Assess bladder for distention.
D. Examine the urinary catheter for abnormal findings.
E. Evaluate intake and output values.
F. Measure vital signs to determine presence of complications.
G. Assess patency of shunts.
H. Assess all body systems for potential alterations as a result of kidney problems.
  1. Peripheral edema.
  2. Hypertension.
  3. Eye disorders.
  4. Anemia.
  5. Lethargic or irritable condition.
  6. Congestive heart failure.
I. Observe for signs and symptoms of fluid and electrolyte imbalances.
J. Evaluate urinary test results for signs of renal abnormalities.
K. Assess client's feelings about body image.
L. Assess for type of imbalance:

Metabolic Alkalosis			Compensation
pH:	↑	>7.40	7.40
$HCO_3{}^-$:	↑	> 24	
BE:	↑	> 0	
pCO_2: normal		40	↑ >40

Metabolic Acidosis			Compensation
pH:	↓	<7.40	7.40
$HCO_3{}^-$:	↓	< 24	
BE:	↓	< 0	
pCO_2: normal		40	↓ <40

Respiratory Alkalosis		Compensation
pH: ↑	>7.40	7.40
pCO$_2$: ↓	< 40	
HCO$_3^-$: normal	24	↓ <24

Respiratory Acidosis		Compensation
pH: ↓	<7.40	7.40
pCO$_2$: ↑	> 40	
HCO$_3^-$: normal	24	↑ >24

DIAGNOSTIC PROCEDURES

Renal Function Tests

A. PSP test indicates the functional ability of the kidney to:
   1. Excrete waste products.
   2. Concentrate and dilute urine.
   3. Carry on absorption and excretion activities.
   4. Maintain body fluids and electrolytes.
B. Renal concentration tests.
   1. Underlying principles.
      a. Evaluate the ability of the kidney to concentrate urine.
      b. As kidney disease progresses, renal function decreases. Concentration tests evaluate this process.
      c. Renal concentration is measured by specific gravity readings (normal range is 1.003 to 1.035, usually 1.010 to 1.025).
      d. If specific gravity is 1.018 or greater, it may be assumed that the kidney is functioning within normal limits.
      e. Specific gravity that stabilizes at 1.010 indicates kidney has lost ability to concentrate or dilute.
   2. Concentration and dilution tests.
      a. Fishberg concentration test—high protein dinner with 200 cc fluid is ordered. Next A.M. on arising, client voids q 1/hr. One specimen should have specific gravity more than 1.025.
      b. Dilution test—n.p.o. after dinner. Morning voiding discarded. Client drinks 1000 ml in 30 to 45 minutes. Four specimens at one hour intervals are collected. One specimen will fall below 1.003.

c. Specific gravity—urine 1.003 to 1.030. Increased solutes cause increased specific gravity.
C. Glomerular filtration test (endogenous creatinine clearance).
   1. Kidney function is assessed by clearing a substance from the blood (filtration in the glomerulus).
   2. Common test is the amount of blood cleared of urea per minute.
   3. Test done on 12-hour or 24-hour urine specimen.
   4. Normal range is approximately 125 ml/minute (male) and 110 ml/minute (female).
D. Electrolyte tests.
   1. Kidney function is essential to maintain fluid and electrolyte balance.
   2. Tests for electrolytes (sodium, potassium, chloride, and bicarbonate) measure the ability of the kidney to filter, reabsorb, or excrete these substances.
   3. Impaired filtration leads to retention, and impaired reabsorption leads to loss of electrolytes.
   4. Tests are performed on blood serum, so venous blood is required.

Analysis of Urine

A. Urinalysis is a critical test for total evaluation of the renal system and for indication of renal disease.
B. Specific gravity shows the degree of concentration in urine.
   1. Indicates the ability of the kidney to concentrate or dilute urine.
   2. Change from normal range indicates diabetes mellitus (greater than 1.030) or kidney damage (less than 1.010).
   3. Renal failure—specific gravity constant at 1.010.
C. Analysis of the pH of urine.
   1. pH is the symbol for the logarithm of the reciprocal of the hydrogen ion concentration.
   2. A measurement of hydrogen ion concentration is taken: the lower the number the higher the acidity of urine.
      a. Normal urine pH is 6 to 7.
      b. Lower than 6 is acidic urine, and higher than 7 is alkaline urine.
   3. Regulation of urine pH is important for treatment of certain conditions.

a. Above pH 6.
  (1) Treatment of hypertension with mecamy-lamine hydrochloride (Inversine).
  (2) Management of blood transfusions.
  (3) Streptomycin and sulfonamide therapy.
  (4) Management of renal calculi.
b. Below pH 6—treatment of urinary tract infections.

D. Chemical analysis of urine.
  1. Protein or albumin: zero is normal for a 24-hour specimen.
    a. Presence may indicate renal disease, such as nephritis or nephrosis.
    b. Inflammatory processes any place in the body may result in proteinuria.
    c. Toxemia of pregnancy yields a finding of proteinuria.
    d. Renal calculi indicate positive test results.
    e. Appearance in urine may be due to dehydration, strenuous exercise, high protein diet.
  2. Glucose: normal range is zero.
    a. Presence of glucose may indicate head injury or diabetes.
    b. Test is usually done by test strips or tablets; change in color indicates presence of glucose.
  3. Ketone bodies: normal range is zero.
    a. Ketonuria primarily indicates diabetic acidosis but is also present with starvation and pernicious vomiting.
    b. Test usually by strip or powder mixed with urine; purple color indicates positive test.
  4. Bilirubin: normal range is zero.
    a. Presence in urine may indicate liver disease and may appear before the clinical symptom of jaundice.
    b. Detected in the urine by qualitative methods, such as inspection of color.
  5. Blood: normal range is zero.
    a. If red blood cells present, may indicate disease of kidney or urinary tract, and the source of hemorrhage must be determined.
    b. Specific diagnosis is made by complete urine analysis for casts and epithelial cells.

E. Microscopic examination of urine.
  1. Evaluation of urinary sediment is important for diagnostic purposes.
  2. Test for cellular elements (epithelial cells, white and red blood cells).
  3. Test for casts, fat bodies, and crystals.

F. Levels of albuminuria.
  30 mg/100 ml = 1 +   300 mg/100 ml = 3 +
  100 mg/100 ml = 2 +   1000 mg/100 ml = 4 +

GU Examination

Male Examination
A. Testicular self-exam (TSE).
  1. Instruct client to perform monthly. (Between ages 15–25, 3rd highest cause of cancer deaths.)
  2. Rotate each testicle between thumb and forefinger, feeling for a firm surface.
  3. If painless lump is felt (*not* the epididymis), notify physician immediately.
B. Prostate Evaluation.
  1. Rectal exam annually at age 40.
  2. Blood chemistry for cancer.
    a. Prostatic acid phosphate (PAP)—elevated.
    b. Prostate specific antigen (PSA)—elevated.
    c. May be false positive readings.
  3. Ultrasound with biopsy if indicated.

Female Gynecological Examination
A. Pelvic examination.
  1. Inspection of external genitalia for signs of inflammation, bleeding, discharge, and epithelial cell changes.
  2. Visualization of vagina and cervix.
  3. Bimanual examination.
  4. Rectal examination.
B. Papanicolaou smear.
  1. Diagnosis for cervical cancer.
  2. Vaginal secretions and secretions from posterior fornix are smeared on a glass slide.
  3. Pathological classifications.
    a. Class I: no abnormal or atypical cells present.
    b. Class II: atypical or abnormal cells present but no malignancy found; repeat pap smear and follow-up if necessary.
    c. Class III: cytology, suggests malignancy; additional procedures: biopsy, D and C.
    d. Class IV: cytology, strongly suggestive of malignancy; additional procedures indicated (biopsy, D and C).
    e. Class V: cytology conclusive of malignancy.
C. Breast examination may also be given.
D. Mammography.
  1. X-ray of soft tissue to detect nonpalpable mass.
  2. Baseline (one time) 35–39; biannual 40–49; annual after 50.

System Planning and Analysis

A. Signs and symptoms of bladder dysfunction are identified readily and interventions initiated promptly.
B. Interventions are planned to preserve renal function as long as possible for clients in renal failure.
C. Lab values and diagnostic tests are reviewed and abnormal findings reported to physician.
D. Appropriate diet is ordered and client is able to tolerate change in altered nutritional state.
E. Hemodialysis and/or peritoneal dialysis treatments are provided on routine basis according to each client's needs.
F. Professional assistance is obtained for clients with chronic disease and/or altered body image.

System Implementation

A. Monitor fluid intake at least every shift for clients with renal dysfunction.
   1. Force fluids.
      a. Urinary tract infection.
      b. Cystitis.
      c. Pyelonephritis.
      d. Urolithiasis.
   2. Restrict fluids.
      a. Glomerulonephritis.
      b. Renal failure.
      c. Nephrotic syndrome.
B. Provide appropriate diet for renal dysfunction.
   1. Pyelonephritis—high calorie, vitamins and protein; if oliguria is present, change diet to low protein.
   2. Glomerulonephritis—40 g protein, low sodium.
   3. Nephrotic syndrome—high protein, high calorie, low sodium.
   4. Renal failure—limited protein, low in nitrogen, potassium, sodium, phosphate, and sulfate.
C. Monitor client for complications associated with renal dysfunction, especially congestive heart failure, pulmonary edema, and hypertension.
D. Provide good skin care; edematous areas are easily broken down.
E. Encourage bed rest for clients in an acute stage of the disease.
F. Administer medications on time to keep blood levels stable and in therapeutic range.
G. Monitor vital signs for early detection of changes in client status.

H. Provide shunt care to maintain patency and prevent infection.
I. Instruct client on diet, fluid alteration, and shunt care as needed.
J. Encourage client to express feelings and concerns with altered body image.

System Evaluation

A. Client remains on therapeutic diet.
B. Fluid overload is avoided through accurate monitoring and recording of intake and output.
C. Skin remains clear and free of breakdown.
D. Complications are identified early and treatment instituted quickly.
E. Bedrest is maintained throughout the acute course of the disease.
F. Blood level of medications is maintained at a stable therapeutic level.
G. Vital signs are routinely monitored and complications are detected rapidly.
H. Shunt remains patent and free of infection.
I. Client adapts to altered body image.

Injuries to the Kidney

Definition: Injury to the kidney includes any trauma that bruises, lacerates, or ruptures any part of the kidney organ.

Assessment

A. Assess for hematuria.
B. Assess for shock, if hemorrhage has occurred.
C. Evaluate pain over costovertebral area.
D. Observe for gastrointestinal symptoms of nausea and vomiting.

Implementation

A. Promote bed rest.
B. Monitor vital signs frequently for possible hemorrhage.
C. Monitor blood work and laboratory examination of urine to assess for hematuria.
D. Prevent infection.
E. Frequently monitor the total status of the client following injury.
   1. Observe for pain and tenderness.
   2. Observe any sudden change in status.

F. Prepare for surgery (nephrectomy) if health status deteriorates (shock indicating severe hemorrhage).

Nephrectomy

Definition: Nephrectomy is the surgical removal of a kidney.

Assessment

A. Evaluate possible cause.
1. Polycystic kidneys.
2. Stones.
3. Preparation for transplantation.
4. Injury.
5. Infection which has destroyed kidney function.

B. Assess urine output for hematuria, cells, pus.

C. Observe for signs of hemorrhage and shock.

D. Evaluate intake and output (anuria can result if remaining kidney is damaged).

E. Check for bowel sounds (paralytic ileus may be a complication).

Implementation

A. Obtain urine specimens as ordered to detect renal function of remaining kidney.

B. Force fluids.

C. Turn, cough, and hyperventilate every two hours (turn to operative side and back).

D. Administer IPPB if necessary.

E. Begin range-of-motion exercises immediately.

F. Encourage early ambulation.

G. Observe that Foley or suprapubic catheter is draining adequately.
1. Tape catheter to leg or abdomen to prevent trauma to bladder.
2. Position catheter bag below bed level to facilitate drainage.

H. If nephrostomy tube is inserted, measure drainage and record characteristics of drainage (drains kidney after surgery).
1. Do not clamp tubes unless ordered.
2. Do not irrigate tubes unless ordered.

Urinary Tract Infections

Definition: A term that refers to a wide variety of conditions affecting the urinary tract in which the common denominator is the presence of microorganisms.

Characteristics

A. Urine is sterile until it reaches the distal urethra.

B. Any bacteria can be introduced into the urinary tract resulting in infection, which may spread to any other part of the tract. Escherichia coli is most frequent organism.

C. The most important factor influencing ascending infection is obstruction of free urine flow.
1. Free flow, large urine output, and pH are antibacterial defenses.
2. If defenses break down, the result may be an invasion of the tract by bacteria.

D. Microscopic examination is completed for an accurate identification of the organism (especially important in chronic infections).

Assessment

A. Evaluate urine cultures and chemical tests to determine presence and number of bacteria.

B. Evaluate urine colony count. Colony count over 100,000/ml indicates urinary tract infection.

C. Assess for location, type, and precipitating factor leading to pain.

D. Observe urine for color, consistency, specific gravity.

Implementation

A. Force fluids to 3000 cc.

B. Administer urinary antiseptics as ordered.
1. Antibacterial effects occur in genitourinary tract and are not systemic.
2. Common drugs—ciprofloxacin (Cipro), norfloxacin (Noroxin), iomefloxacin (Maxaquin), Gantanol, Furadantin.
3. Usual side effects—nausea, vomiting, diarrhea, abdominal pain.

C. Administer aminoglycosides (antibiotics) as ordered.
1. Specific for causative bacteria (given one to two weeks).
2. Common drugs—streptomycin, kanamycin, neomycin, gentamicin.
3. Usual side effects—vertigo, nausea, vomiting, rash.

D. Obtain sterile urine specimens.

E. Provide warm sitz baths.

Cystitis

Definition: Inflammation of bladder from infection or obstruction of the urethra is the most common cause.

Assessment

A. Observe for frequency, urgency, and burning sensation on urination.
B. Evaluate lower abdominal discomfort.
C. Observe for dark and odorous urine (often a manifestation).
D. Assess laboratory findings for presence of bacteria and hematuria.

Implementation

A. Assist physician in identifying and removing the cause of the condition (infection, obstruction, etc.).
B. Administer antibiotics on time.
C. Instruct client on how to prevent infection.
D. Instruct client on measures for symptomatic relief of chronic conditions.
E. Collect an uncontaminated urine specimen (midstream specimen) for laboratory test.
F. Maintain adequate fluid intake.
   1. Force fluids only if specifically ordered.
   2. Check and record intake and output.
G. Encourage bed rest or a decrease in activity during the acute stage.
H. Maintain acid urine (pH 5.5).
I. Instruct client in follow-up urinary tests for pH.

Cystoscopy

Definition: The inspection of the bladder by means of a cystoscope.

Assessment

A. Inspect bladder for stones, etc.
B. Evaluate results of tissue examination obtained from biopsy.
C. Measure vital signs.
D. Observe for urethral bleeding.

Implementation

A. Chart intake and output and consistency of urine.
B. Monitor for signs of infection.
   1. Frequency.
   2. Urgency.
   3. Burning during urination.
C. Monitor for perforation of bladder.
   1. Sharp abdominal pain.
   2. Anuria.
   3. Board-like abdomen.

D. Maintain client on bed rest for four to six hours; then ambulate if no complications.
E. Monitor vital signs for shock and infection.

Pyelonephritis

Definition: An acute or chronic infection and inflammation of one or both kidneys that usually begins in the renal pelvis. Women are more commonly affected. Gram-negative organisms are most often responsible, especially E. coli.

Assessment

A. Observe for attacks of chills, fever, malaise, gastrointestinal upsets.
B. Evaluate for tenderness and dull, aching pain in back.
C. Identify frequent and burning urination (more common in lower tract involvement).
D. Evaluate pus and bacteria in urine.
E. Evaluate renal function. May have normal renal function except for inability to concentrate urine.
F. Evaluate for renal insufficiency.
   1. Progressive destruction of renal tubules and glomeruli.
   2. Inability of kidneys to excrete large amounts of electrolytes.
G. Assess for hypertension in presence of bacterial pyelonephritis.
H. Identify if overt symptoms disappear in a few days but urine is still infected.

Implementation

A. Administer and monitor drug therapy.
   1. Antibiotic therapy (organism-specific for infection).
   2. Urinary antiseptics.
   3. Analgesics and sedatives as needed.
B. Maintain bed rest until asymptomatic.
C. Force fluids to maintain urine output of 1500 cc/day.
D. Continue monitoring for presence of bacteria.
E. Instruct client in methods to prevent chronic renal insufficiency.
F. Monitor urinalysis.
   1. Check urine concentration.
   2. Check electrolytes.
G. Provide diet high in calories and vitamins and low in protein if oliguria is present.

H. Give fluid intake sufficient to maintain adequate urine volume.

I. Observe for edema and signs of renal failure.

J. Instruct client in good hygiene to prevent further infections.

Glomerulonephritis

Definition: Nephritis caused by inflammation of the capillary loops in the glomeruli of the kidney.

Characteristics

A. The kidney's glomeruli are affected by an immunological disorder.

B. Most frequently follows infections with group A beta-hemolytic streptococcus.

C. Upper respiratory infections, skin infections, other autoimmune processes (systemic lupus), and acute infections predispose to glomerulonephritis.

D. Glomerulonephritis symptoms appear seven to fourteen days after original infection.

Assessment

A. Assess for pharyngitis, fever, malaise (initial symptoms).

B. Observe for weakness, anorexia, mild anemia.

C. Evaluate edema—leg, face, or generalized.

D. Observe for oliguria.

E. Assess abdominal pain nausea, vomiting.

F. Identify if hypertension, headache, or convulsions are present.

G. Observe for hypoalbuminemia due to increased loss via urine. (Proteinuria 2 to 8 g daily.)

H. Evaluate hematuria.

I. Assess specific gravity for high values.

J. Assess for congestive heart failure.

K. Evaluate presence of increased BUN.

Implementation

A. Administer penicillin for residual infection.

B. Administer diuretics and antihypertensives if necessary.

C. Provide appropriate diet.

1. Protein restriction if oliguria is severe, otherwise protein allowed at low normal range (normal 40–60 gm/day).

2. BUN level watched for protein determination.

3. Protein should be of the complete type (milk, eggs, meat, fish, poultry).

4. High carbohydrate to spare protein.

5. Potassium usually restricted.

6. Sodium restriction for hypertension and CHF. If diuresis is great, sodium replacement may be necessary.

7. Fluid restriction: replacement is based on insensible loss plus measured sensible loss of previous day or hour.

8. Vitamin replacement.

D. Encourage complete bed rest during acute stage of disease.

1. Continue until clinical signs abate.

2. Start activity when blood pressure and blood urea nitrogen (BUN) normal for one to two weeks.

3. If sedimentation rate increases or urinary findings indicate, return to bed rest regimen.

E. Monitor vital signs continuously.

F. Allow client to verbalize feelings on body image changes (due to edema), loss of health, fear of death.

G. Monitor fluid intake.

1. Measure fluids according to urinary output.

2. Record intake and output.

3. Weigh daily.

H. Monitor for signs of overhydration.

I. Take blood pressure frequently and observe for hypertension.

J. Evaluate for symptoms of renal failure.

1. Oliguria.

2. Azotemia.

3. Acidosis.

Nephrotic Syndrome

Definition: A term that refers to renal disease characterized by massive edema and albuminuria.

Characteristics

A. The syndrome is seen in any renal condition that has damaged glomerular capillary membrane: glomerulonephritis, lipoid nephrosis, syphilitic nephritis, amyloidosis, or systemic lupus erythematosus.

B. A specific form of intercapillary glomerulosclerosis is associated with diabetes mellitus (Kimmelstiel-Wilson syndrome).

C. Occurrence thought to be related to thyroid function.

Assessment

A. Evaluate edema (at first, dependent; later, generalized).
B. Identify if proteinuria (20 to 30 g/day) is present.
C. Identify if decreased serum albumin is present.
D. Identify if elevated serum cholesterol, triglycerides, hyperlipemia are present.
E. Assess hypertension (related to function of renin angiotensin system).
F. Evaluate decreased cardiac output (secondary to fluid loss).
G. Observe for pallor.
H. Observe for malaise, anorexia, lethargy.

Implementation

A. Provide nursing care directed toward control of edema.
   1. Sodium restriction in diet.
   2. Avoidance of sodium-containing drugs.
   3. Diuretics (Lasix and Edecrin) that block aldosterone formation.
   4. Salt-poor albumin.
B. Provide dietary instruction.
   1. High protein (100 g) to restore body proteins.
   2. High calorie.
   3. 500 mg sodium.
C. Administer drug therapy.
   1. Adrenocortical therapy (prednisone promotes sodium retention).
   2. Immunosuppressives.
      a. Cyclophosphamide, drug of choice.
      b. Side effects: alopecia, hemorrhagic cystitis, increased susceptibility to infection.
D. Maintain bed rest until edema has reached stable minimum.
E. Instruct client in the maintenance of general health status, as the disorder may persist for months or years.
   1. Avoiding infections.
   2. Nutritious diet (low sodium, high protein).
   3. Activity as tolerated.
F. Maintain fluid balance.
   1. Daily weights.
   2. Intake and output.

Tuberculosis of the Kidney

Definition: Tuberculosis of the kidney is an infection caused by Mycobacterium tuberculosis which is usually blood-borne from other foci such as the lungs, lymph nodes, or bone.

Assessment

A. Identify frequency and pain on urination.
B. Evaluate burning, spasm, and hematuria.
C. Assess for fatigue and weight loss.
D. Evaluate findings of physical examination. Tuberculosis nodules may be present in the prostate.
E. Evaluate outcome of diagnostic studies.
   1. Urine cultures to isolate the tubercle bacilli.
   2. X-ray to reveal lesions.
   3. Cystoscopic examination.

Implementation

A. Administer medications on time.
   1. Drug therapy aimed at treating the original focus of infection as well as the genitourinary involvement.
   2. Isoniazid, streptomycin, ethambutol, or rifampin.
   3. Usually given together in a single daily dose.
   4. Observe for side effects.
B. Instruct client on methods to improve general health status.
   1. Good dietary habits.
   2. Adequate rest.
C. Prepare the client for possible nephrectomy.

SURGICAL INTERVENTIONS FOR URINARY SYSTEM

Cystostomy

Definition: An opening into the bladder for suprapubic drainage.

Characteristics

A. Diverts urine flow from urethra
B. Empties bladder (similar for Foley catheter, but catheter is inserted in suprapubic area rather than through urinary meatus).
C. Provides less risk of infection for client.
D. Used for:
   1. Urethral stricture.
   2. Following vaginal surgery.
   3. Neurogenic bladder.
   4. Following surgery on prostate and bladder.

Implementation

A. Provide care the same as for any client with indwelling catheter.
B. Clamp catheter and then client is allowed to void on his or her own (through urinary meatus).
C. Remove when able to void on own.

Urolithiasis

Definition: The presence of stones in any portion of the urinary system.

Characteristics

A. Causes: dehydration, immobilization, hypercalcemia, excessive uric acid excretion, obstruction and urinary stasis.
B. Surgical interventions.
   1. Ureterolithotomy: removal of stone from ureter.
   2. Pyelolithotomy: removal of stone from kidney pelvis.
   3. Extracorporeal shock wave lithotripsy (ESWL): under general anesthesia, client is immersed in water and shock waves disintegrate stones that are then excreted in urine.

Assessment

A. Evaluate pain (starts low in back and radiates around front and down the ureter).
B. Observe for nausea, vomiting, and diarrhea.
C. Observe for hematuria.
D. Assess for chills and fever.

Implementation

A. Force fluids to at least 3000 cc/24 hours.
B. Record intake and output.
C. Strain all urine for stones.
D. Send stones to laboratory for chemical analysis.
E. Administer appropriate antibiotics (infections occur especially when stones block off a portion of kidney).
F. Provide diet therapy, depending on chemical composition of stones.
G. Place heating pad on affected area.
H. Watch vital signs for signs of infection.
I. Instruct client in methods to prevent urolithiasis.
   1. Provide adequate fluid intake.
   2. Immediately treat urinary tract infection with appropriate antibiotics.
   3. Ambulate clients to prevent urinary stasis (or reposition in bed frequently).

Urinary Diversion

Definition: Anastomosis of the ureters into a loop of ileum which is then brought through the abdominal wall. Procedure follows removal of bladder for cancer.

Characteristics

A. Cancer of neck of bladder or ureters.
B. Cancer of pelvic area.
C. Neurogenic bladder.

Assessment

A. Assess client's fluid balance.
   1. Intake and output.
   2. Daily weights.
B. Observe characteristics of urine.
C. Observe for complications related to surgical intervention.
   1. Urinary fistula (urine around incision).
   2. Bowel fistula (feces from incision).
   3. Wound complications (dehiscence or evisceration).
D. Assess skin.

MEDICAL IMPLICATIONS

A. Superficial low-grade tumors—TUR.
B. Monthly bladder instillations of thiotepa for one year for superficial tumors.
C. Radon seeds for vesical tumors.
D. Cystectomy for extensive tumors that are curable.
E. High voltage radiotherapy in conjunction with radical surgery.
F. Radiotherapy and chemotherapy (fluorouracil) for inoperable tumors.

Implementation

A. If nasogastric tube is inserted, irrigate when necessary.
B. Provide routine abdominal postoperative care.
C. Provide psychological support for altered body image, change in life style, chronic disease.
D. Refer to enterostomal therapist or cancer society for help with ostomy care.
E. Provide range-of-motion exercise.
F. Ensure tight-fitting ostomy bag around opening to prevent skin irritation.

RENAL FAILURE

Acute Renal Failure

Definition: The sudden loss of kidney function caused by failure of renal circulation or damage to the tubules or glomerulus. Condition reversible with spontaneous recovery in days to several weeks.

Etiology

A. Prerenal—conditions decreasing blood flow.
    1. Severe dehydration; diuretic therapy.
    2. Circulatory collapse: hypovolemia, shock.
B. Renal—disease process, ischemic or toxic conditions.
    1. Acute glomerulonephritis.
    2. Vascular disorders.
    3. Toxic agents (e.g., carbon tetrachloride, sulfonamides, arsenic, etc.).
    4. Severe infection.
C. Postrenal obstruction to urine flow.

Assessment

A. Period of oliguria followed by period of diuresis.
    1. Evaluate urine output often when less than 20ml/hour—at least every two to four hours.
    2. Observe lab reports for increased BUN and creatinine.
B. Evaluate serum levels of potassium, sodium, pH, pCO_2, and HCO_3—indication of complications.
C. Observe urinalysis for proteinuria, hematuria, casts.
D. Evaluate change in mental status.
E. Note if specific gravity fixed at 1.010–1.016
F. Evaluate for potassium intoxication; hyperkalemia.
G. Assess for signs of infection—client may not demonstrate fever or increased WBC.

Implementation

A. Monitor urinary output.
    1. Record intake and output (oliguria followed by diuresis).
    2. Weigh daily (lack of weight loss—1/2 to 1 pound daily—indicates retention of too much fluid).
B. Monitor fluid intake (observe for signs of CHF).
C. Monitor for complications of electrolyte imbalances: acidosis (treated with sodium bicarbonate).
D. Monitor serum potassium levels (above 6 mEq/liter together with peaking T waves and shortening QT interval) for hyperkalemia .
E. Allow client to verbalize concerns and effect of altered body image.
F. Encourage the prescribed diet: moderate protein restriction; high carbohydrate; restrict foods high in K+ (coffee, bananas, juices) .
G. Be cautious when using antibiotics and other drugs.
H. Continually assess status of client for potential complications: dyspnea, tachycardia, increased blood pressure.
I. Evaluate slow return of decreased serum BUN, creatinine, phosphorous, and potassium to normal after diuresis phase begins.

Chronic Renal Failure

Definition: The progressive loss of kidney function that occurs in four stages and, without intervention, ends fatally in uremia.

Characteristics

A. First stage: diminished renal reserve.
    1. Abnormal renal function tests.
    2. No accumulation of metabolic waste.
    3. Presence of polyuria, nocturia, and polydipsia.
B. Second stage: renal insufficiency.
    1. Metabolic waste begins to accumulate.
    2. Increase in BUN and creatinine (10:1 ratio) .
    3. Stress poorly tolerated (e.g., infection).
    4. Chemical abnormalities resolve slowly.
C. Third stage: renal failure.
    1. Hypertension; edema.
    2. Poor urine output.
    3. Severe alterations of electrolytes.
    4. Moderately increased BUN and creatinine.
    5. Anemia common with this condition.
    6. Metabolic acidosis.
D. Uremia.

Assessment

A. Assess for weakness, fatigue and headaches.
B. Assess for anorexia, nausea and vomiting.
C. Evaluate for hypertension and heart failure.
D. Evaluate for anemia, azotemia (nitrogen retention in the blood), and acidosis.
E. Observe for personality changes (e.g., anxiety, irritability, hallucinations, convulsions, and coma).
F. Evaluate for low and fixed specific gravity of urine.

Implementation

A. Provide diet and fluids (low protein with supplemented amino acids) for acute renal failure.
B. Provide electrolyte replacement.
    1. Sodium supplements provided.
    2. Potassium and phosphorus restricted.
    3. Acidosis replacement of bicarbonate stores.

C. Monitor and plan nursing care for hypertension and heart failure.

D. Prepare client for dialysis or kidney transplant.

E. Administer medications with caution—impaired renal function may require adjustment.

Uremia

Definition: The accumulation of nitrogenous waste products in blood due to inability of kidneys to filter out waste products.

Characteristics

A. May occur after acute or chronic renal failure.

B. Increased urea, creatinine, uric acid.

C. Extensive electrolyte imbalances (increased K^+, increased Na, decreased $Cl-$, decreased Ca^{++}, increased phosphorous).

D. Acidosis—bicarbonate cannot be maintained at adequate level.

E. Urine concentration ability lost.

F. Anemia.

G. Metabolic acidosis accumulation affects all body systems.

Assessment

A. Observe for signs of oliguria for one to two weeks (produces less than 400 cc/day).

B. Assess changes in urine characteristics.
   1. Urine contains protein, red blood cells, casts.
   2. Specific gravity of 1.010.
   3. Rise in urine solutes (e.g., urea, uric acid, potassium, magnesium) .

C. Assess for metabolic acidosis.

D. Observe for hypotension or hypertension.

E. Assess for gastrointestinal problems: stomatitis, nausea, vomiting, and diarrhea or constipation.

F. Assess for respiratory complications.

G. Identify if wound healing impaired.

H. Evaluate coma—with alterations of blood chemistry and acid load.

Implementation

A. Monitor restoration of blood volume.

B. Monitor fluid and electrolyte balance.

C. Provide dietary regulation.
   1. Limit protein (20 to 60 g) unless on peritoneal dialysis.
   2. Reduce nitrogen, potassium, phosphate, and sulfate.
   3. Limit sodium intake.
   4. Provide glucose to prevent ketosis.

   5. Control potassium balance to prevent hyperkalemia.
   6. Carbohydrate intake 100 g daily.

DIALYSIS

Peritoneal Dialysis

Definition: A method of separating substances by interposing a semipermeable membrane. The peritoneum is used as the dialyzing membrane and substitutes for kidney function during failure.

Principles of Peritoneal Dialysis

A. Usually temporary; can be used for clients in acute, reversible renal failure.

B. Basic goals of dialysis therapy.
   1. Removal of end products of protein metabolism, such as creatinine and urea.
   2. Maintenance of safe concentration of serum electrolytes.
   3. Correction of acidosis and blood's bicarbonate buffer system.
   4. Removal of excess fluid.

C. Renal perfusion is compromised when increased size of the intravascular compartment and redistribution of blood volume result from:
   1. Gram-negative sepsis.
   2. Overdoses of some drugs.
   3. Anaphylactic shock.
   4. Electrolyte disturbances, such as acidosis.

D. Drugs are used to check for renal failure before client is placed on dialysis.
   1. In most cases, Mannitol is tried before dialysis.
      a. Not reabsorbed by kidney.
      b. Has great osmotic effect and increases urinary flow.
      c. Administration.
         (1) Given quickly in order to get higher blood level and then, in turn, filtered load.
         (2) If infusion is too slow, changes in the urinary flow rate will be delayed as urine flow depends on the amount of Mannitol filtered.
         (3) Give 12.5 g of a 25 percent solution in three minutes; if flow rate can be increased to 40 cc/hour, the client is in reversible renal failure.
         (4) Keep urine at 100 cc/hour with Mannitol.
   2. Drugs such as Lasix (furosemide) and Edecrin (ethacrynic acid) may be used if Mannitol is not effective.

Peritoneal Dialysis Function

A. Works on diffusion and osmosis, similar to hemodialysis; however, in this instance, the peritoneum is the semipermeable membrane.

B. Peritoneum is impermeable to large molecules (proteins).

C. Permeable to low molecular weight molecules (urea, glucose, electrolytes).

D. Cannot be used with clients who have the following conditions:
   1. Peritonitis.
   2. Recent abdominal surgery.
   3. Abdominal adhesions.
   4. Impending renal transplant.

E. Dialysate.
   1. Contains electrolytes but no urea, creatinine.
      a. Common electrolytes in dialysate in mEq/liter.
         Na^+ 140 to 145
         Cl^- 101 to 110
         Ca^{++} 3.5 to 4.0
         Mg^{++} 1.5
         Lactate/acetate (base) 43 to 45
      b. Osmolarity.
         1.5% = 365 mOsm
         4.25% = 504 mOsm
   2. Sterile.
   3. Solutions vary in dextrose concentration.
      a. Solution of 1.5 percent: used for drug intoxication and acute renal failure if large amounts of fluid are not required to be removed.
      b. Solution of 4.25 percent: used for removal of excessive fluid.
   4. If hyperkalemia is not a problem, 4 mEq of potassium chloride is added to each solution.
   5. Heparin is added to bottles to prevent clotting of the catheter.

CAPD Continuous Ambulatory Peritoneal Dialysis

A. A variation of peritoneal dialysis developed to allow the client to be dialyzed while ambulatory.

B. Procedure for CAPD.
   1. Peritoneal catheter is inserted.
   2. 500–1000 ml of dialysate infused through catheter by gravity (10–20 minutes).
   3. The catheter is clamped, bag folded and placed in waistband of client's clothes.
   4. Every 4 hours client drains fluid from peritoneal cavity.
      a. Unclamp catheter.
      b. Place pouch to allow drainage by gravity—below level of abdomen.
      c. Drain for approximately 20 minutes.
      d. Reclamp catheter and remove bag with drainage.
      e. Examine drainage—a change in color may indicate infection (glucose in dialysate predisposes client to infection.)
   5. Aseptically attach a new bag of dialysate and repeat procedure.
   6. Repeat procedure 4 times daily.
   7. Instruct client to change tubing every 24 hours using strict aseptic technique.

C. Be alert for possible complications: peritonitis, fluid and electrolyte imbalances, dehydration, catheter infection, abdominal pain and tenderness, and hemorrhage.

Dialysis Procedure

A. Client preparation.
   1. Client voids before catheter insertion to prevent bladder damage.
   2. Abdominal skin is prepped.
   3. The area between the umbilicus and the pubic bone near the midline is most often used for catheter insertion.
   4. Client is weighed before procedure.
   5. Baseline vital signs (including weight).

B. Dialysis process.
   1. Dialysis fluid instilled in abdominal cavity.
   2. Occurrence of osmosis, diffusion, and filtration via peritoneal membrane (called equilibration).
   3. Fluid drained from abdominal cavity.
   4. Process repeated with a time sequence allowed for each step. Period of time and number of cycles will vary according to client problem, tolerance, response, and type of solution.

C. Duration of dialysis depends on the following factors:
   1. Client's size and weight.
   2. Severity of uremia.
   3. Physical state of client.
   4. Usual time period for dialysis is 24 to 72 exchanges or runs.

D. Monitoring the procedure.
   1. Client's electrolyte status is monitored during the process.
   2. Periodic samples of the return dialysate are sent for culture.

3. Compare client's weight before and after procedure to assess effectiveness.

4. Vital signs must be monitored closely.

E. Care of equipment during procedure.

1. Tubing should be changed every eight hours when the procedure continues for days.

2. Warming the dialysate not only improves urea clearance but also maintains client's body temperature and comfort.

3. Avoid getting air into tubing as this is uncomfortable for the client and impedes smooth and easy return of flow.

F. Quality and quantity of return.

1. Initial few outflows may be slightly bloody due to insertion process.

2. Cloudy fluid is usually an indication of peritonitis.

3. Bowel perforation should be suspected if flow is brown.

4. Record amount and type of solution for each inflow. This includes the medications added (e.g., potassium chloride, heparin, antibiotics).

5. Record outflow amount and characteristics.

6. Duration of each phase of the process should be recorded.

7. Keep a total net balance (difference between input and output for each exchange) and cumulative net balance.

8. Inform physician if client loses or retains large volumes of fluid.

   a. Periodically test urine for presence of sugar which may be absorbed from dialysate.

   b. Heparin helps prevent drainage problems.

G. Procedures to check when drainage slows.

1. Check proper position of clamps.

2. Look for kinking in tubes.

3. Milk the drainage tube.

4. Observe air vent in drainage bottle for patency.

5. Flush catheter.

6. Reposition direction of catheter within means.

7. Have client change positions.

8. Have physician change catheter.

Peritoneal Clearance Rates

- Peritoneal membrane only about 50 percent as efficient as normal kidney function.
- Flow rate of dialysate affects peritoneal clearance.
- Optimal flow rate suggested is 2.5 l/hour.
- Usual cycle to maintain 2.5 l/hour flow: 5 to 10 minutes in-flow time, 20 minutes of equilibration, and 20 minutes for drainage (when using 2 liters of dialysate).
- Increased levels of glucose in dialysate increase urea clearance.
- Dialysate perfused at body temperature increases urea clearance by 35 percent.

Implementation

A. Each morning, send culture on returning dialysate solution to observe for signs of infection.

B. Each day at the same time, weigh client with abdomen empty of solution.

C. Monitor vital signs to observe for complications.

D. Monitor dialysis exchange.

1. Keep exchange on time.

2. Maintain aseptic technique when changing bottles and tubing.

3. Record accurate intake and output on flow sheet.

E. Try the following interventions to assist in returning dialysate from peritoneal cavity.

1. Turn client on side and prop with pillows.

2. Place in Fowler's position after solution is infused into abdomen.

3. Ambulate and/or have client sit in chair if client is able.

4. Palpate abdomen.

5. Place pillow or bath blanket under small of back (this also assists in relieving hiccoughs).

F. Test urine for sugar.

G. Monitor for complications of peritoneal dialysis.

1. Peritonitis.

   a. Diffuse abdominal pain.

   b. Abdomen tender on palpation.

   c. Abdominal wall rigidity.

   d. Cloudy outflow.

2. Hypertension.

3. Pulmonary edema.

4. Hyperglycemia (insulin may be needed).

5. Hyperosmolar coma.

6. Protein loss (0.5 to 1.0 g per liter of drainage).

7. Intestinal perforation.

Hemodialysis

Definition: The diffusion of dissolved particles from one fluid compartment into another across a semipermeable membrane. In hemodialysis, the blood is one fluid compartment while the dialysate is another.

Principles of Hemodialysis

A. The semipermeable membrane is a thin, porous cellophane.
B. The pore size of the membrane permits the passage of low molecular weight substances such as urea, creatinine, and uric acid to diffuse through the pores of the membrane.
C. Water molecules are also very small and move freely through the membrane.
D. Most plasma proteins, bacteria, and blood cells are too large to pass through the pores of the membrane.
E. The difference in the concentration of the substances in the two compartments is called the concentration gradient.
F. The blood, which contains the waste products, flows into the dialyzer where it comes in contact with the dialysate.
G. A maximum gradient is established so that movement of these substances occurs from the blood to the dialysate.
H. Dialysate (bath).
    1. Composed of water and major electrolytes.
    2. Tap water can be used (need not be sterile because bacteria are too large to pass through membrane).

Hemodialysis Function

A. Removes byproducts of protein metabolism: urea, creatinine, and uric acid.
B. Removes excessive fluid by:
    1. Changing osmotic pressure (by adding more dextrose to dialysate).
    2. Negative or positive hydrostatic pressure.
C. Maintains or restores body buffer system.
D. Maintains or restores level of electrolytes in the body.

Dialysis Management

Implementation

A. Take vital signs to observe for shock and hypovolemia.
    1. Hypotension is caused by:
        a. Fluid loss initially.
        b. Decreased blood volume, especially if hematocrit is low.
        c. Use of antihypertensive drugs between dialysis procedures.
    2. Plasma or volume expanders can be used to increase blood pressure; sometimes blood is used while the client is on dialysis.
B. Check serum electrolytes frequently (pre-, mid-, and post-dialysis).
C. Weigh client before and after dialysis to determine fluid loss.
D. Watch for leakage around shunt site.
E. Observe for dialysis disequilibrium syndrome.
    1. Cerebral dysfunction symptoms.
        a. Nausea and vomiting.
        b. Headache.
        c. Hypertension leading to agitation.
        d. Twitching, mental confusion, and convulsions.
    2. Syndrome is caused by rapid, efficient dialysis, resulting in shifts in water, pH, and osmolarity between fluid and blood.
    3. In acutely uremic clients, avoid this syndrome by dialyzing slowly, for short periods of time over two to three days.
    4. Use Dilantin to prevent this syndrome in new clients.
F. If client is heparinized while on dialysis machine.
    1. Take clotting time about one hour before client comes off the machine. If less than 30 minutes, do not give protamine (heparin antagonist).
    2. Keep clotting time at 30 to 90 minutes while on dialysis (normal six to ten minutes).
G. Shunt care.
    1. Temporary vascular access.
        a. Percutaneous cannulation of subclavian vein.
        b. Catheters are single or double lumen.
        c. Internal jugular and subclavian vein catheters in place 3–12 weeks, femoral catheter 2–3 days.
        d. Assess for signs of infection, thrombosis with pulmonary emboli, and hematoma.
        e. Maintain patency with intermittent heparin injection.
    2. Arterial-venous fistula.
        a. Anastomosis of an artery and vein creates a fistula.
        b. Arterial blood flow into the venous system results in marked dilation of veins which

are then easily punctured with a 14-gauge needle.

   c. Two venipunctures are made at the time of dialysis.
     (1) One for blood source.
     (2) One for return.
     (3) Arterial needle is inserted to within 2.5 to 3.8 cm (1 to 1-1/2 inches) from fistula, and venous needle is directed away from fistula.
   d. Observe for patency of graft site.
     (1) Check for bruit with stethoscope.
     (2) Observe for signs of infection.
     (3) Check pulses distal to shunt.
   e. No B/Ps or blood drawing on shunt arm.
  3. Bovine graft.
   a. Graft from neck of cow.
   b. Venipuncture same as for A-V fistula.

Guidelines for Dialysis Management

A. Limit fluid intake (400 cc over previous day's output); provide accurate intake and output.

B. Provide diet low in sodium, low protein, high carbohydrate, high fat, and low in potassium.
  1. Dietary protein should be of animal source.
  2. Chronic peritoneal dialysis requires greater protein intake (1 gm/kg).

C. Check vital signs for hypovolemia; check temperature for infection.

D. Auscultate lungs for signs of pulmonary edema.

E. Provide shunt care for clients on hemodialysis.

F. Observe level of consciousness—indicative of electrolyte imbalance or thrombus.

G. Administer antihypertensive drugs between dialysis if ordered.

H. Administer diuretics if ordered.

I. Administer blood if ordered (cellular portion only is needed because of low hematocrit).

J. Weigh daily to assess fluid accumulation.

K. Prevent use of soap (urea causes dryness and itching, and soap will just add to this problem).

J. Provide continued emotional support.
  1. Allow for expression of feelings about change in body image.
  2. Encourage expression of fears of death especially during dialysis.
  3. Encourage family cooperation.
  4. Support required change in life style.

SURGICAL INTERVENTIONS FOR MALE GENITAL DISORDERS

Prostatic Surgery

Characteristics

A. Benign prostatic hypertrophy (BPH).
  1. Enlargement of prostate gland from normal tissue; causes narrowing of urethra which may result in obstruction.
  2. Clinical manifestations.
   a. Recurring infection and urinary stasis.
   b. Nocturia, frequency, dysuria, urgency, dribbling, retention, and hematuria.

B. Cancer of the prostate.
  1. Type: androgen dependent adenocarcinoma.
  2. Clinical manifestations.
   a. Early symptoms similar to BPH.
   b. Urinary obstruction late in disease.
   c. Pain radiating from lumbosacral area down legs strongly indicative of cancer.

MEDICAL IMPLICATIONS

A. Medical regimen.
  1. Estrogen therapy or luteinizing hormone antagonist (Lupron) may be given to slow rate of growth and extension of tumor.
  2. Orchiectomy decreases androgen production.
  3. Radiation to local lesion to reduce tumor: external beam radiation or implant.

B. Surgical options.
  1. Transurethral resection (TUR) most common intervention—removal of prostatic tissue by instrumentation through urethra.
  2. Suprapubic prostatectomy—removal of prostate by abdominal incision with bladder incision.
  3. Retropubic prostatectomy—abdominal incision without opening bladder.
  4. Perineal prostatectomy—perineal incision between scrotum and anus.

Assessment

A. Observe for signs of hemorrhage and shock.

B. Assess for fluid and electrolyte balance.

C. Observe for complications.
  1. Epididymitis (most frequent).
  2. Gram negative sepsis.

Implementation

A. Maintain adequate bladder drainage via catheter.
1. Suprapubic catheter used following suprapubic prostatectomy.
2. Continuous bladder irrigation (or triple lumen catheter) is used following transurethral resection.
   a. One lumen is used for inflating bag (usually 30 cc bag), one for outflow of urine, and one for instillation of irrigating solution.
   b. Function:
      (1) Continuous antibacterial irrigation of solution to prevent infection.
      (2) Continuous saline irrigation to rid the bladder of tissue and clots following surgery.
   c. Nursing management
      (1) Run solution in rapidly if bright red drainage or clots are present; when drainage clears, decrease to about 40 drops/minute.
      (2) If clots cannot be rinsed out with irrigating solution, irrigate with syringe as ordered.
B. Provide fluids to prevent dehydration (2 to 3 liters).
C. Provide high-protein, high-vitamin diet.
D. Traction is applied to Foley catheter (if not connected to three-way drainage) to help in hemostasis.
1. Catheter is pulled on and taped to leg.
2. Traction not released without order (traction released after bright red drainage has diminished).
E. Instruct client in perineal exercises to regain urinary control.
1. Tense perineal muscles by pressing buttocks together; hold for as long as possible.
2. Repeat this process ten times every hour.
F. Ambulate early (after urine has returned to nearly normal color).
G. Administer urinary antiseptics or antibiotics to prevent infection.
H. Administer anticholinergics, if necessary, to relieve smooth muscle spasms.
I. Provide wound care for suprapubic and retropubic prostatectomies (similar to that for abdominal surgery).
J. Provide sitz bath and heat lamp treatments to promote healing.

CONDITIONS OF THE FEMALE REPRODUCTIVE TRACT

Menstruation

Definition: The sloughing off of the endometrium, which occurs at regular monthly intervals if conception fails to take place. The discharge consists of blood, mucus, and cells, and it usually lasts for four to five days.

Characteristics

A. Menarche—onset of menstruation—usually occurs between the ages of eleven and fourteen.
B. Abnormalities of menstruation.
1. Dysmenorrhea (painful menstruation).
   a. May be caused by psychological factors: tension, anxiety, preconditioning (menstruation is a "curse" or painful).
   b. Physical examination is usually done to rule out organic causes.
   c. May subside after childbearing.
   d. Treatment.
      (1) Oral contraceptives: produce anovulatory cycle.
      (2) Mild analgesics such as aspirin.
      (3) Client urged to carry on normal activities to occupy her mind.
2. Amenorrhea (absence of menstrual flow).
   a. Primary: over the age of seventeen and menstruation has not begun.
      (1) Complete physical necessary to rule out abnormalities.
      (2) Treatment aimed at correction of underlying condition.
   b. Secondary: occurs after menarche; does not include pregnancy and lactation.
      (1) Causes include psychological upsets or endocrine conditions.
      (2) Evaluation and treatment by physician is necessary.
3. Menorrhagia (excessive menstrual bleeding). May be due to endocrine disturbance, tumors, or inflammatory conditions of the uterus.
4. Metrorrhagia (bleeding between periods). Symptom of disease process, benign tumors, or cancer.

Assessment

A. Assess characteristics of the menstrual cycle.
B. Evaluate cycle pattern.
C. Evaluate discomforts associated with menstruation.
   1. Breast tenderness and feeling of fullness.
   2. Temperament and mood changes because of hormonal influence. Levels of estrogen and progesterone drop sharply.
   3. Discomfort in pelvic area, lower back, and legs.
   4. Retained fluids and weight gain.

Implementation

A. Educate client about the physiology of normal menstruation. Answer questions about the myths and cultural beliefs associated with menstruation.
B. Educate client about abnormal conditions associated with menstruation: absence of bleeding, bleeding between periods, etc.
C. Educate client about normal hygiene during menstruation.
   1. Importance of cleanliness.
   2. Use of perineal pads and tampons.
   3. Continuing normal activities.

Menopause

Definition: The cessation of menstruation caused by physiologic factors; ovulation no longer occurs. Menopause usually occurs between the ages of forty to fifty.

Characteristics

A. Ovaries lose the ability to respond to pituitary stimulation and normal ovarian function ceases.
   1. Gradual change due to alteration in hormone production.
      a. Failure to ovulate.
      b. Monthly flow becomes smaller, irregular, and gradually ceases.
   2. Menopause is accompanied by changes in reproductive organs: The vagina gradually becomes smaller; uterus, bladder, rectum, and supporting structures lose tone, leading to uterine prolapse, rectocele, and cystocele.
B. Atherosclerosis and osteoporosis are more likely to develop at this time.

Assessment

A. Clinical manifestations vary from mild to severe.
B. May be accompanied by psychological symptoms, i.e. feelings of loss, children grown, aging process occurring.
C. May be accompanied by hot flashes and nervous symptoms, such as headache, depression, insomnia, weakness and dizziness.

Implementation

A. Instruct client in use of estrogen therapy. Usually given on cyclic basis: one pill daily except for five days during the month when medication is not taken.
B. Suggest treatment for psychological problems if present.

Conditions of the Vulva

Vulvitis

Definition: An inflammation of the vulva, which usually occurs in conjunction with other conditions such as vaginal infections and venereal disease.

Assessment

A. Evaluate burning pain during urination.
B. Assess for itching.
C. Observe for red and inflamed genitalia.
D. Observe for discharge.
E. Evaluate for related conditions, psychological factors, endocrine disorders, and reactions to chemical substances that the client may be using.

Implementation

A. Give soothing compresses, colloidal baths.
B. Apply medicated creams.
C. Administer antihistamines for sedation.

Vaginal Conditions

Vaginal Infections

A. Vagina normally protected from infection by acidic environment.
B. Leukorrhea (whitish vaginal discharge) normal in small amounts at ovulation and prior to menstruation.
C. Trichomoniasis vaginalis (overgrowth of protozoan normally present in vaginal tract)—normal pH altered and overgrowth occurs.
D. Candida albicans—fungal infection caused by yeast, also called monilia.

1. 500,000 Americans get this infection—majority are women.
2. Widespread use of antibiotics increasing epidemic—these destroy protective organisms normally present.
3. Candida thrives in sugar-carbohydrate-rich environment.
4. Symptoms: itching, swelling, white, cheesy discharge from vagina or thrush in mouth; may have systemic symptoms of fatigue, allergies, depression, flatus.
5. Nystatin drug of choice systemically; vaginal inserts and ointment.

Conditions of Ovaries and Pelvic Cavity

Endometriosis

Definition: The abnormal growth of endometrial tissue outside the uterine cavity. A common cause of infertility.

Characteristics

A. Embryonic tissue that remains dormant until ovarian stimulation after menarche.
B. Endometrial tissue transported from the uterine cavity through the fallopian tubes during menstruation.
C. Endometrial tissue transported by lymphatic tissue during menstruation.
D. Accidental transfer of endometrial tissue to pelvic cavity during surgery.

Assessment

A. Evaluate lower abdominal and pelvic pain during menstruation. Due to distention of involved tissue and surrounding area by blood; symptoms are acute during menstruation.
B. Assess for dysmenorrhea: usually steady and severe.
C. Assess for abnormal uterine bleeding.
D. Ask about pain during intercourse.
E. Assess for back and rectal pain.

Implementation

A. Explain to client that pregnancy may delay growth of lesions. Symptoms usually recur after pregnancy.
B. Instruct that hormone therapy with oral contraceptives usually eliminates menstrual pain and controls endometrial growth.
C. Prepare client for surgical intervention; total hysterectomy may be indicated.

Pelvic Inflammatory Disease (PID)

Definition: An inflammatory condition of the pelvic cavity that may involve ovaries, fallopian tubes, vascular system, or pelvic peritoneum.

Assessment

A. Assess for cause of disease.
   1. Staphylococcus or streptococcus.
   2. Venereal disease.
   3. Tubercle bacilli.
B. Assess for elevated temperature.
C. Evaluate for nausea and vomiting.
D. Assess for abdominal and low back pain.
E. Observe for purulent, foul-smelling vaginal discharge.
F. Evaluate for leukocytosis.

Implementation

A. Instruct client on controlling spread of infection.
B. Place in semi-Fowler's position: dependent drainage.
C. Apply heat to abdomen for comfort.
D. Administer warm douches to improve circulation.
E. Take and record vital signs every four hours.
F. Administer antibiotics as ordered.
G. Note nature and amount of vaginal discharge.
H. Instruct to avoid use of tampons and urinary catheterization to prevent spread of infection.
I. Instruct on good nutrition and fluid intake.

Toxic Shock Syndrome

Definition: An uncommon but serious illness reported by menstruating women, usually under age of 30, who use tampons. TSS may also occur in women using sanitary napkins.

Assessment

A. Assess for two primary symptoms: sudden high fever (may be as high as 103–105°F) and rash that looks like a sunburn.
B. Other symptoms commonly observed: vomiting and diarrhea; dizziness, fainting or near fainting when standing up, headache and sore throat.

Implementation

A. When toxic shock suspected, client is hospitalized— the development of severe circulatory compromise cannot be predicted.

B. Blood, urine and vaginal cultures determine sites of focal Staphylococcus aureus infection; a B-lactamase resistant antibiotic with bactericidal activity is administered; when there is no focal infection site, betadine vaginal douches are given 3 times a day for 2–3 days.

C. Monitor blood pressure and administer IV colloids and vasopressor agents as ordered.

D. Administer sodium bicarbonate for acidosis.

Conditions of the Uterus

Assessment

A. Assess for displacements.
 1. Retroversion and retroflexion: backward displacement of the uterus.
 2. May cause difficulty in becoming pregnant.

B. Assess for prolapse.
 1. Weakening of uterine supports causes the uterus to slip down into the vaginal canal; the uterus may even appear outside the vaginal orifice.
 2. Prolapse may cause urinary incontinence or retention.

Implementation

A. Instruct in good perineal hygiene if pessary is used.

B. Follow nursing care for hysterectomy clients.

Fibroid Tumors

A. Fibroid tumors are benign.

B. Occur in 20 to 30 percent of all women between the ages of twenty-five to forty.

C. Symptoms include menorrhagia, back pain, urinary difficulty, and constipation.

D. Fibroid tumors may cause sterility.

E. Treatment.
 1. Removal of tumors, if they are small.
 2. Hysterectomy if tumors are large.

SURGICAL INTERVENTIONS

Tumors of the Breast

Assessment

A. Assess for lump in upper outer quadrant of breast, usually nontender, but may be tender.

B. Observe for dimpling of breast tissue surrounding nipple or bleeding from nipple.

C. Check for presence of asymmetry with affected breast being higher.

D. Evaluate types of surgery to be done.
 1. Lumpectomy—removal of tumor and small amount of normal tissue.
 2. Simple mastectomy—removal of breast. No lymph nodes removed.
 3. Radical mastectomy—removal of breast and muscle layer down to chest wall. Lymph nodes in axillary region also removed.

Implementation

A. Begin emotional support preoperatively and continue in postoperative period.
 1. Client may have altered body image.
 2. Client may be extremely depressed.

B. Place in semi-Fowler's position with affected arm elevated to prevent edema.

C. Turn, cough, and deep breathe to prevent respiratory complications.

D. Turn only to back and unaffected side.

E. Hemovac may be placed postoperatively.

F. Prevent complications of contractures and lymphedema by encouraging range-of-motion exercises early in postoperative period.

G. Provide IV fluids. Should not be administered in affected arm.

H. Monitor vital signs for prevention of complications such as infection and hemorrhage. Take blood pressure on unaffected arm only.

I. Reinforce pressure dressings. Observe for signs of restriction from dressing.
 1. Impaired sensation.
 2. Color changes of skin.

J. If skin grafts were applied, provide nursing care as for any other graft.

K. Encourage visit from Reach for Recovery Group.

L. Instruct to perform self-breast exam monthly at a regular time, seven days after start of menstruation.

Tumors of the Reproductive System

Definition: Tumors or neoplasms are composed of new and actively growing tissue. They are classified in many ways, the most common according to origin and whether they are malignant or benign. The second highest cause of death in the female is malignant tumors of the reproductive system.

Characteristics

A. Cancer of the cervix.
 1. Most common type of cancer in the reproductive system.

2. Usually appears in females between the ages of thirty to fifty.
3. Signs and symptoms include bleeding between periods—may be noted especially after intercourse or douching; leukorrhea.
4. May become invasive and include tissue outside the cervix, fundus of the uterus, and the lymph glands.
5. Treatment—depends upon extent of the disease.
    a. Hysterectomy.
    b. Radiation.
    c. Radical pelvic surgery in advanced cases.
B. Cancer of the endometrium, fundus, or corpus of uterus.
    1. Usually not diagnosed until symptoms appear—Pap smear inadequate for diagnosis.
    2. Progresses slowly—metastasis occurs late.
    3. Treatment.
        a. Early—hysterectomy.
        b. Late—radium and x-ray therapy.
C. Cancer of the vulva.
    1. Long-standing pruritus (itching) and local discomfort.
    2. Foul-smelling and slightly bloody discharge.
    3. Early lesions. May appear as chronic vulval dermatitis.
    4. Surgical interventions.
        a. Vulvectomy is the preferred treatment.
        b. Radiation therapy is used in the inoperable lesions.

Implementation

A. Provide immediate postoperative care.
    1. Observe dressings for signs of hemorrhage.
    2. Check vital signs until stable.
    3. Assist client to turn, cough, and deep breathe every two hours.
    4. Give pain medications as ordered.
    5. Observe drainage and empty Hemovac as necessary.
    6. Record intake and output.
    7. Maintain IV.
    8. Maintain catheter care to reduce incidence of infection.
    9. Position for comfort.
B. Provide convalescent care.
    1. Encourage verbalization regarding change in body image.

2. Irrigate wound as ordered, using solution as prescribed (usual solution is either sterile saline or hydrogen peroxide), which cleans area and improves circulation.
3. Prevent wound infection.
C. Instruct client on discharge teaching.
    1. Signs of infection—foul-smelling discharge, elevated temperature, swelling.
    2. Nutritious diet and planned rest periods.
    3. Wound irrigation and dressing change.
    4. Importance of follow-up care by physician.

Hysterectomy

Characteristics

A. Total hysterectomy—removal of the entire uterus; fallopian tubes and ovaries remain.
B. Panhysterectomy—involves removal of the entire uterus, ovaries, and fallopian tubes.
C. Radical hysterectomy—wide removal of vaginal, cervical, uterosacral and other tissue along with the uterus.

Assessment

A. Observe for hemorrhage—vaginal and at the incision site.
B. Observe for signs of infection—elevated temperature, foul-smelling vaginal discharge, and pelvic congestion.
C. Assess for changes in body image—feelings of loss.
D. Evaluate for pneumonia.
E. Auscultate for paralytic ileus.
F. Observe for thrombophlebitis.

Implementation

A. Immediate postoperative care.
    1. Observe incision site for bleeding and reinforce dressings as needed.
    2. Monitor vital signs frequently.
    3. If client has nasogastric tube to suction, keep n.p.o. and observe amount, color, and consistency of drainage.
    4. Administer pain medications as ordered.
    5. Administer IV fluids as ordered.
    6. Provide for hygienic care.
    7. Give catheter care to prevent infection—observe amount and color of drainage.
    8. Assist client to cough, turn, and deep breathe.
    9. Promote methods to decrease pelvic congestion.

(1) Apply antiembolic stockings.

(2) Avoid high-Fowler's position.

(3) Promote range of motion.

B. Provide convalescent care.

1. Increase activity as tolerated.

2. Ambulate with assistance.

3. Auscultate chest for breath sounds.

4. Auscultate abdomen for bowel signs.

5. Allow client to verbalize feelings of loss of feminity, childbearing ability, disfigurement, fear of cancer.

6. Provide for emotional support.

7. Increase diet as tolerated.

8. Administer laxatives and stool softeners as ordered and rectal tubes or Harris flush for flatus.

C. Prepare client for discharge.

1. Encourage expression of feelings with significant other.

2. Explain that menstruation will no longer occur.

3. Explain that estrogen therapy may be ordered by the physician if the ovaries were removed to control menopausal symptoms.

4. Instruct the client to observe for signs of complications.

a. Elevation of temperature.

b. Foul-smelling vaginal discharge.

c. Redness, swelling, or drainage from the incision site.

d. Abdominal cramping.

5. Explain the importance of follow-up visits with the physician.

6. Explain the importance of taking medications as ordered.

7. Douching and coitus are usually avoided for six weeks.

Anterior and Posterior Colporrhaphy

Characteristics

A. Repair of cystocele—downward displacement of the bladder towards the vaginal entrance, caused by tissue weakness, injuries in childbirth, and atrophy associated with aging.

B. Repair of rectocele—anterior sagging of rectum and posterior vaginal wall caused by injuries to the muscles and tissue of the pelvic floor during childbirth.

Assessment

A. Observe for foul-smelling discharge from vaginal area or operative site.

B. Observe for urinary retention and catheterize as necessary.

Implementation

A. Provide postoperative care to decrease discomfort.

B. Provide care of perineal sutures—two methods:

1. Sutures left alone until healing begins, thereafter daily vaginal irrigations with sterile saline.

2. Sterile saline douches twice daily, beginning with the first postoperative day.

C. Preparation of client for discharge. Client should be instructed in perineal hygiene (no douching or coitus until advised by physician), and to watch for signs of infection.

Pelvic Exenteration

Definition: A surgical procedure that is performed when cancer is widespread and cannot be controlled by other means.

Characteristics

A. Anterior pelvic exenteration—the removal of the reproductive organs, pelvic lymph nodes, adnexa, pelvic peritoneum, bladder, and lower ureter. Ureters are implanted in the small intestines or the colon.

B. Posterior pelvic exenteration—removal of the reproductive organs, vagina, adnexa, colon, and rectum. Pelvic lymph nodes may be removed.

C. Total pelvic exenteration—removal of the reproductive organs, pelvic floor, pelvic lymph nodes, perineum, bladder, rectum, and distal portion of sigmoid colon. A substitute bladder is made from a segment of the ileum. Client will have a permanent colostomy.

Implementation

A. Provide general postoperative procedures.

B. Observe surgical site for drainage and reinforce dressings as necessary; client may have drainage tubes connected to suction from incision area.

C. Apply antiembolic stockings.

D. Encourage client to express feelings.

MUSCULOSKELETAL SYSTEM

The musculoskeletal system provides the support and protective mechanism of the body. Bones, joints, and skeletal muscles comprise the system.

ANATOMY AND PHYSIOLOGY

Bone Structure

A. Types of bones.
  1. Long: legs, arms.
  2. Short: wrists, ankles.
  3. Flat: skull, shoulder blades.
  4. Irregular: vertebrae, face.
B. Bone surfaces.
  1. Grooves and holes provide passage for nerves and blood vessels.
  2. Protrusions at the ends of the bone form parts of the joints.
  3. Shallow depressions and ridges are attachment points for fibrous tissue.
C. Bone function.
  1. Support and protect structures of the body skeleton.
  2. Provide attachments for muscles that move the skeleton.
  3. Central cavity of some bones contain hematopoietic tissue (connective tissue), which forms blood cells.
  4. Assist in regulation of calcium and phosphate concentrations.

Long Bones

A. Diaphysis: long, central shaft.
B. Epiphysis: the end of a long bone.
  1. Covered by hyaline cartilage.
  2. Auricular surface: the part of the epiphysis that contacts other bones.

C. Periosteum: adhering sheath of connective tissue covering bone.
D. Internal structures.
  1. Central medullary cavity: contains yellow marrow composed of fat.
  2. Surface layer: an ivory-like, dense, compact bone.
  3. Cancellous bone: a spongy layer below the surface layer. It contains small cavities that merge with large central cavity.
  4. Red marrow: consists of hemopoietic tissue, macrophages, and fat cells. Fills the spaces between spongy bone.

Joints

A. Classification.
  1. Synarthrosis: fibrous or fixed joints.
  2. Amphiarthrosis: cartilaginous or slightly movable joint.
  3. Diarthrosis: synovial or freely movable joint.
    a. Ball and socket.
    b. Condyloid.
B. Function.
  1. Articulation is the meeting place of two or more joints.
  2. Assist in type and range of movement between bones.
C. Synovial fluid.
  1. Function
    a. Lubricate the cartilage.
    b. Cushion shocks.
    c. Provide a nutrient source.
  2. Structure
    a. Fluid formed by the synovial membrane.
    b. Synovial membrane lines the joint capsule, which contains the fluid.

Fracture Healing

A. Occurs over several weeks.
B. New bone tissue occurs in region of break.
C. Repair is initiated by migration of blood vessels and connective tissue from periosteum in break area.
D. Dense fibrous tissue fills in the break and forms a callus (temporary union).
E. Types of cells.
  1. Osteoblast: near the broken area.

2. Chondroblast: further away from broken area.
F. Cells deposit cartilage between broken surfaces.
G. Cartilage is slowly replaced by mineralized bone tissue, which completes repair.

System Assessment

A. Observe for signs of a fracture.
  1. Cardinal signs of a fracture.
    a. Pain or tenderness over involved area.
    b. Loss of function of the extremity.
    c. Deformity.
      (1) Overriding.
      (2) Angulation: limb is in an unnatural position.
  2. Crepitation: sound of grating bone fragments.
  3. Ecchymosis or erythema.
  4. Edema.
  5. Muscle spasm.
B. Assess for specific types of fracture.
  1. Greenstick.
    a. A crack; the bending of a bone with incomplete fracture. Only affects one side of the periosteum.
    b. Common in skull fractures or in young children when bones are pliable.
  2. Comminuted.
    a. Bone completely broken in a transverse, spiral, or oblique direction (indicates the direction of the fracture in relation to the long axis of the fracture bone).
    b. Bone broken into several fragments.
  3. Open, or compound.
    a. Bone is exposed to the air through a break in the skin.
    b. Can be associated with soft tissue injury as well.
    c. Infection is common complication due to exposure to bacterial invasion.
  4. Closed, or simple.
    a. Skin remains intact.
    b. Chances are greatly decreased for infection.
  5. Compression.
    a. Frequently seen with vertebral fractures.
    b. Fractured bone has been compressed by other bones.
  6. Complete: bone is broken with a disruption of both sides of the periosteum.
  7. Impacted: one part of fractured bone is driven into another.
  8. Depressed fracture.
    a. Usually seen in skull or facial fractures.
    b. Bone or fragments of bone are driven inward.
  9. Pathological: break caused by disease process.
C. Identify whether break is intracapsular: bone broken inside the joint or extracapsular: fracture outside the joint.
D. Observe all extremities for edema, pain and obvious deformities.
E. Assess for possible complications associated with a cast.
F. Evaluate client for complications associated with joint disorders.
G. Observe for presence of phantom limb pain.
H. Assess stump dressings for bleeding and/or signs of infection.
I. Observe position in bed of clients with hip fractures to identify potential complications associated with hip flexion.
J. Assess for signs of shock and hemorrhage following surgery.
K. Evaluate need for client instruction on exercises, positioning, and crutch-walking.
L. Evaluate client's need for rehabilitation program.
M. Observe circulation, movement, and sensation (CMS) for all orthopedic clients.

System Planning and Analysis

A. Signs of infection or bleeding are recognized early and interventions started immediately.
B. Allocations in body alignment are identified and changes in body position, traction, or new cast are instituted.
C. Positioning and constant assessment of affected areas prevent circulatory, sensation, or movement impairment.
D. Plan for increasing muscle strength is developed preoperatively and carried out postoperatively.

System Implementation

A. Maintain alignment through proper care of traction.
  1. Ensure that weights hang freely and do not touch the floor.

2. Ensure that pulleys are not obstructed.
3. Check that ropes in the pulley move freely.
4. Secure knot in rope to prevent slipping.
5. Maintain proper body alignment (up in bed, in direct line with traction) and proper counter-traction.
6. Do not remove or lift weights without specific order. (Exceptions are pelvic and cervical traction that clients can remove at intervals.)
7. Cover sharp edges on traction apparatus with hollowed out rubber balls to prevent injury to personnel.

Cast Care

A. After application of cast, allow 24 to 48 hours for drying.
   1. Cast will change from dull to shiny substance when dry.
   2. Heat can be applied to assist in drying process.
B. Do not handle cast during process as indentation from fingermarks can cause skin breakdown under cast.
C. Keep extremity elevated to prevent edema.
D. Provide for smooth edges surrounding cast.
   1. Smooth edges prevent crumbling and breaking down of edges.
   2. Stockinet can be pulled over edge and fastened down with adhesive tape to outside of cast.
E. Observe casted extremity for signs of circulatory impairment. Cast may have to be cut if edematous condition continues.
F. Always observe for signs and symptoms of complications: pain, swelling, discoloration, tingling or numbness, diminished or absent pulse, paralysis, pain, cool to touch.
G. If there is an open, draining area on affected extremity, a window (cut out portion of cast) can be utilized for observation and/or irrigation of wound.
H. Keep cast dry.
   1. Breaks down when water comes in contact with plaster.
   2. Use plastic bags or plastic coated bed chux during the bath or when using bedpan, to protect cast material.
I. Utilize isometric exercises to prevent muscle atrophy and to strengthen the muscle. Isometrics prevent joint from being immobilized.
J. Position client with pillows to prevent strain on unaffected areas.
K. Turn every two hours to prevent complications. Encourage to lie on abdomen fours hours a day.

Complications of Immobilization

A. Prevent respiratory complications.
   1. Have client cough and deep breathe every two hours.
   2. Turn every two hours if not contraindicated.
   3. Provide suction if needed.
B. Prevent thrombus and emboli formation.
   1. Apply antiembolic stockings.
   2. Initiate isometric and isotonic exercises.
   3. Start anticoagulation therapy, if indicated.
   4. Turn every two hours.
   5. Observe for signs and symptoms of pulmonary and/or fat emboli.
C. Prevent contractures.
   1. Start range-of-motion exercises to affected joints q.i.d., all joints b.i.d.
   2. Provide foot board and/or foot cradle.
   3. Position and turn every two hours.
D. Prevent skin breakdown.
   1. Massage with lotion once a day to prevent drying.
   2. Use alcohol for back care to toughen skin.
   3. Massage elbows, coccyx, heels b.i.d.
   4. Turn every two hours.
   5. Alternate pressure mattress, sheepskin.
   6. Use stryker boots or heel protectors.
   7. Use elbow guards.
E. Prevent urinary retention and calculi.
   1. Encourage fluids.
   2. Monitor intake and output.
   3. Administer urinary antiseptic (Mandelamine, etc.).
   4. Offer bedpan every four hours.
F. Prevent constipation.
   1. Encourage fluids.
   2. Provide high fiber diet.
   3. Administer laxative or enema as ordered.
   4. Offer bedpan at same time each day—encourage to establish good bowel habits.
G. Provide pychological support.
   1. Allow client to ventilate feelings of dependence.
   2. Encourage independence when possible (bathing, self-feeding, etc.).
   3. Encourage visitors for short time periods.
   4. Provide diversionary activities (television, newspapers, etc.).

System Evaluation

A. Client does not experience complications of immobility.
B. Fracture heals with bone in alignment.
C. Rehabilitation program is individualized and completed by client.
D. Circulation, motion, and sensation are not impaired for clients in traction, cast, or surgical intervention.

JOINT DISEASES

Rheumatoid Arthritis

Definition: Chronic, systemic, autoimmune, inflammatory disease affecting the joints. Usual onset is from 20 to 40 years of age.

Assessment

A. Evaluate for bilateral joint involvement (erythema, warm, tender, painful).
B. Assess for insidious onset of malaise, weight loss, paresthesia, stiffness.
C. Assess pain and stiffness early in morning (subsides with moderate activity).
D. Observe for subcutaneous nodules.
E. Assess low-grade temperature.
F. Observe for anemia with fatigue and weakness.

Implementation

A. Instruct client on medications and side effects. Chemotherapy reduces inflammation and relieves pain.
  1. Salicylates.
    a. ASA most common.
    b. Side effects include tinnitus, GI upset, prolonged bleeding time.
  2. Nonsteroidal, anti-inflammatory drugs (NSAIDS).
    a. Phenylbutazone, indomethacin, Motrin, Naprosyn.
    b. Side effects include GI disturbances, CNS manifestations, skin rashes.
  3. Antimalarials.
    a. Remission-inducing agents.
    b. May cause ocular toxicity—opthalmic exam twice yearly indicated.
  4. Gold salts (chrysotherapy).
    a. Three to four months before effective.
    b. Toxicity can be severe.
  5. Antimetabolics—for clients who don't respond to NSAIDS.
    a. Methotrexate.
    b. Azathioprine (Imuran).
  6. Corticosteroids: adjunct therapy only.
    a. Used during exacerbations or severe involvement.
    b. Low dose to prevent toxicity.
B. Instruct client how to preserve joint function.
C. Provide rest periods throughout day.
D. Instruct client in diet control.
E. Provide psychological support for altered body image and living with chronic disease.
F. Prevent flexion contractures and promote exercise.
  1. Initiate ROM exercises.
  2. Avoid weight bearing for inflamed joints.
  3. Give warm baths and exercises.
G. Prepare for surgery if severe joint involvement.
  1. Synovectomy.
  2. Joint replacement.

Osteoarthritis

Definition: Hypertrophic degeneration of joints that is part of the normal aging process. The cartilage that covers the ends of the bones disintegrates.

Characteristics

A. Strikes the joints that receive the most stress, e.g., knees, toes, lower spine. Distal finger joint involvement is usually seen in women.
B. Pain and stiffness in the joints.

Implementation

A. Instruct client on well-balanced diet.
B. Prevent permanent disability.
  1. Plan exercise to prevent joint fixation.
  2. Provide exercise periods to increase muscle tone.
  3. Control exercise periods to prevent fatigue.
C. Maintain proper positioning.
  1. Align and frequently change position to prevent complications.
  2. Encourage and support client as frequent movements cause pain.
D. Apply heat for relief of pain.
  1. Dry heat with a heat lamp to relieve stiffness.
  2. Moist heat with hot tubs, hot towels, or paraffin baths for the hands.
E. Provide adequate rest—10 to 12 hours a day.

F. Administer medications as ordered and teach about side effects.
  1. Salicylates most common for relief of pain.
  2. Side effects of ASA include tinnitus, nausea, and prolonged bleeding time.
  3. Anti-inflammatory drugs (cortisone) reduce the effect of inflammation thus decreasing pain, swelling and stiffness.
G. Provide psychological support and/or psychotherapy.

Gout

Definition: A disease caused by a defect in purine metabolism marked by urate deposits which cause painful arthritic joints. Affects men over fifty years.

Assessment

A. Assess joints (especially big toe) for pain, inflammation, tenderness, presence of urate deposits, and warm to touch.
B. Assess for low grade temperature.
C. Evaluate serum uric acid and elevated urinary uric acid.

Implementation

A. Maintain bedrest during acute attack.
B. Immobilize inflamed, painful joints.
C. Administer ordered medications:
  1. Analgesics for pain.
  2. Antiinflammatory agents.
    a. Colchicine po or IV q l hr × 8 hr until pain subsides or nausea, vomiting, cramping or diarrhea occurs.
    b. Phenylbutazone or indomethacin may be used.
    c. Corticosteroids.
  3. Allopurinol to decrease serum uric acid levels.
  4. Uricosuric agents to promote uric acid excretion and inhibit uric acid accumulation (Probenecil, Sulfin pyrazone).
D. Instruct client on low purine diet and avoidance of alcohol. If client is obese, place on weight reduction diet.
E. Force fluids to at least 2000 cc to prevent stone formation.
F. Maintain urine pH above 6 with alkalinizing agent.

BONE ALTERATIONS

Osteoporosis

Definition: Decrease in the amount of bone capable of maintaining structural integrity of the skeleton. Etiology is unknown.

Assessment

A. Assess for backache with pain radiating around trunk.
B. Evaluate for skeletal deformities.
C. Assess for pathologic fractures.
D. Evaluate lab findings.
  1. Serum calcium, phosphorus and alkaline phosphatase are usually normal.
  2. Parathyroid hormone may be elevated.

Implementation

A. Provide pain control.
B. Prevent fractures.
  1. Instruct in safety factors—watch steps, avoid use of scatter rugs.
  2. Keep side rails up to prevent falls.
  3. Move gently when turning and positioning.
  4. Assist with ambulation if unsteady on feet.
C. Administer medications.
  1. Estrogen—decreases rate of bone resorption.
  2. Calcium and vitamin D—support bone metabolism.
D. Instruct in regular exercise program.
  1. Range-of-motion exercises.
  2. Ambulation several times per day.
E. Instruct in good use of body mechanics.
F. Provide diet high in protein, calcium, vitamin D; avoid excesses of alcohol and coffee.

Fractures

Definition: A break in the continuity of bone caused by trauma, twisting, or as a result of bone decalcification.

Assessment

A. Assess for type of fracture.
B. Evaluate cause of fracture.
  1. Fatigue—muscles are less supportive to bone and therefore cannot absorb the force being exerted.
  2. Bone neoplasms—cellular proliferations of

malignant cells replace normal tissue causing a weakened bone.

3. Metabolic disorders—poor mineral absorption and hormonal changes decrease bone calcification which results in a weakened bone.

4. Bedrest or disuse—atropic muscles and osteoporosis cause decreased stress resistance.

C. Evaluate type of treatment used for fracture.

1. Traction.

2. Reduction (restoring bone to proper alignment).

   a. Closed reduction.

      (1) Manual manipulation.

      (2) Usually done under anesthesia to reduce pain and relax muscles, thereby preventing complications.

      (3) Cast is usually applied following closed reduction.

   b. Open reduction.

      (1) Surgical intervention.

      (2) Usually treated with internal fixation devices (screws, plates, wires, etc.).

      (3) Following surgery, client can be placed in traction; however, client is usually placed in cast.

3. Cast.

D. Assess for complications of immobility.

Implementation

A. Provide emergency care of fractures.

1. Immobilize affected extremity to prevent further damage to soft tissue or nerve.

2. If compound fracture is evident, do not attempt to reduce it.

   a. Apply splint.

   b. Cover open wound with sterile dressing.

3. Splinting.

   a. External support is applied around a fracture to immobilize the broken ends.

   b. Materials used: wood, plastic (air splints), magazines.

4. Function of splinting.

   a. Prevent additional trauma.

   b. Reduce pain.

   c. Decrease muscle spasm.

   d. Limit movement.

   e. Prevent complications, such as fat emboli if long bone fracture.

B. Provide specific care for fracture treatment.

1. Traction.

2. Cast.

3. Surgical intervention.

Traction

Definition: Force applied in two directions to reduce and/or immobilize a fracture, to provide proper bone alignment and regain normal length, or to reduce muscle spasm.

Assessment

A. Evaluate skeletal traction used.

1. Mechanical applied to bone, using pins (Steinmann), wires (Kirschner), or tongs (Crutchfield).

2. Most often used in fractures of femur, tibia, humerus.

3. Balanced suspension traction.

   a. Thomas's splint with Pearson attachment is used in conjunction with skin or skeletal traction (used particularly with skeletal traction for fractured femur).

   b. Balanced suspension traction is produced by a counterforce other than the client.

B. Evaluate if skin traction is used.

1. Traction applied by use of elastic bandages, moleskin strips, or adhesive.

2. Used most often in alignment or lengthening (for congenital hip displacement, etc.) or to relieve muscle spasms in preop hip clients.

3. Most common types.

   a. Russell traction.

   b. Buck's extension.

   c. Cervical traction (used for whiplashes and cervical spasm).

      (1) Pull is exerted on one plane.

      (2) Used for temporary immobilization.

   d. Pelvic traction (used for low back pain).

C. Assess for complications of immobility.

D. Assess for signs and symptoms of infection with skeletal traction.

E. Assess condition of skin for possible breakdown.

Implementation

A. Provide nursing interventions for clients in traction.

1. Maintain correct alignment.

2. Maintain counterbalance or correct pull.

a. Pull is exerted against traction in opposite direction (balanced suspension).

b. Pull is exerted against a fixed point.

c. Bed is elevated under area involved to provide the countertraction.

3. Provide firm mattress or bedboards.

4. Monitor for complications.
   a. Osteomyelitis (infections of bone).
   b. Bone deformities.
   c. Circulatory impairment.
   d. Skin breakdown.

5. Provide range-of-motion exercises for unaffected extremities.

6. Prevent footdrop.
   a. Provide footplate.
   b. Encourage dorsiflexion exercises.

7. Provide overhead trapeze to allow client to assist in activities (turning, moving up in bed, using bedpan, etc.).

8. Prevent postoperative complications.

B. Provide nursing interventions for clients in all types of traction.

Balanced Skeletal Traction

A. Maintain proper alignment.

B. Protect skin from excoriation.
   1. Check around top of Thomas splint.
   2. Pad with cotton wadding or ABDs.

C. Prevent pressure points around the top of Thomas splint by keeping client pulled up in bed.

D. Provide pin site care.
   1. Observe pin or tong insertion site for migration or drainage, odors, erythema, edema (usually indication of inflammatory process or infection).
   2. Watch for skin breakdown if bandage is used to apply traction.
   3. Cover ends of pins or wires with rubber stoppers or cork to prevent puncture of nursing personnel or client.
   4. Cleanse area surrounding insertion site of pin or tongs with hydrogen peroxide or Betadine. Some physicians order antibiotic ointments to be applied to area or order no pin site care.

E. Maintain at least 20-degree angle from thigh to the bed.

F. Provide footplate to prevent footdrop.

G. Keep heels clear of Pearson attachment to prevent skin breakdown and pressure sores.

H. Position client frequently from side to side (as ordered). Place table on unaffected side.

I. Unless contraindicated, elevate head of bed for comfort and to facilitate adequate respiratory functions.

Skin Traction

A. Buck's extension.
   1. Apply foam boot appliance with velcro fastener.
   2. Attach a foot block with a spreader and rope which goes into a pulley.
   3. Attach weight to pulley and hang freely over edge of bed (not more than eight to ten pounds of weight can be applied).
   4. Observe and readjust bandages for tightness and smoothness (can cause constriction that leads to edema or even nerve damage).

B. Cervical traction.
   1. Use head harness (or halter).
      a. Pad chin.
      b. Protect ears from friction rub.
   2. Elevate head of bed and attach weights to pulley system over head of bed.
   3. Observe for skin breakdown.
      a. Powder areas encased in the halter.
      b. Place back of head on padding.

C. Pelvic traction.
   1. Apply girdle snugly over client's pelvis and iliac crest; attach to weights.
   2. Observe for pressure points over iliac crest.
   3. Keep client in good alignment.
   4. May raise foot of bed slightly (30 cm) to prevent client from slipping down in bed.

Fractured Ribs

Assessment

A. Assess lung sounds for pneumothorax or hemothorax.

B. Examine chest excursion for asymmetry.

C. Assess for shock.
   1. Monitor vital signs every hour until stable.
   2. Check color and warmth every two hours.
   3. Check LOC.
   4. Observe for restlessness.

D. Evaluate pain and need for analgesic.

E. Evaluate need for chest tubes.

Implementation

A. Provide nursing interventions for shock.
  1. Administer oxygen as indicated.
  2. Administer IV if signs of shock present.
  3. Keep lightly covered.
  4. Have chest tube insertion tray available.
B. Relieve pain from muscle spasms and fractures.
  1. Give pain medication one-half hour before any movement.
  2. Change position every two hours.
  3. Use pillows for support.
  4. Place client in semi-Fowler's position.
C. Prevent complications of immobility.
  1. Cough and deep breathe every two hours to prevent hypostatic pneumonia.
  2. Turn to unaffected side and back every two hours.
  3. Maintain skin care to prevent decubiti and circulatory impairment.
    a. Back care.
    b. Heel, elbow, coccyx massage.
  4. Institute leg exercises to prevent circulatory impairment.
  5. Prevent constipation and flatus.
    a. Insert rectal tube (no more than 20 minutes at a time).
    b. Provide stool softener.
    c. Maintain diet high in bulk.
    d. Force fluids.

Hip Conditions

Assessment

A. Evaluate types of fracture.
  1. Intracapsular (neck): bone broken inside the joint.
    a. Treated by internal fixation—replacement of femoral head with Austin Moore prosthesis.
    b. Occasionally, primary total hip replacement.
    c. Usually placed in skin traction first for immobilization and relief of muscle spasm.
    d. Client can be out of bed without weight-bearing in one to two days postoperatively (depending on other physical problems).
  2. Extracapsular: trochanteric fracture outside the joint.
    a. Fracture of greater trochanter.
      (1) Can be treated by balanced suspension traction if little displacement of bone. Full weight-bearing usually in six to eight weeks, when healing takes place.
      (2) Surgical intervention is necessary if large displacement or extensive soft tissue damage; usually internal fixation with wire.
    b. Intertrochanteric fracture.
      (1) Extends from medial region of the junction of the neck and lesser trochanter toward the summit of the greater trochanter.
      (2) Treated initially by balanced suspension traction.
      (3) Surgically treated early due to debilitated physical condition of most of these clients (usually seventy years and older with other system diseases like diabetes, hypertension, etc.).
      (4) Internal fixation used with nail-plate, screws, and wire.
    c. Not allowed to flex hip to the side, on the side of the bed, or in a low chair. When hip is flexed displacement can occur.
B. Assess for complications of immobility.

Implementation

FOR CLIENTS OTHER THAN HIP PROSTHESIS

A. Hemovac will usually be in place to drain off excessive blood and fluid accumulation.
  1. Compute intake and output.
  2. Keep Hemovac compressed to facilitate drainage.
B. Have client perform bed exercises at least four times a day.
  1. Flex and extend foot, tense muscles, and straighten knee.
  2. Tighten buttocks, straighten knee, and push leg down in bed.
  3. Tighten stomach muscles by raising neck and shoulders.
  4. Stretch arms to head of bed and deep breathe.
C. Change positions by raising head of bed.
  1. Gatch knees slightly to relieve strain on hips and back.
  2. Turn to unaffected side.
  3. Pivot into chair within one to two days post-

operatively.

4. Have client avoid full weight-bearing until fracture has healed.

D. Perform routine postoperative nursing interventions (respiratory care, etc.).

E. Observe for adequate bowel and bladder function.

F. Observe for complications (pulmonary embolism, infection, hemorrhage).

HIP PROSTHESIS

A. Replacement of head of femur by Austin Moore prosthesis.

B. Keep affected leg abducted and externally rotated with abductor splints, pillows, or sandbags.

C. Make sure hip flexion angle does not exceed 60 to 80 degrees.

D. Forbid client to flex hip while getting out of bed; forbid client sitting in low chair.

1. Use high stools.

2. Use wheelchairs with adjustable backs.

3. Use commode extenders.

E. Elevate head of bed 30 to 40 degrees for meals only.

F. Turn client to unaffected side with pillow support between legs.

G. Ambulate in two to four days with partial weight-bearing.

TOTAL HIP REPLACEMENT

A. Replacement of both the acetabulum and the head of the femur with metal or plastic implants.

B. Used in degenerative diseases or when fracture of head of femur has occurred with nonunion.

C. Keep operative leg in abduction to prevent flexion by use of pillows or abductor splints.

1. Positioning is important (every 2 hours).

2. Turn client about 45° with aid of trapeze and pillows. Do not elevate bed more than 30° to 45°.

3. Do not turn to affected side unless specific orders.

D. Keep Hemovac in place until drainage has substantially decreased (24 to 96 hours).

1. Check dressing to ensure patency of Hemovac.

2. Observe drainage for signs of hemorrhage or infection.

E. Prevent edema.

1. Readjust antiembolic stockings at least every four to eight hours.

2. Change position frequently by raising and lowering head of bed. When ordered, tilt bed to change positions.

F. Continuous passive motion (CPM) first day post-op with increasing degrees of flexion to 90°.

G. Ambulate client carefully at bedside—first or second postoperative day.

1. Do not allow client to bear weight on affected hip.

2. Up with walker second postoperative day.

3. Avoid positions with greater than 90° flexion such as sitting straight up in a chair.

H. Prevent thrombus formation from venous stasis.

1. Have client wear antiembolic stockings.

2. Promote leg exercises—flexing feet and ankles.

I. Start physical therapy after 5–6 days.

J. Instruct client not to use low chairs or to sit on edge of bed.

1. Use extended commode.

2. Use wheelchair that tilts back.

3. Use high stools.

4. No bending-over activities.

KNEE INJURIES

Arthroscopy

Definition: Small incision in knee joint through which cartilage fragments are removed.

Assessment

A. Assess for pain, tenderness, decreased range of motion, clicking noise—torn cartilage (meniscus).

B. Assess for joint instability and pain—torn ligaments.

Implementation

A. Instruct client in surgical procedure for postoperative care.

1. Arthroscopic meniscectomy—removal of torn cartilage fragments through small incision in knee joint using arthroscope.

2. Open meniscectomy—direct surgical technique to knee joint for repair.

B. Elevate leg to minimize swelling.

C. Start client on quad-setting, straight-leg raising exercises. Should be done for five minutes every half hour.

1. Quad-setting: tightening or contracting the muscles of anterior thigh (knee cap is drawn up toward thigh).

2. Straight-leg raising: lifting leg straight off the bed, keeping knee extended and foot in neutral position.

D. Apply ice bags to knee to reduce edema.
E. Ambulate first postoperative day without weight-bearing (use three-point, crutch-walking gait).
F. In addition, give routine postoperative care.

Total Knee Replacement

Definition: Implantation of a metallic upper portion that substitutes for the femoral condyles and a high polymer plastic lower portion that substitutes for the tibial joint surfaces.

Assessment

A. Assess incisional area for drainage.
B. Observe for infection.
C. Observe for circulation, sensation, movement.

Implementation

A. CPM may be ordered post-op—moderate flexion and extension.
B. Have client perform quad-setting and straight-leg-raising exercises every hour.
C. Have client perform general ROM exercises.
D. Splint is usually applied. (Nursing care is same as for any client in a splint).
E. To prevent dislocation, leg is not to be dangled.
F. Hemovac should be inserted to drain excessive blood and drainage.
   1. Maintain accurate intake and output.
   2. Observe for hemorrhage and infection.
G. Instruct client in crutch walking.
H. Client will be out of bed in two to three days.
I. Provide general postoperative care.

CRUTCH WALKING

A. Measure client for crutches.
   1. Distance between axilla and arm pieces on crutches should be two finger widths in axilla space—incorrect measurement could damage brachial plexus.
   2. Elbows should be slightly flexed when walking.
B. Teach gait sequence.
   1. Four-point; crutch-foot sequence.
      a. Move right crutch; move left foot; move left crutch; move right foot.
      b. Gait is slow, but stable; client can bear weight on each leg.
   2. Three-point gait.
      a. Client can bear little or no weight on one leg—two crutches support affected leg.
      b. Move both crutches and affected leg forward; then move unaffected leg forward.

SPINAL SURGERY

Laminectomy and Discectomy

Definition: The excision of vertebral posterior arch. Performed for removal of herniated intervertebral disc.

Assessment

A. Evaluate for circulatory impairment.
   1. Check blanching.
   2. Observe color.
   3. Check warmth of lower or upper extremities (depends on surgical site).
B. Observe for sensation and motion in lower extremities (nerve root damage).
   1. Assess sensation.
   2. Check client's ability to wiggle toes and move feet; record ability to do plantar flexion, dorsiflexion of feet, toes, and ankles.
C. Observe dressings for spinal fluid leak, hemorrhage, and infection.
D. Note bowel sounds (BS) and bladder function.

Implementation

A. Change client's position every two hours by log-rolling for at least 48 hours.
   1. Turn client as one piece by using drawsheet (or pull sheet), placing pillows between legs.
   2. Turn client to either side and back (unless contraindicated). Use support mechanisms when on side.
B. Keep npo until flatus and bowel sounds.
C. Promote general ROM exercises.
D. Ambulate client or have client lie in bed, as sitting puts strain on surgical site.
E. Ambulate in one to two days postoperatively, unless contraindicated.
F. Provide general postoperative care.
G. Administer stronger pain medicines if on medication for a long time preoperative (at least 48 hours postoperative).

Spinal Fusion

Definition: The fusion of spinous processes—stabilizing the spine by removing bony chips from iliac crest and grafting them to fusion site.

Assessment

A. Assess for spinal fluid leak or hemorrhage.
B. Measure vital signs; identify symptoms of infection.
C. Evaluate for circulatory, motion, sensation impairment.
D. Evaluate bladder and bowel function.

Implementation

A. Maintain postoperative positioning.
   1. Some physicians keep client supine for first eight hours to reduce possibility of compression.
   2. Most physicians keep client off back for first 48 hours.
B. Provide ambulation. Start of ambulation varies with physicians, from three to four days to eight weeks, depending on extent of fusion.
   1. Brace is applied when client is ambulated.
   2. Spine should be immobilized for early healing of bone graft and for new callus to form.
C. Instruct client to not lift, bend, stoop, or sit for prolonged periods for at least three months.
D. Inform client grafts are stable by one year.
E. Explain there are some limitations to flexion of spine, depending on extent of fusion.
F. Provide additional interventions same as for laminectomy.

Harrington Rod Fusion

Assessment

A. Observe for circulatory impairment.
B. Evaluate pain.
C. Assess for signs of fluid and electrolyte imbalance.
D. Observe for clinical manifestations of immobility.

Implementation

A. Keep client flat in bed (no leg dangling or head elevation).
B. Provide cast care for full body cast.
C. Log roll every hour, 30 degrees to either side, for at least four days.
D. Assist in pain tolerance.
   1. Severe pain first few days.
   2. Pain for several weeks.
   3. Pain medication routinely every three to four hours for five days.
   4. Positioning.
   5. Relaxation exercises.
E. Provide necessary care for complications of immobility.
F. Monitor signs of fluid and electrolyte imbalance, and record intake and output.
G. Provide diet high in protein, iron, and thiamin and low in calcium.

REMOVAL OF A LIMB

Amputation

Definition: The surgical removal of a limb, a part of a limb, or a portion of a bone elsewhere than at the joint site. Removal of a bone at the joint site is termed disarticulation.

Assessment

A. Evaluate dressings for signs of infection or hemorrhage.
B. Observe for signs of a developing necrosis or neuroma in incision.
C. Evaluate for phantom limb pain.
D. Observe for signs of contractures.

Implementation

A. Provide preoperative nursing management.
   1. Have client practice lifting buttocks off bed while in sitting position.
   2. Provide range of motion to unaffected leg.
   3. Inform client about phantom limb sensation.
      a. Pain and feeling that amputated leg is still there.
      b. Caused by nerves in the stump.
      c. Exercises lessen sensation.
B. Provide postoperative nursing management.
   1. Observe stump dressing for signs of hemorrhage and infection.
      a. Keep tourniquet at bedside to control hemorrhage if necessary.
      b. Mark bleeding by circling drainage with pencil and marking date and time.
      c. Elevate foot of bed to prevent hemorrhage and to reduce edema first 24 hours. (Elevating the stump itself can cause a flexion contracture of hip joint.)
   2. Observe for symptoms of a developing necrosis or neuroma in incision.
   3. Provide stump care.
      a. Rewrap ace bandage three to four times daily.
      b. Wash stump with mild soap and water.
      c. If skin dry, apply lanolin or Vaseline to stump.
   4. Teaching related to stump care.
      a. Below knee amputation—prevent edema formation.

(1) Do not hang stump over edge of bed.

(2) Do not sit for long periods of time.

  b. Above-the-knee amputation—prevent external or internal rotation of limb.

    (1) Place rolled towel along outside of thigh to prevent rotation.

    (2) Use low Fowler's position to provide change in position.

  c. Position client with either type of amputation in prone position to stretch flexor muscles and to prevent flexion contractures of hip. Done usually after first twenty-four to forty-eight hours postoperative.

    (1) Place pillow under abdomen and stump.

    (2) Keep legs close together to prevent abduction.

  d. Teach crutch-walking and wheelchair transfer.

  e. Prepare stump for prosthesis.

    (1) Stump must be conditioned for proper fit.

    (2) Shrinking and shaping stump to conical form by applying bandages or an elastic stump shrinker.

    (3) A cast readies stump for the prosthesis.

  f. Provide care for temporary prosthesis, which is applied until stump has shrunk to permanent state.

5. Recognize and respond to client's psychological reactions to amputation.

  a. Feelings of loss.

  b. Lowered self-image.

  c. Depression.

  d. Phantom limb pain.

TYPES OF TRACTION

Type	Position	Purpose
Skin Traction		
Cervical	Head of bed elevated 30°–40°	Relieve muscle spasms and compression in upper extremities and neck
Buck's	Foot of bed elevated	Immobilize hip when fractured, relieve muscle spasms before hip surgery
Bryant's	Flat with 90° hip flexion	Stabilize fractured femur; correct congenital hip in young children
Russell's	Foot of bed slightly elevated	Stabilize fractured femur prior to surgery
Pelvic	Head of bed elevated, knee gatch elevated to same level (William's position)	Relieve low back, hip, or leg pain; reduce muscle spasm
Skeletal Tongs		
(Blackburn, Gardner-Wells, Crutchfield, Vinke Tongs)	Spine immobilized	Provide for hyperextension; traction allows vertebrae to slip back into position
Halo Vest	Flat, low-Fowler's in bed, ambulate, or sit up	Stabilize fractured or dislocated cervical vertebrae
Balanced Suspension		
Steinmann pin, Kirschner wires, used with Thomas splint and Pearson attachment	Low-Fowler's, either side or back	To approximate fractures of femur, tibia, fibula

INTEGUMENTARY SYSTEM

The integumentary system comprises the enveloping membrane, or skin, of the body and includes the epidermis, the dermis, and all the derivatives of the epidermis, such as hair, nails, and various glands. It is indispensable for the body as it forms a barrier against the external environment and participates in many vital body functions.

ANATOMY AND PHYSIOLOGY

Skin

Definition: The organ that envelops the body. It comprises about 15 percent of the body weight and forms a barrier between the internal organs and the external environment.

Characteristics

A. Consists of three layers: epidermis, dermis, and subcutaneous.
B. It is the largest sensory organ, equipped with nerves and specialized sensory organs sensitive to pain, touch, pressure, heat, and cold.
C. Chief pigment is melanin, produced by basal cells.
D. Functions of skin.
    1. Protection.
    2. Temperature regulation.
    3. Sensation.
    4. Storage.

Bacterial Flora on the Skin

A. Normally present in varying amounts are coagulase positive staphylococcus, coagulase negative staphylococcus, mycobacterium, Pseudomonas, diphtheroids, nonhemolytic streptococcus, hemolytic streptococcus (group A).
B. The organisms are shed with normal exfoliation of skin; bathing and rubbing may also remove bacteria.
C. Normal pH of skin (4.2 to 5.6) retards growth of bacteria.
D. Damaged areas of skin are potential points of entry for infection.

Hair

Definition: A threadlike structure developed from a papilla in the corium layer.

A. Hair goes through cyclic changes: growth, atrophy, and rest.
B. Melanocytes in the bulb of each hair account for color.
C. All parts of the body except the palms, soles of the feet, distal phalanges of fingers and toes, and penis are covered with some form of hair.

Sweat Glands

Definition: Aggregations of cells that produce a liquid (perspiration) having a salty taste and a pH that varies from 4.5 to 7.5.

A. Eccrine sweat glands.
    1. Located in all areas of the skin except the lips and part of the genitalia.
    2. Open onto the surface of the skin.
    3. Activity controlled by the sympathetic nervous system.
    4. Secrete sweat (perspiration).
        a. The chief components of sweat are water, sodium, potassium, chloride, glucose, urea, and lactate.
        b. Concentrations vary from individual to individual.
B. Apocrine sweat glands.
    1. Located in the axilla, genital, anal, and nipple areas.
    2. Located in ear and produce ear wax.
    3. Develop during puberty.
    4. Respond to adrenergic stimuli.
    5. Produce an alkaline sweat.

Sebaceous Glands

A. Develop at base of hair follicle.

B. Secrete sebum.

C. Hormone controlled. Increased activity with androgens; decreased activity with estrogens.

System Assessment

A. Assess color.
   1. Assess color of skin, including deviations from the normal range within the individual's race.
      a. Use a nonglare daylight or 60-watt bulb.
      b. Note especially the bony prominences.
      c. Observe for pallor (white), flushing (red), jaundice (yellow), ashen (gray), or cyanosis (blue) coloration.
      d. Check mucous membranes to be accurate.
   2. Observe for increased or decreased areas of pigmentation.
   3. Observe for various skin discolorations: ecchymosis, petechiae, purpura, or erythema.
B. Evaluate skin temperature.
   1. Palpate skin (especially areas of concern) for temperature.
   2. Note changes in different extremities.
C. Assess turgor.
   1. Observe skin for its ease of movement and speed of return to original position.
   2. Observe for excessive dryness, moisture, wrinkling, flaking and general texture.
   3. Observe for a lasting impression or dent after pressing against and removing finger from skin—indicates edema or fluid in the tissue.
D. Assess skin sensation.
   1. Observe the client's ability to detect heat, cold, gentle touch, and pressure.
   2. Note complaints of itching, tingling, cramps, or numbness.
E. Observe cleanliness.
   1. Observe general state of hygiene. Note amount of oil, moisture, and dirt on the skin surface.
   2. Note presence of strong body odors.
   3. Investigate hair and scalp for presence of body lice.
F. Assess integrity (intactness of skin).
   1. Note intactness of skin. Observe for areas of broken skin (lesions) or ulcers.
   2. Assess any lesion for its location, size, shape, color(s), consistency, discomfort, odor, and sensation associated with it.
G. Assess skin conditions.

   1. Macule: a flat, circumscribed, discolored lesion less than 1 cm in diameter.
   2. Papule: a raised, solid lesion less than 1 cm in diameter.
   3. Nodule: similar to a papule except greater depth.
   4. Vesicle: an elevated lesion of skin or mucous membrane filled with fluid.
   5. Pustule: a pus-filled vesicle.
   6. Wheal: an irregularly shaped and elevated lesion of skin or mucous membrane due to edema.
   7. Plaque: a collection of papules.
   8. Erosion: a moist depressed area due to partial or full loss of epidermis.
   9. Ulcer: the complete loss of dermis leaving irregular depression; scars on healing.
H. Evaluate onset of symptoms.
   1. Local onset and course.
   2. Systemic onset.

System Planning and Analysis

A. The optimum skin condition is reestablished.
B. Nutritional and hydration status of the skin is maintained.
C. The external environment is controlled so as not to contribute to skin problems.
D. Personal hygiene practices promote optimal skin condition.
E. Health status is reflected in condition of the skin.
F. Skin integrity remains constant.
   1. Skin remains intact without signs of ischemia, hyperemia, or necrosis.
   2. Skin shows no signs of dryness, flaking, itching, or burning.

System Implementation

A. Monitor client's most vulnerable body areas for ischemia, hyperemia, or broken areas.
B. Encourage a well-balanced diet, especially protein-rich foods.
C. Promote high-fluid intake to maintain hydration status.
D. Change the client's body position at least every two hours to rotate weight bearing areas.
   1. Observe all vulnerable areas at this time.

2. Include right and left lateral, prone, supine, and swimming-type positioning if possible.
E. Massage skin to increase circulation.
F. Hydrate dry skin to prevent breakdown.
G. Keep skin clean.
H. Protect healthy skin from drainage and environmental pollutants.
I. Encourage active exercise or range of motion to promote circulation.
J. Monitor medications for various skin conditions or lesions.
K. Instruct clients about appropriate skin care.

System Evaluation

A. Client's skin remains intact without signs of ischemia, hyperemia, or necrosis.
B. Client's skin shows no signs of dryness, flaking, itching, or burning.
C. Skin maintains hydration status and adequate fluid is ingested.
D. Temperature of skin remains within normal limits.
E. Various conditions have been treated and skin returns to healthy state.
1. Ulcer evidences a healing process.
2. Healthy tissue is not contaminated.
3. Client is not uncomfortable.
F. Infection of skin is prevented by careful handwashing and skin care.
G. Overall skin condition is healthy.
H. Public is educated about preventative measures.

COMMON SKIN LESIONS

Paronychia

Definition: Infection and inflammation of the tissue around the nailplate.

Characteristics

A. High incidence in middle-age women.
B. High incidence in diabetics.

Assessment

A. Evaluate acute infection from a hangnail.
B. Observe for cellulitis.

Implementation

A. Implement warm soaks.
B. Apply antibiotic or fungicidal ointment.
C. Care for incision and drainage of affected area.

Acne Vulgaris

Definition: A disorder of the skin with eruption of papules or pustules primarily due to increased production of sebum from the sebaceous glands. Affects adolescents and young adults.

Characteristics

A. Noninflammatory type composed of whiteheads and blackheads in the follicular duct.
B. Inflammatory acne pustules with possible scarring.
C. Affected by hormone levels (androgen).

MEDICAL IMPLICATIONS
A. Estrogen therapy.
B. Desquamation preparations, which allow free flow of sebum.
C. Complete cleansing with regular or Neutrogena soap and clean towels.
D. Mild facial erythema via sunlight or lamp.
E. Removal of blackheads and whiteheads.
F. Topical antibiotics.
G. Systemic tetracycline for some cases.
H. Dermabrasion for selected cases.

Implementation

A. Teach good skin and scalp hygiene.
B. Have client avoid squeezing, rubbing, picking.
C. Have client avoid greasy cleansing creams and cosmetics.
D. Support a high-protein, low-fat diet.
1. Fatty foods, white sugar, nuts, and chocolate should be avoided.
2. Diet not as important a therapy as in the past.
E. Encourage client to get adequate rest and sunshine.
F. Provide emotional support for body image and relationship problems.

Impetigo

Definition: A bacterial disease caused by streptococcus or staphylococcus or both.

Characteristics

A. Lesions are intraepidermal vesicles.
B. Lesions progress to pustules, which become crusted.

Implementation

A. Instruct client that the most important intervention is the prevention of the spread of the disease: complete cleansing with hexachlorophene soap and other hygienic care materials; separate towels.
B. Instruct that lesions dry by exposure to air; use compresses of Burow's solution to remove the crusts to allow faster healing.
C. Apply antibiotic ointments; bland emollients to prevent cracking and fissures.

Furuncle (Boil)

Definition: A bacterial disease caused by staphylococcus pyrogen infection of a hair follicle.

Assessment

A. Evaluate furuncle. Onset is sudden; the skin becomes red, tender, and hot around the hair follicle.
B. Observe furuncle. The center forms pus, and the core may be extruded spontaneously or by excision and manipulation.
C. Check for presence of diabetes mellitus. Should be ruled out only after tests prove negative.
D. Instruct client in necessity of scrupulous cleanliness: isolation of towels, soap, and clothing.
E. Administer systemic antibiotics if a series of carbuncles occur.

Herpes Simplex

Definition: A viral disease (coldsore) caused by herpes virus, hominis types I and II.

Characteristics

A. Herpes I.
 1. Most common type.
 2. Causes burning, tingling, and itching, soon followed by tiny vesicles.
 3. Most frequently occurs on lips, but can occur on the face and around the mouth.
B. Herpes II. (See pg. 381.)
 1. Most often the cause of genital infection.

2. Transmitted primarily through sexual contact.
3. Difficult to treat and to prevent recurrence.

Implementation

A. Herpes Simplex Virus, Type I
 1. Keep area dry; apply drying agent (ether).
 2. L-lysine amino acid: 1 gm daily for 6 months.
B. Herpes Genitalis, Type II.
 1. Avoid sexual contact with active lesion.
 2. Use Acyclovir cream; recurrence give Acyclovir 200 mg p.o. × 5 for 5 days.

Herpes Zoster (Shingles)

Definition: Acute invasion of the peripheral nervous system due to reactivation of varicella zoster virus.

Assessment

A. Evaluate eruption with fever, malaise and pain.
B. Assess vesicles (exudate contains virus) that appear in 3–4 days.
C. Assess client's status—if immunosuppressed, condition can be life-threatening.

Implementation

A. Isolate client.
B. Apply drying lotions—calamine.
C. Administer drugs: analgesics for pain; antiviral agents, (Acyclovir) and NSAIDS.
D. Instruct client on preventative measures.

VENEREAL DISEASES AND CUTANEOUS LESIONS

Syphilis

Definition: A contagious venereal disease that leads to many structural and cutaneous lesions. Caused by the spirochete *Treponema pallidum.* The disease is transmitted by direct, intimate contact or in utero.

Characteristics

A. Transmitted commonly by sexual intercourse, but infants may become infected during birth process.
B. No age or race is immune to the disease.
C. Diagnosed by serum studies and/or dark field examination of secretions of the chancre.
 1. Wassermann test.
 2. Kahn test.
D. No immunity develops and reinfection is common.
E. Types of syphilis.
 1. Early syphilis—two stages.
 a. Primary stage.
  (1) Incubation period is 10 days to 3 weeks.

(2) Characteristic lesion is red, eroded, indurated papule; the sore or ulcer at the site of the invasion by the spirochete is called a *chancre.*

(3) Accompanied by enlarged lymph node in drainage area of chancre.

(4) May be painless or painful.

(5) This stage is highly infectious.

b. Secondary stage.

   (1) Develops if the individual is not treated in the primary stage. Occurs in two to six months and may last two years.

   (2) May be mild enough to pass unnoticed or may be severe, with a generalized rash on skin and mucous membrane.

   (3) Headache, fever, sore throat, and general malaise are common.

   (4) Disappears by itself if untreated in three to twelve weeks.

2. Late syphilis—tertiary stage.

a. Symptoms may develop soon after secondary stage or lie hidden for years.

b. Blood test may be negative.

c. Less contagious but very dangerous to individual.

d. If untreated, cardiovascular problems may ensue.

e. Blindness or deep ulcers may occur.

f. May be treated with antibiotics but cure is more difficult.

Implementation

A. Advise client that strict personal hygiene is an absolute requirement.

B. Educate client in prevention: symptoms, mode of transmission, and treatment.

C. Assist in case finding; encourage use of clinics for diagnosis and treatment.

D. Administer long-acting Bicillin (still primary treatment in the early stages).

E. Instruct client to avoid sexual contact until clearance is given by physician.

ALLERGIC RESPONSES

Eczema

Definition: A superficial inflammatory process involving primarily the epidermis.

Characteristics

A. Eczema is a chronic condition with remissions and exacerbations.

B. Eczema occurs at all ages, and is common in infancy.

C. Treatment is dependent on cause (foods, emotional problems, familial tendencies).

D. Child is isolated from recently vaccinated children; child is *not* vaccinated.

Assessment

A. Assess for eruptions that are erythematous, papular, or papulovesicular.

   1. May be edematous, weeping, eroded, and/or crusted.

   2. Chronic form may cause skin to be thickened, scaling, and fissured.

B. Assess if regional lymph nodes are swollen.

C. Assess if irritability is present.

Implementation

A. Have clients keep fingernails short; restrain or provide gloves to prevent scratching.

B. Apply wet dressings or therapeutic baths (no soaps during acute stages).

C. Apply mild lotion (calamine) when no oozing or vesiculation is present.

D. Use cornstarch paste to remove crusts.

E. Rub cornstarch into bed linen, and do not use woolen blankets.

Contact Dermatitis

Definition: A skin reaction caused by contact with an agent to which the skin is sensitive.

Characteristics

A. Causes.

   1. Clothing (especially woolens).

   2. Cosmetics.

   3. Household products (especially detergents).

   4. Industrial substances (i.e., paints, dyes, cements).

B. Treatment

   1. Avoidance of irritant or removal of irritating clothing.

   2. Avoidance of contact with detergent (use of rubber gloves for household chores).

3. Avoidance of contact with industrial agent (use of protective clothing or, for highly sensitive individuals, change of job locations).

Poison Oak or Poison Ivy

Definition: Dermatitis caused by contact with poison oak, poison ivy, or poison sumac, which contain urushiol, a potent skin-sensitizing agent.

Assessment

A. Assess for papulovesicular lesions.
B. Assess for severe itching.

Implementation

A. Cleanse skin of plant oils.
B. Apply lotion.
C. Administer steroids for severe reactions.
D. Apply cold, wet dressings of Burow's solution to relieve itching.

Malignant Skin Tumors

Assessment

A. Evaluate lesion that starts as a papule and spreads; central area may become depressed and ulcerated.
B. Assess extent of local invasion or extensive local destruction.
C. Evaluate lesions that enlarge rapidly (may indicate basal-cell epithelioma, and can metastasize).
D. Assess for any nodular tumor that appears, usually on the lower lip, tongue, head, or neck.
E. Assess for specific type of skin tumor.
   1. Basal-cell epithelioma is a tumor arising from the basal layer of the epidermis formed because of basal cell keratinization. The typical lesion is a small, smooth papule with telangiectasis and atrophic center.
   2. Melanoma is the most malignant of all cutaneous lesions. It arises from melanocytes and is often fatal. It occurs most frequently in light-skinned people when they are exposed to sunlight.
   3. Squamous cell carcinoma is a tumor of the epidermis that frequently comes from keratosis and is considered an invasive cancer. The lesion begins as erythematous macules or plaques with indistinct margins, and the surface often becomes crusted.

Implementation

A. Assist with surgical excision, the most effective treatment.
B. Administer cancer drugs if ordered.
C. Assist with irradiation if ordered.
   1. Counsel client in side effects of treatment.
   2. Offer emotional support throughout treatment.
D. Advise client to prevent occurrence of skin cancer by using sunscreening devices.
E. Advise client to avoid prolonged exposure to sun.
F. Educate client to observe any changes in color or form of moles.
G. Watch for potential malignancy in other locations.

COLLAGEN DISEASES

Definition: Disorders that have common wide-spread immunological and inflammatory alteration of connective tissue.

Characteristics

A. Skin changes occur.
B. Joint and muscle involvement becomes noticeable.
C. Etiology.
   1. Possible autoimmune disturbance.
   2. Hereditary predisposition.

Lupus Erythematosus

Definition: A collagen disease of the connective tissue that may involve any organ of the body.

Assessment

A. Assess for discoid eruption—a chronic, localized scaling erythematous skin eruption over the nose, cheeks, and forehead, giving a characteristic "butterfly" appearance.
B. Evaluate for fever, malaise and weight loss.
C. Observe for exacerbation and remission of symptoms.
D. Assess for sensitivity to sunlight.
E. Systemic (disseminated) lupus erythematosus may have multiple organ involvement that can lead to death.

Implementation

A. Instruct client to avoid sunlight and local antibiotic ointments that spread the lesions.
B. Administer steroid treatment to prevent progression of the disease.
C. Apply topical sunscreen preparations (i.e., Covermark, Pabanol, etc.).
D. Advise client of possible side effects of prescribed medications; advise client to notify physician promptly if side effects occur so drugs may be discontinued before serious complications.

E. Cover up disfigurement from scarring with opaque or tinted cosmetics as recommended by physician.

BURNS

Definition: Destruction of layers of the skin by thermal, chemical, or electrical agents.

Assessment

A. Assess degree of burn—determined by layers involved.
   1. First degree–superficial partial thickness.
      a. Involves epidermis.
      b. Area is red or pink.
      c. Moderate pain.
      d. Spontaneous healing.
   2. Second degree–partial thickness.
      a. Involves epidermis and dermis to the basal cells.
      b. Blistering.
      c. Severe pain.
      d. Regeneration in one month.
      e. Scarring may occur.
   3. Third degree–full thickness.
      a. Involves epidermis, dermis, and subcutaneous tissue and may extend to the muscle in severe burns.
      b. White, gray, or black in appearance.
      c. Absence of pain.
      d. Edema of surrounding tissues.
      e. Eschar formation.
      f. Grafting needed due to total destruction of dermal elements.
   4. Fourth degree.
      a. Involves muscle and bone.
      b. Increased destruction of RBCs.
B. Assess for extent of burn.
   1. Rule of Nines—good for rapid estimation.
      a. Head and neck   9%
      b. Anterior trunk   18%
      c. Posterior trunk   18%
      d. Arms (9% each)   18%
      e. Legs (18% each)   36%
      f. Perineum   1%
   2. Lund/Browder Method.
      a. More accurate and appropriate to use when calculating fluid replacement.
      b. A chart is necessary to compute percentages assigned to body areas.
      c. Percentages vary for different age groups.

C. Assess associated factors which determine seriousness of burn.
   1. Age.
      a. Below eighteen months.
      b. Above sixty-five years.
   2. General health.
   3. Site of burn.
   4. Associated injuries (fractures).
   5. Causative agents.
D. Assess for category of burn classification.
   1. Classification according to the percentage of body area destroyed.
      a. Critical burns: 30 percent or more of the body has sustained second degree burn, and 10 percent has sustained third degree burn; further complicated by fractures, respiratory involvement and smoke inhalation. Burns of feet, hands, face and genitalia.
      b. Moderate burns: less than 10 percent of the body has sustained third degree burn, and 15 to 30 percent has sustained second degree burn.
      c. Minor burns: less than 15 percent of the body has sustained second degree burn, and less than 2 percent has sustained third degree burn.
   2. Classification according to cause.
      a. Thermal burns: flame burns, scalding with hot liquids, or radiation.
      b. Chemical burns: strong acids or strong alkali solutions.
      c. Electrical burns.
         (1) Most serious type of burn.
         (2) Body fluids may conduct an electrical charge through body (look for entrance and exit area).
         (3) Cardiac arrhythmias may occur.
         (4) Toxins are created postburn that injure kidneys.
         (5) Voltage and ampere information important in history taking.

MEDICAL IMPLICATIONS
A. Immediate care.
   1. Cold water for brief duration in second degree burn if seen within 10 minutes of injury.
   2. No ointments.
   3. Burns covered with sterile or clean cloth.
B. Emergency room care.

1. Patent airway is established.
2. 100 percent oxygen if burn occurred in en-closed area.
3. Degree and extent of burn is determined.
4. Fluid balance is maintained.
   a. First day give lactated Ringer's solution according to percent of body burn and weight plus 2000 cc D$_5$W.
   b. Second day give colloids with solutions.
   c. Urine output is maintained at least 50 cc/hour
   d. Vital signs—CVP line usually inserted.
5. Nasogastric tube (inserted to prevent par-alytic ileus).
6. Tetanus toxoid.
7. Escharotomy or fasciotomy if needed.
C. Long-term care.
   1. Wound debridement.
   2. Wound care: ointment and/or dressing.
   3. Skin grafting.
      a. Homograft or Allograft: from cadaver or other person.
      b. Xenograft: from an animal.
      c. Autografts: from self.
D. Op-Site.

Implementation

A. Maintain patent airway.
B. Maintain aseptic area.
C. Provide fluid replacement therapy.
   1. Shock phase.
      a. First 24 to 48 hours postburn, fluid shifts from plasma to interstitial space.
      b. Potassium levels rise in plasma.
      c. Blood hemoconcentration and metabolic acidosis occur.
      d. Fluid loss is mostly plasma.
      e. Nursing responsibilities.
         (1) Monitor vital signs frequently.
         (2) Monitor urinary output (50 to 100 cc/hour).
         (3) Give one half of total fluids in first eight hours.
   2. Postshock phase (diuretic phase).
      a. Capillary permeability stabilizes and fluid begins to shift from interstitial spaces to plasma.
      b. Hypokalemia, hypernatremia, hemodilu-tion, and pulmonary edema are potential dangers.

   c. Nursing responsiblities.
      (1) Monitor CVP.
      (2) Observe lab values.
      (3) Maintain adequate urine output.
D. Relieve pain with morphine sulfate, IV as ordered. Give small doses frequently.
E. Assess peripheral circulation.
F. Provide adequate heat to maintain client's tem-perature.
G. Promote good body alignment: begin range of mo-tion early.
H. Administer antacids to prevent stress ulcer.
I. Maintain reverse isolation.
J. Maintain wound care.
   1. Initial excision: mainly for electrical burns.
   2. Occlusive dressings.
      a. Painful and costly.
      b. Decreases water loss.
      c. Limits range-of-motion exercises.
      d. Helps to maintain functional position.
      e. Advent of topical antibiotics has led to de-creased use.
   3. Exposure method.
      a. Allows for drainage of burn exudate.
      b. Eschar forms protective covering.
      c. Use of topical therapy.
      d. Skin easily inspected.
      e. Range-of-motion exercises easier to per-form.
K. Apply topical preparations to wound area.
   1. Mafenide (Sulfamylon).
      a. Exerts bacteriostatic action against many organisms.
      b. Penetrates tissue wall.
      c. Dressings not needed when used.
      d. Breakdown of drug provides heavy acid load. Inhibition of carbonic anhydrase com-pounds situation. Individual compensates by hyperventilating.
      e. Alternate use with Silvadene.
   2. Silvadene.
      a. Broad antimicrobial activity.
      b. Effective against yeast.
      c. Inhibits bacteria resistant to other anti-microbials.
         (1) Not usually used prophylactically.
         (2) Given for specific organism.
         (3) Not helpful first 48 hours due to vessel thrombosis.
      d. Can be washed off with water.

3. Silver nitrate.
   a. Used for many years but decreasing in popularity.
   b. Controls bacteria in wound and reduces water evaporation.
   c. Disadvantages are that it acts only on surface organisms, dressings are messy and must be kept wet, and bulk of dressing decreases ROM.
4. Gentamicin is no longer recommended as a topical agent.

L. Administer systemic antibiotics.

M. Debridement and eschar removal daily.

N. Provide long-term care.

1. Maintain good positioning to prevent contractures.
2. Prevent infection.
3. Maintain adequate protein and caloric intake to promote healing.
4. Monitor hydration status.
5. Protect skin grafts.
6. Provide psychological support (as important as physical care).
   a. Deal with the client's fear of disfigurement and immobility from scarring.
   b. Provide constant support, as plastic repair is lengthy and painful.
   c. Involve the family in long-term planning and day-to-day care.

Table 1. ISOLATION PROTOCOL

Protocol for Entering Isolation Room	Protocol for Leaving Isolation Room	
1. Put on cap.	1. Untie gown at waist.	6. Pull gown off and place in laundry hamper.
2. Put on and tie mask.	2. Take off gloves.	7. Take off mask.
3. Put on gown and tie.	3. Wash hands.	8. Leave room and wash hands.
4. Wash hands and put on gloves.	4. Take off cap.	
	5. Untie gown at neck.	

LYME DISEASE

Definition: An infection acquired through ticks who live in wooded areas and survive by attaching themselves to animal and human hosts. This disease has many and varied symptoms and is difficult to diagnose because it masquerades as other illnesses.

Assessment

A. Following a tick bite, the first symptoms occur several days to a month following the bite.
   1. Assess for a small red pimple that spreads into a ringed-shaped rash. Rash may be large or small, or not occur at all (making diagnosis difficult).
   2. Assess for flu-like symptoms: headache, stiff neck, muscle aches, and fatigue.

B. Assess for the second stage occurring several weeks following the bite: joint pain and neurological complications (about 15%) or heart disease symptoms (8%).

C. Assess for third stage symptoms: arthritis progresses and large joints are usually involved (50%).

Implementation

A. Blood test may detect the disease but is usually negative during the early phases. Once confirmed, administer antibiotics—dosage depends upon severity of symptoms.

B. Prevention is the best treatment.
   1. Avoid areas that contain ticks—those that are wooded, grassy, especially in the summer months.
   2. Wear tight-fitting clothing and spray body with tick repellent.
   3. Examine entire body for ticks when you return home; if tick is located, remove with tweezers and wash skin with antiseptic, and preserve tick for examination.

DISORDERS OF THE BLOOD AND SPLEEN

The circulatory system, a continuous circuit, is the mechanical conveyor of the body constituent called blood. Blood, composed of cells and plasma, circulates through the body and is the means by which oxygen and nutritive materials are transported to the tissues and carbon dioxide and metabolic end products are removed for excretion.

BLOOD AND BLOOD FACTORS

Blood Components

Plasma

A. Plasma accounts for 55 percent of the total volume of blood.
B. It is comprised of 92 percent water and 7 percent proteins.
1. Proteins include serum, fibrinogen, albumin, gamma globulin.
2. Less than one percent organic salts, dissolved gases, hormones, antibodies, and enzymes.

Solid Particles

A. Comprise 45 percent of the total blood volume.
B. Blood cells.
1. Erythrocytes (red blood cells).
a. Normal count in an adult is five to five and one-half million cells per cu mm.
b. They contain hemoglobin, which carries oxygen to cells and carbon dioxide from cells to lungs.
c. Red blood cells originate in bone marrow and are stored in the spleen.
d. Average life span is 10 to 120 days.
2. Leukocytes (white blood cells).
a. Normal count in an adult is five to eight thousand per cu mm.
b. Primary defense against infections.

c. Neutrophils play an active role in the acute inflammatory process and have phagocytic action.
d. Macrophages—both fixed and wandering cells—act as scavengers and phagocytize foreign bodies, cellular debris, and more resistant organisms, i.e., fungi and *Mycobacterium tuberculosis.*
e. Lymphocytes play an important role in immunologic responses.
f. Monocytes are the largest of the leukocytes and are less phagocytic than macrophages.
3. Platelets (thrombocytes). 250,000 to 450,000/cu mm needed for clot retraction.

Blood Coagulation

A. Clotting takes place in three phases.
1. Phase I: prothrombin activator formed in response to ruptured vessel or damage to blood.
2. Phase II: prothrombin activator catalyzes conversion of prothrombin into thrombin.
3. Phase III: thrombin acts as an enzyme to convert fibrinogen into fibrin thread.
B. Types of clotting factors.
1. Calcium ions.
a. Cofactor in coagulation.
b. Does not enter into reaction.
c. If absent, neither extrinsic or intrinsic system will operate.
2. Phospholipids.
a. Necessary for formation of final prothrombin activator.
b. Thromboplastin is phospholipid in extrinsic system.
c. Platelet factor III is phospholipid for intrinsic system.
3. Plasma protein—all clotting factors from V to XIII.
C. Coagulation mechanisms.
1. Extrinsic mechanisms.
a. Extract from damaged tissue is mixed with blood.
b. Trauma occurs to tissue or endothelial surface of vascular wall, releasing thromboplastin.
2. Intrinsic mechanisms.
a. Blood itself comes into contact with roughened blood vessel wall.

Table 1. BLOOD COAGULATION

Intrinsic Mechanism	Extrinsic Mechanism
Platelet Factor III	Tissue Thromboplastin
Thromboplastin Release	Release

Thromboplastin Release

+

Thromboplastin Release

+

Factor VII

Factor XII
Factor XI
Factor IX
Factor VII

Factor V
Factor X
+
Calcium

Phase I   Prothrombin Activator
_____

+

Prothrombin

+

Calcium

Phase II   Thrombin
_____

+

Fibrinogen

Phase III Fibrin Thread (Matrix of Clot)
_____

    b. Platelets adhere to vessel and disintegrate, which releases blood factor III containing thromboplastin.

D. Fibrinolytic system.
    1. Adequate function is necessary to maintain hemostasis.
    2. Dissolves clots through formation of plasmin.

Blood Grouping

Major Blood Groups

A. ABO blood group.
    1. A.
    2. AB.
    3. B.
    4. O.

B. Rh blood group.
    1. Positive (85 percent of the population).
    2. Negative (15 percent of the population).

Antigens and Antibodies

A. Based on type of antigens present in red blood cells as well as type of antibodies in the serum.
B. A and B antigens.
    1. Clients with type A blood have antigen A present; clients with type B blood have antigen B present.
    2. Clients with type AB blood have both A and B antigens present.
    3. Clients with type O blood have no antigens present.
C. Anti-A and anti-B antibodies present.
    1. Clients with type A blood do not have anti-A antibodies because the blood cells would be destroyed by agglutination.
    2. They have anti-B antibodies.
    3. Type B blood has anti-A antibodies.

System Assessment

A. Assess onset of symptoms, whether insidious or abrupt.
B. Assess for petechiae, ecchymosis.
C. Evaluate bleeding time.
D. Assess for fatigue and general weakness.
E. Assess for chills or fever.
F. Assess for dyspnea.
G. Observe for ulceration of oral mucosa and pharynx.
H. Assess for pruritus.
I. Check skin color—pallor, yellow-cast, or reddish-purple hue.
J. Assess for visual disturbances.
K. Palpate for hepatomegaly or splenomegaly.
L. Assess for dietary deficiencies—ask questions about daily intake of foods.
M. Assess for neurological symptoms.
    1. Numbness and tingling in the extremities.
    2. Personality changes.
N. Evaluate cardiovascular signs and symptoms.
    1. Hypotension or hypertension.
    2. Character of pulse.
    3. Capillary engorgement.
    4. Venous thrombosis.
O. Assess for gastric distress and weight loss.

Table 2. SUMMARY OF ABO BLOOD GROUPING

Blood Type	Antigen in RBC's	Antibodies in Plasma	Incompatible Donor Blood	Compatible Blood Donor
A	A	Anti-B	AB and B	A and O
B	B	Anti-A	A and AB	B and O
AB	A and B	None	None	All blood groups
O	None	Anti-A and Anti-B	All blood groups	O

System Planning and Analysis

A. Blood disorder is identified and treatment instituted.
B. The primary function of blood—to transport oxygen—is not disrupted.
C. Deficiency of circulating red blood cells is corrected.
D. Bleeding, if present, is controlled.
E. Drugs, if responsible for blood disorder, are identified and discontinued.
F. Iron deficiency is corrected through diet or medication.
G. Hemoglobin is maintained at viable level.
H. Infection is prevented.
I. Dietary deficiencies are corrected.

System Implementation

A. Prevent infections.
   1. Maintain reverse isolation and meticulous medical asepsis.
   2. Suggest bed rest.
   3. Provide high-protein, high-vitamin, and high-caloric diet.
   4. Administer antibiotics as ordered.
B. Promote rest for fatigue and weakness.
   1. Conserve the client's strength.
   2. Suggest frequent rest periods.
   3. Ambulate as tolerated.
   4. Decrease disturbing activities and noise.
   5. Provide optimal nutrition.
C. Provide care for hemorrhagic tendencies.
   1. Provide rest during bleeding episodes.
   2. Apply gentle pressure to bleeding sites.
   3. Apply cold compresses to bleeding sites when indicated.
   4. Do not disturb clots.
   5. Use small-gauge needles to administer medications by injection.
   6. Support the client during transfusion therapy.
   7. Observe for symptoms of internal bleeding.
   8. Have a tracheostomy set available for the client who is bleeding from the mouth or the throat.
D. Give care for ulcerative lesions of the tongue, the gums, and/or the mucous membranes.
   1. Provide nonirritating foods and beverages.
   2. Give frequent oral hygiene with mild, cool mouthwash and solutions.
   3. Use applicators or soft-bristled toothbrush.
   4. Lubricate the lips.
   5. Give mouth care both before and after meals.
E. Monitor and treat oxygen deficit.
   1. Elevate the head of the bed.
   2. Support the client in the orthopneic position.
   3. Administer oxygen when indicated.
   4. Prevent unnecessary exertion.
F. Provide measures to alleviate bone and joint pain.
   1. Use cradle to relieve pressure of bedding.
   2. Apply hot or cold compresses as ordered.
   3. Immobilize joints when ordered.
G. Apply cool sponges if fever present.
H. Administer antipyretic drugs as ordered.
I. Encourage fluid intake unless contraindicated.
J. Provide care for pruritus and/or skin eruptions.
   1. Keep the client's fingernails short.
   2. Use soap sparingly, if at all.
   3. Apply emollient lotions in skin care.
K. Attempt to decrease anxiety of the client.
   1. Explain the nature, the discomforts, and the limitations of activity associated with the diagnostic procedures and treatments.
   2. Listen to the client.
   3. Treat the client as an individual.
   4. Allow the family to participate in the client's care.
   5. Encourage the family to visit with the client; provide privacy for the family and client.

Table 3. LABORATORY TESTS FOR BLOOD DISORDERS

Test	Purpose	Normal Values
Red Blood Cell Count	Determines actual number of formed blood elements in relation to volume. Identifies abnormalities.	Males: 4.5–6.2 million/cu mm Females: 4.0–5.5 million/cu mm Children: 3.2–5.2 million/cu mm
Hematocrit (HCT)	Measures percentage of red blood cells per fluid volume of whole blood.	Males: 40–54/100 ml Females: 37–47/100 ml Children: 29–54/100 ml
Hemoglobin (Hgb)	Measures the amount of hemoglobin per 100 ml of blood to determine oxygen-carrying capacity.	Males: above 12 g/100 ml Females: above 10.2 g/100 ml
Platelet Count	Determines number of platelets.	Adults: 150,000–350,000/cu mm
Prothrombin Time (PT)	Evaluates thrombin generation. Detects deficiencies in extrinsic clotting mechanism.	11–15 seconds
Partial Thromboplastin Time (PTT)	Evaluates adequacy of plasma-clotting factors—intrinsic clotting mechanism.	30–45 seconds Prolonged values indicate coagulation factor deficiency
Thrombin Time	Screening test to detect abnormalities in thrombin fibrinogen reaction. (Conversion to fibrin in stage 3 of clotting sequence.)	10–15 seconds
White Blood Cell Count (WBC)	Establishes quantity and maturity of white blood cell elements.	Adults: 4500–11,000/cu mm Children: 5000–13,000/cu mm Neutrophils: 3000–7500/cu mm Band Neutrophils: 150–700/cu mm Basophils: 25–100/cu mm Eosinophils: 50–400/cu mm Lymphocytes: 1500–4500 cu/mm Monocytes: 100–500/cu mm

Erythrocyte Sedimentation Rate (ESR)	Measures rate of red blood cells settling from plasma—reflects infections.	Wintrobe Method
		  Males: 9 mm/hr
		  Females: 0–15 mm/hr
		  Children: 0–13 mm/hr
		
		Westergren Method
		  Males: 0–15 mm/hr
		  Females: 0–20 mm/hr
		  Children: 0–20 mm/hr

Schilling Test	Determines absorption of vitamin B_{12} necessary for erythropoiesis. Definitive test for pernicious anemia.	7% of radioactive B_{12} excreted in urine in first 24 hours Diagnosis is made when less than 3% excreted

System Evaluation

A. Infection is prevented.

B. Fatigue and weakness are minimized and client is able to carry on activities of daily living.

C. Bleeding episodes are minimized.

D. Transfusions are completed with no untoward reactions.

E. Bone and joint pain is alleviated.

F. Skin problems (pruritus or skin eruptions) are reversed.

G. Client's anxiety is decreased.

H. Side effects of medication administration are minimized.

I. Healthy diet is maintained and iron deficiency corrected.

DISORDERS OF THE BLOOD

Purpuras

Definition: The extravasation of blood into the tissues and mucous membranes.

Characteristics

A. Idiopathic thrombocytopenic purpura is characterized by platelet deficiency due to either hypoproliferation, excessive destruction, or excessive pooling of platelets in the spleen.

B. Vascular purpura is characterized by weak, damaged vessels, which rupture easily.

Assessment

A. Observe for petechiae.

B. Assess postsurgical bleeding.

C. Evaluate increased bleeding time.

D. Evaluate abnormal platelet count.

E. Assess for ecchymosis.

Implementation

A. Identify underlying cause if possible.

B. Complete steps to control bleeding.

C. Monitor transfusion of platelets.

D. Monitor administration of corticosteroids.

E. Monitor client with postsurgical splenectomy for idiopathic thrombocytopenia.

Agranulocytosis

Definition: An acute, potentially fatal blood disorder characterized by profound neutropenia and most commonly caused by drug toxicity or hypersensitivity.

Assessment

A. Assess for chills and fever.

B. Assess for sore throat.

C. Assess for exhaustion and depletion of energy.

D. Observe for ulceration of oral mucosa and throat.

Implementation

A. Discontinue suspected chemical agents or drugs.

B. Isolate the client to reduce exposure to infections.

C. Administer corticosteroids only if the client appears to be toxic.

Polycythemia Vera

Definition: A chronic disease of unknown etiology characterized by overactivity of bone marrow with overproduction of red cells and hemoglobin.

Assessment

A. Assess skin.
   1. Reddish-purple hue.
   2. Pruritus.

B. Assess cardiovascular system.
   1. Increased blood volume.
   2. Capillary engorgement.
   3. Hemorrhage.
   4. Venous thrombosis.
   5. Hypertension.

C. Assess for hepatomegaly and splenomegaly.

D. Assess for visual disturbances and congestion of conjunctiva.

E. Assess for gastric distress and weight loss.

Implementation

A. Monitor administration of radiophosphorus in dosages based on body weight; initially IV, then orally.

B. Assist with phlebotomy to remove 500 to 2000 ml of blood per week until hematocrit reaches 50 percent; procedure is repeated when hematocrit rises.
   1. Monitor blood pressure, pulse, and respirations for tachycardia during procedure and postprocedure.

2. Promote client comfort by positioning in prone position to prevent vertigo and syncope.

C. Monitor for complications (impending CVA, thrombocytosis).

D. Instruct client to monitor symptoms of iron deficiency.

E. Instruct client to watch common bleeding sites (nose, skin) and report immediately.

Anemia

Definition: A condition that occurs when there is a decrease in either quantity or quality of blood. The deficiency may be a decrease in erythrocytes or a reduction in hemoglobin.

Characteristics

A. Common causes of anemia.
   1. Blood loss.
   2. Destruction of red blood cells (hemolysis).
   3. Abnormal bone marrow function.
   4. Decreased erythropoietin due to renal damage.
   5. Inadequate maturation of red blood cells.
B. Classifications.
   1. Normocytic normochromic.
      a. Chronic infection.
      b. Cancer.
      c. General debilitation.
   2. Macrocytic normochromic.
      a. Vitamin B_{12} deficiency.
      b. Folic acid deficiency.
   3. Microcytic hypochronic.
      a. Chronic blood loss.
      b. Iron deficiency.

Assessment

A. Assess for signs related to tissue hypoxia.
   1. Weakness and fatigue.
   2. Need for sleep and rest.
   3. Lethargy.
   4. Dyspnea.
   5. Tachycardia and tachypnea.
   6. Pallor.
   7. Cold extremities.
B. Assess for signs related to the central nervous system.
   1. Vertigo.
   2. Irritability.
   3. Depression.
C. Evaluate poor wound healing.
D. Assess for dietary deficiencies.

Implementation

A. Provide diet high in protein, iron, and vitamins to increase production of erythrocytes; remember that client is sensitive to hot, cold, and spicy foods.

B. Maintain adequate fluid intake.

C. Protect from infection.

D. Provide complete bed rest.

E. Promote good skin care to prevent decubiti.

F. Protect from falls and injury (due to vertigo).

G. Avoid extremes of heat and cold (due to disturbance in sensory perception).

H. Provide good mouth care with diluted mouthwash and soft toothbrush.

I. Provide emotional support for long-term therapy.

Iron Deficiency Anemia (Microcytic Hypochromic)

Characteristics

A. A common, slowly progressive anemia.
B. Occurs most often in infants, adolescents, pregnant females, alcoholics, and the elderly.
C. Results from chronic blood loss, inadequate intake, defective absorption, improper utilization of iron, prolonged drug therapy, or improper cooking of foods.

Assessment

A. Assess for cheilosis—fissured condition of the lips.
B. Assess for dysphagia.
C. Check glossitis.
D. Assess for papillae atrophy of tongue.
E. Check for pica syndrome (abnormal craving for sand, clay, ice).
F. Observe for signs of anaphylactic shock, particularly with IV medications.
   1. Headache.
   2. Urticaria.
   3. Hypotension.

Implementation

A. Provide diet high in iron: liver, lean meats, egg yolk, dried fruit, whole wheat bread, wheat germ, red beans, asparagus.
B. Administer iron preparations.
   1. Oral.
      a. Administer ferrous sulfate, 300 mg t.i.d.
      b. Give liquid iron with straw to avoid staining of teeth.

c. Administer oral iron on empty stomach to increase absorption.

d. Give iron with orange juice since iron absorption is aided by vitamin C.

e. Watch for side effects: epigastric distress, abdominal cramps, nausea, and diarrhea or constipation.

2. Parenteral.

a. Administer Imferon (IV, IM), Sorbitex (IM).

b. Use Z-track to prevent pain and discoloration.

C. Monitor fluid and electrolyte balance.

D. Provide frequent rest periods for intense fatigue.

Pernicious Anemia

Definition: A chronic and, if untreated, progressive macrocytic anemia caused by the failure of gastric mucosa to produce an intrinsic factor essential for absorption of vitamin B_{12}. RNA is altered.

Characteristics

A. Causes

1. Total gastrectomy.
2. Surgical resection of small intestine.
3. Atrophy of gastric mucosa.
4. Malabsorption disease—sprue.
5. Bacterial or parasitic infections.

B. May be autoimmune difficulty.

C. Genetic predisposition (especially in northern Europe).

Assessment

A. Assess for neurological disturbance—tingling of extremities.

B. Assess for symptoms of spinal cord degeneration—alterations in gait.

C. Check any loss of finger movement.

D. Evaluate personality and behavioral changes.

E. Assess for glossitis—beefy, red tongue.

F. Assess for anorexia.

G. Assess for fatigue, weakness, pallor.

H. Observe yellow cast to skin.

Implementation

A. Obtain blood work for RBC count and megaloblastic maturation.

B. Prepare client for the following treatment:

1. Bone marrow aspiration (assist physician during test).
2. Upper GI series (administer bowel prep).
3. Schilling test (maintain n.p.o. for 12 hours; collect 24-hour urine).
4. Gastric analysis—insertion of nasogastric tube, collection of aspirant, injection of histamine.

C. Provide emotional support during bone marrow aspiration.

D. Provide safety measures if a neurological deficiency is present—assist with ambulation.

E. Avoid pressure on lower extremities due to circulatory changes (foot cradle, etc.).

F. Avoid extremes of heat and cold.

G. Provide support and explain behavior changes to client and family.

H. Administer B_{12} deep IM.

I. Instruct in administration of B_{12}—lifelong therapy.

Aplastic Anemia

Definition: Deficiency of circulating RBCs resulting from bone marrow suppression. Pancytopenia frequently accompanies RBC deficiency.

Characteristics

A. Etiology.

1. Toxic action of drugs (Chloromycetin, sulfonamides, Dilantin, alkylating, and antimetabolites).
2. Exposure to radiation.
3. Diseases that suppress bone marrow activity (leukemia and metastatic cancer).

B. Treatment.

1. Bone marrow transplant and WBC transfusion are becoming more prevalent.
2. Splenectomy (especially in severe thrombocytopenia).

Assessment

A. Assess for increased fatigue.

B. Assess for lethargy.

C. Assess for dyspnea.

D. Watch for cutaneous bleeding.

E. Evaluate blood for low platelet and leukocyte count.

Implementation

A. Avoid use of toxic chemical agents—DDT, carbon tetrachloride, etc.
B. Administer androgens and/or corticosteroids as ordered.
C. Monitor transfusion of fresh platelets (RBC transfusion may be introduced also).
D. Administer antibiotics when infection occurs.
E. Carry out reverse isolation procedure.
F. Protect from infections.
G. Provide for adequate rest periods.
H. Observe for complications.
I. Provide physical comfort measures.
J. Provide emotional support for client and family, especially while in isolation.
K. Educate public in use of toxic pesticides and chemicals.

SPLEEN

Definition: A glandlike organ located in the upper left part of the abdominal cavity; it is a storage organ for red corpuscles and, because of a large number of macrophages, acts as a blood filter.

Characteristics

A. Functions as a blood reservoir.
B. Purifies blood by removing waste and infectious organisms.
C. Destroys old red blood cells.
D. Is the primary source of antibodies in infants and children.
E. Produces lymphocytes, plasma cells, and antibodies in adults.
F. Produces erythrocytes in fetus.
G. Destroys erythrocytes when they reach the end of their life span.

Hypersplenism

Definition: The premature destruction of erythrocytes, leukocytes, and platelets.

Characteristics

A. The most common form of hypersplenism is congestive splenomegaly, usually due to portal hypertension secondary to cirrhosis.
B. Other causes are idiopathic thrombocytopenia, thrombosis, stenosis or atresia.
C. Secondary hypersplenism occurs in association with leukemias, lymphomas, Hodgkin's disease, and tuberculosis.
D. Treatment: correct underlying condition and/or splenectomy.

Rupture of the Spleen

Definition: Traumatic rupture following violent blow or trauma to the spleen.

Assessment

A. Assess weakness due to blood loss.
B. Evaluate abdominal pain and muscle spasm particularly in the left upper quadrant.
C. Assess for rebound tenderness.
D. Assess for referred pain to left shoulder.
E. Palpate for tenderness.
F. Check leukocytes (well over 12 thousand).
G. Assess for progressive shock with rapid, thready pulse; drop in blood pressure; and pallor.

Implementation

A. Prepare for surgical intervention—splenectomy.
B. Prevent infection.
C. Monitor vital signs closely.

Splenectomy

Definition: Excision of the spleen.

Assessment

A. Evaluate indications for surgical intervention.
   1. Trauma.
   2. Hypersplenism.
   3. Idiopathic thrombocytopenia.
   4. Hodgkin's disease.
   5. Lymphoma.
   6. Preceding renal transplantation (reduces rejection).
B. Observe for signs of infection.
C. Assess vital signs for baseline data.

Implementation

A. Prevent thrombus formation.
   1. Initiate bed exercises.
   2. Ambulate early.

3. Provide adequate hydration.
B. Prevent respiratory complications due to reduced expansion of left lung and location of spleen near diaphragm.
   1. Turn, cough, and deep breathe every two hours.
   2. Maintain IPPB if prone to URI.
C. Prevent infection if rupture occurs.
   1. Observe for signs of infection.
   2. Administer antibiotics.

NEOPLASTIC BLOOD DISORDERS

Leukemia

Definition: A disorder of blood-forming tissue characterized by neoplastic proliferation of hematopoietic cells or their precursors.

Characteristics

A. The increased proliferation process alters the cell's ability to mature and/or function correctly.
B. In acute processes the predominant cell is poorly differentiated but in chronic processes the leukemic cell is well defined.
C. Anemia results from an increased number of white blood cells that are immature and do not function normally and a decreased number of red blood cells, hemoglobin, and platelets.
D. Diagnostic tests.
   1. Bone marrow aspiration/biopsy.
   2. Differential count.
E. Etiology.
   1. Excess radiation exposure.
   2. Viral factors.
   3. Immune alteration.
   4. Noxious chemicals and drugs.
   5. Bone marrow alterations.

Assessment

A. Assess for sudden high fever with abnormal bleeding.
B. Assess for nosebleeds, purpura, ecchymosis, petechiae, or prolonged menses.
C. Evaluate general nonspecific symptoms such as weakness, lethargy, low-grade fever.
D. Evaluate recurrent infections if any of the above symptoms are present.

Chemotherapy Principles

A. Combination of drugs used.
   1. Limits toxicity of individual drugs.
   2. Increases destruction of cells sensitive to various agents.
B. Induction therapy used after initial diagnosis.
C. Maintenance therapy used during remission.

Implementation

A. Administer chemotherapeutic agents as ordered.
   1. Antimetabolites: interfere with cellular metabolic process, thereby stopping synthesis of cell protein.
      a. Common drugs: cytosine arabinoside, thioguanine, 6-mercaptopurine, fluorourail (5-FU), methotrexate.
      b. Toxic effects: anorexia, nausea, vomiting, diarrhea, skin rash, alopecia, hyperuricemia, stomatitis, depression of bone marrow.
   2. Alkylating agents damage DNA production of cells.
      a. Common drugs: thiotepa, nitrogen mustard, Cytoxan Leukeran, busulfan, Alkeran, Myleran.
      b. Toxic effects: stomatitis, alopecia, anorexia, nausea, vomiting, bone marrow depression, skin reactions.
   3. Antibiotic agents: interfere with synthesis of RNA.
      a. Common drugs: Adriamycin, daunorubicin, dactinomycin, bleomycin, mithramycin, mitomycin.
      b. Toxic effects: nausea, vomiting, alopecia, stomatitis, skin rash, bone marrow depression, fever.
   4. Plant alkaloids.
      a. Common drugs: vincristine, vinblastine.
      b. Toxic effects: nausea, vomiting, alopecia, stomatitis, bone marrow depression, paralytic ileus, peripheral neuritis.
   5. Enzymes
      a. Common drug: L-asparaginase.
      b. Toxic effects: nausea, vomiting, hyperglycemia, hypersensitivity reactions, bone marrow depression.
   6. Hormones
      a. Common drugs.
         (1) Estrogens: DES, Estinyl.

(2) Progestins: Delalutin, Megace, Provera.

(3) Androgens: testosterone.

(4) Adrenocorticosteroids: Meticorten.

(5) Dexamethasone: Decadron.

   b. Toxic effects: edema, increased susceptibility to infection, sex characteristic alterations, electrolyte alterations.

  7. Combination drugs.

    a. VAMP: vincristine, amethopterin, 6-MP, prednisone.

    b. POMP: prednisone, Oncovin, methotrexate, 6-MP.

    c. COAP: Cytoxan, Oncovin, Ara-C, prednisone.

B. Prevent complications related to the side effects of drugs.

  1. Proper mouth care (ulcerations and bleeding).

  2. Anorexia.

C. Maintain fluid and electrolyte balance.

D. Administer allopurinol to combat problems associated with increased serum uric acid (from rapid destruction of body tissue).

E. Provide high-calorie, high-vitamin diet to prevent weight loss, weakness, debilitation.

F. Provide emotional support.

  1. Alopecia.

  2. Altered body image.

  3. Fear of dying.

  4. Depression.

  5. Financial burden.

G. Provide client education.

  1. Drugs—dosage and side effects.

  2. Associated treatments.

  3. Disease process.

H. Prevent infections, ulcerations, hemorrhage.

Acute Myelogenous Leukemia (AML)

Characteristics

A. Incidence: occurs more commonly after forty years of age, slightly higher incidence in males. Onset can be insidious or rapid.

B. Pathophysiology: stem cell of WBC proliferates, decreasing stem cells availability for RBCs and platelets.

Assessment

A. Assess for anemia and symptoms of dyspnea, fatigue, pallor, palpitations.

B. Assess for symptoms of platelet deficiency: epistaxis, gingival bleeds, purpura, petechiae, or bleeding in major systems.

C. Assess for symptoms of local abscesses, elevated temperature, chills.

D. Palpate for splenomegaly.

E. Assess for lymph node enlargement and difficulty with respiration and swallowing.

F. Assess for bone pain.

G. Evaluate CNS involvement with signs of increased ICP.

H. Check for hyperuricemia.

Implementation

A. Administer medications.

  1. Cytarabine and thioguanine.

  2. COAP.

B. Monitor local irradiation for lymph node enlargement and bone pain.

C. Administer antibiotics for increased temperature.

D. Monitor platelet administration when bleeding occurs.

E. Administer allopurinol when hyperuricemia occurs.

Chronic Myelocytic Leukemia (CML)

Characteristics

A. Incidence: primarily a disease of young adults. Thought to have a genetic origin. Philadelphia chromosome is involved.

B. Pathophysiology: marked increase of granulocytes and megakaryocyte (platelet cell). The mature neutrophil is the cell that is predominant.

Assessment

A. Assess for fatigue and malaise.

B. Palpate for splenomegaly.

C. Observe skin for pallor, purpura, nodules.

D. Assess for abdominal discomfort.

E. Evaluate fever, heat intolerance, or increased perspiration.

F. Assess for retinal hemorrhage.

G. Assess for bone pain.

H. Assess anemia.

I. Evaluate increased uric acid level.

Implementation

A. Administer oral alkylating agent (Myleran).
B. Prepare for splenectomy or irradiation.
C. Instruct client and family in preventative principles.
  1. Good nutrition.
  2. Prevention of infection.
  3. Complicating signs.
  4. Skin care.
  5. Adequate rest to minimize weakness.

Chronic Lymphocytic Leukemia (CLL)

Characteristics

A. Incidence—insidious onset, most common in ages fifty to seventy.
B. Pathophysiology—the small lymphocyte (B cell) is the predominant cell type and eventually leads to decreased production of other hematopoietic cells.

Assessment

A. Assess classic signs.
  1. Anemia.
  2. Weight loss.
  3. Abdominal discomfort with hepatomegaly/splenomegaly.
  4. Palpable lymph nodes.
B. Assess less common signs.
  1. Excessive diaphoresis.
  2. Malaise and fatigue.
  3. Infection.

Implementation

A. Administer drugs: chlorambucil (Leukeran), cyclophosphamide (Cytoxan).
B. Prepare for splenectomy in some cases.
C. Prevent infection, be especially oriented toward maintaining clean skin.
D. Observe for complications: thrombocytopenia.
E. Provide emotional support.

Acute Lymphocytic Leukemia (ALL)

Characteristics

A. Incidence—usually appears before age fifteen but is highest in three- to four-year-olds. Males slightly more at risk.
B. Pathophysiology—the lymphoblasts are most responsible for the pathogenesis with eventual reduction of other blood cells.

Assessment

A. Assess for malaise, fatigue, and fever.
B. Assess bone involvement and lymph and spleen alterations.
C. Check for bleeding gums, skin and nose.
D. Evaluate CNS symptoms, especially stiff neck and headache.

Implementation

A. Prepare for induction chemotherapy.
B. Maintain therapy when in remission.
C. Administer drugs: methotrexate, daunomycin, Oncovin.

MALIGNANCY OF THE LYMPH SYSTEM

Hodgkin's Disease

Definition: A chronic, progressive, neoplastic, invariably fatal reticuloendothelial disease involving the lymphoid tissues of the body. It is most common between the ages of twenty and forty. While the exact etiology is unknown, the suspected sources are viral, environmental, genetic, and immunologic. Onset is often insidious.

Assessment

A. Assess for painless enlargement of cervical lymph nodes.
B. Assess for severe pruritus.
C. Evaluate irregular fever, night sweats.
D. Palpate for splenomegaly and hepatomegaly.
E. Observe for jaundice, weight loss.
F. Assess edema and cyanosis of the face and neck.
G. Evaluate pulmonary symptoms including dyspnea, cough, chest pain, cyanosis, and pleural effusion.
H. Assess for fatigue, malaise, and anorexia, which indicates progressive anemia.
I. Evaluate bone pain and vertebral compression.
J. Assess nerve pain and paraplegia.
K. Assess laryngeal paralysis.
L. Evaluate increased susceptibility to infection.
M. Assess degree of staging.
  1. Stage I: disease is restricted to single anatomic site, or is localized in a group of lymph nodes; asymptomatic.
  2. Stage II(a): two or three adjacent lymph nodes in the area on the same side of the diaphragm are affected.

MEDICAL IMPLICATIONS

A. Radiation is used for stages I, II, and III in an effort to eradicate the disease.
B. Wide-field megavoltage radiation with doses of 3500 to 4000 roentgens over a four- to six-week period.
C. Chemotherapy with Cytoxan, nitrogen mustard, thiotepa, TEM, Velban, Oncovin, prednisone, and Matulane.
D. Diagnostic laparotomy.

3. Stage II(b): symptoms appear.
4. Stage III: disease is widely disseminated on both sides of diaphragm into the lymph areas and organs.
5. Stage IV: involvement of bone, bone marrow, pleura, liver, skin, gastrointestinal tract, central nervous system, and gradually the entire body.

Implementation

A. Provide supportive relief from effects of radiation and chemotherapy.
   1. Side effects include nausea and vomiting.
   2. Controlled by premedication of sedatives and antiemetic agents.
B. Assist client to maintain as normal a life as possible during course and treatment of disease.
   1. Counsel client and family to accept process of treatment.
   2. Provide supportive assistance in dealing with feelings of anger, depression, fear, and loneliness.
C. Prevent infection as body's resistance is lowered.
D. Continually observe for complications: pressure from enlargement of lymph glands on vital organs.

ENDOCRINE SYSTEM

The endocrine system consists of a series of glands that function individually or conjointly to integrate and control innumerable metabolic activities of the body. These glands automatically regulate various body processes by releasing chemical signals called hormones.

ANATOMY AND PHYSIOLOGY

Function

A. Maintenance and regulation of vital functions.
  1. Response to stress or injury.
  2. Growth and development.
  3. Reproduction.
  4. Fluid, electrolyte, and acid-base balance.
  5. Energy metabolism.
B. Endocrine glands.
  1. Have specific functions.
  2. Influence one another.
  3. Secrete hormones.
  4. Controlled by autonomic nervous system.
  5. Located in various parts of body.
C. Hormones.
  1. Proteins or steroids.
  2. Chemical messengers that stimulate or inhibit life processes.
  3. Transmitted via the bloodstream to target tissues.
  4. Regulated through negative feedback control system (hypothalamic-pituitary axis). For example, the TSH-releasing hormone (TRH) is secreted by the hypothalamus, which causes the pituitary to secrete TSH. TSH stimulates the thyroid to secrete thyroxine. Thyroxine feeds back on the pituitary and inhibits production of TSH.
  5. Also regulated by renin-angiotensin-aldosterone, insulin-glucose, and calcium-parathormone.
  6. Endocrine disorders caused by a deficit or excess in hormone production.

Structure

A. Hypothalamus connects pituitary gland to central nervous system.
B. Pituitary gland divided into three lobes.
  1. Anterior pituitary control (master gland).
     a. Tropic hormones exert effect through regulation of other endocrine glands—ACTH, TSH, FSH, LH.
     b. Target tissues: hormones have direct effect on tissues—growth hormone, prolactin, MSH.
  2. Posterior lobe (neurohypophysis)—ADH, oxytocin, melanophore stimulating hormone.
  3. Intermediate lobe.

System Assessment

A. Assess for growth imbalance.
  1. Excessive growth.
     a. Pituitary or hypothalamic disorders.
     b. Excess adrenal, ovarian, or testicular hormone.
  2. Retarded growth.
     a. Endocrine and metabolic disorders; difficult to distinguish from dwarfism.
     b. Hypothyroidism.
B. Evaluate obesity.
  1. Sudden onset suggests hypothalamic lesion (rare).
  2. Cushing's syndrome (with characteristic buffalo hump).
C. Assess abnormal skin pigmentation.
  1. Hyperpigmentation may coexist with depigmentation in Addison's disease.
  2. Thyrotoxicosis may be associated with spotty brown pigmentation.
  3. Pruritus is a common symptom in diabetes.
D. Check for hirsutism.
  1. Normal variations in body occur on nonendocrine basis.
  2. First sign of neoplastic disease.
  3. Indicates changes in adrenal status.
E. Evaluate appetite changes.
  1. Polyphagia is a common sign of uncontrolled diabetes.

Table 1. ENDOCRINE SYSTEM

Endocrine Gland	Hormones Produced	Function	Endocrine Disorder

Pituitary
 	
Location: Base of the brain
	Anterior Lobe
	  Adrenocorticotropic hormone (ACTH)
	  Thyrotropic hormone (TSH)
	  Somatotropic growth stimulating hormone (STH)
	  Gonadotropic hormones (FSH, LH, LTH)
	Posterior Lobe
	  Vasopressin (ADH)
	  Oxytocin
	  Melanophore stimulating hormone (MSH)
		Termed "master gland" as it directly affects the function of other endocrine glands.
		Controls sexual development and function.
		Promotes growth of body tissues.
		Influences water absorption by kidney.
		Influenced by hypothalamus.
			Anterior pituitary
			  Giantism
			  Acromegaly
			  Dwarfism
			Posterior pituitary
			  Diabetes insipidus

Adrenal
 	
Location: On top of each kidney
	Cortex
	  Glucocorticoids
	    Cortisol
	    Cortisone
	    Corticosterone
	  Mineralocorticoids
	    Aldosterone
	    Deoxycorticosterone
	    Corticosterone
	  Sex hormones
	    Androgens
	    Estrogens
	Medulla
	  Epinephrine
	  Norepinephrine
		Regulates sodium and electrolyte balance.
		Affects carbohydrate, fat, and protein metabolism.
		Influences the development of sexual characteristics.
		Stimulates "fight or flight" response to danger.
			Addison's disease
			Cushing's syndrome
			Pheochromocytoma
			Primary aldosteronism

Thyroid Location: Anterior part of the neck	Thyroxine Triiodothyronine Thyrocalcitonin	Controls rate of body metabolism, growth, and nutrition.	Goiter Cretinism Myxedema Hyperthyroidism (Graves' disease)
Parathyroid Location: Near thyroid	Parathormone (PTH)	Controls calcium and phosphorus metabolism.	Hypoparathyroidism Hyperparathyroidism
Pancreas Islets of Langerhans Location: Posterior to liver	Insulin Glucagon	Influences carbohydrate metabolism. Indirectly influences fat and protein metabolism.	Diabetes mellitus Hyperinsulinism
Ovaries Location: Pelvic cavity Testes Location: Scrotum	Estrogen and progesterone Testosterone	Controls development of secondary sex characteristics.	Lack of acceleration or regression of sexual development

Table 2. HORMONE PHYSIOLOGY

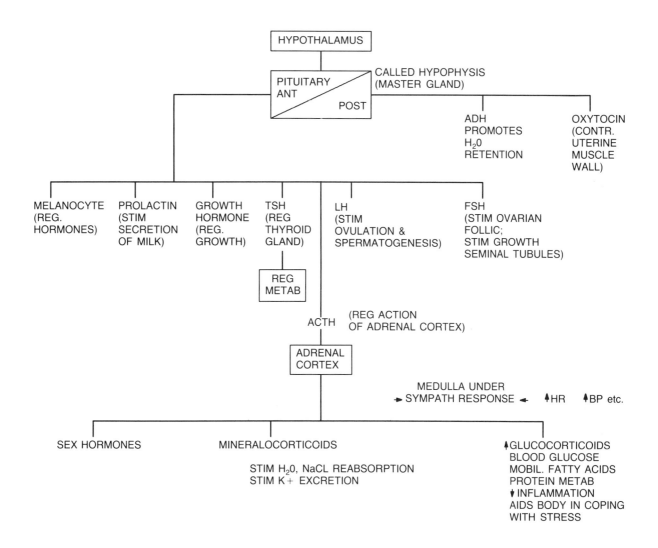

2. Indicates thyrotoxicosis.

3. Nausea and weight loss may indicate addisonian crisis or diabetic acidosis.

F. Check for polyuria and polydipsia.

1. Symptoms usually of nonendocrine etiology.

2. If sudden onset, suggest diabetes mellitus or insipidus.

3. May be present with hyperparathyroidism or hyperaldosteronism.

G. Assess mental changes.

1. Though often subtle, may be indicative of underlying endocrine disorder.

   a. Nervousness and excitability may indicate hyperthyroidism.

   b. Mental confusion may indicate hypopituitarism, Addison's disease, or myxedema.

2. Mental deterioration is observed in untreated hypoparathyroidism and hypothyroidism.

H. Assess for coma state.

1. Drowsiness.

2. Hypernea.

3. Tachycardia.

4. Subnormal temperature.

5. Fruity odor to breath.

6. Acetone in urine (test done if over 2+ sugar in urine).

7. Stupor leading to coma.

Diagnostic Procedures

Radioactive Iodine (RAI) Uptake (Radioiodine ^{131}I)

A. Purpose: measures the absorption of the iodine isotope to determine how the thyroid gland is functioning.

B. Principles.

1. The use of ^{123}I rather than ^{131}I is now preferred because of its lower radiation hazard. (^{123}I can be used on pregnant women while ^{131}I is contraindicated.)

2. The amount of radioactivity is measured 2, 6, and 24 hours after ingestion of the capsule.

3. ^{131}I (as does ^{123}I) evaluates the storage of iodine and gives a distribution pattern.

C. Results.

1. Normal values: 5 to 35 percent in 24 hours (recently lowered values in United States due to increased ingestion of iodine).

2. Elevated values indicate: hyperthyroidism, thyrotoxicosis, hypofunctioning goiter, iodine lack, excessive hormonal losses.

3. Depressed values indicate: low T_4, antithyroid drugs, thyroiditis, myxedema, or hypothyroidism.

T_3 and T_4 Resin Uptake Tests

A. Purpose: both of these *in vitro* tests are used as screening tests for diagnosis in thyroid disorders. T_4 is 90 percent accurate in diagnosing hyperthyroidism and hypothyroidism.

B. Principles.

1. Levels of T_3 and T_4 in the blood regulate thyroid stimulating hormone (TSH).

2. These levels alter according to a balancing system of negative feedback.

3. Venous blood sample is obtained to directly measure concentration of unsaturated thyroxine-binding globulin in the serum.

4. Thyroid function tests should be interpreted according to the clinical situation.

C. Results.

1. Normal values.

   a. T_4: 3.8 to 11.4%.

   b. T_3: 25 to 35%.

2. T_4.

   a. Elevated: hyperthyroidism, early hepatitis, exogenous T_4.

   b. Decreased: hypothyroidism, abnormal binding, exogenous T_3.

3. T_3.

   a. Elevated: hyperthyroidism, T_3 toxicosis.

   b. Decreased: advancing age.

Thyroid Stimulation Test

A. Purpose: differentiates primary from secondary hypothyroidism and assesses level of thyroid gland activity.

B. Principles.

1. Administration of IM TSH (thyrotropin) measures the responsiveness of the thyroid gland.

2. Blood samples are obtained at intervals.

C. Results.

1. Normal values less than $10\mu U/ml$ (may vary with laboratory).

2. Increased values indicate primary hypothyroidism.

3. Decreased values indicate hyperthyroidism, large doses of glucocorticoids, secondary hypothyroidism.

Glucose Tolerance Test

A. Purpose: primary aim is to diagnose or rule out diabetes, but also important for unexplained hypoglycemia and malabsorption syndrome.

B. Principles.
1. This test determines rate of removal of a concentrated dose of glucose from the bloodstream.
2. Test is indicated when there is sugar in the urine or when fasting blood sugar is elevated.
3. This is a timed test done in the morning after fasting for at least 12 hours. Blood and urine samples are taken at intervals up to three hours.
4. This test is contraindicated for recent surgical clients or clients with history of myocardial infarctions.

C. Results.
1. Normal values are between 60 to 125 mg fasting and no sugar in the urine.
2. Increased values indicate hyperinsulinism, Addison's disease, hypothyroidism, or celiac disease.
3. Decreased values indicate diabetes, hyperthyroidism, hyperplasia, anemia, or certain central nervous system disorders.

System Planning and Analysis

A. Specific endocrine disorder is identified.
B. Regulating effect of organs is reestablished.
C. Hormone production remains equalized and deficit or excess is corrected.
D. Clinical manifestations of endocrine disorders are corrected.
E. Fluid, electrolyte, and acid-base balance are maintained.
F. Energy metabolism is stabilized.

System Implementation

A. Administer hormone replacement on time to keep blood level stable.
B. Monitor for side effects of hormone replacement therapy.

C. Identify clinical manifestations indicating hyperfunction or hypofunction of endocrine glands.
D. Monitor for fluid and electrolyte imbalances due to hormone imbalance.
E. Provide appropriate diet specific for endocrine disorder.
F. Promote rest and reduce stress.
G. Prepare client physically and psychologically for surgical removal of endocrine gland.
H. Instruct client on methods to prevent infection.
I. Differentiate diabetic coma from other causes.
1. Urinalysis for sugar and acetone.
2. Blood sugar level.
3. Eyeballs—soft due to loss of intracellular fluid.
4. Undigested food is found in stomach if Levin tube is inserted.

System Evaluation

A. Imbalances in hormone production (either deficits or excess) are corrected by replacement hormones.
B. Side effects of replacement hormones are minimal.
C. Vital functions directed by endocrine glands are preserved.
D. Fluid and electrolytes remain balanced.
E. Diagnostic studies reveal no irreversible hyperfunction or hypofunction of endocrine glands.
F. Side effects of hormone imbalance diminish after treatment.
G. Nutritional status is maintained.
H. Infectious processes are prevented.

Conditions Associated with Hormonal Imbalances

A. Tumors of the glands.
1. Benign (common).
2. Malignant (rare).
3. Ectopic.
B. Absence of gland.
C. Autoimmune factors.
D. Infections.
E. Side effects of replacement hormones.
F. Dysfunction of the pituitary gland, which affects functioning of the target glands.

PITUITARY GLAND DISORDERS

Acromegaly (Anterior Pituitary Hyperfunction)

Definition: The hypersecretion of growth hormone by the anterior pituitary. Occurs in adulthood after closure of the epiphyses of the long bones.

Assessment

A. Assess for excessive growth of short, flat bones.
  1. Large hands and feet.
  2. Thickening and protrusion of the jaw and orbital ridges that cause teeth to spread.
  3. Increased growth of soft tissue.
  4. Coarse features.
  5. Pain in joints.
B. Evaluate voice which becomes deeper.
C. Assess increased diaphoresis.
D. Assess for oily, rough skin.
E. Assess increased hair growth over the body.
F. Evaluate menstrual disturbances; impotence.
G. Assess for symptoms associated with local compression of brain by tumor.
  1. Headache.
  2. Visual disturbances; blindness.
H. Check any related hormonal imbalances.
  1. Diabetes mellitus (growth hormone is insulin antagonist).
  2. Cushing's syndrome.
I. Evaluate laboratory values—increased growth hormone level.

Implementation

A. Provide emotional support.
  1. Encourage client's expression of feelings.
    a. Loss of self-image and self-esteem.
    b. Fears about brain surgery.
    c. Consequences of surgery (sterility and lifetime hormone replacement).
  2. Have client avoid situations that may be embarrassing.
  3. Encourage support of and communication with family.
B. Provide frequent skin care.
C. Position and support painful joints.
D. Test urine for sugar and acetone.
E. Administer supportive care for irradiation of pituitary.
F. Provide preoperative and postoperative care for hypophysectomy.

Giantism (Anterior Pituitary Hyperfunction)

Definition: The hypersecretion of growth hormone by the anterior pituitary. Occurs in childhood prior to closure of the epiphyses of the long bones.

Assessment

A. Assess for symmetrical overgrowth of the long bones.
B. Evaluate increased height in early adulthood (may be eight to nine feet).
C. Check for deterioration of mental and physical processes, which may occur in early adulthood.
D. Assess for other tissue response similar to acromegaly.

Implementation

A. Supportive care for irradiation of pituitary.
B. Provide preoperative and postoperative care for hypophysectomy.

Hypophysectomy

Definition: The removal of the pituitary gland because of tumor formation.

Surgical Procedures

A. Craniotomy.
B. Microsurgery.
C. Cryohypophysectomy.
D. Hormone replacement.

Implementation

A. Preoperative care.
  1. Provide general preoperative care.
  2. Provide emotional support.
B. Postoperative care.
  1. Administer corticosteroids on time.
  2. Monitor fluid and electrolyte balance.
    a. Hypernatremic due to ADH disturbance leading to fluid imbalance.
    b. Avoid water intoxication.
  3. Carefully monitor vital signs.
  4. Monitor blood gas determinations.
  5. Provide routine care for craniotomy. Observe for:

a. Vital signs.
b. Increased intracranial pressure.
c. Shock.
d. LOC.
6. Initiate client education.
a. Compensate for altered stress response.
b. Avoid contact with infectious individuals.
c. Carry emergency adrenal hormone drugs.
d. Use medic-alert arm band.
C. Monitor for complications.
1. Craniotomy—bleeding in acromegaly (due to excessive growth of frontal bones).
2. Microsurgery—rhinorrhea and meningitis (due to interruption of CSF during surgery).
3. Cryohypophysectomy—probe hits other vital structures.

Dwarfism (Anterior Pituitary Hypofunction)

Definition: Dwarfism is the hyposecretion of growth hormone by the anterior pituitary. Growth is symmetrical but decreased.

Assessment

A. Assess for retarded physical growth.
B. Evaluate premature body-aging processes.
C. Assess for pale, dry, smooth skin.
D. Check poor development of secondary sex characteristics and external genitalia.
E. Evaluate slow intellectual development.

Implementation

A. Administer human growth hormone (HGH) injections if the imbalance is diagnosed and treated in early stage.
B. Monitor for complications.

Diabetes Insipidus (Posterior Pituitary Hypofunction)

Definition: An antidiuretic hormone (ADH) deficiency, usually seen in young adults, resulting from damage or tumors in the posterior lobe of the pituitary gland. May develop following brain surgery or head injury.

Assessment

A. Assess for severe polyuria and polydipsia.
B. Evaluate fatigue and muscle pain.
C. Assess for dehydration.

D. Assess weight loss, muscle weakness, headache.
E. Check laboratory values—low urinary specific gravity (<1.006).
F. Evaluate for inability to concentrate urine.

Implementation

A. Maintain adequate fluids.
B. Measure intake and output and weight.
C. Stress importance of medic-alert band.
D. Avoid liquids or foods with diuretic-type action.
E. Provide comfort measures if client is on radiation therapy.
F. Provide preoperative and postoperative care for hypophysectomy.
G. Administer vasopressin tannate (Pitressin Tannate), IM, or nasal spray if ordered.
H. Administer benzthiazide diuretics for mild cases.
I. Give Diabinese to potentiate vasopressin or act as antidiuretic.
J. Give supportive care for irradiation of tumor.

ADRENAL CORTEX DISORDERS

Addison's Disease (Adrenocortical Hypofunction)

Definition: The hypofunction of the adrenal cortex of the adrenal gland, resulting in deficiency of the steroid hormones. It often has a slow and insidious onset and is eventually fatal if left untreated.

Assessment

A. Assess normal dietary intake.
B. Assess for lassitude, lethargy, and generalized weakness.
C. Check out any gastrointestinal disturbances, nausea, diarrhea, and anorexia.
D. Assess for hypotension.
E. Evaluate increased pigmentation of the skin of nipples, buccal mucosa, and scars. This condition occurs in 15 percent of clients.
F. Evaluate emotional disturbances.
G. Assess weight loss.
H. Assess laboratory values.
1. Elevated potassium; decreased sodium; elevated BUN levels due to decreased glomerular filtration rate.
2. Low blood sugar.

3. Lack of normal rise in urinary output of 17-ketosteroids and 17-hydroxycorticosteroids following IV administration of ACTH over eight hours.
4. Lack of normal rise in blood level of plasma cortisol following IM injection of ACTH.

Implementation

A. Take daily weight and keep accurate intake and output records.
B. Take vital signs q.i.d.
C. Check for inadequate or overdosage of hormones.
   1. Cortisone and hydrocortisone.
      a. Sodium and water retention.
      b. Potassium depletion.
      c. Drug-induced Cushing's syndrome.
      d. Gastric irritation (give medication with meal or antacid).
      e. Mood swings.
      f. Local abscess at injection site when given IM (inject deeply into gluteal muscle).
      g. Addisonian crisis, which might be produced by sudden withdrawal of medication.
   2. Fludrocortisone acetate (Florinef)—the same side effects as cortisone and hydrocortisone, particularly sodium retention and potassium depletion.
   3. Desoxycorticosterone (Cortate, Doca Acetate)—sodium retention and potassium depletion.
D. Protect from exposure to infection and from stress.
E. High-protein, high-carbohydrate diet in small, frequent feedings.
F. Provide emotional support.
G. Provide client education.
   1. Safe self-administration of replacement hormones. Lifelong replacement therapy with synthetic corticosteroid drugs is necessary.
   2. Avoidance of over-the-counter drugs.
   3. Care to avoid infections; report promptly to physician if infections appear.
   4. Medic-alert band.
   5. Regular exercise; avoid strenuous activity, particularly in hot weather.
   6. Importance of continuous medical supervision.
   7. Avoidance of stress.

Addisonian Crisis

Definition: A condition caused by adrenal insufficiency, which may be precipitated by infection, trauma, stress, surgery, or diaphoresis with excessive salt loss. Death may occur from shock, vascular collapse, or hyperkalemia.

Assessment

A. Assess for severe headache and abdominal, leg, and lower back pain.
B. Assess for extreme, generalized muscular weakness.
C. Evaluate for severe hypotension and shock.
D. Assess for irritability and confusion.

Implementation

A. Administer parenteral fluids for restoration of electrolyte balance.
B. Administer adrenocorticosteroids; do not vary dosage or time from that ordered.
C. Continually monitor vital signs and intake and output until crisis passes.
D. Protect client from infection.
E. Keep client immobile and as quiet as possible; avoid unnecessary nursing procedures.

Cushing's Syndrome (Adrenocortical Hyperfunction)

Definition: Clinical condition resulting from the combined metabolic effects of persistently elevated blood levels of glucocorticoids.

Characteristics

A. Etiology.
   1. Overactivity of adrenal cortex.
   2. Benign or malignant tumor of adrenal gland.
B. Cause may be iatrogenic—drug therapy for other conditions.

Assessment

A. Assess for abnormal adipose tissue distribution.
   1. Moon face.
   2. Buffalo hump.
   3. Obese trunk with thin extremities.
B. Assess skin—color and texture.
   1. Florid facies.
   2. Red striae of skin stretched with fat tissue.
   3. Fragile skin, easily bruised.
C. Assess for osteoporosis—susceptible to fractures, renal stones.
D. Assess for hyperglycemia—may eventually develop diabetes mellitus.

E. Evaluate mood swings—euphoria to depression.

F. Check for high susceptibility to infections; diminished immuno-response to infections once they occur.

G. Evaluate lassitude and muscular weakness.

H. Assess for masculine characteristics in females.

I. Check for thin extremities.

J. Assess for hypertension.

K. Evaluate electrolyte imbalance.
   1. Potassium depletion.
   2. Sodium and water retention.

L. Assess laboratory values.
   1. Elevated blood sugar and glycosuria.
   2. Elevated white blood count with depressed eosinophils and lymphocytes.
   3. Elevated plasma cortisone levels.
   4. Elevated 17-hydroxycorticosteroids in urine.

Implementation

A. Protect from infections.

B. Protect from accidents or falls.

C. Provide meticulous skin care, avoiding harsh soaps.

D. Provide low-calorie, high-protein, high-potassium diet.

E. Provide emotional support.
   1. Allow for ventilation of client's feelings.
   2. Avoid reactions to client's appearance.
   3. Anticipate the needs of the client.
   4. Explain that changes in body appearance and emotional liability should improve with treatment.

F. Measure intake and output and daily weights; test for urinary sugar.

G. Follow specific nursing measures posthypophysectomy.

H. Provide comfort measures during radiation therapy, usually cobalt irradiation of the pituitary.

I. Provide postsurgery care for adrenalectomy, unilateral or bilateral.
   1. Bilateral—lifetime replacement of steroids.
   2. Unilateral—temporary steroid replacement (6 to 12 months).

J. Administer chemotherapy for inoperable, cancerous tumors (Mitotane).

K. Provide client teaching.
   1. Importance of continuous medical supervision.
   2. Safe self-administration of replacement hormones.
   3. Side effects of medications.

4. Avoidance of infections and stress.

5. Need for adequate nutrition and rest.

Primary Aldosteronism

Definition: A disorder due to the hypersecretion of aldosterone from the adrenal cortex of the adrenal gland. It is usually caused by tumors. Females are more at risk.

Assessment

A. Assess for hypokalemia.
   1. Weakness of muscles.
   2. Excessive urine output (polyuria); excessive thirst (polydipsia).
   3. Metabolic alkalosis.

B. Assess for hypertension, postural hypotension, headache.

C. Check for positive Chvostek's sign (muscle twitching when area over facial nerves is tapped).

D. Assess laboratory values
   1. Lowered potassium level.
   2. Elevated serum sodium level.
   3. Increased urinary output of aldosterone.
   4. Alkalosis.

Implementation

A. Provide quiet environment.

B. Measure intake and output and daily weights.

C. Check muscular strength and presence of Chvostek's sign.

D. Measure blood pressure in supine and standing positions.

E. Provide same postoperative care as for adrenalectomy.

F. Monitor administration of potassium salts and spironolactone.

ADRENAL MEDULLA DISORDERS

Pheochromocytoma (Hyperfunction)

Definition: A small tumor in the adrenal medulla of the adrenal gland that secretes large amounts of epinephrine and norepinephrine. Familial autosomal dominant.

Assessment

A. Observe that condition occurs primarily in children and middle-aged women.

B. Assess for hypertension—primary manifestation.

C. Observe for sudden attacks that resemble overstimulation of the sympathetic nervous system.

   1. Hypertension.

   2. Severe headache.

   3. Excessive diaphoresis.

   4. Palpitation, tachycardia.

   5. Nervousness and hyperactivity.

   6. Nausea, vomiting, and anorexia.

   7. Dilated pupils.

   8. Cold extremities.

   9. Cardiac failure or cerebral hemorrhage leading to death if not treated.

D. Assess for increased rate of metabolism and loss of weight.

E. Evaluate hyperglycemia.

F. Assess laboratory values.

   1. Findings common to hypertension, cardiac disease, and loss of kidney function.

   2. Elevated vanillymandelic acid (VMA) and catecholamine levels in urine.

   3. Elevated blood levels of catecholamines.

   4. Elevated blood sugar and glycosuria.

   5. Presence of tumor on x-rays.

Implementation

A. Monitor for evidence of hypertensive attacks; keep Regitine at bedside for hypertensive crisis.

B. Monitor for normal vital signs and absence of glycosuria after a-adrenegic blocking agents (phenoxybenzamine) are given.

C. Test urine daily for glucose and acetone.

D. Provide high-calorie, nutritious diet omitting stimulants.

E. Promote rest and reduce stress.

F. Provide preoperative care for surgical excision of tumor.

   1. Give Regitine one to two days before surgery to counteract hypertensive effects of epinephrine and norepinephrine.

   2. Closely monitor blood pressure during interval of phentolamine administration.

G. Provide postoperative care—observe for precipitous shock, hemorrhage, persistent hypertension.

H. Administer drugs if ordered: alpha blocker; phentolamine, phenoxybenzamine.

Adrenalectomy

Definition: Surgical removal of an adrenal gland when overproduction of adrenal hormone is evident (Cushing's syndrome, pheochromocytoma) or in metastatic breast or prostatic cancer.

Assessment

A. Assess test results that indicate whether radiation, drug therapy, or surgery is appropriate to reverse Cushing's syndrome or restore hormone balance.

B. Surgical intervention requires special management.

   1. Assess hypertension.

   2. Assess degree of edema.

   3. Evaluate for signs of diabetes.

   4. Assess for cardiovascular manifestations.

C. Assess client's knowledge of disorder and understanding of management.

D. Assess all laboratory reports before surgery.

   1. Check for signs of hypernatremia and hypokalemia.

   2. Assess for hyperglycemia or glycosuria.

E. Assess dietary intake and fluid intake and output.

F. Assess for complications.

   1. Wound infections.

   2. Hemorrhage.

   3. Peptic ulcers.

   4. Pulmonary disorders.

Implementation

A. Preoperative care.

   1. Provide general preoperative care.

   2. Administer exogenous glucocorticoids.

B. Postoperative care.

   1. Monitor vital signs and intake and output.

   2. Administer parenteral fluids.

   3. Strictly adhere to sterile techniques when changing dressings.

   4. Observe for shock, hypoglycemia.

   5. Maintain hydrocortisone therapy.

THYROID GLAND DISORDERS

Cretinism (Thyroid Hypofunction)

Definition: A condition caused by severe hypofunction of the thyroid gland in the fetus, in utero, or soon after birth.

Assessment

A. Assess for severe retardation of physical development, resulting in grotesque appearance, sexual retardation.
B. Assess for severe mental retardation, apathy.
C. Check for dry skin; coarse, dry, brittle hair.
D. Assess for constipation.
E. Evaluate slow teething.
F. Evaluate poor appetite.
G. Observe for large tongue.
H. Observe for pot belly with umbilical hernia.
I. Evaluate sensitivity to cold.
J. Assess for yellow skin.
K. Assess laboratory values.
 1. T_4 under 3 μg/100 ml.
 2. Elevated serum cholesterol.
 3. Low radioactive iodine uptake.

Implementation

A. Administer desiccated thyroid or Synthroid.
B. Administer Cytomel, which is used when rapid response is needed.

Myxedema (Adult Hypothyroidism)

Definition: The decreased synthesis of thyroid hormone in adulthood, resulting in a hypothyroid state. Occurs primarily in older age group, five times more frequent in women than in men.

Assessment

A. Assess for slowed rate of body metabolism.
 1. Lethargy, apathy, and fatigue.
 2. Intolerance to cold.
 3. Hypersensitivity to sedatives and barbiturates.
 4. Weight gain.
 5. Cool, dry, rough skin.
 6. Coarse, dry hair.
B. Assess for personality changes.
 1. Forgetfulness and loss of memory.
 2. Complacency.
C. Assess for anorexia, constipation, and fecal impactions.
D. Observe for interstitial edema.
 1. Nonpitting edema in the lower extremity.
 2. Generalized puffiness.
E. Observe decreased diaphoresis.
F. Check for menstrual disturbances.
G. Assess for cardiac complications.
 1. Coronary heart disease.
 2. Angina pectoris.
 3. MI and congestive heart failure.
H. Evaluate anemia.
I. Assess laboratory findings.
 1. Low serum thyrotoxin concentration.
 2. Hyponatremia.

Implementation

A. Allow time for client to complete activities.
B. Provide warm environment: extra blankets, etc.
C. Provide meticulous skin care.
D. Orient client as to date, time, and place.
E. Prevent constipation.
F. If sedatives or narcotics are necessary, give one-half to one-third normal dosage, as ordered by physician.
G. Monitor thyroid replacement (initial small dosage, increased gradually).
H. Maintain individualized maintenance dosage.
 1. Desiccated thyroid.
 2. Thyroxine (Synthroid).
 3. Triiodothyronine (Cytomel).
I. Monitor for overdosage symptoms of thyroid preparations.
 1. Myocardial infarction and angina and cardiac failure, particularly in clients with cardiac problems.
 2. Restlessness and insomnia.
 3. Headache and confusion.

Myxedema Coma

Definition: A condition resulting from persistent low thyroid production.

Assessment

A. Assess for hypoventilation.
B. Observe for hypotension leading to cardiac abnormalities.
C. Evaluate cold sensitivity leading to severe hypothermia.
D. Evaluate mood swings.

Implementation

A. Provide total hygienic care.
B. Provide psychological support.
 1. Body image change.
 2. Complete dependency.
 3. Mental depression.

C. Closely observe hormone replacement.

D. Provide low-calorie diet.

E. Provide ventilatory support if needed.

F. Measure vital signs frequently, especially temperature.

G. Monitor fluid intake to prevent dilutional hyponatremia.

H. Avoid use of sedatives and hypnotics.

Thyrotoxicosis/Hyperthyroidism Graves' Disease

Definition: A condition that results from the increased synthesis of thyroid hormone. When associated with ocular signs and a diffuse goiter, it is called Graves' Disease. Occurs four times more frequently in women than in men; usually occurs between twenty to forty years of age.

Assessment

A. Assess increased rate of body metabolism.
   1. Weight loss despite ravenous appetite and ingestion of large quantities of food.
   2. Intolerance to heat.
   3. Nervousness, jitters, and fine tremor of hands.
   4. Smooth, soft skin and hair.
   5. Tachycardia and palpitation.
   6. Diarrhea.
   7. Diaphoresis.

B. Assess personality changes.
   1. Irritability and agitation.
   2. Exaggerated emotional reactions.
   3. Mood swings—euphoria to depression.
   4. Quick motions, including speech.

C. Assess any enlargement of the thyroid gland (goiter).

D. Observe for exophthalmos.
   1. Fluid collects around eye sockets, causing eyeballs to protude.
   2. Not always present.
   3. Usually does not improve with treatment.

E. Assess for cardiac arrhythmias.

F. Evaluate difficulty focusing eyes.

G. Assess laboratory values.
   1. Above normal test results: PBI, ^{131}I, and T_3 and T_4.
   2. Relatively low serum cholesterol.

MEDICAL IMPLICATIONS

A. Antithyroid drugs.
   1. Propylthiouracil.
   2. Methimazole (Tapazole).
   3. Side effect: agranulocytosis.

B. Iodine preparations.
   1. Saturated solution of potassium iodide (SSKI).
   2. Lugol's solution.

C. Propranolol.
   1. Rapidly reverses toxic manifestations.
   2. Used preoperatively.

D. Radioiodine therapy.
   1. Useful in clients who are poor surgical risks.
   2. Uptake of ^{131}I by thyroid gland results in destruction of thyroid cells.
   3. Myxedema may occur as complication.

E. Thyroidectomy.

Implementation

A. Provide adequate rest.
   1. Bed rest.
   2. Diversionary activities.
   3. Sedatives.

B. Provide cool, quiet, stable environment.

C. Maintain high calorie, protein, carbohydrate, vitamin diet without stimulants.

D. Take daily weights.

E. Provide emotional support.
   1. Be aware that exaggerated emotional responses are a manifestation of hormone imbalance.
   2. Be sensitive to needs.
   3. Avoid stress-producing situations.

F. Adhere to regular schedule of activities.

G. Provide client education.
   1. Protection from infection.
   2. Safe self-administration of medications.
   3. Importance of adequate rest and diet.
   4. Avoidance of stress.

Thyroidectomy

Definition: Removal of thyroid gland for persistent hyperthyroidism.

Assessment

A. Assess type of surgery to be done: total resection or subtotal resection of the gland.
B. Assess vital signs and weight for baseline data.
C. Assess serum electrolytes for hyperglycemia and glycosuria.
D. Assess level of consciousness.
E. Evaluate for signs of thyroid storm.

Implementation

A. Preoperative care—prevent thyrotoxicosis.
  1. Administer antithyroid drugs to deplete iodine and hormones (five to seven days).
  2. Administer iodine to decrease vascularity and increase size of follicular cells (five to seven days).
  3. Provide routine preoperative teaching.
  4. Reassure client.
  5. Maintain nutritional status.
B. Postoperative care.
  1. Check frequently for respiratory distress—keep tracheostomy tray at bedside.
  2. Maintain semi-Fowler's position to avoid strain on suture line.
  3. Observe for bleeding.
    a. Vital signs—tachycardia, hypotension.
    b. Pressure on larynx.
    c. Hematoma around wound.
  4. Observe for damage to laryngeal nerve.
    a. Respiratory obstruction.
    b. Dysphonia.
    c. High-pitched voice.
    d. Stridor.
    e. Dysphagia.
    f. Restlessness.
  5. Observe for signs of hypoparathyroidism (causes an acute attack of tetany).
    a. Chvostek's sign.
    b. Convulsions.
    c. Irritability and anxiety.
    d. Stridor, wheezing and dyspnea.
    e. Photophobia, diplopia.
    f. Muscle and abdominal cramps.

Thyroid Storm or Thyroid Crisis

Definition: An acute, potentially fatal hyperthyroid condition that may occur as a result of surgery, inadequate preparation for surgery, severe infection, or stress.

Characteristics

A. Cause not known; symptoms reflect exaggerated thyrotoxicosis.
B. Infrequent due to premedication of iodine and antithyroid drugs.
C. Can be precipitated by stressors.
  1. Infection.
  2. Abrupt withdrawal of medication.
  3. Metabolic causes.
  4. Emotional stress.
  5. Pulmonary embolism.

Assessment

A. Assess for increased temperature (>100° F).
B. Assess diaphoresis.
C. Assess for dehydration.
D. Evaluate cardiopulmonary symptoms.
  1. Tachycardia (>120).
  2. Arrhythmias.
  3. Congestive heart failure.
  4. Pulmonary edema.
E. Assess gastrointestinal symptoms.
  1. Abdominal pain.
  2. Nausea, vomiting, and diarrhea.
  3. Jaundice.
F. Assess central nervous system symptoms.
  1. Tremors.
  2. Severe agitation, restlessness, and irritability.
  3. Apathy leading to delirium and coma.

MEDICAL IMPLICATIONS

A. Large doses IV propranolol to control thyroid storm.
B. Adrenergic and catecholamine blocking agents to decrease heart activity.
C. Glucocorticoids to allay stress effects.
D. Sodium iodide to slow IV infusion.
E. SSKI p.o.
F. Antithyroid drugs.

Implementation

A. Do not palpate thyroid gland (stimulus increases symptoms).
B. Decrease temperature: ASA, external cold (ice packs, cooling blanket).
C. Protect from infection, especially pneumonia.
D. Monitor vital signs.
E. Maintain fluid and electrolyte balance.
  1. Electrolyte shifts cause brittle situation of over and under hydration.

2. Maintain adequate output.
3. Observe for sodium and potassium imbalance due to vomiting and diarrhea.
4. Observe for signs of overhydration if cardio-pulmonary complications are evident.
F. Monitor ECG for arrhythmias if:
1. Adrenergic blockers are used.
2. Diuretics are given.
3. Electrolyte imbalance is present.
4. Cardiovascular medication is given.
G. Administer IV glucose diet with glucose and large doses of vitamin B complex.
H. Protect for safety if agitated or comatose.
I. Provide calm, quiet environment.
J. Reassure client and family.

PARATHYROID GLAND DISORDERS

Hypoparathyroidism

Definition: A condition caused by acute or chronic deficient hormone production by the parathyroid gland. Usually occurs following thyroidectomy.

Assessment

A. Assess for acute hypocalcemia.
1. Numbness, tingling, and cramping of extremities.
2. Acute, potentially fatal tetany.
   a. Painful muscular spasms.
   b. Seizures.
   c. Irritability.
   d. Positive Chvostek's sign.
   e. Positive Trousseau's sign.
   f. Laryngospasm.
   g. Cardiac arrhythmias.
B. Assess for chronic hypocalcemia.
1. Poor development of tooth enamel.
2. Mental retardation.
3. Muscular weakness with numbness and tingling of extremities.
4. Loss of hair and coarse, dry skin.
5. Personality changes.
6. Cataracts.
7. Cardiac arrhythmias.
8. Renal stones.
C. Assess laboratory values.

1. Low serum calcium levels.
2. Increased serum phosphorus level.
3. Low urinary calcium and phosphorus output.
4. Increased bone density on x-ray examination.

MEDICAL IMPLICATIONS

A. Acute.
1. Slow drip of IV calcium gluconate or calcium chloride.
2. Anticonvulsants and sedatives (phenytoin and phenobarbital).
3. Parathyroid hormone IM or sub q.
4. Aluminum hydroxide (decreases phosphate level).
5. Rebreathing bag to produce mild respiratory acidosis.
6. Tracheostomy if laryngospasm causes obstruction.
B. Chronic.
1. Oral calcium carbonate (OS CAL).
2. Vitamin D preparations (Calciferol).
3. High-calcium, low-phosphorus diet.

Implementation

A. Same as for convulsions and epilepsy.
B. Frequently check for increasing hoarseness.
C. Observe for irregularities in urine.
D. Force fluids as ordered.
E. Observe for dystonic reactions if on phenothiazines.
F. Provide psychological support.
1. Altered body image.
2. Emotional instability.
3. Extreme weakness.

Hyperparathyroidism

Definition: A condition caused by excessive hormone production of the parathyroid gland.

Assessment

A. Assess for bone demineralization with deformities; pain; high susceptibility to fractures.
B. Assess for hypercalcemia.
1. Calcium deposits in various body organs: eyes, heart, lungs, and kidneys (stones).
2. Gastric ulcers.
3. Personality changes, depression, and paranoia.
4. Nausea, vomiting, anorexia, and constipation.

5. Polydipsia and polyuria.
C. Assess laboratory values.
1. Elevated serum calcium level.
2. Low to normal serum phosphorus levels.
3. Elevated urinary calcium and phosphorus levels.
4. Evidence of bone changes on x-ray examinations.
5. Normal to increased alkaline phosphatase.

Implementation

A. Force fluids. Include juices to make urine more acidic.
B. Provide normal saline IV infusion.
C. Observe for electrolyte imbalance with Lasix administration.
D. Measure intake and output.
E. Closely observe urine for stones and gravel.
F. Observe for digitalis toxicity if client is taking digitalis.
G. Provide a high-phosphorus, low-calcium diet.
H. Prevent accidents and injury through safety measures.
I. Provide surgical care if subtotal surgical resection of parathyroid glands is done.
J. Administer additional oral calcium for bone rebuilding processes (several months).

Parathyroidectomy

Definition: Removal of one or more of the parathyroid glands, usually as a result of thyroidectomy.

Assessment

A. Assess for positive Chvostek's and Trousseau's signs.
B. Assess for CNS signs of psychomotor or personality disturbances.
C. Evaluate laboratory results for baseline data.
1. Serum potassium, calcium, phosphate, and magnesium.
2. Renal magnesium function tests (renal damage from hyperplasia).
D. Evaluate urine for presence of stones.
E. Assess lung sounds for prevention of pulmonary edema.
F. Assess muscle weakness, ability to walk, and range of movement for minimizing bone stress.

Implementation

A. Observe for tetany and treat accordingly.
B. Maintain patent airway.
1. Observe for respiratory distress.
2. Keep a tracheostomy tray at the bedside.
C. Provide diet high in calcium, vitamin D, and magnesium salts.
D. Increase fluids to prevent formation of urinary stones—monitor intake and output for low levels of calcium, magnesium and phosphate.
E. Monitor IV administration of calcium gluconate if given for postoperative emergency.
F. Monitor for postoperative complications.
1. Renal colic.
2. Laryngeal nerve damage.
3. Acute psychosis (look for listlessness).
G. Position client in semi-Fowler's and support head and neck to decrease edema.
H. Ambulate client as soon as possible to speed up recalcification of bones.

PANCREAS DISORDERS

Diabetes Mellitus (Type I, Type II)

Definition: A group of disorders that have a variety of genetic causes, but have glucose intolerance as a common thread.

Characteristics

A. Classifications.
1. Type I—insulin dependent diabetes mellitus (IDDM).
2. Type II—noninsulin dependent mellitus (NIDDM).
3. Gestational (GDM)—increased blood glucose levels during pregnancy.
4. Impaired glucose tolerance (IGT). Plasma glucose levels vacillate between normal or increased (formerly latent, borderline, and subclinical diabetes).
B. Etiology.
1. Genetic factors.
a. Presence of HLA antigens.
b. Individual genes located on "shortarm" of sixth chromosome.
2. Viruses.
a. Type I diabetes occurs at time viral diseases are prevalent—autumn and spring.

b. Type I onset often preceded by viral attack.

c. Coxsackie B_4 is found in pancreas.

d. Twenty viruses associated with diabetes.

C. Pathophysiology.

  1. Type I (IDDM, insulin dependent), formerly Juvenile type.

    a. Rapid onset—requires insulin due to absence of circulating insulin.

    b. Autoimmune response.

    c. Presence of anti-islet cell antibodies.

    d. Pancreatic beta cells die.

    e. Ketosis unless treated.

  2. Type II (NIDDM, noninsulin dependent), formerly Adult Onset type.

    a. Gradual onset—may be controlled by diet.

    b. 90 percent diabetes is this type.

    c. Impaired beta cell response to glucose (client usually nonobese).

    d. Tissues insensitive to insulin (client usually obese).

      (1) Extrapancreatic defect.

      (2) Normal or high levels of circulating insulin.

D. Somogyi effect: hypoglycemia usually at night followed by compensatory rebound hyperglycemia in the morning (lasts 12–72 hours).

  1. Usually caused by too much insulin or an increase in insulin sensitivity.

  2. Client may be stabilized by gradual lowering of insulin dose and increase in diet at the time of the hypoglycemia reaction.

E. Dawn phenomenon.

  1. Blood sugar normal until 3 A.M.—begins to rise in early morning hours.

  2. Common problem—glucose released from liver in early A.M.—needs to be controlled.

  3. Algorithm for hyperglycemia—altering time and dose of insulin (NPH or ultralente) by one or two units will stabilize client.

Table 3. COMPARISON OF TYPE I AND TYPE II DIABETES

	IDDM–Child Insulin-Dependent Diabetes Mellitus	NIDDM—Adult Noninsulin-Dependent Diabetes Mellitus
Etiology	Heredity prominent factor; autoimmune process involved.	Heredity more relevant (100% children contract NIDDM when both parents have it).
Cause	Absence of circulating insulin. (In some cases disease is mild and benign.)	Insulin insufficient, not totally deficient; defective glucose-mediated insulin secretion.
Onset	Usually abrupt—under 35.	Insidious, often over 35.
Weight	History of failure to gain despite voracious appetite.	Obese or overweight.
Sex	Found in girls and boys equally.	Most common in females.
Cardinal signs	Polydipsia, polyphagia, polyuria.	Polyphagia, polyuria and polydipsia.
Other signs	Bed-wetting, weight loss, irritability, overly tired, sores slow to heal.	Overweight, fatigue, frequent infections.
Stability	Unstable; brittle—difficult to control.	Stable with compliance; less difficult to control.
Distinguishing feature	Honeymoon phase—symptoms decrease with a short remission.	No honeymoon phase.
Complications	Hyperglycemia, diabetic ketosis and ketoacidosis.	Neuropathy, retinopathy, uropathy.
Treatment	Insulin and ADA diet.	ADA diet alone; ADA and insulin, or ADA and oral hypoglycemic agents.

MEDICAL IMPLICATIONS

A. Diet.
1. The cornerstone of management, interdependent with medication and exercise.
2. Attainment of normal weight may clear symptoms in NIDDM.
3. Total calories are individualized.
4. Focus of diet.
   a. High complex carbohydrates, high-soluble fiber foods (oat bran cereals, beans, peas, fruits with pectin) assist in controlling blood glucose. Few simple or refined sugars.
   b. Protein—60 to 85 grams according to calorie intake.
   c. Fat—70 to 90 grams or 20–30%. Emphasize low saturated fats and mono- and polyunsaturated fats.
5. ADA exchange diet; seven exchange lists.
   a. Prescribed as to total calories and number of exchanges from each group.
   b. Calories divided into: CHO–60%; fat–20%; and protein–20%.
6. Metoclopramide (Reglan) given to stimulate GI motility. Used to treat gastric stasis.

B. Medications.
1. Insulin types: see chart on pg. 306.
2. Oral hypoglycemic drugs.
   a. Effective for those with some functioning beta cells in Islets of Langerhans.
   b. Used for older clients, noninsulin dependent with normal weight, and diet will not control hyperglycemia.
   c. Sulfonylureas.
      (1) Thought to stimulate beta cells to increase insulin release.
      (2) Tolbutamide (Orinase), short acting (6–10 hours).
      (3) Chlorpropamide (Diabinese), long acting (36–60 hours).
      (4) Acetohexamide (Dymelor), intermediate acting (10–20 hours).
      (5) Tolazamide (Tolinase), intermediate acting (12–24 hours).
   d. Second generation sulfonylureas.
      (1) Glyburide, intermediate acting (12–24 hours).
      (2) Glipizide, short acting (10–18 hours).

C. Exercise.
1. Decreases body's need for insulin.
2. Moderate activity recommended.
3. Administer 10 gm CHO before exercise.

Insulin Pump

A. Continuous delivery of fixed small amounts of diluted insulin—mimics release of insulin by pancreas.
B. Uses regular insulin: 50 percent continuous delivery and 50 percent divided into three premeal bolus doses.
C. Amount calculated by blood glucose monitoring done 2–4 times per day.
D. Usually pump and syringe with needle placed in abdomen and taped in place.
E. Method useful for conscientious, active person who does not want to adjust life to coincide with insulin peaks.
F. Client disadvantages.
1. Requires conscientious client commitment to understand and learn pump use.
2. Requires extensive client teaching.
3. Regimen is complicated and may require more time than client can spend.

Nasal Spray Insulin

A. Intranasal insulin may soon replace regular insulin for mealtimes.
1. Single puff of 30 units will replace 8 units sub q insulin.
2. Short-acting and will not replace the need for insulin injections.
B. Advantages—has rapid physiological action and can be used either before or after meals.
C. Disadvantages—will require higher doses and thus be more expensive—potential side effect may be nasal irritation.

Assessment

A. Assess for early symptoms.
1. Common to both Type I and Type II.
   a. Polyuria.
   b. Polydipsia.
   c. Polyphagia.
   d. Blurred vision.
   e. Fatigue.
   f. Abnormal sensations (prickling, burning).
   g. Infections (vaginitis).
2. Type I.
   a. Postural hypotension.
   b. Decreased muscle mass.
   c. Weight loss in spite of increased appetite.
3. Type II.
   a. Often asymptomatic.
   b. Often obese.
   c. Slow wound healing.

Table 4. INSULIN TREATMENT

Category	Types	Onset	Peak	Duration	Time and Symptoms of Untoward Reaction
Short acting	Regular Semilente Humulin R	1/2–1 hour 1–2 hours 1/2–1 min.	2–5 hours 3–8 hours 2–3 hours	6–8 hours 10–16 hours 5–7 hours	15 minutes to 4–5 hours: hunger, trembling, visual disturbance, cold perspiration, weakness, coma
Intermediate acting	NPH Lente 70/30	1–2 hours 1–3 hours 1/2–1 hour	6–12 hours 6–12 hours 2–12 hours	16–26 hours 18–24 hours 18–24 hours	4–6 hours: majority of attacks occur in early morning or evening—extreme fatigue may be the only symptom
Long acting	Protamine Zinc (PZI) Ultralente	4–8 hours 4–6 hours	10–20 hours 8–24 hours	36 hours 24–36 hours	12–24 hours: usually early morning, gradual onset, sleeplessness, nausea, headache, mental confusion

B. Assess for distinguishing features of Type I and Type II diabetes.

C. Assess for risk factors.
  1. Client history—hereditary predisposition.
  2. Weight—presence of obesity.
  3. High stress levels.

D. Assess results of laboratory values.
  1. Fasting blood sugar >140, postprandial blood sugar >200 and at least once between meals at 2 hrs. p.c.; abnormal glucose tolerance test or tolbutamide (Orinase) tests.
  2. Clinitest and Testape.
    a. Indicate presence of sugar in urine, i.e., 1+ to 4+.
    b. Clinitest: 2-drop and 5-drop method: from no sugar (blue) to 4+ or 2 percent (orange-rust).
    c. Values of the two tests are not interchangeable. (Usefulness of both tests as a reflection of blood sugar is limited.)
  3. Acetest and Ketostix—may be positive for presence of acetone in urine.
  4. Elevated cholesterol and triglyceride levels.
  5. Capillary blood glucose (finger stick).
  6. Glycosylated hemoglobin test (Hgb A).
    a. Reflects glycemic state over preceding 8–12 weeks.
    b. Abnormally high in diabetics with chronic hyperglycemia.
    c. Values: normal 3.5–6.2%—good control less than 7.5%—fair control 7.6–8.9%—poor control more than 9.0%.

Implementation

A. Give IV fluids and medications as ordered.

B. Test urine (second voided specimen).

C. Adhere to procedures for other laboratory tests.

D. Provide meticulous skin care, particularly lower extremities.

E. Protect from infection, injury, stress.

F. Observe for signs of insulin reactions and ketoacidosis.

G. Measure intake and output.

H. Provide emotional support.
  1. Allow for verbalization of client's feelings.
    a. Necessary changes in lifestyle, diet, and activities.
    b. Change in self-image and self-esteem.
    c. Fear of future and complications.
  2. Encourage involvement of family.

I. Provide client education (key to effective self-management).
  1. Assessment.
    a. Level of knowledge.
    b. Cultural, socioeconomic, and family influences.
    c. Daily dietary and activity patterns.
    d. Emotional and physical status and effect on client's current ability to learn.
  2. Insulin and insulin injections.
    a. Keep insulin at room temperature; refrigerate extra supply of insulin.
    b. Rotate insulin bottle gently prior to drawing up insulin.
    c. Use sterile injection techniques.

d. Rotate injection sites to prevent injection in dystrophied areas.

e. Watch for signs of under- and over-dosage.

3. Current trends in insulin administration.

   a. Abdominal injection sites preferred for consistent and rapid rate of absorption.

   b. Rotating injection areas is not recommended, due to variation in insulin absorption and action.

      (1) One body area may be used consistently.

      (2) Injection site should be one inch from the previous injection site.

   c. Wait 30 seconds after slowly injecting insulin to prevent insulin leakage.

   d. Aspirating before and massaging after injection is no longer recommended.

4. New approach—target glucose level.

   a. Balancing blood glucose levels result in fewer complications.

      (1) Premeal: 90–140 mg/dl.

      (2) Two hours pp: under 180 mg/dl.

      (3) 2 A.M. to 4 A.M.: over 100 mg/dl.

   b. Protocol is taking blood glucose levels 2–4 times/day.

   c. Pattern control is goal—adjust one insulin dose at a time (action has domino effect).

      (1) Blood sugar lower than target level—cut insulin by 2–4 units.

      (2) Blood sugar higher than target level—raise insulin by 1–2 units at a time.

   d. Use algorithms as guidelines for amount of insulin.

5. Oral medications.

   a. Take medications regularly.

   b. Watch for hypoglycemic reactions occurring with sulfonylureas.

   c. Remember that alcohol ingestion in conjunction with sulfonylureas causes an Antabuse-like reaction.

6. Avoidance of infection and injury.

   a. Report infection or injury promptly to physician.

   b. Maintain meticulous skin care.

   c. Maintain proper foot care.

      (1) Wash with mild soap—dry well.

      (2) Use lanolin to prevent cracking.

      (3) Cut toenails straight across.

      (4) Use clean cotton socks.

      (5) Inspect feet daily—report skin breaks.

      (6) Avoid "bathroom surgery" for corns and calluses.

   d. Be aware that insulin requirements may increase with infections.

   e. Be prepared for healing process impairment.

f. Avoid tight-fitting garments and shoes.

7. Diet.

   a. Do not vary meal times.

   b. Incorporate diet with individual needs, life style, cultural, and socioeconomic patterns.

   c. Most adults require 30 calories/kg of ideal body weight.

8. Exercise.

   a. Regulate time and amount.

   b. Avoid sporadic, vigorous activities; use aerobic exercise.

   c. Give 10 gms CHO before exercise and every hour during exercise.

   d. Do not exercise during peak action time of insulin.

   e. Rigorous exercise while blood sugar is 240–300% may precipitate ketoacidosis.

9. Medic-alert band.

10. Provide constant availability of concentrated sugar.

COMPLICATIONS

Ketoacidosis (DKA)

Definition: The two major metabolic problems that are the source of this condition are hyperglycemia and ketoacidemia, both due to insulin lack associated with hyperglucagonemia.

Characteristics

A. Without insulin, carbohydrate metabolism is affected.

B. Hyperglycemia results from increased liver production of glucose and decreased glucose uptake by peripheral tissues.

C. The liver oxidizes fatty acids into:

   1. Acetoacidic acid (increased ketone bodies lead to ketoacidosis).

   2. Beta-hydroxybutyric acid (acetone is volatile and is blown off by lungs).

   3. As glucose levels increase, there is osmotic overload in kidney resulting in dehydration and electrolyte losses.

   4. As ketone bodies increase, acidosis and comatose states occur.

Assessment

A. Assess for ketoacidotic coma—usually preceded by a few days of polyuria and polydipsia with associated symptoms.

B. Assess for ill appearance.

C. Assess for anorexia, nausea and vomiting.

D. Assess for drowsiness, confusion and mental stupor.

E. Assess for dehydration, deep, rapid breathing, and fruity odor of acetone to breath.

F. Observe for complications of circulatory collapse or respiratory distress.

Implementation

A. Maintain fluid and electrolyte balance.
   1. Normal saline IV until blood sugar reaches 250 to 300 mg%; then a dextrose solution is started.
   2. Potassium added to IV after renal function is evaluated and hydration is adequate.

B. Provide insulin management.
   1. Give one-half dose IV during acute phase and one-half dose sub q.
   2. Give with small amounts of albumin as insulin to IV tubing.
   3. Hourly dosage depends on S & A and blood levels.
   4. Watch for onset of insulin reaction.

C. Provide patent airway and adequate circulation to brain (cardiac monitoring if status indicates).

D. Monitor vital signs.

E. Monitor urine frequently for sugar and acetone.

F. Test blood sugar level q 1 to 2 hours.

G. Perform hourly urine measurements.

H. Maintain personal hygiene.

I. Keep client warm.

J. Protect from injury if comatose.

Insulin Reaction/Hypoglycemia

Definition: An abnormally low blood glucose, usually below 50 mg, resulting from too much insulin, not enough food, or excessive activity.

Assessment

A. Assess for symptoms, especially before meals.

B. Assess for sweating, tremors, pallor, tachycardia, palpitations, or nervousness.

C. Evaluate for headache, confusion, emotional changes, memory lapses, slurred speech, numbness of lips and tongue, alterations in gait, loss of consciousness.

D. Evaluate lab tests.
   1. Blood glucose, usually below 50–60 mg/dl.
   2. Urine for acetone (usually negative).

Implementation

A. Administer oral sugar in form of dextrosol tablet, unsweetened orange juice or 8 oz. of skim milk if client is alert; administer glucagon (sub q or IV) if client is not alert.

B. Administer carbohydrates by mouth when client awakens.

C. Provide client teaching.
   1. Maintain regimen of diet, medications and exercise.
   2. Treat the symptoms early to prevent complications.
   3. Instruct client to always carry simple carbohydrates for treatment of early symptoms.
   4. Take 200 calorie snack one-half hour before peak time of insulin to prevent hypoglycemia.
   5. Extra food should be taken before engaging in heavy physical exercise.

D. Prevent compensatory rebound hyperglycemia (Somogyi effect).
   1. Caused by the body's attempt to oppose the excessive action of insulin through liver glycogenolysis.
   2. Insulin dose is reduced and client returned to stabilized rate.

E. Provide instruction in use of portable insulin pump if ordered.

F. Provide instruction in use of blood sugar monitors.
   1. Prick finger and smear drop of blood on reagent strip.
   2. Compare results with monitor or chart.

Chronic Complications

Definition: Chronic complications of diabetes are becoming more common as diabetics live longer. Included in this category are blindness, renal disease and vascular conditions.

A. *Retinopathy:* progressive impairment of retinal circulation that eventually causes vitreous hemorrhage with vision loss.
   1. Assessment.
      a. Duration and degree of disease (incidence increases with length of time disease is present).
      b. Impaired vision.
      c. Ability to carry out daily tasks: blood glucose testing and insulin injections.
      d. Need for assistance from others.
   2. Implementation.
      a. Assist in ways to maintain independence and self-esteem.
      b. Support client when treatment is implemented: photocoagulation or vitrectomy.
      c. Instruct in actions that prevent or reduce complications: stable blood glucose levels.

B. *Nephropathy:* the specific renal disease, intercapillary glomerulosclerosis, is called Kimmelstiel-Wilson syndrome. It is the result of chronic diabetes.

1. Assessment.
   a. Urine alterations; proteinuria, azotemia, frequent urinary tract infections, neurogenic bladder.
   b. Serum lab values; BUN, creatinine.
   c. Thirst and fatigue.
2. Implementation.
   a. Administer medications to prevent urinary tract infections.
   b. Instruct client to keep blood glucose levels within normal limits.
   c. Maintain adequate fluid intake.
   d. Instruct in 20–40 gm protein diet.
   e. Restrict sodium and potassium in diet.
   f. Prepare patient for dialysis therapy if appropriate.

C. *Neuropathy:* general deterioration that affects the peripheral and autonomic nervous systems.
   1. Assessment.
      a. Peripheral neuropathy.
         (1) Pain in the legs.
         (2) Aching and burning sensations in lower extremities.
      b. Alterations in bowel and bladder function.
         (1) Bowel dysfunction: constipation, diarrhea, nocturnal fecal incontinence.
         (2) Urinary dysfunction: infrequent voiding, weak stream, dribbling, signs of urinary infection.
      c. Autonomic nervous system impairment.
         (1) Sexual dysfunction.
         (2) Orthostatic hypotension.
         (3) Pupillary changes.
      d. Circulatory abnormalities.
         (1) Skin breakdown and signs of infection.
         (2) Thick toenails: suggestive of circulatory impairment.
         (3) Low temperature and poor color in feet; athlete's feet.
         (4) Thin, shiny, atropic skin.
         (5) Poor peripheral pulses.
   2. Implementation.
      a. Assist client to deal with pain.
         (1) Encourage walking for exercise.
         (2) Provide foot cradle when in bed.
      b. Assist client to deal with bladder-bowel problems.
         (1) Provide privacy for toileting.
         (2) Provide psychological support.
         (3) Administer Lomotil as ordered for diarrhea.
         (4) Administer neomycin as ordered to prevent bacterial growth in an atonic bowel.
         (5) Administer Urecholine as ordered.

      (6) Establish two hour voiding schedule to prevent urinary stasis.
      (7) Encourage fluids.
   c. Counsel client who has sexual dysfunction.
      (1) Allow client to ventilate feelings about sexual impotence.
      (2) Observe for depression (sexual impotence is usually permanent).
   d. Provide excellent foot care.
      (1) Wash with soap and warm water, dry thoroughly.
      (2) Massage feet with lanolin or mineral oil to prevent scaling or cracking.
      (3) File or cut toenails across nail. Do not injure soft tissue around nail (check hospital policy for nail care).
      (4) Prevent moisture from accumulating between toes.
      (5) Instruct in well-fitting shoes. Do not go barefoot.
      (6) Wear loose-fitting socks.
      (7) Exercise feet daily.
      (8) See podiatrist regularly.
      (9) Notify physician if cuts, pain or blisters appear on feet.

Functional Hyperinsulinism/ Hypoglycemia

Definition: A condition that occurs as the result of excess secretion of insulin by the beta cells of the pancreas gland.

Characteristics

A. May be associated with "dumping syndrome" following gastrectomy.
B. May occur prior to development of diabetes mellitus.

Assessment

A. Assess personality changes.
   1. Tenseness.
   2. Nervousness.
   3. Irritability.
   4. Anxiousness.
   5. Depression.
B. Assess for excessive diaphoresis.
C. Assess for excessive hunger.
D. Evaluate muscle weakness and tachycardia.
E. Assess laboratory values—low blood sugar during hypoglycemic episodes.

Implementation

A. High-protein, low-carbohydrate diet.
B. Counseling may reduce anxiety and tenseness.

Table 5.   COMPLICATIONS ASSOCIATED WITH DIABETES

Clinical Manifestations	Hypoglycemia	Diabetic Ketoacidosis (DKA)	Hyperglycemic Hyperosmolar Nonketotic Coma (HHNK)
	Type I	Type I	Type II
Cause	Too much insulin or too little food	Absence or inadequate insulin	Uncontrolled diabetes or oral hypoglycemic drugs
Onset	Rapid (within minutes)	Slow (about eight hours)	Slow (hours to days)
Appearance	Exhibits symptoms of fainting	Appears ill	Appears ill
Respirations	Normal	Rapid and deep, shortness of breath	Rapid and deep; absence of Kussmaul's
Breath odor	Normal	Sweetish due to acetone	Normal
Pulse	Tachycardia	Tachycardia	Tachycardia
Blood pressure		Hypotension	Hypotension
Hunger	Hunger pangs in epigastrium	Loss of appetite	Hunger
Thirst	None	Increased	Increased, dehydration
Vomiting	Nausea; vomiting rare	Common	Common
Eyes	Staring, double vision	Appear sunken	Visual loss
Headache	Common	Occasionally	Occasionally
Skin	Pallor, perspiration, chilling sensation	Hot, dry skin	Hot, dry skin
Muscle action	Twitching common, unsteady gait	Twitching absent	Twitching absent
Pain in abdomen	None	Common	Common
Mental status	Confusion, erratic, change in mood, unable to concentrate	Malaise, drowsy, confusion, coma	Confused, dull, coma
Lab findings			
Sugar in urine	None after residual is discarded	Present	Present
Blood sugar	Below 50–70 mg/dl blood	High, 350–900 mg/dl	Very high, 800 mg/dl up to 2400 mg/dl
Ketones	Absent	High	Absent
Ketones in blood plasma	Absent	4+ present	Absent

PERIOPERATIVE CARE CONCEPTS

The term perioperative refers to all phases of surgical care: preoperative, intraoperative and postoperative. This section outlines the nursing care measures for surgical clients and covers the principles of care, anesthesia, postoperative complications and fluid replacement therapy.

PREOPERATIVE AND POSTOPERATIVE CARE

Routine Preoperative Care

Psychological Support

A. Reinforce the physician's teaching regarding the surgical procedure.
B. Identify client's anxieties; notify physician of extreme anxiety.
C. Listen to client's verbalization of fears.
D. Provide support to the client's family (where family can wait during surgery, approximately how long the surgery takes, etc.).

Preoperative Teaching

A. Postoperative exercises: leg, coughing, deep breathing, etc.
B. Equipment utilized during postoperative period: intermittent positive pressure breathing machine (IPPB), NG tube for suctioning, etc.
C. Pain medication and when to ask for it.
D. Explanation of n.p.o.

Physical Care

A. Completed night before surgery.
   1. Observe and record client's overall condition.
      a. Nutritional status.
      b. Physical defects, such as loss of limb function, skin breakdown.
      c. Hearing or sight difficulties.

   2. Obtain chest x-ray, ECG, and blood and urine samples, as ordered.
   3. Take preoperative history and assess present physical condition.
   4. Determine if any drug allergies.
   5. Perform skin prep and shave when necessary; have client shower with antibacterial soap, if ordered.
   6. Give enema, if ordered.
B. Completed one to two hours before surgery.
   1. Insert indwelling catheter, nasogastric tube, IV.
   2. Administer preoperative medications.
   3. Provide quiet rest with siderails up and curtains drawn.

Nurse's Responsibility

A. Perform or supervise skin prep and shave.
B. Carry out preoperative nursing interventions.
C. Notify physician of drug allergies, overwhelming anxiety, unusual ECG findings, abnormal lab findings.
D. See that consent form is signed.
E. Administer preoperative medications on time.
F. Complete preoperative checklist.
G. Check if history and physical examination findings are on chart.
H. Chart preoperative medications.
I. Check Identaband, provide quiet environment.
J. Remove dentures, nail polish, hairpins, etc.

Recovery Room

Assessment

A. Assess patent airway.
B. Assess need for oxygen.
C. Check gag reflex.
D. Observe for adverse signs of general anesthesia or spinal anesthesia.
E. Assess vital signs.
   1. Pulse rate, quality and rhythm.
   2. Blood pressure.
   3. Respirations, rate, rhythm, and depth.
F. Evaluate temperature for heat control.
G. Observe dressings and surgical drains.
   1. Mark any drainage on dressings and note time by drawing a line around the drainage.
   2. Note color and amount of drainage on dressings and in drainage tubes.

312

3. Ensure that dressing is secure.
4. Reinforce dressings as needed.
H. Observe client's overall condition.
   1. Check skin for warmth, color, and moisture.
   2. Check nailbeds and mucous membranes for color and blanching; report if cyanotic.
   3. Observe for return of reflexes.
I. Assess client for return to room.
   1. Be sure vital signs are stable and within normal limits for at least one hour.
   2. See if client is awake and reflexes are present (gag and cough reflex). Check for movement and sensation in limbs of clients with spinal anesthesia.
   3. Take oral airway out (if not out already). Observe for cyanosis.
   4. Be sure dressings are intact and there is no excessive drainage.

Implementation

A. Maintain patent airway.
B. Administer oxygen by mask or nasal cannula.
C. Check gag reflex. Leave airway in place until client pushes it out.
D. Position client for adequate ventilation.
E. Observe for adverse signs of general anesthesia or spinal anesthesia.
   1. Level of consciousness.
   2. Movement of limbs.
F. Monitor vital signs every ten to fifteen minutes.
   1. Pulse—check rate, quality, and rhythm.
   2. Blood pressure—check pulse pressure and quality as well as systolic and diastolic pressure.
   3. Respiration—check rate, rhythm, depth, and type of respiration (abdominal breathing, nasal flaring).
   4. Vital signs are sometimes difficult to obtain due to hypothermia.
   5. Movement from operating room table to guerney can alter vital signs significantly, especially with cardiovascular clients.
G. Maintain temperature (operating room is usually cold)—apply warm blankets.
H. Maintain patent IV.
   1. Check type and amount of solution being administered.
   2. Adjust correct flow rate.
   3. Check IV site for signs of infiltration.

4. Check blood transfusion.
   a. Blood type and blood bank number. Time transfusion started.
   b. Client's name, identification number, expiration date.
   c. Amount in bag upon arrival in recovery room. Color and consistency of blood.
I. Monitor dressings and surgical drains for drainage.
J. Administer medications.
   1. Begin routine drugs and administer all STAT drugs.
   2. Pain medications are usually administered sparingly and in smaller amounts.
K. Discharge client from recovery-room.
   1. Call anesthesiologist to discharge client from recovery room (if appropriate).
   2. Give report on client's condition to floor nurse receiving client.
   3. Ensure IV is patent.
   4. Reinforce or change dressings as needed.
   5. Ensure all drains are functioning.
   6. Record amount of IV fluid remaining and amount absorbed.
   7. Record amount of urine in drainage bag.
   8. Record all medications administered in recovery room.
   9. Clean client as needed (change gown, wash off excess surgical scrub solution).

Surgical Floor

Assessment

A. Assess for patent airway; administer oxygen as necessary.
B. Assess vital signs—usual orders are q 15 minutes until stable; then q ½ hour × 2, q hour × 4; then q 4 hours for 24–48 hours.
C. Check IV site and patency frequently.
D. Observe and record urine output.
E. Assess intake and output.
F. Observe skin color and moisture.

Implementation

A. Maintain patent airway. Position client for comfort and maximum airway ventilation.
B. Turn every two hours and p.r.n.
C. Give back care at least every four hours.

D. Encourage coughing and deep breathing every two hours (may use IPPB or blow bottles).

E. Keep client comfortable with medications.

F. Check dressings and drainage tubes every two to four hours; if abnormal amount of drainage, check more frequently.

G. Give oral hygiene at least every four hours; if nasogastric tube, nasal oxygen, or endotracheal tube is inserted, give oral hygiene every two hours.

H. Bathe client when temperature can be maintained—bathing removes the antiseptic solution and stimulates circulation.

I. Keep client warm and avoid chilling, but do not increase temperature above normal.
   1. Increased temperature increases metabolic rate and need for oxygen.
   2. Excessive perspiration causes fluid and electrolyte loss.

J. Irrigate nasogastric tube every two hours and p.r.n. with normal saline to keep patent and to prevent electrolyte imbalance.

K. Maintain dietary intake—type of diet depends on type and extent of surgical procedure.
   1. Minor surgical conditions—client may drink or eat as soon as he is awake and desires food or drink.
   2. Major surgical conditions.
      a. Maintain n.p.o. until bowel sounds return.
      b. Clear liquid advanced to full liquid as tolerated.
      c. Soft diet advanced to full diet within three to five days (depending on type of surgery and physician's preference).

L. Place on bedpan two to four hours postoperatively if catheter not inserted.

M. Start activity, as tolerated and dictated by surgical procedure. Most clients are dangled within first twenty-four hours.

ANESTHESIA

Preoperative Medications

General Action

A. Decreases secretions of mouth and respiratory tract.

B. Depresses vagal reflexes—slows heart and prevents complications with excitation during intubation.

C. Produces drowsiness and relieves anxiety.

D. Allows anesthesia to be induced more smoothly and in smaller amounts.

Types of Drugs

A. Barbiturates.
   1. Short-acting barbiturate at bedtime (seconal or nembutal).
   2. Short-acting barbiturate one hour preoperatively (decreases blood pressure and pulse and relieves anxiety).

B. Belladonna alkaloids.
   1. General action.
      a. Decreases salivary and bronchial secretions.
      b. Allows inhalation anesthetics to be administered more easily.
      c. Prevents postoperative complications such as aspiration pneumonia.
   2. Scopolamine is used in conjunction with morphine or Demerol to produce amnesic block.
   3. Atropine blocks the vagus nerve response of decreased heart rate, which can occur as a reaction to some inhalation anesthetics.

PREOPERATIVE MEDICATIONS: TYPE AND ACTION

Hypnotic or opiate—given night before surgery
   Decreases anxiety
   Promotes good night's sleep
Hypnotic or opiate—preoperative medication
   Decreases anxiety
   Allows smooth anesthetic induction
   Provides amnesia for immediate perioperative period
Anticholinergic—preoperative medication
   Decreases secretions
   Counteracts vagal effects during anesthesia

C. Nonnarcotic analgesic.
   1. Actions.
      a. Stadol used as component of balanced anesthesia.
      b. Given IM.
      c. Does not cause dependence or respiratory depression with increased dose.
      d. Contraindicated in narcotic addiction.
   2. Side effects.
      a. Sedation, lethargy.
      b. Headache, vertigo.

c. Nervousness, palpitations, diplopia.

d. Nausea, dry mouth.

Anesthetic Agents

A. Anesthesia produces insensitivity to pain or sensation.

B. Dangers associated with anesthesia depend on overall condition of client.

1. High risk if associated cardiovascular, renal, or respiratory conditions.

2. High risk for unborn fetus and mother.

3. High risk if stomach full (chance of vomiting and aspiration).

C. Types of anesthesia.

1. General—administered IV or by inhalation. Produces loss of consciousness and decreases reflex movement.

2. Local—applied topically or injected regionally. Client is alert, but pain and sensation are decreased in surgical area.

General Anesthesia

A. Balanced anesthesia (combination of two or more drugs) is used to decrease side effects and complications of anesthetic agents.

B. Goals of general anesthesia.

1. Analgesia.

2. Unconsciousness.

3. Skeletal muscle relaxation.

C. Stages of general anesthesia.

1. Stage one: early induction—from beginning of inhalation to loss of consciousness.

2. Stage two: delirium or excitement.

a. No surgery is performed at this point—dangerous stage.

b. Breathing is irregular.

3. Stage three: surgical anesthesia.

a. Begins when client stops fighting and is breathing regularly.

b. Four planes, based on respiration, pupillary and eyeball movement, and reflex muscular responses.

4. Stage four: medullary paralysis—respiratory arrest.

D. Classifications of general anesthesia.

1. Potent (halothane, ether, chloroform)—capable of achieving all three goals of general anesthesia but with severe side effects.

2. Nonpotent (nitrous oxide).

a. If given in large dose, can achieve all three

goals of general anesthesia but produces toxicity.

b. When given in smaller doses, lacks analgesia or skeletal muscle relaxation.

3. Basal anesthesia (thiopental, Pentothal).

a. Ultra short-acting barbiturate: high doses are needed for prolonged deep anesthesia, which can lead to respiratory depression.

b. Used for induction: effects are rapid, allowing for less inhalation anesthesia.

4. Dissociative anesthesia (ketamine HCl and Innovar).

a. Used with nitrous oxide and oxygen for short anesthesia.

b. Client is awake but unaware of what is actually happening.

c. Useful for burn dressings.

E. Adjuncts for general anesthesia.

1. Preoperative medications.

2. Neuromuscular blocking agents (Anectine, Pavulon, Flaxedil) used to facilitate intubation.

Local Anesthesia

A. Topical anesthetics.

1. Poorly absorbed through skin but usually rapid through mucous membranes (mouth, gastrointestinal tract, etc.).

2. Systemic toxicity is rare but local reactions common, especially if used for long periods of time on clients allergic to chemicals.

3. Used for hemorrhoids, episiotomy, nipple erosion, and minor cuts and burns.

4. Used on eye procedures extensively—removing foreign bodies and tonometry.

B. Infiltrated local anesthesia (or field block).

1. Anesthesia directly applied to surgical area.

2. Drug is injected into tissue.

3. Can have systemic effects if injected into highly vascular area.

C. Regional anesthetics (central nerve blocks).

1. Types: spinal, caudal, saddle, epidural.

2. Precautions.

a. Spinal and epidural anesthesia: position client with head and shoulders elevated (prevents diffusion of anesthesia to the intercostal muscles which could produce respiratory distress).

b. Epidural (continuous anesthesia used in obstetrics): make sure catheter is securely fastened to prevent it from slipping out.

POSTANESTHESIA

Implementation

A. General anesthesia.
1. Maintain patent airway.
2. Promote adequate respiratory function (position client for lung expansion).
3. Have client deep breathe and cough frequently, especially if inhalation anesthesia used, to promote faster elimination of gases.
4. Turn frequently to promote lung expansion and to prevent hypostatic pneumonia and venous stasis.

B. Spinal and epidural anesthesia.
1. Take precautions to prevent injury to lower extremities (watch heating pad, position limb correctly, etc.).
2. Provide gentle passive range of motion to prevent venous stasis.
3. Keep head flat or slightly elevated to prevent spinal headache (client may turn head from side to side).
4. Increase fluid intake, if tolerated, to increase cerebral spinal fluid.

Postoperative Medications

A. Evaluate need for pain relief.
B. Provide nonmedication measures for relief of pain such as relaxation techniques, back care, positioning.
C. Identify the pharmacological action of the medication.
D. Review the general side effects of the medication.
1. Drowsiness.
2. Euphoria.
3. Sleep.
4. Respiratory depression.
5. Nausea and vomiting.
E. Administer medications as ordered, usually at three to four hour intervals for first 24 to 48 hours for better action and pain relief. Assess for pain relief.
F. Know the action of the following drugs.
1. Opiates.
2. Synthetic opiate-like drugs.
3. Nonnarcotic pain relievers.
4. Narcotic antagonists.
5. Antiemetics.

Narcotic Analgesics

A. Pharmacological action—reduces pain and restlessness.
B. General side effects.
1. Drowsiness.
2. Euphoria.
3. Sleep.
4. Respiratory depression.
5. Nausea and vomiting.
C. Given at three- to four-hour intervals for first 24 to 48 hours for better action and pain relief.
D. Types of analgesics.
1. Opiates.
   a. Morphine sulfate—potent analgesic.
      (1) Specific side effects: miosis (pinpoint pupils) and bradycardia.
      (2) Usual dosage: ¼ to ⅙ gr IM q 3–4 hours p.r.n.
   b. Dilaudid—potent analgesic.
      (1) Specific side effects: hypotension, constipation, euphoria.
      (2) Usual dosage: 2 to 4 mg p.o., IM or IV q 4–6 hours.
   c. Numorphan—potent analgesic.
      (1) Specific side effects: urinary retention, ileus, euphoria.
      (2) Usual dosage: 1–1.5 mg sub q or IM q 4–6 hours; 0.5 mg IV q 4–6 hours.
   d. Codeine sulfate—mild analgesic.
      (1) Specific side effect: constipation.
      (2) Usual dosage: 30 mg to 60 mg q 3–4 hours IM.
2. Synthetic opiate-like drugs.
   a. Demerol (meperidine)—potent analgesic.
      (1) Specific side effects: miosis or mydriasis (dilatation of pupils), hypotension, and tachycardia.
      (2) Usual dosage: 25 mg to 100 mg q 3–4 hours IM.
   b. Talwin (pentazocine)—potent analgesic.
      (1) Specific side effects: gastrointestinal disturbances, vertigo, headache, and euphoria.
      (2) Usual dosage: 50 mg oral tablets q 3–4 hours; 30 mg IM q 3–4 hours p.r.n.
3. Nonnarcotic pain relievers.
   a. Salicylates (aspirin).
      (1) Decrease pain perception without causing drowsiness and euphoria. Act at point of origin or pain impulses.

316

(2) Side effects.
  (a) Gastrointestinal irritation (give client milk and crackers).
  (b) Gastrointestinal bleeding.
  (c) Increased bleeding time (watch if client is on anticoagulants).
  (d) Hypersensitivity reactions to aspirin.
  (e) Tinnitus indicates toxic level reached.
  (f) Thrombocytopenia can occur with overdose (especially in children).
(3) Usual dosage: 300 to 600 mg q 3–4 hours, orally or rectally.
b. Nonsalicylate analgesics (acetaminophen).
  (1) Action similar to aspirin.
  (2) Side effects: hemolytic anemia and kidney damage.
  (3) Usual dosage: 325–650 mg q 3–4 hours orally.
c. Nonsteroid antiinflammatory.
  (1) Action: analgesic and antipyretic for moderate to severe pain.
  (2) Side effects: nausea, gastrointestinal disturbances, vertigo, drowiness, rash.

Antiemetics

A. Pharmacological action.
  1. Reduces the hyperactive reflex of the stomach.
  2. Makes the chemoreceptor trigger zone of medulla less sensitive to nerve impulses passing through this center to the vomiting center.
B. General side effects.
  1. Drowsiness.
  2. Dry mouth.
  3. Nervous system effects.
C. Common drugs.
  1. Phenothiazines.
    a. Compazine (prochlorperazine).
      (1) Specific side effects: amenorrhea, hypotension, and vertigo.
      (2) Normal dosage: 5 to 10 mg q 3–4 hours IM.
    b. Phenergan (promethazine).
      (1) Specific side effects: dryness of mouth and blurred vision.
      (2) Normal dosage: 12.5 to 50 mg q 4 hours p.r.n.
  2. Nonphenothiazines.
    a. Dramamine (dimenhydrinate).
      (1) Specific side effect: drowsiness.
      (2) Normal dosage: 50 mg IM q 3–4 hours.
    b. Tigan (trimethobenzamide).
      (1) Specific side effects (rare); hypotension and skin rashes.
      (2) Normal dosage: 200 mg (2 cc) t.i.d. or q.i.d. IM.

COMMON POSTOPERATIVE COMPLICATIONS

Respiratory Complications

Assessment

A. Evaluate complaint of tightness or fullness in chest.
B. Assess for cough, dypsnea, or shortness of breath.
C. Evaluate increased vital signs, particularly temperature and respiratory rate.
D. Observe for restlessness.
E. Assess for decreased breath sounds, crackles.

Implementation

A. Turn, cough, hyperventilate at least every two hours.
B. Have client use incentive spirometer to provide motivation and evaluation of sustained inspiration.
  1. Inhale deeply and hold 3 seconds.
  2. Repeat hourly.
  3. Yawning also accomplishes same goal of stimulating surfactant and opening collapsed alveoli.
C. Provide pharmacological therapy (through nebulization or oral route).
  1. Antibiotics—to fight infection by causative organism.
  2. Bronchodilators—act on smooth muscle to reduce bronchial spasm.
    a. Sympathomimetics (beta$_2$ agonists preferred).
    b. Anticholinergics (atropine sulfate inhalant).
    c. Theophyllines.
  3. Adrenocorticosteroids—to reduce inflammation (prednisone).
  4. Enzymes—to liquefy thick, purulent secretions through digestion.
    a. Dornavac.
    b. Varidase.
  5. Expectorants—to aid in expectoration of secretions.

a. Mucolytic agents reduce viscosity of secretion (Mucomyst).

b. Detergents liquefy tenacious mucus (Tergemist, Alevaire).

D. Medicate for pain to facilitate TCH and use of mechanical devices.

Pneumonia (see page 174)

Atelectasis

Definition: Collapse of pulmonary alveoli caused by mucus plug or inadequate ventilation.

Assessment

A. Assess for clinical manifestations that usually develop 24 to 48 hours postoperatively. (Most common cause of early postoperative temperature increase).

B. Observe for asymmetrical chest movement.

C. Auscultate lung sounds. Decreased or absent breath sounds over affected area; crackles; bronchial breathing over affected area.

D. Evaluate shortness of breath.

E. Assess for painful respirations; splinting of diaphragm.

G. Assess for increased vital signs: temperature, respiration, pulse.

H. Observe for anxiety and restlessness.

Implementation

A. Auscultate breath sounds every two to four hours and report unusual occurrences.

B. Encourage sustained inspiration exercises.

C. Instruct in proper cough technique (splint incision).

D. Turn frequently and position to facilitate expectoration.

E. Do clapping, percussion, vibration, if ordered.

F. Do postural drainage every four hours.

G. Administer expectorants and other medications, as ordered.

H. Suction as necessary.

I. Encourage oral fluid intake to reduce tenacious sputum and to facilitate expectoration.

J. Place client in cool room with mist mask or vaporized steam.

K. Mobilize client as soon as possible.

L. Medicate for pain to allow for respiratory ventilation.

Deep Vein Thrombophlebitis (see page 158)

Pulmonary Embolism

Definition: The movement of a thrombus from site of origin to lung.

Assessment

A. Assess for mild condition (involves smaller arteries).
1. Signs mimic pleurisy or bronchial pneumonia.
2. Transient dyspnea.
3. Mild pleuritic pain.
4. Tachycardia.
5. Increased temperature.
6. Cough with hemoptysis.

B. Assess for severe condition (involves pulmonary artery).
1. Chest pain.
2. Severe dyspnea leading to air hunger.
3. Shallow, rapid breathing.
4. Sharp substernal chest pain.
5. Vertigo leading to syncope.
6. Hypovolemia.
7. Cardiac arrhythmias.
8. Generalized weakness.
9. Feelings of doom.
10. Hypotension.

Implementation

A. Provide patent airway.
1. Place in semi- to high-Fowler's position if vital signs allow.
2. Administer oxygen as needed (nasal cannula).
3. Assist with intubation as needed.
4. Auscultate breath sounds every one to two hours.
5. Obtain arterial blood gases to ascertain acid-base imbalance.
6. Check sputum for presence of blood or blood-tinged mucus.
7. Administer diuretics or cardiotonics, as necessary.
8. Observe for signs of shock.

318

B. Administer anticoagulants (check lab values each day before administering medication, following initial anticoagulation).
C. Give narcotics for pain (watch for respiratory depression).
D. Take vital signs every two to four hours.
E. Turn as directed by physician; do not do percussion or clapping or administer back rubs.
F. Encourage client to cough and deep breathe every one to two hours.
G. Maintain bed rest; have client avoid sudden movements.
H. Give emotional support and prepare for lung scan.
I. Observe for possible extension of emboli or for occurrence of other emboli.
   1. Check urine for hematuria or oliguria.
   2. Check legs, especially calf.
J. Prepare for surgical intervention.
   1. Surgical intervention carries high risk.
   2. Types of surgery.
      a. Femoral vein ligation.
      b. Ligation of inferior vena cava.
      c. Pulmonary embolectomy.

Fat Embolism

Definition: Release of medullary fat droplets into bloodstream following trauma.

Characteristics

A. Embolism occurs after long bone or sternum fractures (particularly from mishandling of client or incorrect splinting of fracture).
B. Fat droplets that are released from the marrow enter the venous circulation and usually become lodged in the lungs. If the fat droplets become lodged in the brain, the embolism is severe and usually fatal.
C. Usually occurs within first 24 hours following injury.
D. Major cause of death from fractures.
E. Prevent by adequate splinting at accident scene.

Assessment

A. Assess for classical sign: petechiae from fat globule deposits across chest, shoulders, and axilla. Petechiae do not blanch, but fade out within hours. Can involve conjunctiva.

B. Evaluate related pulmonary signs: shortness of breath, leading to pallor, cyanosis, and hypoxemia.
C. Evaluate related brain involvement: restlessness, memory loss, confusion, headache, hemiparesis.
D. Observe for related cardiac involvement.
   1. Tachycardia.
   2. Right ventricular failure.
   3. Decreased cardiac output.
E. Assess for other signs and symptoms.
   1. Diaphoresis.
   2. Change in level of consciousness.
   3. Shock.
   4. Increased temperature (if involvement of hypothalamus).

Implementation

A. Position client in high-Fowler's position to allow for respiratory exchange. Maintain bed rest.
B. Administer oxygen to decrease anoxia and to reduce surface tension of fat globules (IPPB may be needed).
C. Obtain arterial blood gases to maintain sufficient pO_2 levels.
D. Physician may intubate and place on respirator if respirations are severely compromised.
E. Institute preventive treatment to avoid further complications, such as shock and heart failure.
F. Monitor administration of medications.
   1. Alcohol drip.
   2. Cortisone therapy to reduce inflammation.
   3. Decholin to emulsify fat.
   4. Antihyperlipemic drugs.
   5. Heparin to decrease platelet aggregation.
   6. Dextran to improve blood flow.

Shock Lung (Adult Respiratory Distress Syndrome, or Wet Lung)

Characteristics

A. Can be secondary to viral pneumonia.
B. Massive trauma and hemorrhagic shock.
C. Fat emboli.
D. Neurological injuries.
E. Sepsis.
F. Pathophysiology—damage to pulmonary capillary membrane that produces a leak, diffuse interstitial edema, and intra-alveolar hemorrhage.
G. Decrease in surfactant.

H. Intrapulmonary shunting with decreased oxygen saturation—hypoxia.

I. Decreased lung compliance.

Assessment

A. Assess for clinical manifestations. Usually seen within first 24 hours following shock.

B. Observe for extreme dyspnea, tachypnea, and cyanosis.

C. Assess for pulmonary edema.

D. Auscultate lungs for atelectasis (many small emboli throughout lungs).

E. Evaluate blood gas alterations.
  1. pO_2 decreased.
  2. pCO_2 normal or decreased due to tachypnea.
  3. pH normal to slightly alkalotic.

Implementation

A. Prevent overhydration in severe trauma cases.

B. Provide early treatment of severe hypoxemia.

C. Keep clients "dry," as they have excess fluids in their lungs. (Restrict fluid intake.)

D. Administer medications.
  1. Corticosteroids to reduce inflammation and to prevent further capillary membrane deterioration.
  2. Diuretics to decrease fluid overload.
  3. Sedatives to prevent client from resisting respirator.
  4. Heparin to reduce platelet aggregation.
  5. Antibiotics.

E. Maintain adequate ventilation and oxygenation.
  1. Provide intubation and mechanical ventilation with volume respirator.
  2. Obtain frequent arterial blood gases.
  3. Suction frequently with "bagging." Ambu bag increases alveolar expansion.

F. Provide tracheostomy care, if necessary, every four hours.

G. Provide oral hygiene every four hours.

H. Prevent further complications, such as shock and septicemia.

I. Provide adequate nutrition.

Wound Infections

Characteristics

A. Usual causative agents.
  1. Staphylococcus.
  2. Pseudomonas aeruginosa.
  3. Proteus vulgaris.
  4. Escherichia coli.

B. Usually occur within five to seven days of surgery.

PATIENTS AT RISK FOR POSTOPERATIVE INFECTION

Uncontrolled diabetes
Renal failure
Obesity
Receiving corticosteroids
Receiving immunosuppressive agents
Prolonged antibiotic therapy
Protein and/or ascorbic acid deficiencies
Marked dehydration and hypovolemia
Decreased cardiac output
Edema and fluid and electrolyte imbalances
Anemia
Preoperative infection

Assessment

A. Observe for slowly increasing temperature and tachycardia.

B. Evaluate pain and tenderness surrounding surgical site.

C. Observe for edema and erythema surrounding suture site.

D. Feel for increased warmth around suture site.

E. Observe for purulent drainage.
  1. Yellow if staphylococcus.
  2. Green if pseudomonas.

Implementation

A. Take all cultures before starting medication.

B. Administer specific antibiotics for causative agent.

C. Irrigate wound with solution as ordered (usually hydrogen peroxide and normal saline).

D. Keep dressing and skin area dry to prevent skin excoriation and spread of bacteria.

E. Use sterile technique in changing dressings.

F. If excoriation occurs, use karaya powder and drainage bags around area of wound.

Wound Dehiscence and Evisceration

Definition: Dehiscence is the splitting open of wound edges. Evisceration is the extensive loss of pinkish fluid (purulent if infection is present) through a wound and the protrusion of a loop of bowel through an open wound. Client feels like "everything is pulling apart."

Assessment

A. Observe for usual causes.
  1. General debilitation.
    a. Poor nutrition.
    b. Chronic illness.
    c. Obesity.
  2. Inadequate wound closure.
  3. Wound infection.
  4. Severe abdominal stretching (by coughing or vomiting).
B. Evaluate wound daily. Condition occurs about seventh postoperative day.

Implementation

A. Wound dehiscence.
  1. Apply butterfly tapes to incision area.
  2. Increase protein in diet.
  3. Observe for signs of infection and treat accordingly.
  4. Apply scultetus binder when ambulating.
B. Evisceration.
  1. Lay client in supine position.
  2. Cover protruding intestine with moist, sterile, normal saline packs; change packs frequently to keep moist.
  3. Notify physician.
  4. Take vital signs for baseline data and detection of shock.
  5. Notify operating room for wound closure.
  6. Provide patent IV.

Disseminated Intravascular Coagulation (DIC)

Definition: Simultaneous activation of the thrombin (clotting) and fibrinolytic system.

Characteristics

A. Excessive intravascular thrombin is produced, which converts fibrinogen to fibrin clot.
B. After fibrinogen is used up, circulating thrombin continues to be present and will continue to convert any form of fibrinogen to fibrin.
C. Fibrinogen enters system by transfusion or by body production of fibrinogen. This process intensifies the hemorrhagic state.
D. DIC is associated with extracorporeal circulation and obstetric complications.

E. Arterial hypotension results in arterial vasoconstriction and capillary dilatation; this causes a shunting of blood which leads to acidotic blood formed from blood stagnation.
F. Stress is the primary cause of increased fibrinolysis.

Assessment

A. Observe for excessive bleeding (caused by depletion of clotting factors) through genitourinary tract, following injections, etc.
B. Evaluate lab results for low hemoglobin, low platelets.
C. Evaluate arterial blood gases for acidosis.
D. Observe for skin lesions, such as petechiae, purpura, subcutaneous hematomas.

Implementation

A. Treat cause of DIC symptomatically.
  1. Antibiotics for infections.
  2. Fluids and colloids for shock.
  3. Steroids for endotoxins.
  4. Dialysis for renal failure.
B. Administer heparin IV to stop cycle of thrombosis—hemorrhage.
  1. Neutralizes free circulating thrombin.
  2. Inhibits blood clotting in vivo, due to effect on factor IX.
  3. Prevents extension of thrombi.
  4. Keep clotting time two to three times normal.
  5. Give 10,000 to 20,000 units every two to four hours.
C. Give transfusion of platelets and fresh-frozen plasma to replace clotting factors.
D. Administer oxygen as needed.
E. Take precautions to prevent additional hemorrhage.
  1. Avoid chest tube "milking."
  2. Take temperature orally or axillary, not rectally.
  3. Avoid administration of parenteral medications if possible.
  4. Avoid trauma to mucous membranes.
  5. If nasogastric tube inserted, prevent bleeding by administering antacids and keeping NG tube connected to low suction. Do not irrigate unless absolutely necessary.

Table 1. TRANSFUSION REACTIONS

Type	Clinical Manifestations	Nursing Interventions
Bacterial	Sudden increase in temperature	Stop transfusion immediately.
	Hypotension	Maintain IV site; change tubing as soon as possible.
	Dry, flushed skin	Observe for shock. Monitor vital signs every 15 minutes until stable.
	Abdominal pain	Obtain urine specimen. Insert Foley if necessary.
	Headache	Notify physician and obtain order for broad spectrum antibiotic.
	Lumbar pain	Draw blood cultures before antibiotic administration.
	Sudden chill	Send blood tubing and bag to lab for culture and sensitivity.
		Control hyperthermia.
Allergic	Urticaria and hives, pruritus	Stop transfusion immediately if symptoms are severe.
	Respiratory wheezing, laryngeal edema	Monitor vital signs for possible anaphylactic shock.
	Anaphylactic reaction	If symptoms are mild, slow down transfusion and obtain order for antihistamine.
		Monitor for signs of progressive allergic reaction as transfusion continues.
Hemolytic	Severe pain in kidney region and chest	Stop transfusion immediately.
	Pain at needle insertion site	Change IV tubing as soon as possible, maintaining patent IV. If necessary, disconnect IV tubing from needle and run normal saline through IV tubing into emesis basin. Reconnect tubing to needle and obtain new tubing as soon as possible.
	Fever (may reach 105°F), chills	Administer oxygen.
	Dyspnea and cyanosis	Send two blood samples, from different sites, urine sample (cath if necessary), blood, and transfusion record to lab.
	Headache	Obtain orders for IV volume expansion and diuretic (mannitol) to ensure flushing of kidneys to prevent acute renal tubular necrosis.
	Hypotension	Monitor vital signs every 15 minutes for shock.
	Hematuria	Monitor urine output hourly for possible renal failure. Foley catheter may need to be inserted.

POSTOPERATIVE COMPLICATIONS

POTENTIAL COMPLICATION	PATIENTS AT RISK	INDICATIVE FINDINGS

Atelectasis: collapse of alveoli; may be diffuse and involve a segment or lobe, or lung
 	
Potential Onset:
First 48 hours
	All with general anesthesia
	Special risk clients:
	Smokers
	Chronic bronchitis
	Emphysema
	Obesity
	Elderly
	Upper abdominal surgery
	Chest surgery
	Abdominal distention
		Fever to 102°F
		Tachycardia
		Restlessness
		Tachypnea 24–30 min
		Altered breath sounds
		  Dullness to percussion
		  Diminished or absent breath
		    sounds
		  Rales
		ABGs: decreased PaO_2

Pneumonia: inflammatory process in which alveoli are filled with exudate
 	
Potential onset:
First 36 to 48 hours
	Clients with unresolved atelectasis
	Following aspiration
	Smoker
	Elderly
	Chronic bronchitis
	Emphysema
	Heart failure
	Debilitated
	Alcoholic
	Immobile
	Cough suppressant medications
	Respiratory depressant medications
		Client complains of dyspnea; tachycardia; increasing temperature; productive cough and increasing amount of sputum becoming tenacious, rusty, or purulent
		Tactile fremitus
		Dullness to percussion
		Bronchial breath sounds
		Increased wet rales or rhonchi
		Voice sounds present
		  Bronchophony
		    Egophony
		      Whispered pectoriloquy
		ABGs: decreased PaO_2

Pulmonary embolism: foreign object has migrated to branch of pulmonary artery *Potential onset:* Seventh to tenth day *Massive embolism:* Pulmonary hypertension, dyspnea, right heart failure, shock, ABGs: decreased PaO_2, increased $PaCO_2$	Superficial vein thrombosis: rare Deep vein thrombosis: 40 to 60 percent Air emboli: intraperitoneal surgery Fat emboli: long bone fracture, split sternum	Only 10 percent recognized clinically Pain sharp and stabbing, occurs with breathing; localized (right lower lobe most frequent) Increased respiratory rate Increased heart rate Restlessness
Pulmonary infarction: necrosis of lung tissue due to occlusion of blood supply (less than 10 percent develop) *Potential onset:* 2 to 72 hrs. after arterial obstruction	Pulmonary embolism	Hemoptysis Cough Fever 101° to 102°F Pleural friction rub Pleuritic pain

PREVENTION	INTERVENTION	DRUG THERAPY
Preoperative: have client practice turning, coughing, and deep breathing Discuss importance of exercises *Postoperative clients at risk:* Turn q30 min. Deep breathe and cough *Other clients:* Initiate turning and deep breathing exercises q1–2 hrs. Ambulate as soon as possible Medicate to reduce pain, splinting, and resistance to treatment	Increase effectiveness of pulmonary toilet Administer supplemental oxygen as ordered Monitor response to treatment Monitor for onset of pneumonia If entire lobe of lung is involved, prepare for bronchoscopy to remove plug	*Analgesics:* pain control Bronchodilators (nebulized through IPPB): liquefy secretions Water or saline (nebulized through IPPB): liquefy secretions
Provide vigorous treatment of atelectasis Prevent aspiration	Turn, cough, and deep breathe q1 hr. May need to stimulate cough with nasotracheal suctioning Send sputum for culture and sensitivity Frequent mouth care for comfort Administer oxygen as ordered Increase fluid intake Monitor for response to treatment	Antibiotics: Cephalosporin or ampicillin prophylactically for 48 hours for high risk patients Cephalosporin IV or parenteral for infections Antipyretics: decrease temperature
Provide range of motion Encourage early ambulation Prevent thrombophlebitis Do not massage a potential or suspected thrombophlebitic area	Administer oxygen to relieve hypoxia Reduce anxiety Position client on left side with head dependent to prevent air embolus Prevent recurrent embolization; prepare for fibrinolysis; prepare for anticoagulation Prepare for x-ray, angiography, and/or ventilation/perfusion scan	Anticoagulation therapy: low-dose heparin or warfarin Sodium prophylactically for high risk patients Streptokinase: thrombolytic effect (24 hours) Heparin therapy: decrease clotting time Analgesics: pleuritic pain control
Prevent thromboembolic pulmonary artery occlusion. See prevention of thrombophlebitis	Describe indicative findings to physician Institute relaxation techniques to decrease client's anxiety Administer oxygen Support and comfort client	Antibiotics: infection control

POTENTIAL COMPLICATION	PATIENTS AT RISK	INDICATIVE FINDINGS
Thrombophlebitis: inflammation of vein with clot formation *Potential onset:* Seventh to fourteenth day	*Abnormal vein walls:* Varicose veins Previous thrombophlebitis Trauma to vein wall Tight strap on operating room table Surgery on hips or in pelvis Age more than 60 (arteriosclerosis) *Venous stasis:* Immobility Casts, restrictive dressings Constant Fowler's position Prolonged dependent lower extremities Knee-gatch elevated Pillows under knees Pillows under calves Obesity Abdominal distention Shock Heart failure *Hypercoagulability:* Surgical stress repsonse Stress and anxiety Infection Anesthesia Decreased circulation Hypovolemia Malignant neoplasms Postpartum Oral contraceptives	*Superficial vein thrombophlebitis:* Pain, redness, tenderness, and induration along course of vein Palpable "cord" corresponding to course of vein History of trauma including IV site *Deep small-vein thrombophlebitis:* Increased muscle turgor and tenderness over affected vein Deep muscle tenderness Most frequent site: vessels at calf Affected limb warm to touch with occasional swelling Client complains of tightness or stiffness in affected leg Positive Homan's sign (dorsiflexion of foot leads to calf pain) Fever rarely more than 101°F *Major deep-vein thrombophlebitis:* No superficial signs of inflammation Homan's sign unreliable *Femoral vein thrombosis:* Pain and tenderness in distal thigh and popliteal region. Swelling extends to level of knee *Iliofemoral vein:* Often massive swelling, pain and tenderness of entire lower extremity Cyanosis of extremity when dependent Superficial veins sometimes visibly dilated Circumference differential more than 15 mm in males and more than 12 mm in females; most reliable for diagnosis
Gastric distention: accumulation of swallowed air and gastric juices in presence of ileus *Potential onset:* First 24 to 36 hours	All surgical clients	Increased abdominal circumference (measured) Client's complaining of fullness and/or "gas pains" Tympanic abdominal percussion sounds

PREVENTION	INTERVENTION	DRUG THERAPY
Avoid injury to vein wall: Use care when strapping to operating room table Avoid IVs in lower extremities Pad side rails for restless, convulsive, and/or combative client Avoid restraints *Avoid venous stasis:* Encourage early ambulation Provide feet and leg exercises: 10 min. q1–2 hr. while in bed Increase frequency of exercise for client at risk Prevent client's sitting with legs in dependent position Place pillow between legs while client is lying on side to prevent pressure from upper leg on lower Provide deep breathing exercise Provide active and passive range of motion Prevent restrictive dressings, casts, and positions Increase velocity of blood flow: No standing Steady IV flow Antiembolic stockings (controversial) Decrease hypercoagulability: Provide adequate hydration Prevent infections Maintain circulation Decrease stress/anxiety	*Superficial vein thrombophlebitis:* Treat symptoms Local heat Continue ambulation unless accompanied by deep venous involvement Monitor for progression toward saphenafemoral junction (may need ligation) *Deep vein thrombophlebitis:* Provide adequate bed rest Elevate foot of bed with 6–8″ blocks Administer warm moist compresses to relieve venospasm and help resolve inflammation Monitor for pulmonary embolism	Streptokinase: thrombolytic effect (24 hours) Heparin IV or Sub q.: decrease clotting time (short term) Coumadin p.o.: decrease clotting time (long term) Analgesics: pain control
Encourage client to avoid air swallowing Do not use straws Early ambulation	Provide frequent turning to move air and secretions Have client sit up in chair or ambulate if appropriate Insert nasogastric tube and connect to low suction Monitor abdominal circumference by measuring q1 hr. Monitor for return of bowel sounds Monitor for passage of flatus Insert rectal tube	IV Electrolyte therapy: potassium Lactated Ringer's or Physiologic Saline IV solution

POTENTIAL COMPLICATION	PATIENTS AT RISK	INDICATIVE FINDINGS
Ileus: failure of peristalsis *Potential onset:* First 24 to 36 hours	All surgical clients Stress response to surgical trauma	No bowel sounds or fewer than 5/min. (normal: 5–35 clicks or gurgles/min.) Vomiting Abdominal distention

Paralytic ileus: paralysis of intestinal
  peristalsis
 	
Potential onset:
First three to four days
	Intraperitoneal surgery
	Peritonitis
	Kidney surgery
	Decreased cardiac output
	Pneumonia
	Electrolyte imbalance
	Wound infection
		No bowel sounds
		Abdominal distention
		No passage of flatus
		Nasogastric drainage green to yellow,
		  1–2 liters in 24 hrs.

Intestinal obstruction: adhesions,
  trap or kink in segment of intestine
 	
Potential onset:
Third to fifth day
	Abdominal surgery	No postoperative bowel movement
		Abdominal distention
		Client complains of periodic sharp,
		  colicky pains
		Hyperactive, high-pitched, tinkling
		  bowel sounds
		Abdominal tenderness
		Nasogastric drainage: dark brown or
		  black
		The lower the obstruction the more
		  gradual the onset

Urinary tract infection
 	
Potential Onset:
Third to fifth day or 48 hrs. after
  removal of catheter
	Decreased resistance:
	History of bladder distention
	History of urinary retention
	Previous urinary tract infection
	History of prostatic hypertrophy
	History of catheterization
	Diabetic
	Debilitated
	Immobile
		Dysuria
		Frequency
		Urgency
		High fever: up to 104°F with fewer
		  systemic toxic symptoms than would
		  be expected
		Change in urine odor
		Pus in urine
		Sediment
		May be asymptomatic

PREVENTION	INTERVENTION	DRUG THERAPY
Do not feed until bowel sounds return Offer only sips of water until return of bowel sounds Maintain normal serum potassium level	Monitor for return of normal bowel sounds Monitor for distention Monitor for passage of flatus signaling return of peristalsis Monitor signs of hypokalemia	
Maintain electrolyte balance Maintain cardiac output Prevent pneumonia Prevent wound infection Provide early ambulation	Same as for gastric distention Maintain nasogastric suction until peristalsis returns Monitor for intestinal obstruction	Potassium chloride if serum level is low
None	Identify condition early Report to physician immediately Reduce client anxiety Maintain patent nasogastric tube Prepare for insertion of intestinal tube (Miller-Abbott, Canton, or Harris) Prepare for surgery if necessary	Antibiotic therapy: for prevention of infection (optional) Analgesics: pain control Never give laxative or purgative if obstruction is suspected
Maintain sterile technique with catheterization and catheter removal Provide competent indwelling catheter care Encourage early ambulation to decrease retention and stasis	Encourage fluid intake; cranberry juice to decrease urine pH Increase activity to enhance bladder emptying Encourage voiding q2 hrs. while awake Send specimen for culture and sensitivity Monitor for residual urine of more than 100 cc	Urinary antiseptics (sulfonamides): bacterial suppression Antibiotics (ampicillin, tetracycline): bacterial suppression Anticholinergics: antispasmodic Topical urinary analgesic: pain relief

POTENTIAL COMPLICATION	PATIENTS AT RISK	INDICATIVE FINDINGS
Wound infection *Potential onset:* Streptococcal: 24 to 48 hrs. after contamination Staphylococcus gram-negative rods, etc.: five to seven days postoperatively	*Slow to heal:* Obese Diabetic *Poor nutrition:* Debilitated Elderly Ulcerative colitis *Poor circulation:* Elderly Hypovolemic Heart failure *Lack of oxygen to wound:* Vasoconstriction Severe anemia Depressed immunity Cancer Renal failure Preoperative steroid therapy Prolonged complex surgery (stress response leading to increased ACTH) Malnutrition Elderly At risk for transmission Proximity of another client with infection Transmission by hands of personnel	Initial inflammation: 36–48 hrs. Wound tender, swollen, warm, increased redness Increasing heart rate Increasing temperature Increasing or recurring serous drainage There may be no local signs if infection is deep

SHOCK STATES

Definition: An abnormal physiological state in which there is insufficient circulating blood volume for the size of the vascular bed, thereby resulting in circulatory failure and tissue anoxia.

Classifications of Shock States

A. Hypovolemic.
  1. Definition: decreased intravascular fluid volume.
  2. Etiology.
    a. Blood loss (hematogenic)—from trauma, surgery, etc.
    b. Plasma and/or fluid loss.
      (1) Plasma loss—burns.
      (2) Fluid loss—diarrhea, vomiting, diabetes.
B. Neurogenic.
  1. Definition: massive vasodilation and pooling of blood due to failure of sympathetic nerve impulses to produce vasoconstriction.
  2. Etiology.
    a. Drug overdose, especially narcotics.
    b. Severe pain.
    c. Damage to medulla.
    d. Deep anesthesia.
C. Vasogenic.
  1. Definition: massive vasodilation and pooling of blood due to failure of peripheral vessels to react to neural stimuli.
  2. Etiology.
    a. Antigen—antibody reaction causes anaphylactic shock.
      (1) Insect stings.
      (2) Allergies to drugs, particularly antibiotics.
      (3) Blood transfusions.
      (4) Vaccines.
    b. Bacterial invasion causes gram negative sepsis (septic shock).
      (1) Following urinary tract instrumentation.

PREVENTION	INTERVENTION	DRUG THERAPY
Maintain nutrition	Maintain nutrition	Anticholinergics: antispasmodic
Maintain good circulation	Maintain oxygenation	Topical urinary analgesic: pain relief
Maintain normal blood volume	Maintain circulation and blood volume	
Provide nonrestrictive dressings, casts, etc.	Maintain pulmonary toilet	
Provide frequent turning	Send wound drainage specimen for culture and sensitivity	
Have client sit up in chair or ambulate as soon as possible	Cleanse wound or irrigate as ordered	
Maintain PaO$_2$	Monitor for systemic response to infection, fever, malaise, headache, anorexia, nausea	
Treat atelectasis	Treat symptoms	
Prevent pulmonary complications		
Monitor ABGs if necessary		
Prevent severe anemia: replace lost RBCs		
Increase attention to prevention for clients with depressed immunity		
Prevent transmission:		
Practice effective handwashing		
Practice aseptic technique in wound care		
Separate postoperative from infected clients		
Maintain dry dressings		
Use special caution for a new wound, easily contaminated		

(2) Overwhelming bacterial invasion of an "at risk" client.

D. Cardiogenic.
  1. Definition: left ventricular pump failure which results in circulatory inadequacy.
  2. Etiology.
    a. Myocardial infarction.
    b. Congestive heart failure.
    c. Cardiac arrest.

Assessment

Assessment of Early Shock

A. Assess early stages, regardless of cause.
  1. Decreased tissue perfusion.
  2. Cellular hypoxia.
  3. Increased sympathetic nervous system activity.
B. Observe for oliguria—usually the first sign of shock.
  1. Decreased blood volume through kidneys.

  2. Decreased urine output; hyperkalemia can be a problem.
C. Observe for hypotension.
  1. Due to compensatory peripheral vasoconstriction (not evident initially, but it does appear in late shock).
  2. Narrowing pulse pressure—due to systolic pressure falling and diastolic pressure being maintained.
  3. Traditional criteria—systolic blood pressure below 70 mm Hg.
D. Assess for tachycardia—due to heart's responding to increased sympathetic activity.
E. Assess for tachypnea.
  1. Medulla is stimulated by buildup in lactic acid through anaerobic metabolism.
  2. As blood pH is lowered, the respiratory rate increases in an effort to blow off excess carbon dioxide and return body to acid-base balance.
F. Evaluate if cool, dry, or moist skin is present.
  1. Caused by peripheral vasoconstriction.
  2. Blood is supplied to vital organs rather than to skin.

G. Assess sensorium changes—due to brain cell hypoxia.
   1. Restlessness.
   2. Apprehension and anxiety.
   3. Lethargy.
   4. Confusion.
   5. Semiconsciousness to coma.
H. Observe if excess thirst is present due to loss of fluids or blood volume as well as peripheral vasoconstriction, which decreases salivary secretions.
I. Evaluate fatigue and muscle weakness—result of shift from aerobic to anaerobic metabolism leading to lactic acid buildup.

Assessment of Severe Shock

A. Assess blood pressure: below 70 mm Hg and narrowing of pulse pressure (body loses ability to compensate and blood pressure drops rapidly).
B. Observe for shallow, irregular respirations.
C. Observe for tachycardia.
D. Evaluate level of unconsciousness: progresses to coma as blood supply to brain cell decreases.
E. Observe for dilated, fixed pupils due to decreased oxygen to brain.
F. Observe for anuria as blood supply to kidneys decreases sharply.
G. Evaluate cyanotic skin, mucous membranes, and nailbeds.

Hypovolemic Shock

Degrees of Shock

A. Slight: approximately 20 percent of blood volume is lost.
B. Moderate: approximately 35 percent of blood volume is lost.
C. Severe: approximately 45 percent of blood volume is lost.

Implementation

A. Prepare client for IV fluid, plasma expanders, blood replacement, and drugs (vasodilator).
B. Start IV fluid with D_5W. When adequate kidney function is assessed, change to Ringer's lactate (this is more isotonic).

C. Place client in supine position with legs elevated, and head on pillow. (Trendelenburg's position compromises ventilation and baroreceptor mechanisms).
D. Provide oxygen via nasal catheter, mask, or cannula.
E. Record vital signs every fifteen minutes. Changes take place slowly except in massive hemorrhage.
   1. Blood pressure.
      a. Decreased BP is usually late sign of shock.
      b. Orthostatic hypotension develops before systemic hypotension.
      c. Systolic BP below 80 mm Hg indicates inadequate coronary artery blood flow.
      d. Progressive drop in BP with a thready, increasing pulse indicates fluid loss.
      e. Decreased BP with strong, irregular pulse indicates heart failure.
   2. Respirations.
      a. Become rapid and shallow early in shock (compensation for tissue anoxia).
      b. Slow breathing (below four per minute) appears late in shock after compensatory failure.
      c. Emergency respiratory equipment (ventilator, trach tubes, etc.) should be available.
   3. Temperature.
      a. Below normal with hemorrhagic shock.
      b. Gradually increasing temperature indicates sepsis.
   4. Central venous pressure.
      a. CVP line should be inserted in subclavian vein.
      b. If below 5 cm, H_2O indicates shock condition.
      c. If CVP decreases early, it is usually a sign of shock.
F. Insert Foley catheter for hourly urine volumes.
   1. Record intake and output.
   2. Notify physician if total urine output is below 30 cc/hour.
G. Monitor skin changes.
   1. Change in skin temperature and color reflect changes in tissue oxygenation and perfusion.
      a. Cold, clammy skin indicates peripheral vascular constriction.
      b. Flushing and sweating reflects overheating, which indicates increased metabolic rate and the need for oxygen.
      c. Pallor and cyanosis indicate tissue hypoxia.
   2. Observe for restlessness—indicates hypoxia.
H. Place enough light covering over client to prevent

chilling, but not enough to cause vasodilatation.

I. Treat the cause of the shock (stop bleeding, prepare for surgery, etc.).

Cardiogenic Shock

Assessment

A. Identify specific symptoms related to severe shock.

B. Assess for additional common symptoms of shock.
1. Cardiac arrhythmias leading to cardiac arrest.
2. Increased left ventricular pressure.
3. Heart failure symptoms.
   a. Orthopnea.
   b. Cyanosis.
   c. Dyspnea.
   d. Pitting edema.
   e. Distended neck veins.
   f. Pulmonary congestion.
4. Acidosis.
5. Hypokalemia.

Implementation

A. Monitor hemodynamics (PCWP, SVI), vital signs, heart rhythm.

B. Administer vasodilator or pressor agents as ordered.

C. Administer inotropic agents (dopamine, dobutamine).

D. Check arterial blood gases frequently.

E. Utilize intra-aortic balloon counterpulsation.

F. Follow interventions for hypovolemic shock for additional nursing care.

Septic Shock

Assessment

A. Stage I "warm shock" may appear to be mild infection.
1. Mental confusion may be first sign.
2. Assess fever, flushed pink face warm to the touch.
3. Observe for normal blood pressure; pulse and respirations slightly increased.
4. May not appear to be shock.

B. Stage B "cool shock."
1. Assess tachycardia; blood pressure continued normal; PO_2 is dropping.
2. Does not appear pink and warm/cool skin.
3. Observe for hyperventilation; pulmonary congestion.
4. Assess urine output—may drop to 30 cc an hour.
5. Assess thirst.

C. Stage 3 most dangerous.
1. Assess cold and clammy skin—client looks "shocky."
2. Assess hypotension and tachycardia (CVP is increased).
3. Observe urine output—may fall to zero.

Implementation

A. Administer broad spectrum antibiotics as ordered—begin stat (do not wait for regular medication times).
1. Continue to check IV site frequently—if evidence of infection, get a new site.
2. Check BUN level regularly.

B. Take vital signs hourly. Stages can progress rapidly.

C. Observe continually for change in pattern: blood pressure down, pulse and respirations up. Notify physician immediately.

D. Check PO_2 and pH—client may go into metabolic acidosis. Notify physician if pH falls below 7.35.

E. Administer O_2 as ordered—concentration should be moderate.

F. Give frequent skin care to prevent breakdown.

G. Check I & O frequently; pay attention to amount of urine from catheter.
1. Urine output falls below 33cc/hour, notify physician.
2. Prevent fluid overload by calculating previous hourly urine output plus 30cc/hour.

H. Administer aspirin or cooling blanket if necessary to control fever.

I. Provide appropriate psychological support.
1. Client is frightened, so remain in the room.
2. Explain all procedures and attempt to alleviate anxiety.

J. Observe for complications or reversal in improvement of shock state:
1. Respiratory: dyspnea, cyanosis, intercostal retractions (shock lung).
2. Cardiac: heart failure—may require digitalis.
3. Renal: oliguria—may require mannitol.

Vasogenic Shock

ANAPHYLACTIC SHOCK

A. Caused by hypersensitivity to allergen (allergic reaction to medication, bee sting, etc.).

B. Antigen—antibody reaction.

C. Increased cell membrane permeability—histamine is released, causing marked vasodilatation.
D. Bronchiolar constriction.
E. Pooling of blood, causing decreased venous return.
F. Decreased cardiac output and hypoxia.

Assessment

A. Evaluate local edema.
B. Observe for urticaria (occasional).
C. Evaluate flushed face.
D. Evaluate if apprehension is present.
E. Assess for dyspnea, respiratory difficulty, cyanosis, wheezing.
F. Observe for vertigo, decreased blood pressure, increased pulse.

Implementation

A. Identify causative agent.
B. Position client for optimal cerebral perfusion (flat or 30-degree elevation if dyspneic).
C. Maintain patent airway.
D. Administer epinephrine, sub q.
   1. Dilates bronchioles and constricts arterioles.
   2. Side effects: tachycardia, CNS stimulation.
   3. Rapid acting.
E. Administer oxygen.
F. Administer antihistamine (Benadryl).
   1. Relieves itching, wheals, congestion of nasal mucosa.
   2. Side effect: dries mucous membranes.
G. Maintain IV of D₅W—as much as 2000 cc in one hour.
H. Administer corticosteroids.
   1. Reduce formation of cellular proteins and decrease edema.
   2. Side effects: same as any steroids.
I. Administer aminophylline—bronchodilator; controls bronchospasms.

Snake Bite and Bee Sting

Snake Bite

Assessment

A. Assess extent of envenomation.
   1. Rattlesnakes, copperheads, cottonmouths (pitvipers) are responsible for 98 percent of venomous bites.

2. Signs:
   a. Blood oozing from wound.
   b. One or two distinct puncture wounds.
   c. Edema and discoloration.
   d. Numbness around bite within 5 to 15 minutes.
   e. Painful and enlarged lymph nodes.
3. Reactions to poisonous snakes occur within 30 to 60 minutes.
B. Assess advanced signs indicating shock.
   1. Nausea, vomiting.
   2. Ecchymosis, blebs, blisters.
   3. Bleeding.
   4. Weakness, vertigo, clammy skin.

Implementation

A. Emergency treatment: within 30 to 60 minutes of medical help.
   1. Immobilize area with support or sling.
   2. Apply tourniquet.
   3. Do not allow client to physically exert self as this hastens spread of venom.
   4. Seek medical help immediately.
B. Emergency treatment: when medical help is not available within 30 to 60 minutes.
   1. Apply nonocclusive tourniquet or constriction band 5 to 13 cm above wound.
      a. Adjust to allow for venous and lymphatic flow restriction but allow for arterial flow.
      b. Loosen, but do not remove, for 1½ minutes every 15 minutes.
   2. Wash around bite with alcohol, hydrogen peroxide, or soap and water.
   3. Sterilize knife with match flame, alcohol, or soap and water, make longitudinal incision (not cross marks) 0.3 to 0.6 cm long and no more than 0.3 cm deep through each fang mark.
   4. Apply suction over incision site.
   5. Procedure must be done within 10 minutes of bite. After 30 to 60 minutes, little venom will be extractable.
C. In-hospital treatment.
   1. Within 30 to 60 minutes, make incisions and use suction intermittently for at least one hour.
   2. Test for sensitivity to horse serum.
   3. Judge severity of envenomation before giving antivenin.
      a. Minimal pitviper bite: 1 to 5 ampules of

antivenin (Crotalid) IM.
b. Moderate bite: 5 to 9 ampules IV drip.
c. Severe bite: 9 ampules IV drip immediately and up to 20 ampules over next 4 to 24 hours, until edema ceases and symptoms improve.
4. Administer tetanus toxoid.
5. Administer analgesics for pain.
a. ASA for mild pain.
b. Codeine or Demerol for severe pain.
6. Administer antibiotics.
a. Initial dose: ampicillin, erythromycin, or tetracycline 500 mg.
b. Maintain 250 mg every 4 hours for 24 hours.

Bee Sting

Assessment

A. Assess for generalized itching.
B. Check for erythema and hives.
C. Assess for feeling of heat throughout body.
D. Evaluate weakness, vertigo.
E. Assess nausea, vomiting, abdominal cramps.
F. Assess tightness in chest, difficulty swallowing or breathing.

Implementation

A. Remove stinger with tweezers or by scraping motion with fingernail. Do not squeeze venom sac.
B. Immediately administer epinephrine 1:1000 solution sub q.
1. Adult: 0.25 to 0.3 ml at sting site and same amount in unaffected arm.
2. Child: 0.01 ml/kg (maximum 0.25 ml at each site).
C. Repeat injections one to three times at 20-minute intervals until blood pressure and pulse rise toward normal.
1. Adult: 0.3 to 0.4 ml.
2. Child: less than 20 kg, 0.10 to 0.15 ml; over 20 kg, 0.15 to 0.3 ml.
D. Apply tourniquet above sting on an extremity. Loosen every three to five minutes to allow venom to slowly enter circulation.
E. Cleanse sting area and apply ice to relieve pain and edema.
F. Administer pressor agents if blood pressure does

not stabilize following 2 to 3 sub q injections of epinephrine.
1. Aramine or Levophed drugs of choice.
2. Administer IV drip at 30 to 40 drops per minute.
G. Begin IV solution of D_5W with 250 mg aminophylline and 30 to 40 mg Solu-Cortef to support circulation and prevent shock.
H. Observe for signs of laryngospasm or bronchospasm. Be prepared to assist with a tracheostomy.
I. Keep client warm and positioned supine with head and feet slightly elevated.
J. Administer rapid-acting antihistamine: Benadryl 50 mg IM.

FLUID REPLACEMENT THERAPY

Fluid Replacement Solutions

A. Types of IV solutions.
1. Hypertonic solution—a solution with higher osmotic pressure than blood serum.
a. Cell placed in solution will crenate.
b. Used in severe salt depletion.
c. Common types of solution: normal saline, dextrose 10% in saline, dextrose 10% in water, and dextrose 5% in saline.
d. Should not be administered faster than 200 cc/hr.
2. Hypotonic solution—a solution with less osmotic pressure than blood serum.
a. Causes cells to expand or increase in size.
b. Used in diarrhea and dehydration.
c. Common types of solution: dextrose 5% in ½ strength (0.45%) NS, dextrose 5% in ¼ strength (0.2) NS, and dextrose 5% in water.
d. Should not be administered faster than 400 cc/hr.
3. Isotonic solution—a solution with the same osmotic pressure as blood serum.
a. Cells remain unchanged.
b. Used for replacement or maintenance.
c. Common type of solution: lactated Ringer's solution.

B. Choice of fluid replacement solution—depends on client's needs.
   1. Fluid and electrolyte replacement only.
      a. Saline solution.
      b. Lactated Ringer's solution.
   2. Calorie replacement—dextrose solutions.
   3. Restriction of dietary intake, such as low sodium.
   4. IV medications that are insoluble in certain IV fluids.
   5. Rate of administration of IV solution to correct fluid imbalance.
   6. Dextrose plays no part in tonicity. It is metabolized off.
C. Purpose of fluid and electrolyte therapy.
   1. To replace previous losses.
   2. To provide maintenance requirements.
   3. To meet current losses.

Implementation

A. Check circulation of immobilized extremity.
B. Check label of solution against physician's order.
C. Check rate of infusion.
D. Observe vein site for signs of swelling.
E. Take vital signs at least every 15 minutes for replacement fluid administration.

Intravenous Calorie Calculation

A. 1000 cc D_5W provides 50 g of dextrose.
B. 50 g of dextrose provides four calories per gram (actually 3.4 calories).
C. 1000 cc D_5W provides 200 calories.
D. Usual IV total/day is 3000 cc (600 calories/day).

Intravenous Regulation

A. Calculation of drip factor.
   1. Microdrop—60 gtt/cc fluid.
   2. Adult drop factor usually depends on administration set 10–20 gtt/cc fluid.
B. General formula.

$$\text{Drops/min.} = \frac{\text{Total volume infused} \times \text{drops/cc}}{\text{Total time for infusing in minutes}}$$

Example: Ordered 1000 cc D_5W administered over eight-hour period of time.
   1. With microdrip, it is easy to remember that the number of drops per minute equals the number of cc's or ml's to be administered per hour.

Example: $\frac{1000}{8} = 125$ cc/hour

Using Formula: (8×60) $\frac{1000 \times 60}{480} = \frac{60,000}{480} = \frac{125}{\text{gtt/min.}}$

   2. With administration set that delivers 10 gtt/min.

$$\frac{1000 \times 10}{480} = \frac{10,000}{480} = 20.8 \text{ or } 21 \text{ gtt/min.}$$

   3. With administration set that delivers 15 gtt/min.

$$\frac{1000 \times 15}{480} = \frac{15,000}{480} = 31 \text{ gtt/min.}$$

C. Calculation of medication as dose per hour.
   Example: Add 20,000 units heparin to 500 cc D_5W. Give 1,000 units per hour, using a 20 gtt/cc set.

$$\frac{1,000 \text{ units}}{60} \times \frac{500 \text{ cc}}{20,000 \text{ units}} \times \frac{20 \text{ gtts/cc}}{1}$$

$$\frac{\overset{25}{\overset{50}{\cancel{1,000}}}}{\underset{3}{\cancel{60}}} \times \frac{\overset{1}{\cancel{500}}}{\underset{40}{\underset{2}{\cancel{20,000}}}} \times \frac{\overset{1}{\cancel{20}}}{1} = \frac{25}{3} = 8 \text{ gtts/min.}$$

D. Calculation of medication as dose per minute.
   Example: Add 2 Gms lidocaine to 500cc D_5W. Give 2 mg a minute, using a 60 gtt/cc set.

$$\frac{2mg}{1} \times \frac{500cc}{2 \text{ Gm}} \times \frac{60gtt/cc}{1}$$

$$\frac{\overset{1}{\cancel{2}}}{1} \times \frac{\overset{1}{\cancel{500}}}{\underset{4}{\underset{2}{\cancel{2,000mg}}}} \times \frac{\overset{30}{\cancel{60}}}{1} = 30 \text{ gtts/min.}$$

Transfusion Administration

Procedure

A. Check carefully for correct name, ID numbers, blood group donor number (double-check by having another person check the information).
B. Do not warm blood as bacteria thrives in this medium.

C. Do not allow duration of blood infusion to exceed four hours.

D. Use blood filter to prevent fibrin and other materials from entering the bloodstream.

E. Start transfusion with normal saline or another electrolyte solution; blood will agglutinate without the presence of electrolytes.

Implementation

A. Follow rules for preventing transfusion reaction.
 1. Check physician's orders—type and number of units.
 2. Identify client and blood bottle or bag. Check:
  a. ID band number matches transfusion record number.
  b. Name spelled correctly on transfusion record.
  c. Blood bottle number and pilot tube number are the same.
  d. Blood type matches on transfusion record and blood bottle (A, B, O and Rh).

B. Observe blood bag or bottle for bubbles, cloudiness, dark color, or black sediment—indicative of bacterial invasion.

C. Check blood with another RN before infusing. Sign form with another RN according to hospital policy.

D. Ask client about allergy history and report any previous blood reactions.

E. Start infusion within 30 minutes from time it is removed from refrigeration. (Blood should not remain at room temperature for long period of time.)

F. Do not allow duration of blood infusion to exceed four hours.

G. Use blood filter to prevent fibrin and other materials from entering the bloodstream.

H. Maintain aseptic technique during procedure.

I. Use gloves to prevent accidental exposure to body fluids.

J. Start transfusion with normal saline or another electrolyte solution; blood will agglutinate without the presence of electrolytes.

K. Start transfusion slowly at 20 to 40 drops per minute and observe for transfusion reactions—usually occurs during the first 15 minutes.

L. Take baseline vital signs at start of transfusion and again five minutes later.

M. Complete the transfusion in no less than two hours.
 1. Usually administered at a rate of 60 to 80 drops per minute. (Administration set—10 gtt/cc)
 2. Hypovolemic client.
  a. Administered blood at the rate of 500 cc in 10 minutes by use of a blood pump.
  b. Observe for pulmonary edema and hypervolemia.

TRANSFUSION REACTIONS

Hemolytic or Incompatibility Reaction

Characteristics

A. Most severe complication.

B. Caused by mismatched blood.

C. The reaction is caused by agglutination of the donor's red cells.
 1. The antibodies in the recipient's plasma react with the antigens in the donor's red cells.
 2. The clumping blocks off capillaries and therefore obstructs the flow of blood and oxygen to cells.

Assessment

A. Assess for increased temperature.

B. Evaluate for decreased blood pressure.

C. Observe for pain across chest and at site of needle insertion.

D. Assess for chills.

E. Observe for hematuria.

F. Evaluate if backache in the kidney region is present.

G. Assess dyspnea and cyanosis.

H. Observe for jaundice in severe cases.

Implementation

A. Stop transfusion immediately upon appearance of symptoms.

B. Return remaining blood and client's blood sample to the laboratory for type and cross match.

C. Keep IV patent after changing blood tubing with either normal saline or preferably D_5W.

D. Take vital signs every 15 minutes.

E. Insert Foley catheter for a urine sample for red blood cells and an accurate output record.

F. Check for oliguria.

G. Administer medications such as vasopressors if indicated.

H. Administer oxygen as necessary.

Bacterial Contamination

A. Do not use blood that is cloudy or discolored or appears to have bubbles present.
B. If transfusion has been started, discontinue immediately.
C. Send remaining blood to laboratory for culture and sensitivity. It is usually advisable to send client's blood sample as well, if transfusion has been started.
D. Change IV tubing and keep it patent.
E. Check vital signs, including temperature, every fifteen minutes.
F. Insert Foley catheter for accurate output and urine specimen as ordered.
G. Control hyperthermia, if present, with antipyretics, cooling blankets, or sponge baths.

Transmission of AIDS

A. Blood donations are now screened for the AIDS virus.
B. AIDS Antibody Test keeps potentially infectious blood and blood products out of the nation's blood supply.
   1. AIDS antibody is a protein naturally produced in body in response to presence of the AIDS virus.
   2. Positive test indicates the AIDS antibody is in blood.
   3. Blood that tests positive will not be accepted (even if result may be a false positive).
C. Based on the AIDS Antibody Test for all blood and blood products, transfusion-related AIDS will be extremely rare in the future.

Allergic Reactions

Characteristics

A. Allergic response to any type of allergen in the donor's blood.
B. Common reaction, usually mild in nature.

Assessment

A. Assess for hives.
B. Assess for urticaria.
C. Observe for wheezing.
D. Check for laryngeal edema.

Implementation

A. Administer an antihistamine like Benadryl to control itching and to relieve edema.

B. If reaction is severe, discontinue the transfusion and keep vein open with normal saline.

Transmission of Viral Hepatitis

Characteristics

A. Donors are screened to prevent transmission.
   1. If blood shows positive for Australia antigen, donor is rejected.
   2. If donor has had jaundice or hepatitis, donor is rejected permanently.
B. Usually hepatitis transmitted through blood is not fatal.
C. Nursing management is related to the care of clients with hepatitis, based on the seriousness of the condition. (Refer to medical section of this book for specific nursing actions.)

Circulatory Overload

Characteristics

A. Transfusion is administered too rapidly.
B. Quantity is in excess of what the circulatory system can accommodate.
C. Usually occurs when transfusion is administered to debilitated clients, elderly or young clients, and clients with cardiac or pulmonary disease.

Assessment

A. Observe CVP for increased reading.
B. Assess for tachycardia.
C. Evaluate for respiratory difficulty, i.e., dyspnea, shortness of breath, cough, rales, rhonchi.
D. Assess for hemoptysis and/or pink frothy sputum.
E. Evaluate edema, especially pulmonary edema.

Implementation

A. Discontinue transfusion.
B. Provide for patent airway and adequate ventilation.
   1. Administer oxygen p.r.n.
   2. Intubate as needed.
C. Place client in semi- to high-Fowler's position to facilitate respiration.
D. Give diuretics as ordered.
E. If client is in congestive heart failure, may need to digitalize.

Table 2. BLOOD COMPONENT THERAPY

Type	Use	Alerts	Administration Equipment
Fresh Plasma	To replace deficient coagulation factors To increase intravascular compartment	Hepatitis is a risk Administer as rapidly as possible Use within 6 hours	Any straight line administration set
Platelets	To prevent or treat bleeding problems, especially in surgical clients To replace platelets in clients with acquired or inherited deficiencies (thrombocytopenia, aplastic anemia) To replace when platelets drop below 30,000 cu/mm (normal 150,000–350,000 cu/mm)	Administer at rate of 10 minutes a unit (usually come in multiple platelet packs)	Platelet transfusion set with special filter to allow platelets to infuse through filter
Granulocytes	To treat oncology clients with severe bone marrow depression and progressive infections To treat granulocytopenic clients with infections that are unresponsive to antibiotics To treat clients with gram-negative bacteremia or infections where marrow recovery does not develop	Administer slowly, over two to four hours Give one transfusion daily until granulocytes increase or infection clears Use within 48 hours after drawn Give when granulocytes are below 500 Observe for shaking chills and fever (treat with Tylenol before transfusions) Observe for hives and laryngeal edema (treat with antihistamines)	Use Y-type blood filters and prime with physiological saline. A microaggregate filter is not used as it filters out platelets
Serum Albumin	To treat shock	Available as 5% or 25%-solution	Special tubing accompanies solution

BLOOD COMPONENT THERAPY (continued)

Type	Use	Alerts	Administration Equipment
	To treat hypoproteinemia	Infuse 25%-solution slowly 1 ml/minute to prevent circulatory overload Administer 100–200 cc (25% solution) for shock clients and 200–300 cc for hypoproteinemia	
Gamma Globulin	To treat agammaglobulinemia To act as prophylaxis for hepatitis exposure	Pooled plasma contains antibodies to infectious agents Administer 0.25 ml–0.50 ml of immune serum globulin per kg of body weight every two to four weeks	Given IM
Coagulation Factors Factor VIII (cryoprecipitate)	To treat clients with von Willebrand's disease To treat clients with factor VIII, hemophilia A	Made from fresh-frozen plasma Administer one unit cryoprecipitate for each 6 kg of body weight initially, followed by 1 unit per 3 kg of body weight at 6- to 12-hour intervals until treatment discontinued Administer one unit per five minutes Observe for febrile reactions: shaking chills, fever, and headache	Standard syringe or component drip set only
Factor IX	To treat clients with factor IX, hemophilia B	Administer in 12- to 24-hour cycle Preparation for administration is 400 to 500 u/vial. Must reconstitute in 10- to 20-cc diluent One unit/lb. of body weight increases the circulating factor activity by 5% Serum hepatitis can be transmitted	Any straight line set

SURGICAL POSITIONS AND AMBULATION

System	Postop Position	Ambulation
Neurosurgical		
Craniotomy		
Surgery involving: posterior fossa	Supine or low-Fowler's; (10°) side to side only	Evening or first day
Anterior or middle fossa	Low- or semi-Fowler's; side to back to side unless bone flap removed, then nonoperative side and back only	Evening or first day
Ventricolo-peritoneal shunt	Supine, back to unoperative side	First to second day
Respiratory		
Laryngectomy	Semi-Fowler's; side-back-side	First or second day, depends on extent of surgery
Tracheostomy	Semi-Fowler's; side-back-side	Evening of surgery
Nasal surgery Submucous resection Rhinoplasty	Semi-Fowler's; back	First day
Tonsillectomy	Semi-Fowler's if local anesthesia used; modified Trendelenburg, side-lying or prone with head turned to side if general anesthesia used	Evening of surgery
Lung surgery Lobectomy Segmental resection Thoracotomy	Semi- to high-Fowler's; side-back-side	Evening of surgery or first day
Pneumonectomy	Semi- to high-Fowler's; back to operative side	First day
Circulatory		
Open-heart surgery for atrial and ventricular septal defects	Low-Fowler's or supine; turn side-back-side	First to third day
Valve replacement surgery	Supine or low-Fowler's until vital signs stable; turn side-back-side	First to second day
Coronary artery bypass	Supine or low-Fowler's until vital signs stable; turn side-back-side	First to second day
Ear		
Stapedectomy	Low-Fowler's; unoperative side only	Evening of surgery or first day
Eye		
Cataract removal	Low-Fowler's; unoperative side only	Day of surgery; usually within 2-4 hours postop
Repair of detached retina	Varies with site of detachment; unoperative side only or as ordered	Evening of surgery or first day
Enucleation	High-Fowler's; unoperative side only or as ordered	First day
Gastrointestinal		
Gastric resection Ileostomy	Minimum low-Fowler's; turn side-back-side	Evening of surgery or first day

SURGICAL POSITIONS AND AMBULATION (continued)

System	Postop Position	Ambulation
Gastrointestinal (continued)		
Colostomy Colon resection Appendectomy Cholecystectomy		
Small bowel resection Portacaval shunt Partial pancreatectomy	Low-Fowler's; turn side-back-side	First day
Hemorrhoidectomy	Supine; turn side to side	First day
Radical neck	Fowler's, side lying either side	First to second day
Genitourinary		
Nephrostomy	Semi- to high-Fowler's; unoperative side only	Evening of surgery
Nephrolithotomy Nephrectomy Transplant	Semi- to high-Fowler's; side-back-side	Evening of surgery
Ureterolithotomy TURP Orchiectomy	Low-Fowler's; side-back-side	Evening of surgery
Cystectomy and ileal conduit Bladder suspension	Low-Fowler's; side-back-side	First day
Gynecologic		
Hysterectomy Oophorectomy	Low-Fowler's; side-back-side	Evening of surgery
Radical hysterectomy Pelvic exenteration Vulvectomy	Supine or low-Fowler's; side-back-side	Third day
Mastectomy	Fowler's; unoperative side or back	Evening of surgery
Musculoskeletal		
Amputation	Low-Fowler's; unoperative side and back, prone once per shift after first day	Evening of surgery; use adaptive devices, i.e., crutches
Open reduction and internal fixation	Fowler's; side-back-side	Evening of surgery or first day
Hip prosthesis	Low-Fowler's; back or unoperative side only. DO NOT FLEX hips, keep in abduction and external rotation	First or second day, nonweight bearing
Hip nailing Total knee replacement	Low-Fowler's; unoperative side and back only	First day, nonweight bearing
Total hip replacement	Supine or side to side with orders; DO NOT FLEX hips, keep in abduction and external rotation	First to third day, nonweight bearing
Laminectomy	Low-Fowler's; turn side to side, may position on back, log roll	Evening of surgery or first day
Spinal fusion	Flat, side to side only, not on back, log roll	Second or third day with brace

NURSING CARE FOR AIDS

One of the most critical health care problems facing our country today is AIDS. This section reviews immune system physiology to establish the foundation for understanding the HIV-1 infection. AIDS and ARC are described, as well as the HIV antibody test. A thorough assessment of an AIDS client and implementation of nursing interventions is included, together with an approach to psychosocial care.

ACQUIRED IMMUNODEFICIENCY SYNDROME (AIDS)

Definition: An acquired immune deficiency characterized by a defect in natural immunity against disease. With loss of the immune system, the individual is susceptible to a variety of "opportunistic infections."

A. A complex system of organs and cells that work to distinguish foreign invaders from natural components in the body.
   1. The body's skin and mucous membranes provide *the first line of defense* against invading organisms.
   2. When a foreign organism enters the body, it may be destroyed by circulating white blood cells, macrophages and neutrophils—*the second line of defense*.
B. The immune response is triggered when an antigen has not been stopped or destroyed by the body's first and second defense system.
   1. Lymphocytes then mobilize to defend the body against invaders or antigens.
   2. Lymphocytes fall into two classes.
      a. B cells (30 percent of blood lymphocytes) develop in the bone marrow.
      b. T cells (70 percent of blood lymphocytes) originate in the bone marrow but complete development in the thymus gland.

C. Normal vs AIDS immune response.
   1. In the normal immune system, proportion of killer/suppressor and helper/inducer T cells are evenly distributed.
   2. AIDS clients show an acquired defect of immunity.
      a. Helper T cells are depleted which causes a reversal of normal ratio of helper to killer/suppressor T cells.
      b. Client cannot activate effective immune response either to foreign invaders or to cancer cells.
      c. This deficiency leads to the majority of signs and symptoms observed in AIDS clients.

Characteristics

A. HIV is a retrovirus and has a different life cycle from a normal virus.
   1. Genetic information is usually sequenced by DNA being transcribed into RNA, which is then translated into proteins necessary for life.
   2. Retroviruses reverse the sequence: RNA code is transcribed backward into DNA and may be integrated into host cell chromosomes.
B. HIV virus attaches and changes the protein on the surface of the helper T cells.
   1. When helper T cells are affected, they are unable to activate B cells and killer T cells.
   2. The immune system collapses when many helper T cells have been destroyed.
   3. When immune system ceases to function, diseases that may be mild become life-threatening.
      a. Most common illnesses are Pneumocystis carinii pneumonia, a parasitic lung infection and Kaposi's sarcoma, a type of skin cancer.
      b. These illnesses, not AIDS, result in death.
C. Transmission of the HIV virus.
   1. HIV virus does not appear to be highly contagious.
   2. Transfer of the virus occurs through a transfer of body fluids, either through intimate contact or IV injections: semen, blood, breast milk, vaginal/cervical secretions.
   3. Body fluids containing infected lymphocytes must enter the blood stream or body cavity to spread the virus.
   4. The virus exists in tears, saliva, urine, feces, spinal fluid, sputum, pus, and bone marrow;

epidemiological evidence has not confirmed transmission through these body fluids.

   a. High concentrations of HIV virus found in blood, semen and cerebrospinal fluid.

   b. Lower concentrations of HIV virus found in urine, vaginal secretions, saliva, feces, breast milk.

D. ARC and AIDS.

  1. The CDC (Centers for Disease Control) use a strict surveillance definition to establish an AIDS diagnosis because AIDS symptoms can occur in non-AIDS clients.

  2. Dual criteria must be met.

   a. Presence of diagnosed disease at least moderately indicative of underlying cellular immunodeficiency (Pneumocystis carinii pneumonia).

   b. Absence of known causes of reduced resistance to the disease other than that due to the HIV.

E. ARC, or AIDS-related complex, is secondary to HIV caused immunodeficiency, but is not full-blown AIDS.

  1. The CDC definition requires that there be two major clinical findings or one major and two or more minor findings plus one or more immunologic findings plus two or more laboratory findings.

  2. Symptoms of ARC.

   a. Symptoms occur because immune system is damaged and cannot effectively fight off illnesses.

   b. Symptoms last for weeks or months.

   c. Swollen lymph glands usually in neck, arm pits or groin.

   d. Diarrhea.

   e. Severe fatigue, unexplained.

   f. Rapid weight loss, greater than 10 pounds.

   g. Night sweats.

   h. Recurring fever and chills.

   i. Infections such as thrush.

  3. Symptoms of AIDS.

   a. Include symptoms of ARC, plus the following.

   b. Shortness of breath, dry cough indicating presence of Pneumocystis carinii pneumonia (PCP).

   c. Pink or purple spots on the skin indicating presence of Kaposi's sarcoma (KS).

F. Opportunistic conditions: Disease processes that occur as a result of suppressed immune system.

  1. Pneumocystis carinii: a parasitic infection of the lungs. One of the two rare diseases that affect 85 percent of AIDS clients; similar to other types of pneumonia.

  2. Kaposi's sarcoma: a type of cancer usually occurring on the surface of the skin or in the mouth. This disease may also spread to internal organs.

  3. Dementia with the AIDS virus: a clinical syndrome in which there is acquired persistent intellectual impairment; in this case caused by the HIV virus.

G. HIV-1 antibody test.

  1. The ELISA (enzyme-linked immunosorbent assay) test was developed to screen national donor blood.

   a. This test does not test for AIDS, but the antibodies to the HIV virus.

   b. Once exposed to a virus, it takes the body time to produce antibodies. A person may already be infected and if the body has not yet produced antibodies, the ELISA test will be negative.

   c. Test is also imperfect in that it may produce a false positive or false negative.

  2. All positive results must be retested via ELISA.

  3. If second test is positive, the Western blot test is given for final confirmation.

Assessment

A. Assess for chronic fatigue.

  1. Activity level and need for support.

  2. Alterations in sleep patterns.

  3. Pulmonary insufficiency.

  4. Degree of anxiety associated with pulmonary problems.

B. Assess presence of diarrhea.

  1. Intractable or intermittent.

  2. Degree of dehydration.

  3. Electrolyte imbalance; observe blood chemistries.

  4. Malnutrition due to GI malabsorption and intractable diarrhea.

C. Assess for skin breakdown and mucous membrane involvement.

  1. Lesions and Kaposi's sarcoma.

  2. Degree of excoriation or pressure sores.

  3. Presence of Candida or genital/anal herpes.

4. Mouth for bleeding or lesions.

D. Assess for persistent elevated temperature.
   1. Check temperature every 4 hours or more as needed.
   2. Need for cooling measures such as ice packs, alcohol rubs, cooling blankets.

E. Assess for degree of pain.
   1. Character, intensity or dramatic changes in pain.
   2. Need for medication and effects of drug regimen.

F. Assess nutritional status.
   1. Malnutrition.
      a. Severe weight loss.
      b. Weakness and fatigue.
      c. Decreased serum proteins.
      d. Decreased intake of foods and fluids.
   2. Intake and output.
   3. Dehydration.
      a. Decreased skin turgor.
      b. Dry mucous membranes.
      c. Weight loss.
   4. Need for antiemetics.

G. Assess presence of neurologic symptoms.
   1. Memory lapses and confusion.
   2. Seizure activity.
   3. Confusion and disorientation.
   4. Infection of the optic nerve.
      a. Visual changes.
      b. Blindness.
   5. Symptoms of dementia.

H. Assess degree of pulmonary involvement.

I. Assess client for potential injury.
   1. Identify risk factors.
      a. Weakness.
      b. Sedation.
      c. Mental confusion, dementia.
      d. Orthostatic hypotension.
   2. Assess physical status for degree of independence.
      a. Ability to be mobile without assistance.
      b. Amount of medication that interferes with alertness.

Implementation

A. Maintain nutritional status of client.
   1. Administer fluids PO to maintain hydration status, minimum 1500–2000 ml per day.
   2. Provide dietary planning for client.
      a. Allow client to participate in menu planning.
      b. Suggest family members bring in food from home.
   3. Provide dietary supplements—high protein, high calorie, canned nutritional supplements, vitamin supplements.
   4. Administer antiemetics to minimize anorexia and nausea.
   5. Administer IV fluids if necessary.
      a. Examine IV site every shift for infection, inflammation.
      b. Change dressings as needed; do not allow dressing to remain wet.
   6. Provide good oral hygiene.
      a. Use soft toothbrush, lemon glycerine swabs.
      b. Use dilute H_2O_2 several times a day as mouthwash.
   7. Suggest anesthetic solution (viscous lidocaine) before meals to assist in swallowing.
   8. Administer nasogastric tube feedings as ordered.
   9. Evaluate status for Total Parenteral Nutrition (TPN); institute before nutritional status has severely deteriorated.

B. Provide oxygen and maintain pulmonary function.
   1. Monitor pulmonary status from baseline data to determine changes that require medical management.
   2. Maintain bedrest if condition indicates (dyspnea upon any exertion).
   3. Provide oxygen if indicated.
   4. Monitor vital signs; pulse, B/P, respirations, skin color.

C. Provide comfort measures for fatigue.
   1. Periods of rest during the day, especially before meals.
   2. Provide oxygen on exertion or continuously, if indicated.
   3. Administer medications to assist in adequate sleep.
   4. Teach relaxation methods to assist in coping with anxiety (which can be debilitating).
   5. Assist with activities of daily living as necessary.
   6. Increase activity levels as tolerated. Suggest PT, OT, etc.

D. Provide excellent skin care.
   1. Keep skin clean and free of moisture.
   2. Change soiled or wet linen immediately.
   3. Provide bath if condition indicates.

4. Massage with lotion to increase tissue perfusion.

5. Wash and air perineum and anal area regularly.

6. Administer pressure sore treatment as indicated.
   a. Prescribed ointments.
   b. Op-Site treatment.

7. Assist with position changes as necessary; for client on bedrest turn every 2 hours.
   a. Maintain functional body alignment.
   b. Provide appropriate beds: Clinitron, air mattress, etc.

E. Provide supportive care for elevated temperature.
   1. Administer antipyretics (acetaminophen and/or nonsteroidal anti-inflammatory) as ordered.
   2. Monitor temperature every 4 hours; note pattern of temperature spikes.
   3. Change linen for night sweats.
   4. Provide cooling measures as necessary (alcohol rubs, cooling blankets).
   5. Encourage fluid intake; consider need for IV fluids.

F. Administer appropriate care for diarrhea.
   1. Administer prescribed antidiarrheal medications following each loose stool; if not adequate, administer around-the-clock maximum dose.
   2. Monitor for constipation to prevent impaction.
   3. Monitor to avoid complications from intractable diarrhea.
      a. Nutritional depletion.
      b. Electrolyte imbalance.
   4. Provide appropriate diet: bland, low-fiber, low milk products.
   5. Give client incontinent pads to prevent accidents.

G. Provide measures to reduce pain.
   1. Administer analgesics to relieve pain (do not allow client to go for long periods without medication if pain is extensive).
   2. Allow client to monitor own pain medication to increase effectiveness.
   3. Provide alternate pain relief.
      a. Massage and touch help to relieve pain.
      b. Teach visualization techniques to reduce pain.
      c. Give client warm baths.
      d. Provide emotional support—talking, touching, etc.

H. Monitor client to prevent injuries.

1. Evaluate degree of weakness.
   a. Encourage use of call bell.
   b. Assist with ambulation.
   c. Use side rails if necessary.
   d. Keep belongings within reach.
2. Evaluate degree of mental confusion.
   a. Reorient frequently; remind client to call for assistance.
   b. Restrain as appropriate.
3. Provide bedpan or bedside commode and assist.

Psychosocial Care

A. Identify problem area.
   1. Fear of contagion.
      a. Family and friends fear contagion because of lack of knowledge about AIDS transmission.
      b. The AIDS person is actually the most vulnerable to contagion.
   2. Fear of rejection by family.
      a. Disclosing AIDS (and that they are homosexual) to family leads to fears of rejection.
      b. Guilt and shame accompany diagnosis of AIDS.
   3. Planning for terminal care.
      a. Resources and funds may be depleted when terminal care is needed.
      b. Long-term total care is often needed for physical as well as mental debilitation.

B. Provide milieu of individual acceptance.
   1. Use of nonjudgmental attitudes.
   2. Encourage open, honest communication from staff to client.

C. Assist client to clarify fears and concerns of rejection.
   1. Encourage verbalization of fears and feelings but only if client is ready to verbalize.
   2. Encourage honesty when telling others of diagnosis, concerns and needs.

D. Mediate between client, parents and loved ones.
   1. Clarify role client wishes friends, partner and family to take during illness.
   2. Assist client to clarify decisions regarding treatment, finances and caregiving.

E. Assist client to go through grieving process caused by loss (of self-image, independence, identity, and worthiness).

F. Support parents and loved ones who are bereaved at loss of partner or child.

5

MATERNITY NURSING

This chapter, outlined in the nursing process, is designed to give the nurse an understanding of the important phases and processes related to pregnancy. Key topics covered in a comprehensive manner include female anatomy, the health status of the female before and through pregnancy, labor and delivery, complications and postpartum adjustment, fetal development, and care of the newborn.

Consistent with the other chapters, strong emphasis is placed on assessment and implementation. To help the nurse integrate nursing content, the psychosocial aspects of maternal-child nursing are covered in detail.

The nursing content in this chapter is broad in scope. Much technical information is presented in outline format, with the remainder contained in several tables and appendices to facilitate learning and provide convenient reference.

ANATOMY AND PHYSIOLOGY OF FEMALE REPRODUCTIVE ORGANS

Anatomy

Female Reproductive Organs

A. Usually divided into two groups, the external and internal genitalia.

B. External genitalia are collectively called the vulva, which consist of:
   1. Mons veneris or mons pubis.
   2. Labia majora.
   3. Labia minora.
   4. Clitoris.
   5. Vestibule.
   6. Urinary meatus.
   7. Skene's ducts and Bartholin's glands.
   8. Hymen.
   9. Perineum.

C. Internal organs of reproduction are located in the pelvic cavity.
   1. Uterus—muscular organ.
      a. Two major functions.
         (1) Organ in which fetus develops.
         (2) Organ from which menstruation occurs.
      b. Consists of two major parts.
         (1) Corpus (body), which has three layers.
         (a) Perimetrium—external layer.
         (b) Myometrium—middle layer.
         (c) Endometrium—internal layer.
         (2) Cervix, composed of three parts.
         (a) Internal os—opens into body of uterine cavity.
         (b) Cervical canal—located between internal and external os.
         (c) External os—opens into vagina.
   2. Fallopian tubes—two slender muscular tubes that extend laterally from the cornu of the uterine cavity to the ovaries; they are the passageways through which the ova reach the uterus.
   3. Ovaries—two flat, oval-shaped organs located on each side of the uterus. (Correspond to the testes in the male.) Two major functions are:
      a. Development and expulsion of ova.
      b. Secretion of certain hormones.

4. Vagina—a canal that extends from lower part of the vulva to the cervix; serves three functions for the body:
   a. Passageway for menstrual blood.
   b. Passageway for fetus.
   c. Organ of copulation.

Skeletal Features of the Pelvis

A. The pelvis is important in obstetrics because it is the passage through which the baby passes during birth. Disproportions between fetus and size of pelvis may make vaginal delivery difficult or impossible.

B. Four bones form the pelvis—two innominate bones, the sacrum, and the coccyx.

C. Divisions of pelvis.
   1. False pelvis—shallow extended portion above brim that supports abdominal viscera.
   2. True pelvis—portion that lies below pelvic brim and is divided into three sections—the pelvic inlet, the mid-pelvis, and the pelvic outlet.
   3. Four main types of pelves.
      a. Gynecoid—inlet nearly round or blunt, heart-shaped (45 percent of women).
      b. Android—inlet wedge-shaped (15 percent of women).
      c. Anthropoid—inlet oval-shaped (35 percent of women).
      d. Platypelloid—inlet oval-shaped, transversely (5 percent or less of women).

D. Measurements of the pelvis.
   1. Diagonal conjugate (CD)—distance between sacral promontory and lower margin of symphysis pubis. Measurement greater than 11.5 cm adequate.
   2. True conjugate, or conjugate vera (CV)—distance from upper margin of symphysis to sacral promontory. Measurement greater than 11 cm adequate.
   3. Tuberischial diameter (TI)—transverse diameter of outlet. Measurement greater than 8 cm adequate.
   4. Size determination.
      a. X-ray pelvimetry is most accurate means of determining size of pelvis.
      b. X-ray pelvimetry is contraindicated to avoid undue exposure of mother and infant unless pelvic contraction is suspected.

Physiology

Menstruation and the Menstrual Cycle

Definition: The periodic discharge of blood, mucus, and epithelial cells from the uterus.

A. Menstrual cycle—usually lasts 28 days, but may vary from 21 to 35 days with ovulation occurring about 14 days before menstruation begins. Usually occurs between the ages of twelve to forty-five.

B. Hormonal control—depends upon adequate functioning of pituitary, ovaries, and uterus. Hypothalamus exerts control through releasing and inhibiting factors.
  1. Proliferative phase—estrogen.
     a. Follicle stimulating hormone (FSH), released by anterior pituitary, stimulates the development of the graafian follicle.
     b. As graafian follicle develops, it produces increasing amounts of follicular fluid containing a hormone called estrogen.
     c. Estrogen stimulates build-up or thickening of the endometrium.
     d. As estrogen increases in the bloodstream, it suppresses secretion of FSH and favors the secretion of the luteinizing hormone (LH).
     e. LH stimulates ovulation and initiates development of the corpus luteum.
  2. Secretory phase—progesterone.
     a. Follows ovulation, which is the release of mature ovum from the graafian follicle.
     b. Rapid changes take place in the ruptured follicle under the influence of LH.
     c. Cavity of the graafian follicle is replaced by the corpus luteum (mass of yellow-colored tissue).
     d. Main function of the corpus luteum is to secrete progesterone and some estrogen.
     e. Progesterone acts upon the endometrium to bring about secretory changes that prepare it for pregnancy. Also, progesterone maintains the endometrium during the early phase of pregnancy, should a fertilized ovum be implanted.
  3. Menstrual phase.
     a. Corpus luteum degenerates in about eight days unless the ovum is fertilized.
     b. There is a cessation of progesterone and es-

trogen produced by corpus luteum and blood levels drop.
     c. Endometrium degenerates and menstruation occurs.
     d. The drop in blood levels of estrogen and progesterone stimulate production of FSH and a new cycle begins.
     e. Basal body temperature dips then rises around time of ovulation: .5 to 1 degree.

Development of the Fetus

Fertilization

Definition: A gamete is a sex cell—ovum or spermatozoon—that has undergone maturation and is ready for fertilization.

A. Fertilization takes place when two essential cells—sperm and ovum—unite.
B. Each reproductive cell (one gamete) carries 23 chromosomes.
C. Sperm carries two types of sex chromosomes, X and Y, which when united with female X chromosome determine the sex of the child (XY—male; XX—female).
D. The site of fertilization is usually in the outer third of the fallopian tubes, and the fertilized egg then descends to the uterus.

Fetal Development

Definition: Embryo is the fertilized ovum during the first two months of development. Fetus is product of conception from two months to time of birth.

A. Implantation occurs about the seventh day after fertilization—nidation.
B. First eight weeks, when all major organs are developing, is the period of greatest vulnerability.
C. Embryonic development—cells arrange themselves into three layers:
  1. Ectoderm—outer layer—gives rise to skin, salivary and mammary glands, nervous system, and other external parts of the body.
  2. Endoderm—inner layer—gives rise to thymus, thyroid, bladder, and other small organs and tubes.
  3. Mesoderm—layer between the other two—gives rise to urinary and reproductive organs, circulatory system, connective tissue, muscle, and bones.
D. Fetal membranes and amniotic fluid.

1. Fetal membranes—membranes that surround the fetus—are composed of two layers:
   a. Amnion—glistening inner membrane—forms early, about the second week of embryonic development; encloses the amniotic cavity.
   b. Chorion—outer membrane.
2. Amniotic fluid—forms within the amniotic cavity and surrounds the embryo. Usually consists of 500 to 1000 ml of fluid at the end of pregnancy.
   a. Amniotic fluid contains fetal urine, lanugo from fetal skin, epithelial cells, and subaqueous materials.
   b. Function of the fluid is to provide an optimum temperature and environment for fetus and provide a cushion against injury; fetus also drinks the fluid, probably as much as 450 ml a day near term.
   c. Source is uncertain. Probably maternal exudate, fetal urine, or secretion of the amniotic membrane. Replaced continuously at a rapid rate.

E. Placental function.
1. Placenta—organ that provides for the exchange of nutrients and waste products between mother and fetus and acts as an endocrine organ.
   a. Provides oxygen and removes carbon dioxide from the fetal system.
   b. Maintains fetal fluid and electrolyte, acid-base balance.
2. Placenta develops by the third month.
   a. Formed by union of chorionic villi and decidua basalis.
   b. Fetal surface smooth and glistening.
   c. Maternal surface red and fleshlike.
3. Exchange takes place between mother and fetus through diffusion.
4. Placental function is dependent upon maternal circulation.
5. Materials passed through placenta in addition to nutrients are drugs, antibodies to some diseases, and certain viruses. Large particles such as bacteria cannot pass through barrier.
6. Placental transfer of maternal immunoglobulin (G) gives the fetus passive immunity to certain diseases for the first few months after birth.
7. Hormones produced by the placenta.
   a. Chorionic gonadotropin (HCG)—detected in urine fifteen days after implantation. Hormone stimulates the corpus luteum to maintain endometrium and is basis of immunological test of pregnancy.
   b. Human placental lactogen (HPL)—effect similar to growth hormone.
   c. Estrogen and progesterone.
8. The umbilical cord extends from the fetus to the center of the fetal surface of the placenta.
   a. Contains two arteries and one vein.
   b. Is protected by mucoid connective tissue termed Wharton's jelly.

F. Fetal circulation.
1. Arteries carry venous blood.
2. Vein carries oxygenated blood.
3. Fetal circulation bypass.
   a. Bypass due to nonfunctioning lungs: ductus arteriosus (between pulmonary artery and aorta) and foramen ovale (between right and left atrium).
   b. Ductus venosus bypass—due to fetal liver not being used for exchange of waste.
   c. Bypasses must close following birth to allow blood to flow through the lungs for respiration and through the liver for waste exchange.

G. Calculation of expected date of delivery or confinement (EDC).
1. Nägele's rule: Count back three months from first day of last menstrual period and add seven days.

   Example: LMP July 18
            EDC April 25

2. Pregnancy usually does not terminate on the exact EDC. It may vary from one week before to two weeks after the expected date.

H. Multiple pregnancies (uterus contains two or more embryos). May be the result of fertilization of a single ovum or two separate ova. If division takes place very early in monozygotic twins, two placentas and two chorions are formed.

SUMMARY CHART OF
OBSTETRICAL ASSESSMENT

ASSESSMENT	NORMAL	ABNORMAL
INITIAL PHYSICAL ASSESSMENT		
Assess **breasts** and **nipples**		
Contour and size		
Presence of lumps	No lumps	Lumps
Secretions	Colostrum secretions in late first trimester or early second trimester	Secretions, other than colostrum
Assess **abdomen**		
Contour and size		
Changes in skin color	Linea nigra (black line of pregnancy along midline abdomen)	
	Primiparas: coincidentally with growth of fundus	
	Multiparas: after 13 to 15 weeks gestation	
Striae (reddish-purple lines)	On breasts, hips, and thighs during pregnancy	
	After pregnancy, faint silvery-grey	
Scars, rashes, or other skin disturbances	Usually none present	
Fundal height in centimeters (fingerbreadths less accurate): measure from symphysis pubis to top of fundus	Fundus palpable just above symphysis at 8–10 weeks	Large measurements: EDC is incorrect; tumor; ascites; multiple pregnancy; and polyhydramnios
	Halfway between symphysis and umbilicus at 16 weeks	Less than normal enlargement: fetal abnormality, oligohydramnios, placental dysmaturity, missed abortion, fetal death
	Umbilicus at 20–22 weeks	
Perineum: scars, moles, rashes, warts, discharge		
BASELINE DATA		
Evaluate **weight**		
Take **vital signs, blood pressure** (BP), **temperature, pulse,** and **respiration** (TPR)		
Evaluate **lab findings**		
Urine: sugar, protein, albumin	Negative for sugar, protein, and albumin throughout pregnancy	Positive for sugar, protein, and/or albumin
Hematocrit (HCT)	38% to 47%	
Hemoglobin (Hgb)	12 to 16 gm/dl	
Blood type and Rh factor		If Rh negative, father's blood should be typed
		If Rh positive, titers should be followed; possible RhoGAM at termination of pregnancy
Pap smear		
VD smears and screening		

ASSESSMENT	NORMAL	ABNORMAL
ANTEPARTUM ASSESSMENT		
Evaluate **weight** to assess maternal health and nutritional status and growth of fetus	1st trimester: 3 to 4 lbs 2nd trimester: 12 to 14 lbs 3rd trimester: 8 to 10 lbs Minimum weight gain during pregnancy: 24 lbs (2 lbs/week or 5 lbs/month)	Inadequate weight gain: possible maternal malnutrition Excessive weight gain: if sudden at onset, may indicate preeclampsia; if gradual and continual, may indicate overeating
Evaluate **blood pressure**	Fairly constant with baseline data throughout pregnancy	Increased: possible anxiety (Client should rest 20 to 30 minutes before you take BP again) Rise of 30/15 above baseline data: sign of preeclampsia Decreased: sign of supine hypotensive syndrome. If lying on back, turn client on left side and take BP again
Evaluate **fundal height**	Drop around 38th week: sign of fetus engaging in birth canal Primipara: sudden drop Multipara: slower, sometimes not until onset of labor	Large fundal growth: may indicate wrong dates, multiple pregnancy, hydatidiform mole, polyhydramnios, tumors Small fundal growth: may indicate fetal demise, fetal anomaly, retarded fetal growth, abnormal presentation or lie, decreased amniotic fluid
Determine **fetal position,** using Leopold's maneuvers. Complete external palpations of the pregnant abdomen to determine fetal position, lie, presentation and engagement		
First maneuver: to determine part of fetus presenting into pelvis Second maneuver: to locate the back, arms, and legs; fetal heart heard best over fetal back Third maneuver: to determine part of fetus in fundus Fourth maneuver: to determine degree of cephalic flexion and engagement	Vertex presentation	Breech presentation or transverse lie

ASSESSMENT	NORMAL	ABNORMAL
Evaluate **fetal heart rate** by quadrant, location, and rate	120 to 160 beats/minute	More than 160 or less than 120: may indicate fetal distress. *Notify physician*
Check for presence of **edema**	In lower extremities towards end of pregnancy	In upper extremities and face: may indicate preeclampsia
Evaluate **urine** (clean catch midstream)	Negative for sugar, protein, and albumin	Positive for sugar: may indicate subclinical or gestational diabetes Positive for protein and/or albumin: may indicate preeclampsia
Evaluate **levels of discomfort** (See Obstetrical Supplement at end of this section)		

INTRAPARTUM ASSESSMENT

Assess for **lightening** and **dropping** (the descent of the presenting part into the pelvis)	Several days to two weeks before onset of labor Multipara: may not occur until onset of labor Relief of shortness of breath and increase in urinary frequency	No lightening or dropping: may indicate disproportion between fetal presenting part and maternal pelvis
Check if **mucous plug** has been expelled from cervix	Usually expelled prior to onset of labor	
Assess for **"bloody show"**	Clear, pinkish, or blood-tinged vaginal discharge that occurs as cervix begins to dilate and efface	

Steps of Leopold's maneuvers.

ASSESSMENT	NORMAL	ABNORMAL
Assess for ruptured membranes Time water breaks	Before, during, or after onset of labor	Breech presentation: frank meconium or meconium staining
Color of **amniotic fluid**	Clear, straw color	Greenish-brown: indicates meconium has passed from fetus, possible fetal distress Yellow-stained: fetal hypoxia 36 hours or more prior to rupture of membrane or hemolytic disease
Quantity of amniotic fluid	500 to 1000 ml of amniotic fluid, rarely expelled at one time	Polyhydramnios: excessive fluid over 2000 cc Observe newborn for congenital anomalies: craniospinal malformation, orogastrointestinal anomalies, Down's syndrome and congenital heart defects Oligohydramnios: minimal fluid, less than 500 cc Observe newborn for malformation of ear, genitourinary tract anomalies, and renal agenesis
Odor of fluid	No odor	Odor: may indicate infection; deliver within 24 hours
Fetal heart rate	120 to 160 beats/minute Regular rhythm	Decreased: indicates fetal distress with possible cord prolapse or cord compression Accelerated heart rate: initial sign of fetal hypoxia Absent: may indicate fetal demise
Evaluate **contractions** *Frequency:* from start of one contraction to start of next	3 to 5 minutes between contractions	Irregular contractions with long intervals between: indicates false labor
Duration: from beginning of contraction to time uterus begins to relax	50 to 90 seconds	Over 90 seconds: uterine tetany; stop pitocin if running
Intensity: (strength of contraction): measured with monitoring device	Peak 25 mm Hg End of labor may reach 50–75 mm Hg	Over 75 mm Hg: uterine tetany or uterine rupture
LABOR AND DELIVERY ASSESSMENT		
First stage *Latent phase* (0 to 4 cm dilation)	0 to 3–4 cm average 6.4 hrs	Prolonged time in any phase: may indicate poor fetal position, incomplete fetal flexion, CPD, or poor uterine contractions

ASSESSMENT	NORMAL	ABNORMAL
Active phase (4 to 8 cm)		
Transition phase (8 to 10 cm)	Length of time varies	Labor less than 3 hours: indicates precipitous labor, increasing risk of fetal complications, or maternal lacerations and tears
Assess for **blood show**		
Observe for presence of **nausea or vomiting**		
Assess **perineum**	Beginning to bulge	
Evaluate **urge to bear down**		Often uncontrolled Multipara: can cause precipitous delivery "Panting" (can be controlled until safe delivery area established)
Second stage (10 cm to delivery)	Primipara: up to 2 hours Multipara: several minutes to 2 hours	Over 2 hours: increased risk of fetal brain damage and maternal exhaustion
Assess for **presenting part**	Vertex with ROA or LOA presentation	Occiput posterior, breech, face or transverse lie
Assess **caput** (infant head) Multipara: move to delivery room when caput size of dime Primipara: move to delivery room when caput size of half dollar	Visible when bearing down during contraction	"Crowns" in room other than delivery room: delivery imminent (Do not move client)
Assess **fetal heart rate**	120 to 160/minute	Decreased: may indicate supine hypotensive syndrome (Turn client on side and take again.) Hemorrhage (Check for other signs of bleeding; notify physician.) Increased or decreased: may indicate fetal distress secondary to cord progression or compression (Place client in Trendelenburg's or knee-chest position; give oxygen if necessary; inform physician.)
Evaluate **breathing**	Controlled with contractions	Heavy or excessive: may lead to hyperventilation and/or dehydration
Evaluate **pain** and **anxiety**	Medication required after dilated 4 to 5 cm unless using natural childbirth methods	Severe pain early in first stage of labor: inadequate prenatal teaching, backache due to position in bed, uterine tetany

ASSESSMENT	NORMAL	ABNORMAL
Third stage (from delivery of baby to delivery of placenta)	Placental separation occurs within 30 minutes (usually 3–5 minutes)	Failure of placental separation Abnormality of uterus or cervix, weak, ineffectual uterine contraction, tetanic contractions causing closure of cervix Over 3 hours: indicates retained placenta
Fourth stage (first hour postpartum)		Mother in unstable condition (hemorrhage usual cause) Highest risk of hemorrhage in first postpartum hour
Temperature	36.5° to 37.5°C	Over 37.5°C: may indicate infection Slight elevation: due to dehydration from mouth breathing and NPO
Pulse	Pulse: 60 to 100	Increased: may indicate pain or hemorrhage
Respiration	Respirations: 12–22	
Blood pressure	Blood pressure: 140–120/80	Increased: may indicate anxiety, pain, or posteclamptic condition Decreased: hemorrhage

POSTPARTUM ASSESSMENT

ASSESSMENT	NORMAL	ABNORMAL
Assess **vital signs** every 15 minutes for 1 hour, every 30 minutes for 1 hour, every hour for 4 hours, every 8 hours, and as needed	Pulse may be 45–60/minute in stage 4 Pulse to normal range about third day	Decreased BP and increased P: probably postpartum hemorrhage; elevated temperature above 38°C: indicates possible infection Temperature elevates when lactation occurs
Assess **fundus** every 15 minutes for 1 hour, every 8 hours for 48 hours, then daily	Firm (like a grapefruit) in midline and at or slightly above umbilicus Return to prepregnant size in 6 weeks: descending at rate of 1 fingerbreadth/day	Boggy fundus: immediately massage gently until firm; report to physician and observe closely; empty bladder; medicate with pitocin if ordered Fundus misplaced 1 to 2 fingerbreadths from midline: indicates full bladder (Client must void or be catheterized.)

ASSESSMENT	NORMAL	ABNORMAL
Assess **lochia** every 15 minutes for 1 hour, every 8 hours for 48 hours, then daily		
Color	3 days postpartum: dark red (rubra) 4 to 10 days postpartum: clear pink (serosa) 10 to 21 days postpartum: white, yellow brown (alba)	Heavy, bright-red: indicates hemorrhage (Massage fundus, give medication on order, notify physician.) Spurts: may indicate cervical tear No lochia: may indicate clot occluding cervical opening (Support fundus; express clot.)
Quantity	Moderate amount, steadily decreases	
Odor	Minimal	Foul: may indicate infection
Assess **breasts** and **nipples** daily	Day 1 to 2: soft, intact, secreting colostrum Day 2 to 3: engorged, tender, full, tight, painful Day 3+: secreting milk Increased pains as baby sucks: common in multiparas	Sore or cracked (Clean and dry nipples; decrease breast feeding time; apply breast shield between feeding.) Milk does not "let down": help client relax and decrease anxiety; give glass of wine or beer
Assess **perineum** daily	Episiotomy intact, no swelling, no discoloration	Swelling or bruising: may indicate hematoma
Assess **bladder** every four hours	Voiding regularly with no pain	Not voiding: bladder may be full and displaced to one side, leading to increased lochia (Catheterization may be necessary.)
Assess **bowels**	Spontaneous bowel movement 2 to 3 days after delivery	Fear associated with pain from hemorrhoids
Assess mother-infant **bonding**	Touching infant, talking to infant, talking about infant	Refuses to touch or hold infant
Evaluate **Rh-negative status**	Client does not require RhoGAM	RhoGAM administered

MATERNAL HISTORY: DEFINITION OF TERMS

Abortion: pregnancy loss before fetus is viable (usually less than 26 weeks or 660 gm).

Gravida: any pregnancy, including present one.

Primigravida: refers to first-time pregnancy.

Multigravida: refers to second or any subsequent pregnancy.

Para: past pregnancies that continued to viable age (26 weeks); infants may be alive or dead at birth.

Primipara: refers to female who has delivered first viable infant;

born either alive or dead.

Nullipara: refers to female who has never carried pregnancy to viable age for fetus.

Multipara: refers to female who has given birth to two or more children either alive or dead.

ANTEPARTUM PERIOD

ANTEPARTAL MATERNAL CHANGES

Physiological Changes

Reproductive Organs

A. Uterus—increases in weight from 57 grams to about 907 grams at the end of gestation and in size from five to six times larger.
 1. Changes in tissue.
    a. Hypertrophy of muscle cells with limited development of new muscle cells.
    b. Development of connective and elastic tissue, which increases contractility.
    c. Increase in the size and number of blood vessels.
    d. Hypertrophy of the lymphatic system.
    e. Growth of the uterus is brought about by the influences of estrogen during the early months and the pressure of the fetus.
 2. Other changes.
    a. Contractions occur throughout pregnancy, starting from very mild to increased strength.

Table 1. MULTIPLE PREGNANCIES

Double Ovum	Single Ovum
Dizygotic or fraternal twins	Monozygotic or identical twins
Ova from same or different ovaries	Union of a single ovum and a single sperm
Same or different sex	Same sex
Brother or sister resemblance	Identical genetic pattern
Two placentas but may be fused	One placenta
Two chorions and two amnions	One chorion and two amnions

b. As the uterus grows, it rises out of the pelvis displacing intestines and may be palpated above the symphysis pubis.

B. Ligaments—broad ligaments in the pelvis become elongated and hypertrophied to help support and stabilize uterus during pregnancy.

C. Cervix.
 1. Becomes shorter, more elastic, and larger in diameter.
 2. Marked thickening of mucous lining and increased blood supply.
 3. Edema and hyperplasia of the cervical glands and increased glandular secretions.
 4. Mucous plug expelled from cervix as cervix begins to dilate at onset of labor.
 5. Increased vascularity, deepening of color to dark red or purple—Chadwick's sign.

D. Vagina.
 1. Hypertrophy and thickening of muscle.
 2. Loosening of connective tissue.
 3. Increased vaginal discharge.
 4. High pH secretions.

E. Perineum.
 1. Increased vascularity.
 2. Hypertrophy of muscles.
 3. Loosening of connective tissue.

F. Ovaries and tubes.
 1. Usually one large corpus luteum present in one ovary.
 2. Ovulation does not take place.

Breast

A. Changes in tissue.
 1. Extensive growth of alveolar tissue, necessary for lactation.
 2. Montgomery's glands—enlargement of sebaceous glands of primary areola.

B. Other changes.
 1. Breast increases in size and firmness and becomes nodular.
 2. Nipples become more prominent and areola deepens in color.
 3. Superficial veins grow more prominent.
 4. At the end of third month, colostrum appears.
 5. After delivery, anterior pituitary stimulates production and secretion of milk.

Abdomen

A. Contour changes as the enlarging uterus extends into the abdominal cavity.

B. Striae gravidarum usually appear on the abdomen as pregnancy progresses.

Skin

A. Pigmentation increases in certain areas of the body.
   1. Breast—primary areola deepens in color.
   2. Abdomen—linea nigra, dark streak down the midline of abdomen, especially prominent in brunettes.
   3. Face—chloasma, the "mask of pregnancy" pigmentation distributed over the face. Usually disappears after pregnancy.
   4. Face and upper trunk—occasionally spider nevi or palmar erythema develops with the increase in estrogen.
B. Pigmented areas on abdomen and breast usually do not completely disappear after delivery.

Circulatory System

A. Considerable increase (up to 50 percent) in volume as a result of:
   1. Increased metabolic demands of new tissue.
   2. Expansion of vascular system, especially in the reproductive organs.
   3. Retention of sodium and water.
B. Increase in plasma volume is greater than increase in red blood cells and hemoglobin.
   1. Decline in hemoglobin due to hemodilution referred to as "pseudoanemia."
   2. Low hemoglobin in pregnancy, below 11.5 percent, usually caused by iron-deficiency anemia.
C. Iron requirements are increased to meet demands of increased blood supply and growing fetus (need cannot be met by diet alone; supplement usually given).
D. Heart increases in size. Cardiac output is increased (25 to 50 percent).
E. Blood pressure *should not* rise during pregnancy. Slight decline is normal in second trimester.
F. Fibrinogen concentration increases to term.
G. Palpitations may be experienced during pregnancy due to sympathetic nervous disturbance and intraabdominal pressure caused by enlarging uterus.

Respiratory System

A. Thoracic cage is pushed upward and diaphragm is elevated as uterus enlarges.

B. Thoracic cage widens to compensate, so vital capacity remains the same or is increased.
C. Oxygen consumption is increased 15 percent to support fetus and tissue.
D. Shortness of breath may be experienced in latter part of pregnancy due to pressure upon diaphragm caused by enlarging uterus.

Digestive System

A. Nausea, vomiting, and poor appetite are present in early pregnancy because of decreased gastric motility and acidity.
B. Constipation is due to a decrease in gastrointestinal motility, reduced peristaltic activity, and the pressure of the uterus; it may be present in latter half of pregnancy.
C. Flatulence and heartburn may be present, due to decreased gastric acidity and decreased motility of the gastrointestinal tract.

Urinary System

A. Kidneys.
   1. Kidney and renal function increase.
   2. Renal blood flow and glomerular filtration increase.
   3. Renal threshold for sugar is reduced in some women.
B. Bladder and ureters.
   1. Blood supply to the bladder and pelvic organs is increased.
   2. Pressure of the uterus on the bladder causes frequent urination in early and late pregnancy.
   3. Atonia of smooth muscles during pregnancy leads to dilatation of ureters and renal pelvis, and may cause urine stasis.
   4. A decrease in bladder tone is caused by hormonal influences, and a decrease in bladder capacity occurs because of crowding; may lead to complications during pregnancy and in the postpartum period.

Joints, Bones, Teeth, and Gums

A. Softening of pelvic cartilages occurs, probably due to the hormone relaxin.
B. Posture changes as upper spine is thrown forward to compensate for increased abdominal size.
C. Demineralization of teeth does not occur as a result of normal pregnancy but may be related to poor dental hygiene.
D. Increased vascularity of gums due to hormonal changes with tendency to bleed easily.

Endocrine System

A. Placenta produces the hormones human chorionic gonadotropin (HCG) and placental lactogen (HPL).
   1. Production of estrogen and progesterone is taken over from the ovaries by the placenta/fetal unit after the second month.
   2. Normal cycle of production of estrogen and progesterone is suspended until after delivery.
B. Anterior lobe of pituitary gland enlarges slightly during pregnancy.
C. Adrenal cortex enlarges slightly.
D. Thyroid enlarges slightly and thyroid activity increases.
E. Aldosterone levels gradually increase beginning about the fifteenth week.

Metabolism

A. Increase in body weight—an 11 kg weight gain usually recommended.
B. Some of the weight gain is caused by retention of fluid and by deposits of fatty tissue.
C. Water metabolism.
   1. Tendency to retain fluid in body tissues, especially in the last trimester.
   2. Reversal of fluid retention usually takes place in the form of diuresis in the first twenty-four hours postpartum.
D. Basal metabolic rate increases 20 percent.

Psychosocial Changes

Altered Emotional Characteristics

A. Pregnancy may be viewed as a developmental process involving endocrine, somatic, and psychological changes, as a period of increased susceptibility to crises with an altered state of consciousness.
B. Emotional reactions to pregnancy may vary from early rejection to elation.
C. Mother may be puzzled by changes in her feelings.
D. Mother may have fears and worries about the baby and herself.
E. Quick mood changes are common; some emotional instability usually occurs.
F. Mother may experience dependency-independency conflict.

Socialization for Parental Role

A. Pregnant woman may fantasize or daydream to experience the role of mother before the actual birth.
B. Takes on adaptive behaviors that are best suited to her own personality and situation.
C. Experiences a "letting go" of her former role (e.g., as a career woman).
   1. May experience ambivalence about letting go of her old role to take on the new one.
   2. Desire to have a baby influences adjustment.
D. Concerns.
   1. First and second trimester—concerns about body changes; fear of labor and delivery; beginning conceptualization of fetus as separate individual.
   2. Third trimester—more confident about labor and delivery; shows readiness to assume care of infant; incorporation of concept of fetus as a separate individual should be complete.
E. Father may also experience ambivalence at taking on new role, assuming increased financial responsibility, and sharing wife's attention with child.
F. Father may experience physiologic changes, such as weight gain, nausea, and vomiting.

Signs of Pregnancy

Definition: The signs of pregnancy are divided into three groups: presumptive, probable, and positive. Positive signs cannot be detected until after the fourth month.

General Assessment

Presumptive Signs

A. Amenorrhea (cessation of menstruation).
B. Breast changes: increased size and feeling of fullness, nipples more pronounced, areola darker.
C. Nausea and vomiting (morning sickness): appears in about 50 percent of pregnant women and usually disappears at the end of the third month.
D. Frequent urination—frequent desire to void: usually occurs in the first three to four months. Pressure on the bladder from an enlarged uterus gives the sensation of a distended bladder.
E. Quickening—first perception of fetal movement: occurs between sixteenth and eighteenth week.

F. Increased pigmentation of skin, chloasma, linea nigra, and striae gravidarum.

G. Fatigue: periods of drowsiness and lassitude during first three months.

H. Vaginal changes: Chadwick's sign, discoloration, and thickening of vaginal mucosa.

Probable Signs

A. Enlargement of the abdomen: usually occurs after the third month when the fetus rises out of the pelvis into the abdominal cavity.

B. Changes in internal organs.
  1. Change in shape, size, and consistency of the uterus.
  2. Hegar's sign—softening of the isthmus of the uterus: occurs about sixth week.
  3. Goodell's sign—softening of the cervix: occurs beginning of the second month.

C. Braxton Hicks contractions: usually not felt by the mother until seven months, but contractions begin in the early weeks of pregnancy and continue.

D. Ballottement—giving a sudden push to the fetus and feeling it rebound in a few seconds to the original position: usually possible in the fourth to fifth month.

E. Outline of the fetus by abdominal palpation (a probable sign, because a tumor may simulate fetal parts).

F. Pregnancy tests.
  1. Positive test is based upon the secretion of chorionic gonadotropin in the urine; it is usually detectable ten days after the first missed period. Test is 95 percent effective.
  2. Radioimmunoassay (RIA) test.
     a. Test for B = subunit of HCG: most sensitive but not readily available. Pregnancy can be detected before the first period. Test requires 24 hours to complete.
     b. Two-hour tube tests: first void specimen; quite reliable.
     c. Two-minute rapid-slide test: less sensitive and less reliable.
     d. False positive readings: may be due to protein or blood in urine, neoplasms, ingestion of certain drugs (aspirin, methadone).

G. Amenorrhea by week four.

Positive Signs

A. Apparent after eighteenth to twentieth week.

B. Auscultation of fetal heart rates with stethoscope or ultrasonic equipment (rates: 120–160). (With ultrasonic equipment, FH rate may be heard at ten to twelve weeks.)

C. Active fetal movements are perceptible by the physician.

D. X-ray or sonogram examination, showing fetal outline. X-ray not visible until fourteenth week or later, when bone calcification occurs.

General Planning and Analysis

A. The optimum physical, psychological, and social health, comfort, and well-being of the pregnant woman are provided.

B. Optimal growth and development of the fetus is obtained.

C. The pregnant state is identified in a timely manner through physical examination, pregnancy testing, and health history.

D. Pregnant woman is provided prenatal supervision to assess maternal and fetal health status, comfort, and problems; to take action when necessary; and to evaluate the efficacy of those actions.

E. Knowledge, skills, and support are provided to the pregnant woman to assist her to take action to maintain her own health, comfort, and well-being and that of her fetus; to prepare for labor and delivery; and to prevent complications.

F. Early identification and treatment of complications that might lead to morbidity and mortality in the woman and/or fetus are provided.

General Implementation

Physical Examination

A. Initial examination.
  1. Record complete history: past obstetrical history, medical history, family history.
  2. Assist with physical examination: pelvic, breast, chest, abdomen, blood work (CBC), pap smear, rubella titer, slide for gonorrhea, and serology for syphilis.
  3. Establish baseline blood pressure and weight.
  4. Provide client with diet and health instructions.

B. Subsequent examinations: usually once a month until the last trimester, then more frequently. More frequent in high-risk pregnancy.

Table 2. FETAL GROWTH DURING PREGNANCY

Age	Development
End of one month or four weeks	Form of embryonic disc No clearly defined features Body systems rudimentary form Cardiovascular system functioning
End of two months or eight weeks	Head greatly enlarged, about the size of rest of body Some fetal movement due to beginning neuromuscular development Facial features becoming distinct Body covered with thin skin
End of three months or twelve weeks	Teeth forming under gums Center ossification appearing in most bones Fingers and toes are differentiated and bear nails Kidneys able to secrete Eyes have lids that are fused shut until six months Fetus swallows Sex distinguishable
End of four months or sixteen weeks	Lanugo appears over body Meconium in intestines Face has human appearance Size: about 15 cm long; weight: about 100 g
End of five months or twenty weeks	Skeleton begins to harden Buds of permanent teeth develop Vernix caseosa makes appearance Fetal movements stronger and felt by mother Fetal heart rate heard Size: about 25 cm long; weight: about 310 g
End of six months or twenty-four weeks	Fat beginning to deposit beneath skin Body and head better proportioned Eyebrows and eyelashes appear Size: about 30 cm long; weight: about 680 g
End of seven months or twenty-eight weeks	Skin reddish and covered with vernix Size: about 36 cm long; weight: about 1130 g May be viable if born at this time, though still immature
End of eight months or thirty-two weeks	Nails are firm and extend to end of digits Lanugo begins to disappear Size: about 41 cm long; weight: about 1810 g Increased chance for survival if born at this time
End of nine months or thirty-six weeks	Increased fat deposits under skin Increased development Size: about 46 cm long; weight: about 2270 g Good chance of survival
End of ten months or forty weeks	Full term Little lanugo Smooth skin Size: about 50 cm long; weight: 3175–3400 g Optimum time for survival

1. Assess weight, blood pressure, and urine for protein and sugar.
2. Assist with physical examination.
   a. Measure fundal height.
   b. Palpate abdomen.
   c. Auscultate fetal heart rate.
   d. Observe for signs of complications.
   e. Pap smear and smear for GC before delivery.

Client Instruction

A. Provide client with diet and health instructions.
   1. It is important that mother maintain adequate nutrition. (For specific guidelines, refer to appendices following Nutrition chapter.)
   2. Vitamin and iron supplements are usually prescribed.
   3. All drugs can be expected to cross the placenta and affect the fetus.
   4. Greatest danger is first trimester, especially when organs are developing.
   5. Many other effects of drugs on the fetus are unknown and may not be evident for years.
   6. Pregnant women should refrain from taking drugs during pregnancy, even commonly used drugs such as aspirin.
   7. Nicotine: current research indicates that smoking retards the growth of fetus.
      a. Vasoconstriction of mother's vessels, resulting in decreased placental flow.
      b. Increase in carbon dioxide levels in mother's blood and reduction of oxygen-carrying capacity.
   8. Caffeine: may cause malformations. Suggest limited intake or avoidance of sources of caffeine, i.e., coffee, coke, and chocolate.
B. Inform client regarding activities of daily living.
   1. Exercise in moderation is beneficial but should never be carried on past the point of fatigue.
   2. Sports may be participated in if they are part of the mother's usual activity and there are no complications present.
   3. Fatigue is common in early pregnancy.
   4. Frequent rest periods, at ten- to fifteen-minute intervals, are helpful in avoiding needless fatigue.
   5. Dental hygiene should be maintained daily and infections treated promptly.
   6. Tub baths may be taken. Water enters vagina under pressure only. Baths are contraindicated after membranes have ruptured.
   7. Travel.
      a. May travel with physician's permission.
      b. Airlines discourage travel after the eighth month.
      c. When traveling, tell client to elevate feet and walk around periodically to decrease pedal edema.
C. Assess if client is employed and provide instructions as applicable.
   1. May be continued as long as it does not cause overfatigue.
   2. Have client avoid areas where chemicals or gases are used as these may cause congenital malformations in infant.
   3. Have client avoid heavy lifting and individuals with contagious diseases.
D. Provide information to client regarding sexual intercourse.
   1. May be carried on without fear unless bleeding or premature contractions develop.
   2. May need to vary usual positions as pregnancy advances.

Psychosocial Support

A. Reassure client that emotional changes and feelings are normal reactions and that the woman need not feel guilty.
B. Provide supportive atmosphere allowing the woman to express fears and concerns regarding self, baby, changes in family relationship, etc.
C. Inform client's mate that changes in attitudes, feelings, sexuality, and emotions are temporary and are related to pregnancy.

OBSTETRICAL GUIDELINES

ASSESSMENT	NORMAL	ABNORMAL
RECOMMENDATIONS FOR PRENATAL CLIENTS		
Instruct about **nutrition**		
Instruct about intake of **sodium,** which is essential for maintaining increased body fluids needed for adequate placental flow, increased tissue requirements, and adequate renal blood flow		
Instruct about **exercise** 　Exercise is beneficial in moderation 　Continued exercise in familiar sports throughout pregnancy is recommended 　Participation in new or unfamiliar sports is not recommended	Fatigue in early pregnancy: may need to decrease exercise	Excessive fatigue: may indicate too much exercise
Instruct about **rest** 　Frequent rest periods are necessary to prevent fatigue 　Legs should be elevated to promote venous return 　Crossing legs at knees should be avoided to prevent pressure on veins	Venous stasis in legs and feet late in pregnancy: may occur due to weight of fetus on femoral plexus	
Instruct about **clothing** 　Bras should support with wide shoulder straps 　Client may need several sizes during pregnancy 　Shoes should be supportive, with low heels 　Clothing should be loose and comfortable. Client should avoid constrictive clothing, especially on legs		
Instruct about **bathing** 　Tub baths are acceptable if membranes intact and no bleeding 　Client should be helped when getting in and out of the tub		Tub baths avoided: client large and unstable on feet; signs of bleeding, onset of labor
Instruct about **drugs** and **tobacco** 　Tobacco should be eliminated or decreased 　Alcohol should be eliminated		Alcohol use associated with small-for-gestational-age infants (SGA) If mother is allergic to alcohol: fetal alcohol syndrome

ASSESSMENT	NORMAL	ABNORMAL
Instruct about **sexual relations**	Continuation if no bleeding, ruptured membranes, or premature contractions	
Instruct about **preparations for labor and delivery** at about 30th to 32nd week of gestation		
Instruct about **major discomforts** and **relief measures**		
RECOMMENDATIONS FOR POSTPARTUM CLIENTS		
Instruct about **nutrition**		
Instruct about **exercise**	Return to previous level of activity slowly, progressively, with physician's approval	Early, strenuous exercise: may lead to fatigue and hemorrhage
Encourage adequate **rest**		
Inform about **care of baby** Bathing/skin care Diapering/dressing Feeding/burping Sleeping/positioning Temperature/signs of illness Medical check-ups/ immunizations Safety Growth and development		
Instruct about **contraceptives** if necessary	Nursing: use condom, gel, foam for first 6 weeks then method of choice may be used Nonnursing: may use oral contraceptives after delivery	
Instruct about **sexual relations**	Resume when episiotomy healed and lochia stopped	Pain with intercourse: may need water-based jelly for lubrication for four to six months; episiotomy may not be healed

Table 3. INSTRUCTIONS REGARDING MAJOR DISCOMFORTS AND RELIEF MEASURES

Discomfort	Trimester Most Prominent	Relief Measures
Nausea and vomiting	1st	Eat five or six small, frequent meals. In between meals, have crackers without fluid. Avoid foods high in carbohydrates, fried and greasy, or with a strong odor.
Fatigue	1st	Take frequent rest periods during the day.
Frequency	1st, 3rd	Wear perineal pads if there is leakage.
Heartburn	2nd, 3rd	Avoid fatty, fried, and highly spiced foods. Small frequent feedings. *Avoid* sodium bicarbonate.
Abdominal distress	1st, 2nd, 3rd	Eat slowly, chew food thoroughly, take smaller helpings of food.
Flatulence	2nd, 3rd	Maintain daily bowel movement. Avoid gas-forming foods.
Constipation	2nd, 3rd	Drink sufficient fluids. Eat fruit and foods high in fiber and roughage. Exercise moderately. *Do not* use mineral oil.
Hemorrhoids	3rd	Apply ointments, suppositories, warm compresses. Avoid constipation.
Insomnia	3rd	Exercise moderately to promote relaxation and fatigue.
Backaches	3rd	Rest and improve posture; use a firm mattress. Use a good abdominal support; wear comfortable shoes. Do exercises such as squatting, sitting, and pelvic rock.
Varicosities, legs and vulva	3rd	Avoid long periods of standing or sitting with legs crossed. Sit or lie with feet and hips elevated. Move about while standing to improve circulation. Wear support hose; *avoid* tight garters.
Edema of legs and feet	3rd	Elevate feet while sitting or lying down. Avoid standing or sitting in one position for long periods.
Cramps in legs	3rd	Extend cramped leg and flex ankles, pushing foot upward with toes pointed toward knee. Increase calcium intake.
Pain in thighs or aching of perineum	3rd	Alternate periods of sitting and standing. Rest.
Shortness of breath	3rd	Sit up. Lie on back with arms extended above bed.
Breast soreness	1st, 2nd, 3rd	Wear brassiere with wide adjustable straps that fits well.
Supine hypotensive syndrome	3rd	Change position to left side to relieve pressure of uterus on inferior vena cava.
Vaginal discharge	3rd	Practice proper cleansing and hygiene. Avoid douche unless recommended by physician. Observe for signs of vaginal infection common in pregnancy.

General Evaluation

A. Maternal blood pressure, weight gain, and urine tests remain within normal limits.

B. There is no evidence of signs indicative of pregnancy complications such as vaginal bleeding, edema of the face and hands, and premature labor.

C. Expressed relief from discomforts of pregnancy.

D. Continuation by women of normal activities such as exercise, travel, sexual intercourse, and employment.

E. Avoidance of drugs or substances, such as drugs or coffee, that might affect fetal growth and development.

F. Proper nutrition and hydration of the woman as evidenced by a steady but moderate weight gain (11 to 14 kg), adequate energy level, and adequate general health (i.e., no severe anemia, infection, etc.).

G. Expressed confidence by the pregnant women and their mates in their abilities to experience the type of childbirth they desire, express their needs to each other and to health personnel during labor and delivery, and maintain control during the labor and delivery process.

H. Steady growth and development of the fetus as evidenced by progressive and steady maternal weight gain. Normal increments in fundal height (according to McDonald's measurement) and in diameters of fetal skull.

I. Evidence of fetal well-being through maternal reports of fetal movement, FHT that are within the range of 120 to 160, and tests of fetal well-being when indicated.

Childbirth Education and Preparation

A. Theories of childbirth.
   1. Each method varies somewhat but basic underlying concepts are similar. Birth is viewed as a natural occurrence. Knowledge about the birth experience dispels fears and tension, and distraction and concentration during labor and delivery modify the pain experience.
   2. Purpose: to promote relaxation enabling the mother to work with the labor process. Allows parents to take an active part in the birth process, thereby increasing self-esteem and satisfaction.

B. Factors that influence pain in labor.
   1. Preconditioning: by "old wives' tales," fantasies, and fears. Accurate information about the childbirth process can often alleviate effects of preconditioning.
   2. Pain produces stress, which in turn affects the body's functioning. Interpretations of and reactions to pain can be altered by a refocusing of attention and by conditioning.
   3. Feelings of isolation. Social expectations and tension may also include feelings of pain.

C. Goals accomplished by means of:
   1. Education: anatomy and physiology of reproductive system, and the labor and delivery process; replacement of misinformation and superstition with facts. May include classes on nutrition, discomforts of pregnancy, breast-feeding, infant care, etc.
   2. Training: controlled breathing and neuromuscular exercises.
   3. Presence of father or significant other in labor and delivery rooms to serve as coach and lend support.

D. Common methods presently available.
   1. Read method (natural childbirth): introduced by Grantly Dick-Read in England. Believed pain in childbirth was psychological rather than physiological. Pain brought about by fear and tension.
   2. Lamaze method.
   3. Bradley method.
   4. Scientific relaxation for childbirth.

E. LeBoyer technique: used in delivery room to reduce stress of birth upon infant.
   1. Room temperature is increased to a comfortable level for infant, lights are dimmed, noise is controlled.
   2. Infant is placed in skin-to-skin contact on mother's abdomen and gently stroked; cord clamping is delayed until pulsation stops.
   3. Infant is submerged up to head in a bath of warm water until it appears relaxed, then is dried and wrapped snugly in a warm blanket.

F. Instruction for parents on delivery by C-section.

FETAL MATURITY AND PLACENTAL FUNCTION

Studies for Delivery Capability

Assessment

A. Estriol excretion: estrogen metabolism in pregnancy is dependent upon a healthy mother, a healthy fetus, and an intact placenta.
  1. Estriol level increases as the fetus grows and decreases when growth ceases.
  2. Measured by 24-hour urine specimen or serum estriol levels.
  3. Provides guide to normalcy of fetoplacental unit.
     a. Placental functioning.
     b. Fetal well-being.
  4. Excretion of high estriol levels indicates good function; low levels may indicate fetal jeopardy.
  5. Serial assays are usually done, starting at about thirty-two weeks, to assess the fetal condition.
B. Amniotic fluid studies.
  1. Amniocentesis is the introduction of a needle through the abdominal and uterine walls and into the amniotic cavity to withdraw fluid for examination.
     a. Possible after the fourteenth week.
     b. Amniocentesis indicates:
        (1) Sex of baby.
        (2) Certain congenital defects such as Down's Syndrome.
        (3) State of fetus affected by Rh isoimmunization.
        (4) Fetal maturity.
  2. Lecithin/sphingomyelin ratio (L/S Ratio).
     a. Test for fetal maturity by examining amniotic fluid for presence of surfactant.
     b. Lecithin major constituent of surfactant.
     c. At thirteenth week, the concentration of sphingomyelin is higher than lecithin.
     d. Thereafter, lecithin increases slowly until the thirty-fifth week when it is two or more times greater than sphingomyelin. At this time, fetal lungs are said to be mature, and the infant is unlikely to develop respiratory distress syndrome.
  3. Creatinine level.
     a. Progressive rise as fetus approaches term.
     b. Excreted in fetal urine, measures increasing muscle mass.
     c. Values of 2 mg/100 ml amniotic fluid correlates with gestation of about thirty-six weeks.
  4. Bilirubin level.
     a. Amount of bilirubin in amniotic fluid decreases near term of normal fetus. Usually disappears during the last month of gestation.
     b. Exposure of blood sample to light for a period greater than a few seconds invalidates the test.
  5. Cytological studies: sebaceous glands of fetus begin to function and shed near term. Percentage of lipid globules present gives indication of fetal age.
C. Ultrasound.
  1. A diagnostic test of intermittent high frequency sound waves that reflect off tissues according to varying densities.
  2. Advantages—technique is noninvasive, nondamaging and painless.
  3. Purpose—to differentiate tissue mass and do serial studies. Determines fetal movements, breathing, heart valve capability.
  4. Results—detects placental location (amniocentesis, placenta previa) gestational age, presence of twins, fetal growth.
  5. Procedure—client instructed to have a full bladder; test takes 20–30 minutes to complete. Near term, anticipate supine hypotension, nausea and vertigo.
D. Amnioscopy.
  1. Transcervical visualization of amniotic fluid through intact membranes.
  2. Greenish amniotic fluid indicates fetal distress.
  3. Cervix must be dilated to more than 1 cm.

Planning and Analysis

A. Fetal maturity established.
B. Placental function assessed.
C. Delivery capability determined.

Implementation

A. Inform client about procedure, answer all questions, and obtain her signature on appropriate consent forms.
B. Have client empty bladder.
C. Auscultate fetal heart rate and obtain base line vital signs.
D. Make client comfortable.
E. Prepare abdomen with antiseptic solution.
F. Have necessary equipment available and ready for use.
G. Assist physician with collection of specimens.
H. Continue to monitor fetus and client throughout the procedure and for 30 minutes after.
I. Provide emotional support—procedure may create fear for fetus in client.

Evaluation

A. Specimen is obtained.
B. Fetal heart rate and maternal vital signs remain stable.
C. Client does not appear unduly fearful or anxious.

Nonstress Test

Assessment

A. Test designed to measure fetal baseline heart rate and variability. May also include record of fetal movement as reported by the client.
B. Indicated in conditions of known maternal problems such as diabetes, chronic hypertension, and preeclampsia.
C. Usually given after the thirty-second week on a weekly or semi-weekly basis and on an outpatient basis.

Planning and Analysis

A. Baseline fetal heart rate will be ascertained for future evaluation.
B. Heart rate will be normal.

Implementation

A. Place client in semi-Fowler's position.
B. Take baseline vital signs.
C. Place external monitor on maternal abdomen.
D. Instruct client to press recording button each time she feels fetal movement.
E. Normal test time is 20 to 30 minutes.
F. Record fetal heart rate and contractile activity.

Evaluation

A. A healthy fetus with good reserves shows a monitor strip with a normal fetal heart rate pattern and good variability.
B. The acceleration of fetal heart rate occurs with recorded fetal movement.

Oxytocin Challenge Test or Stress Test

Assessment

A. Assess test results to determine status of fetoplacental unit.
   1. If placental flow is normal, fetus remains oxygenated during uterine contractions.
   2. Placental insufficiency produces characteristic late deceleration pattern during contraction. Fetal bradycardia is less than 120 beats/min or persistent drop of 20 beats below baseline.
B. Assess test for:
   1. Persistent late decelerations occurring with at least three contractions (positive).
   2. Three consecutive contractions in a 10-minute period without decelerations (negative). Test may be repeated each week until delivery.
   3. Suspicious—occasional or several nonpersistent decelerations (suspicious).
C. Observe for complications.
   1. Fetal heart rate below 120.
   2. Sustained uterine contractions.
   3. Supine hypotensive syndrome (check maternal blood pressure).

Planning and Analysis

A. Fetoplacental status clearly determined.
B. Complications do not occur.

Implementation

A. Client usually not admitted.
B. Place client in semi-Fowler's or lateral recumbent position to prevent supine hypotensive syndrome.
C. Give liquid nourishment if ordered.
D. Explain procedure to client.
E. Apply external fetal monitor.
F. Observe for uterine activity and fetal heart rate—usually for 10 to 20 minutes to obtain base line.
G. IV solution with oxytocic drug is started; infusion pump usually used to administer more accurate dosage.

H. Dosage is increased every 15 to 20 minutes until client has three good contractions in a 10-minute period. (Oxytocin is discontinued once pattern is established.)

I. Observe client for signs of sensitivity to drug.

J. Record vital signs and oxytocic infusion every 15 minutes on strip.

K. Monitor contractions and fetal heart rate until client returns to pre-oxytocic state.

L. Discontinue IV and prepare client for discharge.

M. Record all information on chart; monitor strip is considered legal document and becomes part of chart.

N. Discontinue drug immediately if fetal heart rate decreases below 120 or sustained uterine contraction develops.

Nipple Stimulation Test

A. Purpose—start contractions without use of oxytocin.

B. Preferred method—non-invasive.

C. Procedure: manual stimulation of mother's nipples to induce contractions.
1. Contractions similar to those with spontaneous labor.
2. Nerve impulses cause release of endogenous oxytocin.
3. Contractions begin within 15–30 minutes.
4. Assess FHR for prolonged decelerations.
5. Perform test in or near delivery room.

COMPLICATIONS OF PREGNANCY

Definition: High-risk pregnancy occurs when there is an increased chance of morbidity and/or mortality to the mother and/or fetus due to the presence of a complicating factor.

Characteristics

A. The development of obstetrically related conditions during the pregnancy such as vaginal bleeding, toxic states, and premature labor.

B. Medical conditions such as cardiac disease, diabetes, or infection.

C. Unfavorable obstetrical history such as high parity—five or more pregnancies, previous infant death, premature birth, or infant with congenital malformations, difficulty in conceiving, less than a year since last pregnancy, and Rh incompatibility and sensitization.

D. Psychosocial conditions such as under 17 years of age, narcotic or alcohol addiction, and poverty.

General Assessment

A. Obtain a general assessment of pregnant client for signs indicative of the development of complications. Include an accurate health history.

B. Observe for presence of danger signals.
1. Bleeding from the vagina.
2. Escape of amniotic fluid denoting premature rupture of the membranes.
3. Contractions increasing in strength, duration, and proximity before term.
4. Dizziness or blurred vision.
5. Edema of the face and fingers.
6. Persistent and severe vomiting.
7. Chills, malaise, and/or elevated temperature.
8. Absence of or significant and consistent decrease in fetal movement.
9. Decrease or absence of fetal heart tones.

General Planning and Analysis

A. The risk-causing condition is identified early.

B. Interventions aimed at controlling the risk-causing condition are instituted thereby containing or reducing the probability of complications to mother and fetus.

C. Education of pregnant women to recognize and report signs indicative of possible complications is accomplished.

D. Knowledge, skills, and support are provided to women with high-risk pregnancy to increase the effectiveness of their efforts to keep and bring the risk-causing condition under control.

E. Fetal well-being and placental function are assessed.

General Implementation

A. Assess, monitor, and control the specific conditions leading to identification of the client as high risk.

B. Refer to following conditions for specific management.

General Evaluation

A. The risk-causing conditions are controlled: cessation of premature labor, temperature and blood pressure within normal limits, laboratory tests within normal limits, etc.

B. The pregnancy progresses to term.

C. The fetus demonstrates signs of growth, development, and well-being as evidenced by patterns of fetal movement, FHT within the range of 120 to 160, tests within normal limits such as a negative OCT, normal estriol levels, etc.

Abortions

Types of Abortions

A. Spontaneous abortion: involuntary expulsion of the fetus before viability.

B. Threatened: some loss of blood and pain without loss of products of conception.

C. Imminent: bleeding profuse, contractions severe, bearing down sensation; without intervention, products of conception will be lost.

D. Inevitable: bleeding, contractions, ruptured membranes, and cervical dilatation.

E. Incomplete: portion of products of conception remain in uterine cavity.

F. Complete: all products of conception expelled.

G. Habitual: abortion in three or more succeeding pregnancies.

Characteristics

A. Abnormalities of fetus: blighted embryo.

B. Abnormalities of reproductive tract.

C. Injuries: physical and emotional shocks.

D. Endocrine disturbances.

E. Acute infectious diseases.

F. Maternal diseases.

G. Psychogenic problems.

Assessment

A. Observe amount of vaginal bleeding: slight, moderate or heavy.

B. Evaluate intermittent contractions, pain (usually beginning in the small of the back), and abdominal cramping.

C. Observe for passage of tissue.

D. Evaluate condition of internal cervical os.

E. Evaluate size of uterus and compare estimated length of pregnancy.

F. Assess psychological state of client.

Planning and Analysis

A. Spontaneous abortion is interrupted before it proceeds to the inevitable stage.

B. All the products of conception have been passed and the bleeding is arrested if spontaneous abortion occurs.

> **MEDICAL IMPLICATIONS**
> - Endocrine disturbances: hormone therapy (estrogen and progesterone), thyroid therapy.
> - Incompetent cervical os: McDonald operation, or Shirodkar procedure: internal os constricted by encircling suture, which is removed when labor begins.
> - Abnormalities and fibromas: surgical correction of abnormalities, if possible, and removal of fibromas.
> - Oxytocic drug may be given to hasten process of abortion, if it is inevitable, and to promote contraction of uterus after abortion.
> - Medication for pain if necessary.
> - Blood transfusion if necessary.
> - Dilation and curettage in incomplete abortion.
> - Administration of RhoGAM to Rh-negative mothers.
> - Antibiotic therapy if infection seems possible.

Implementation

A. Save all perineal pads and expelled tissue for examination.

B. Offer emotional support but do not give false reassurance.

C. Observe for signs of shock and institute emergency measures if necessary (type and cross-match).

D. Maintain client on bed rest.

E. Provide instructions regarding activity restriction.

F. Provide diversional activities while on bed rest.

G. If incompetent cervix is treated with cerclage, provide the following nursing care:
  1. Place woman in Trendelenburg's position to keep pressure off cervix.
  2. Continuously monitor FHT and contractions.
  3. Observe for premature rupture of the membranes.
  4. When woman goes into labor, verify that all sutures are removed and carefully observe labor pattern.

H. Ensure client receives psychotherapy if needed.

I. Have client restrict activities such as climbing stairs and coitus for at least two weeks after bleeding stops.

Evaluation

A. Bleeding ceases and pregnancy continues (if process is interrupted before abortion occurs).
B. No signs of complicating sequelae such as infection, anemia, DIC, etc.
C. The couple is able to express feelings of grief, inadequacy, or guilt.

Extrauterine, or Ectopic, Pregnancy

Definition: Implantation of the fertilized ovum outside the uterus; usually cannot develop longer than 10 to 12 weeks.

Characteristics

A. Although the fertilized ovum usually attaches to the uterine lining, it may become implanted at any point between the graafian follicle and the uterus.
B. Tubal pregnancy is the most common form (95 percent), but the ovum may attach to an ovary, the abdomen, or interligaments.
C. Implantation.
   1. Ovum attaches to tube and erodes into mucosa wall, as it would to the endometrial lining of the uterus.
   2. Tube increases in size and stretches.
   3. Pregnancy usually terminates during the first three months by:
      a. Spontaneous tubal abortion.
      b. Tubal rupture.
      c. Death and disintegration of products of conception within the tube.
D. Abdominal pregnancies have been known to progress to term.
E. Etiology
   1. Progress of ovum through tube is delayed for some reason.
   2. Tubal deformities: congenital or due to disease such as gonorrhea.
   3. Tumors pressing against the tube.
   4. Adhesions from previous surgery.
   5. Tubal spasms.
   6. Migration of ovum to opposite tube.

Assessment

A. Gather history of missed periods and "spotting."
B. Assess early signs of pregnancy. (Woman may or may not know she is pregnant.)
C. Assess for Rh factor.
D. Evaluate enlarged uterus due to hormonal influence.
E. Assess for slight abdominal pain or sudden excruciating pain in lower abdomen—often first indication of ruptured tube.
F. Evaluate fainting and signs of shock from hemorrhage into peritoneal cavity.

Planning and Analysis

A. Bleeding will be controlled and blood loss replaced.
B. Client will maintain healthy status.
C. Removal of affected tube is completed.
D. Treatment for shock is carried out.

Implementation

A. Institute same care as for postsurgical client.
B. Observe for signs of shock and institute treatment for shock as necessary.
C. Protect client against undue fatigue and infection (energy level and resistance will be low because of severe blood loss).
D. Provide emotional support: client may be frightened and feel the loss of the pregnancy.

Evaluation

A. Vital signs are stable; shock is controlled.
B. No signs of infection or other possible complications.
C. Client is able to express feelings regarding loss of pregnancy, fears for future pregnancies.

Hydatidiform Mole

Definition: A benign neoplasm of the chorion, in which chorionic villi degenerate, become filled with a clear viscid fluid, and assume the appearance of grapelike clusters involving all or parts of the decidual lining of the uterus.

Characteristics

A. Incidence is rare—occurs once in every two thousand pregnancies, except in the Orient where it is more common.
B. Usually there is no fetus found.
C. May be pathological ova.
D. High incidence in the Orient may be due to dietary protein deficiency.

Assessment

A. Evaluate bleeding: may vary from spotting to profuse.
B. Assess for intermittent brownish discharge after the twelfth week.
C. Check for enlargement of the uterus; may be out of proportion to duration of pregnancy.
D. Check for nausea and vomiting: appears earlier, is more severe, and lasts longer than normal.
E. Evaluate for severe preeclampsia, which develops in the early part of the second trimester.
F. Evaluate hypertension, which occurs with the rapid expansion of the uterus.
G. Assess for passage of characteristic vesicles.
H. Check fetal heart tones: none may be heard; no fetal parts may be discerned.

Planning and Analysis

A. Evacuation of the uterus is completed.
B. Diagnosis and medical treatment are implemented.

> MEDICAL IMPLICATIONS
> • Test for increased titer of chorionic gonadotropin. A 24-hour specimen is collected for the total daily output.
> • Sonography: gives positive diagnosis in the first trimester.
> • Amniography: x-ray following injection with contrast dye.
> • Evacuation of uterus as soon as positive diagnosis is made: by dilitation and curettage or vacuum curettage suction.
> • Follow-up supervision for one year.
> • Continued high HCG titers indicate a pathological condition.
> • Pregnancy not advised until one year after tests are negative.

Implementation

A. Observe for uterine hemorrhage following evacuation as uterus is very fragile and has little tone.
B. Provide emotional support: client may fear a malignancy or may feel the loss of the baby or repulsion at products of conception.
C. Encourage client to have follow-up treatment because of possibility of development of neoplasm.
D. Have client avoid pregnancy for one year.

Evaluation

A. Pregnancy is terminated.
B. Vital signs are stable, and there is no sign of excessive bleeding.
C. Client is able to express fears and feelings regarding loss of pregnancy and defective products of conception.
D. Client continues with follow-up treatment.

Placenta Previa

Definition: A condition where the ovum implants low in the uterus, toward the cervix, and the placenta develops so that it partially or completely covers the internal os. Occurs once in every 150 to 200 pregnancies.

Characteristics

A. Types:
 1. Complete: os entirely covered.
 2. Partial: only part of os covered.
 3. Marginal: margin overlaps os.
B. Occurs more often in multiparas.
C. Occurs more often with increased age of mother.
D. Scarring or tumor of uterus.

Assessment

A. Observe for painless vaginal bleeding, intermittent or in gushes, after the seventh month without precipitating cause. (As internal os begins to dilate, the part of the uterus that overlies the os separates and leaves gaping vessels, so bleeding occurs.)
B. Evaluate uterine tone and contractibility.
C. Check for signs of hemorrhage.
D. Assess pain if any (generally painless).
E. Assess vital signs.

Planning and Analysis

A. Bleeding will be controlled and a healthy neonate delivered.
B. Diagnosis and medical treatment are implemented.

> MEDICAL IMPLICATIONS
> • History of painless bleeding late in pregnancy.
> • Placenta is localized by ultrasound or radioisotope.

- Sterile vagina or pelvic examinations are conducted when adequate preparation has been made.
- Have blood available for transfusion.
- Set up for possible emergency cesarean delivery.
- Determine whether fetal age is adequate for survival.
- Client is hospitalized immediately and placed on bed rest.
- Blood type is determined and crossmatched for possible transfusion.
- Treatment depends upon type of placenta previa, condition of mother, and viability of baby.
- Mechanical pressure is applied to placental site by bringing down baby's head and occluding blood vessels—usually accomplished by the rupture of membranes; vaginal delivery is possible if bleeding is checked.
- Delivery by cesarean method if bleeding is excessive.
- If baby is small and bleeding stops, delivery is usually postponed.

Implementation

A. Maintain client in bed and provide quiet, restful atmosphere and diversion.
B. Count perineal pads and measure blood amounts on bedding, chux, etc.
C. Give emotional support, explain procedures, and help allay fears.
D. *Do not* perform vaginal examination.
E. Have emergency setup for cesarean delivery available.
F. Carefully monitor fetal heart tones.
G. Client may be externally monitored.

Evaluation

A. Bleeding is minimized.
B. Vital signs are stable.
C. A healthy infant is delivered.

Abruptio Placentae

Definition: A condition that occurs when the placenta separates from the normal implantation site in upper segment of uterus before birth of baby; occurs once in five hundred deliveries.

Characteristics

A. Types.
   1. Complete separation: placenta becomes completely detached from uterine wall.
   2. Partial separation: portion of placenta adheres to uterine wall.
B. Hemorrhage.
   1. External: blood escapes from the vagina.
   2. Concealed: blood is retained in uterine cavity.
C. Etiology.
   1. Trauma.
   2. Chronic vascular renal disease.
   3. High parity.
   4. Cocaine use.
   5. Hypertensive disease.

Assessment

A. External assessment: chief symptom is vaginal bleeding accompanied by abdominal pain.
B. Evaluate concealed condition.
   1. Intense, cramplike uterine pain.
   2. Uterine tenderness and rigidity.
   3. Lack of alternate contraction-relaxation of uterus.
   4. Fetal heart tones—bradycardia or absent.
C. Assess for signs of shock: decreased blood pressure, increased pulse rate, pallor.
D. Continuous evaluation for DIC.

Planning and Analysis

A. Bleeding is controlled.
B. Delivery of fetus occurs as quickly as possible.

MEDICAL IMPLICATIONS
- Treatment depends upon severity and extent of labor.
- Moderate bleeding: membranes are ruptured to hasten delivery and help control bleeding.
- Severe: immediate cesarean delivery.
- Treatment for blood loss and shock.
- Blood drawn for coagulation studies.
- Narcotics may be given for severe pain.
- Oxygen may be given.

Implementation

A. Keep client on bed rest.
B. Observe for signs of shock.
C. Carefully monitor contractions, fetal heart tones, and vital signs.

D. If bleeding is severe, begin administration of intravenous solution: 5 percent dextrose in Ringer's lactate.

E. Order type and crossmatch blood for possible transfusion.

F. Observe for hemorrhage after delivery.

G. Record intake and output and observe for anuria or oliguria. (Anuria may develop as a result of acute tubular necrosis.)

H. Provide emotional support as fetal prognosis is guarded.

Evaluation

A. Vital signs remain stable.

B. No vaginal bleeding.

C. Client is able to express grief over loss of infant.

Hyperemesis Gravidarum

Definition: Pernicious vomiting during pregnancy. Usually develops during first three months of pregnancy.

Characteristics

A. May be caused by the addition of new substances to the body system—a toxicity or maladjustment of the maternal metabolism.

B. Psychological etiology cannot be verified. Current data suggests that this is not the cause.

Assessment

A. Check for persistent nausea and amount of vomiting.

B. Assess for abdominal pain and hiccups.

C. Measure weight loss.

D. Evaluate dehydration status.

E. Assess electrolyte imbalance: depletion of essential electrolytes because of unreplaced loss of sodium chloride and potassium.

F. Assess for metabolic acidosis: acetone odor to breath.

G. Evaluate increase in blood urea nitrogen.

H. Assess for hypoproteinemia and hypovitaminosis.

I. Check amount of food ingested.

Planning and Analysis

A. Vomiting is controlled.

B. Fluid and electrolyte balance maintained.

C. Weight gain promoted.

Implementation

A. Use tact and understanding of the client's problem.

B. Carefully record intake and output; maintain IVs.

C. Provide attractive small meals, and remove dishes as soon as the client finishes eating.

D. Offer frequent small feedings: small amounts every two hours, dry foods preferred.

E. Administer antiemetics, plus a tranquilizer or a sedative as ordered.

F. If vomiting is persistent:
   1. Client is usually hospitalized.
   2. Dehydration and starvation is treated by administration of parenteral fluids.
   3. Rest and sedatives are prescribed.
   4. Psychotherapy if necessary.

G. Provide rest, reduce stimuli, and restrict visitors.

H. Monitor fetal heart tones.

Evaluation

A. Vomiting subsides.

B. No evidence of dehydration or acidosis.

C. Fetal heart tones are stable.

D. Adequate intake and weight gain.

PREGNANCY INDUCED HYPERTENSION

Preeclampsia

Definition: An acute, hypertensive disease that is peculiar to pregnancy. It may be mild or severe.

Assessment

A. Assess period in pregnancy that condition appears: usually after the twentieth week.

B. Evaluate for major symptoms: hypertension, proteinuria, and edema (may appear separately or together). Two of these three symptoms are usually needed for diagnosis.

C. Assess for mild preeclampsia.
   1. Elevation of blood pressure 30/15 mm Hg on two occasions, six hours apart.
   2. Generalized edema.
   3. Proteinuria: 0.3 g/liter, 24-hour specimen.
   4. Weight gain: more than 1360 g per week in second trimester and 450 g per week in third trimester.

D. Assess for severe preeclampsia.
1. Blood pressure 160/110 or above, or systolic 50 mm Hg above normal.
2. Massive edema: excessive weight gain.
3. Proteinuria: 5 g or more in twenty-four hours.
4. Oliguria: 400 cc or less in twenty-four hours.
5. Visual disturbances.
6. Headache.
7. Vasospasms.
8. Hemoconcentration.
9. Epigastric pain (usually a late sign).
10. CNS irritability (hyperreflexia).

Planning and Analysis

A. Further progression of disease is controlled.
B. Client and fetus maintained on healthy status.

MEDICAL IMPLICATIONS

Mild Preeclampsia
• Treatment aimed at preventing further increase in disease.
• Client usually remains at home.
• Extra rest is prescribed.
• Adequate fluid intake.
• Diet: increased protein and carbohydrate, reduced fat, moderate salt.
• Daily weight.

Severe Preeclampsia
• Antihypertensives, sedatives.
• Diet: increased protein, moderate salt.
• Bed rest.
• Efforts to increase diuresis: diuretics not given.
• Observe for signs of central nervous system irritability and hyperactivity.

Implementation

A. Maintain client on bed rest and plan care to promote rest.
B. Monitor magnesium sulfate medication.
C. Monitor fetal heart tones and observe for signs of labor.
D. Carefully monitor vital signs and lab values.
E. Record intake and output; examine urine for protein.
F. Immediately report increases in signs and symptoms.
G. Check daily weight at the same time each day.

H. Examine retina daily for arteriole changes or edema.
I. Limit visitors in severe cases.
J. Maintain seizure precautions.
K. Final resolution is delivery of the fetus.
L. Prepare client for surgery if indicated.

Evaluation

A. Blood pressure is reduced.
B. Output reflects intake.
C. Edema and proteinuria are reduced.
D. No signs of arteriole change in retina.
E. No signs of central nervous irritability: twitching, nervousness, irritability.
F. Client and fetus retain healthy status.

Eclampsia

Definition: A more severe form of hypertensive disease, characterized by convulsions and even coma.

Assessment

A. Observe for severe edema.
B. Check urine output and for urine that contains red blood cells, varied casts, and protein.
C. Assess for blood pressure elevation to 200/110 or above.
D. Check for visual disturbances, blurring, or even blindness caused by edema of the retina.
E. Determine if severe epigastric pain is present.
F. Observe convulsions, both tonic and clonic.
G. Assess for signs of labor. (Labor may begin and fetus may be born prematurely or die.)
H. Assess vital signs: temperature and respiratory status.
I. Observe reflex irritability.
J. Assess level of consciousness.
K. Determine fetal heart tones and uterine contractibility.
L. Assess for necessity of doing emergency cesarean section.

Planning and Analysis

A. The disease process is controlled.
B. Maternal and fetal morbidity and mortality prevented.
C. Convulsions controlled.

D. Vasodilation to combat vasospasms promoted.

E. Diuresis promoted.

F. Blood pressure is controlled.

Implementation

A. Provide a quiet, darkened room with a constant attendant and bed rest.

B. Check client frequently for edema.

C. Maintain seizure precautions.

D. Suction if necessary.

E. Provide oxygen as necessary.

F. Keep record of vital signs and lab values.

G. Check blood pressure frequently.

H. Keep client n.p.o.

I. Maintain IV and give medications.

J. Monitor fetal heart tones and contractions.

K. Observe carefully for 24 hours postpartum for anuria, convulsions, headache, and blurred vision.

L. See Appendix 1 for drugs normally used for pregnancy induced hypertension.

Evaluation

A. Convulsive activity ceases, and central nervous system hyperactivity is reduced.

B. Blood pressure is reduced.

C. Urinary output within normal limits.

D. Edema reduced.

E. A healthy neonate is delivered.

MEDICAL DISEASES COMPLICATING HIGH-RISK PREGNANCY

Cardiovascular Disease

Characteristics

A. Classification.

1. Class I: no alteration of activity.
2. Class II: slight limitation of activity.
3. Class III: marked limitation of activity.
4. Class IV: symptoms present at rest.

B. Pregnancy expands plasma volume, increasing cardiac output and load on heart.

C. Most deaths are caused by cardiac failure, when blood volume is at a maximum in the last weeks of the second trimester.

D. Heart failure occurs infrequently in labor.

E. Over age thirty-five, there is an increase in the incidence of heart failure and death.

Assessment

A. Observe for signs of cardiac decompensation, especially during the second trimester.

1. Cardiac function, such as pulse rate over 110 or respiratory rate over 24.
2. Decreased vital capacity.
3. Dyspnea.
4. Edema.

B. Evaluate for signs of infection, especially respiratory infection.

1. Elevated temperature.
2. Sore throat.
3. Productive cough.
4. Nasal congestion or discharge.

C. Assess for signs of anxiety or stress.

D. Check vital signs and fetal heart tones.

E. Evaluate activity level.

MEDICAL IMPLICATIONS

- With proper management mortality is minimal.
- Client should avoid people with acute infections, especially respiratory infections; antibiotics may be prescribed prophylactically.
- Client should rest frequently.
- Strenuous activities, such as stair climbing, heavy cleaning, and straining, should be avoided.
- Clients in Class III and over may be hospitalized before labor for controlled rest and diet.
- If client decompensates or has distress symptoms with exertion, she should remain on bed rest or in a chair.
- Digitalis treatment when indicated.
- Emotional stress should be avoided and pain and anxiety controlled.

Diet.

- Salt intake may or may not be restricted.
- Diuretics may be prescribed if signs of heart failure occur.
- The use of highly salted foods is discouraged.
- Iron supplement is important.

Planning and Analysis

A. Cardiac client is identified and treated during pregnancy, labor, delivery, and postpartum period.

B. Client is compliant to treatment regimen.

C. Cardiac decompensation is prevented.

D. Client and infant progress through labor and delivery and remain stable.

Implementation

A. Educate client about classifications and effects of pregnancy before conception.

B. Educate client about special needs and danger signals during pregnancy and postpartum.

C. Care for client during labor:
1. Check vital signs every fifteen minutes or more often as needed.
2. Keep client in bed, preferably lying on one side or in semirecumbent position.
3. Administer oxygen as necessary.
4. Provide calm atmosphere and emotional support to alleviate fears.
5. Administer pain medications as ordered to reduce discomfort during labor.
6. Be alert for signs of impending heart failure.
7. Monitor fetal heart tones.

D. Provide careful observation during postpartum period.

E. Counsel client during postpartum to have help at home and planned rest periods.

Evaluation

A. No signs of cardiac decompensation or advancement of disease.

B. No signs of infection.

C. Stress of labor minimized.

D. Healthy infant is delivered and mother's condition is stabilized.

Diabetes

Definition: A chronic metabolic disease caused by a disturbance in normal insulin production.

Characteristics

A. Estimated 2 percent of pregnancies seen in large metropolitan areas will have some degree of diabetes.

B. Women during pregnancy have a tendency to develop gestational diabetes as a result of placental hormones, variations in insulin level, and an increase in free cortisol.

C. Pregnant women should be screened for glucose levels: should remain 100 mg/dl except for brief periods after meals.

D. Screening essential with presence of following signs and symptoms.
1. Obesity—excessive weight gain.
2. Excessive hunger or thirst.
3. Polyuria.
4. Recurrent monilial infections.
5. Maternal hypertension.
6. Family history of diabetes.
7. Previous delivery of large infant or hydramnios.

E. A three-hour glucose tolerance test will confirm diabetes when two or more values are above normal.

F. Sepsis, eclampsia, and hemorrhage, the most common causes of maternal death, are more common in the pregnant diabetic.

White's Classifications

A. Class A: abnormal glucose tolerance test, indicative of latent or gestational diabetes.

B. Class B: diabetes beginning after age twenty.

C. Class C: diabetes at ages ten to nineteen years or beginning in adolescence after age ten.

D. Class D: diabetes of long duration or onset in childhood before the age of ten.

E. Class E: evidence of pelvic vascular disease.

F. Class F: nephropathy, including capillary glomerulosclerosis.

G. Class R: malignant retinopathy.

Implications of Diabetes in Pregnancy

A. Diabetes is more difficult to control.

B. There is a tendency for client to develop acidosis.

C. Client is prone to infection.

D. Pregnancy induced hypertension, hemorrhage, and polyhydramnios are more likely to develop.

E. Gestational diabetes may develop into full-blown diabetes.

F. Insulin requirements are increased.

G. Premature delivery is more frequent.

H. Infant may be overgrown but have functions related to gestational age rather than size.

I. Infant is subject to hypoglycemia, hyperbilirubinemia, respiratory distress syndrome, and congenital anomalies.

J. Stillborn and neonatal mortality rates are high, but may be reduced by proper management and strict control of diabetes.

Assessment

A. Observe for signs of hypoglycemia.

B. Observe for signs of hyperglycemia.

C. Assess for signs of preeclampsia.
1. Hypertension.
2. Proteinuria.
3. Edema.

D. Check for signs of infection.
1. Increased temperature.
2. Erythematous areas.
3. Respiratory problems.

E. Check for signs of premature labor.

F. Assess for signs of polyhydramnios.
1. Respiratory distress.
2. Fluid stasis in legs.

G. Assess insulin needs.

H. Assess fetal status.

Planning and Analysis

A. Blood glucose levels maintained within a normal range.

B. Episodes of hypoglycemia and hyperglycemia prevented.

C. Medical treatment implemented.

MEDICAL IMPLICATIONS

- Strict control of diabetes through insulin and dietary and exercise regulation.
- Frequent, every one to two weeks, prenatal supervision throughout gestation.
- Control of infection: vaginitis, urinary infections.
- Client may be hospitalized at 36 to 37 weeks gestation for evaluation and possible early termination of pregnancy.
- Placental function may be evaluated: placental insufficiency (pathological process in placenta resulting in inefficient exchange of waste and gases between mother and fetus) is common in diabetics due to vascular changes.
- Assessment of fetal growth and maturity if early delivery is indicated.
- Strict control of diabetes is important.
- Oral diabetic agents are contraindicated as they may cause congenital malformation.

Implementation

A. Educate client on the effects of diabetes on her and the fetus during pregnancy and the reasons for adhering to therapy protocol.

1. Bimonthly visits for six months; weekly visits thereafter.
2. Maintenance of blood glucose levels according to gestational week.
3. Frequent monitoring for glycosuria and ketonuria (grave threat to CNS of fetus).
4. Weight control.
5. Dietary control to increase calorie intake with adequate insulin therapy so glucose will go into the cells.
   a. Daily calories of 30–40/kg of body weight. (Severe calorie restriction may lead to ketosis.)
   b. High protein: 60–90 gm/day (or 2 gm/day/kg of body weight).
   c. Carbohydrate: 200 mg/day.
   d. Fat: 60–90 gm—provide 36 percent total calories.
6. Exogenous insulin if diet cannot control blood sugar levels. Oral hypoglycemics contraindicated; may cause fetal hypoglycemia and abnormalities.

B. Provide care if client is hospitalized.
1. Maintain insulin on regular schedule. Insulin may change daily.
2. Test blood for glucose level as ordered.
3. Provide adequate diabetic diet as prescribed by physician.
4. Monitor fetal heart rate.
5. Check vital signs, especially blood pressure q.i.d. and p.r.n.
6. Weigh daily at the same time.
7. Keep accurate records of intake and output.
8. Provide diversion for client.
9. Provide support and explanations to help allay fears and reduce anxiety.

C. In addition, provide following care to client in labor.
1. Monitor fetal status continuously for signs of distress. If noted, prepare client for immediate cesarean section.
2. Carefully regulate insulin and provide IV glucose as labor depletes glycogen.

D. Provide postpartum care.
1. Observe client closely for insulin reaction: precipitous drop in insulin requirements usual; hypoglycemic shock may occur.
   a. May require no insulin for first 24 hours.
   b. Reregulate insulin needs following first day according to blood sugar testing.

c. Diet and exercise must also be re-examined.

2. Observe for early signs of infection.

3. Observe for postpartum hemorrhage.

Evaluation

A. Client follows prescribed diabetic regimen: takes insulin injections as directed, eats controlled diet, performs finger sticks regularly throughout the day for glucose level, and exercises regularly.

B. No complaints of hypoglycemic episodes.

C. Client is able to institute measure to relieve signs of hypoglycemia.

D. Blood sugar levels remain consistently within a normal range, but there may be occasional lapses.

E. Vital signs remain stable.

F. No signs of premature labor.

G. Fetus indicates signs of well-being: movement, FHT within the normal range, negative OCT, etc.

Chronic Hypertension in Pregnancy

Definition: Hypertensive vascular disease is characteristic hypertension that is already present. It may be aggravated by the pregnancy, or clinical symptoms may first manifest with pregnancy.

Assessment

A. Observe for hypertension: evident before the twenty-fourth week; blood pressure is 140/80 at rest.

B. Check for presence of headache; client may otherwise feel well.

C. Evaluate edema (however, proteinuria is usually *not* present).

D. Assess for signs of superimposed preeclampsia.

E. Check for fetal heart rate.

Planning and Analysis

A. Control of blood pressure maintained.

B. Untoward effects on fetus decreased.

C. Rest and limitation of activity reduce symptoms.

D. Fluids and electrolytes remain in balance.

E. Diet provides necessary nutrients.

Implementation

A. Maintain bed rest and create an environment conducive to rest.

B. Provide supportive atmosphere.

C. Accurately record vital signs, check urine for protein, and check weight daily.

D. Monitor fetal heart tones.

E. Keep careful record of intake and output.

F. Provide adequate diet and fluids.

G. Report any unusual symptoms.

H. Observe for signs of heart failure.

I. Maintain on antihypertensive drugs.

MEDICAL IMPLICATIONS

Mild

• Rest and limitation of activity.

• Curtailment of excessive weight gain.

• Prevention of edema.

Severe

• Hospitalization.

• Bed rest.

• Increased protein diet.

• Adequate fluids.

• Close observation of general condition.

• Daily weight.

• Accurate record of intake and output.

• Check urine for protein.

• Frequent check of vital signs.

• Antihypertensives.

• Serial test is NST after the thirty-second week; if non-reactive, OCT's to determine well-being of fetus are completed.

Evaluation

A. Blood pressure is stabilized.

B. Edema decreased and fluids and electrolytes stabilized.

C. Hospitalization not necessary as condition is controlled by treatment regimen.

D. Diet high in protein provided adequate nutrients.

E. Client's positive adherence to treatment regimen resulted in decrease in symptoms.

F. Healthy baby is delivered.

Anemia

Definition: A deficiency in the blood, usually referring to a decrease in the numbers of erythrocytes or a reduction in hemoglobin. The name implies a low red cell count.

Assessment

A. Evaluate iron deficiency status. This is cause of anemia in 90 percent of the cases.

B. Observe for client who looks pale, tires easily, and is lethargic.
C. Assess for headache or dizziness.
D. Assess for shortness of breath.
E. HGB levels 11 g/dl or below or HCT below 37 percent.

Planning and Analysis

A. Iron deficiency is diagnosed and treated successfully.
B. Medical treatment of supplemental iron (ferrous sulfate) 0.3 g t.i.d. is given, or in severe cases, Imferon as a parenteral medication is given.
C. Complications resulting from iron deficiency are reversed.

Implementation

A. Educate client as to the need to take supplements.
B. Encourage client to eat foods high in iron.
C. Instruct client that iron should be taken after meals to minimize gastric upset.
D. Let client know that stools will become dark from iron absorption.
E. Instruct client to use frequent oral hygiene measures to guard against iron deposit on teeth and gums.
F. Administer Imferon as directed.

Evaluation

A. HGB and HCT return to normal levels.
B. Client understands need for iron supplements and complies to dietary regimen.
C. Client's symptoms of deficiency are reversed.
D. Complications do not occur.

Urinary Tract Infection

Characteristics

A. Usually occurs after the fourth month or in early postpartum; affects 10 percent of maternity clients.
B. Causes.
1. Pressure on ureters and bladder.
2. Hormonal effects on tone of ureters and bladder.
3. Displacement of bladder.
4. History of urinary infections, vaginitis.
C. Kidneys as well as ureters may be involved.

Assessment

A. Observe for frequent micturition.

B. Check for paroxysms—pain in kidney.
C. Assess for fever and chills.
D. Evaluate catheterized urine specimen to determine if it contains bacteria and pus.
E. Check for burning on urination.
F. Check for signs of premature labor.

Planning and Analysis

A. Infection treated and contained.
B. Discomfort relieved.
C. Rest promoted.
D. Medical treatment implemented.

Implementation

A. Maintain client on bed rest.
B. Encourage fluid intake by providing client with a variety of fluids.
C. Obtain specimens as ordered.
D. Monitor antibiotic treatment.
E. Monitor urinary antispasmodics and analgesics.

Evaluation

A. No burning on urination.
B. No reported pain in kidney area.
C. Normal temperature; no reports of chills or malaise.
D. Urine is free of bacteria and pus.

Infectious Diseases

Characteristics

A. Diseases such as influenza, scarlet fever, toxoplasmosis, and cytomegalovirus (type of herpes virus causes cytomegalic inclusion disease) may be transmitted to fetus.
B. Diseases may cause abortions or malformations in early pregnancy, premature labor or fetal death.
C. Rubella in first trimester—a teratogen—may cause congenital anomalies.

Assessment

A. Check for elevation in temperature.
B. Observe for productive cough and nasal secretions.
C. Evaluate for sore throat.
D. Assess for skin rash.
E. Check for contact or exposure of client to persons with infectious disease.

Planning and Analysis

A. Infectious diseases in pregnant women are prevented.

MEDICAL IMPLICATIONS
- Rubella vaccine is available and should be given to children from age one to puberty or to the mother in early postpartum while still hospitalized. (Vaccine should not be given if pregnancy is suspected.)
- Rubella titer should be checked on first prenatal visit.
- Gamma globulin may be given to women if exposure to contagious infectious disease has occurred.

Implementation

A. Educate women before pregnancy to have rubella titer and a vaccination.
B. Educate women to avoid contact with people having known or suspected infectious diseases.
C. Educate women to notify their physician immediately should exposure occur.

SEXUALLY TRANSMITTED DISEASES (STDs)

Chlamydia

Characteristics

A. Most common sexually transmitted disease (STD) in the U.S.
B. 3 to 4 million people contract disease each year.
C. High risk women: young, nonwhites with multiple sex partners and women not using barrier contraceptives.
D. Chlamydia is not a reportable disease in 50% of states.
E. Statistics:
   1. 20% men and 40-50% women with gonorrhea also are infected with chlamydia.
   2. 25-50% of pelvic inflammatory diseases (PID) are caused by chlamydia.
   3. 155,000 infants born to mothers with chlamydia are at risk for pneumonia and inclusion conjunctivitis.
   4. Each year 1 billion dollars spent on infection.
F. Chlamydiae are bacteria microorganisms, but have characteristics of both viruses and bacteria.
G. Sensitive to antibiotics.
H. Spread through sexual contact. Incubation period

5-10 days or longer (28 days) (gonorrhea is only 2-10 days).
I. Tests for chlamydia include Chlamydiazyme—enzyme immuno assay test and Microtak—direct fluorescent antibody test.

Assessment

Observe for
A. A discharge—vaginal or urethral.
B. Assess for burning.
C. Check for lower abdominal pain or testicular pain.
D. Assess for bleeding or pain with coitus.
E. Assess for rectal pain or discharge.
F. 33% women report no symptoms.

Implementation

A. Administer antibiotics as ordered.
   1. Tetracycline 500 mg 4x/day for 7 days or Doxycycline 100 mg 2x/day for 7 days.
      a. Take on an empty stomach.
      b. May be sensitive to the sun.
      c. Avoid becoming pregnant.
   2. Erythromycin 500 mg 4x/day for 7 days as second choice (take with meals).
   3. Penicillin does not cure chlamydia.
B. Educate men and women about transmission, symptoms and prevention.
   1. Frequent examinations if people are not monogamous.
   2. If symptoms/signs occur, seek help immediately—teach importance of taking medication as prescribed.
   3. Suggest sexually active people use barrier methods of contraception.
   4. Avoidance of sex until completion of treatment.
C. Provide accurate information about disease, health care and prevention.

Syphilis

Definition: A chronic infectious disease caused by *Treponema pallidum.*

Characteristics

A. Transmission is by intimate physical contact with syphilitic lesions, which are usually found on the skin or the mucous membranes of the mouth and the genitals.
B. Incubation period is two to six weeks following exposure.

C. Primary stage.
   1. Most infectious stage.
   2. Appearance of chancres, ulcerative lssions.
   3. Usually painless, produced by spirochetes at the point of entry into the body.
D. Secondary stage.
   1. Lesions appear about three weeks after the primary stage and may occur anywhere on the skin and the mucous membranes.
   2. Highly infectious.
   3. Generalized lymphadenopathy.
E. Tertiary stage.
   1. The spirochetes enter the internal organs and cause permanent damage.
   2. Symptoms may occur ten to thirty years following the occurrence of an untreated primary lesion.
   3. Invasion of the central nervous system.
      a. Meningitis.
      b. Locomotor ataxia: foot slapping and broad-based gait.
      c. General paresis.
      d. Progressive mental deterioration leading to insanity.
   4. Cardiovascular: most common site of damage is at the aortic valve and the aorta itself.
F. Characteristics relating to pregnancy.
   1. May cause abortion or premature labor.
   2. Infection is passed to the fetus after the fourth month of pregnancy as congenital syphilis.

Assessment

A. Evaluate serum test (STS) for syphilis on first prenatal visit.
B. May repeat just before 4th month, as disease may be acquired after initial visit.

Planning and Analysis

A. Disease is identified and treated.
B. Congenital syphilis is prevented.

Implementation

A. Educate women to recognize signs of syphilis.
B. Educate women to seek immediate treatment if known exposure occurs.
C. Educate women as to the need for simultaneous treatment of partner as reinfection may occur.
D. Monitor treatment: during pregnancy, 4.8 million units of procaine penicillin G with 2 percent aluminum monostearate, IM normally in divided doses.
E. Report all cases of syphilis to health authorities for treatment of contacts.

Evaluation

A. Disease is treated and congenital syphilis is prevented.
B. Infant shows no signs of syphilis.
C. Client is educated about the disease and danger of transmission.

Gonorrhea

Definition: An infection caused by *Neisseria gonorrhoeae,* which causes inflammation of the mucous membrane of the genitourinary tract.

Characteristics

A. Transmission is almost completely by sexual intercourse.
B. Incidence is of epidemic proportions in the United States.
C. Signs and symptoms.
   1. Male.
      a. Painful urination.
      b. Pelvic pain and fever.
      c. Epididymitis with pain, tenderness, and swelling.
   2. Female (usually asymptomatic).
      a. Vaginal discharge.
      b. Urinary frequency and pain.
D. Complications.
   1. Female: pelvic inflammatory disease (PID) with abdominal pain, fever, nausea, and vomiting.
   2. Male: postgonococcal urethritis and spread of infection to posterior urethra, prostate, and seminal vesicles.
   3. PID can lead to sterility.
   4. A secondary infection can develop in any organ.
E. Infection may be transmitted to baby's eyes during delivery, causing blindness.

Assessment

A. Obtain culture for gonorrhea (usually done on first prenatal visit).

B. Repeat later as infection may occur during pregnancy.

Planning and Analysis

A. Infection is treated.

B. Gonococcal opthalmia neonatorum in infant is prevented.

C. Medical treatment is implemented.

Implementation

A. Educate women to recognize signs of gonorrhea and to seek immediate treatment.

B. Administer prophylactic broad spectrum antibiotic, erythromycin, or 1 percent silver nitrate to newborn (still used in some locations).

C. Monitor treatment: same as for syphilis.

D. Important to treat sexual partner, as client may become reinfected.

Herpes Simplex Type 2 (Genital Herpes)

Characteristics

A. Involves external genitalia, vagina, and cervix.

B. Development and draining of painful vesicles.

C. Virus may be lethal to fetus if innoculated during vaginal delivery. Delivery usually by C-section.

D. Safe use of Acyclovir has not been established for pregnant women.

Assessment

A. Evaluate for presence of painful, draining vesicles on external genitals, vagina, and cervix.

B. Check for increased temperature and vital signs.

Planning and Analysis

A. Prevention of transmission of disease to neonate during labor, delivery, and postpartum is accomplished.

B. Maternal discomfort during acute periods is relieved.

Implementation

A. Educate client as to dangers to fetus.

B. Encourage client to report symptoms.

C. Explain to client as to the possibility of a cesarean section should an outbreak occur around the time of delivery. Policy regarding time limit of outbreak in relation to time of delivery varies, but usual policy is an outbreak within two weeks.

D. Maintain precautions during vaginal examinations of client.

E. Maintain isolation precautions during hospitalization if disease is active.

F. Encourage careful handwashing by client.

G. Infant and mother may be separated during active period depending upon hospital policy or other special precautionary measures may be used to avoid transmission of disease to neonate. Encourage mother to express her feelings regarding separation and to talk about baby.

Genital Warts

Characteristics

A. Almost one million Americans develop this disorder—major STD of 1990s. Caused by the human papilloma virus (HPV).

B. The virus affects cervix, uretha, penis, scrotum, and anus.

C. Warts appear after 1 or 2 months after exposure, transmitted through intimate sexual contact.

Assessment

A. Assess for small to large wart-like growths on genitals (no symptoms other than lesions).

B. Assess for cervical cell changes—HPV associated with up to 90 percent of cervical malignancies.

Implementation

A. There is no cure for HPV—treatment is cryotherapy, liquid nitrogen, or electrocautery to remove lesions.

B. Key is prevention—similar to any other STD: limit sexual contacts and use condoms.

C. Suggest Pap test every year (cancer risk).

ASSOCIATED COMPLICATIONS OF PREGNANCY

Pregnancy in Adolescents

Characteristics

A. Crisis of pregnancy compounds the crises of adolescence—physical, social, emotional, social development.

B. Client may be unwed and have no financial resources.

C. Physical development may not be complete.

D. High incidence of prematurity and toxemia.

E. Diet may be inadequate.

Assessment

A. Assess nutritional status of client.

B. Evaluate any signs of emotional problems, conflicts, or crisis.

C. Evaluate financial status.

D. Assess for signs of premature labor and toxemia.

E. Assess knowledge of pregnancy and infant care.

Planning and Analysis

A. Client maintains her health during pregnancy.

B. Client continues her psychological and social development during pregnancy.

C. Client understands the process of pregnancy.

D. Client delivers a healthy baby.

Implementation

A. Encourage early antepartum care.

B. Provide health instruction on pregnancy, nutrition, hygiene, and infant care.

C. Observe frequently for complications.

D. Provide emotional support and counseling.

Evaluation

A. Client takes responsibility for nutrition, hygiene, and health care during pregnancy.

B. Client makes preparations for infant.

C. No signs of complications.

Disseminated Intravascular Coagulation (DIC)

Definition: A condition in the mother's body that results in an exaggerated clotting process.

Characteristics

A. Possible complication of abruptio placenta, missed abortion, fetal death, amniotic fluid embolism.

B. May result in uncontrolled bleeding.
   1. Thromboplastin from placental tissue and clots enters the bloodstream through open vessels at the placental site and initiates an exaggeration of the normal clotting process.
   2. As more thromboplastin is introduced into circulation, more fibrinogen and clotting factors are used up.
   3. In addition, the fibrinolytic process that disintegrates fibrin is initiated, resulting in fibrin degradation products, which in turn further interfere with the clotting process.

Assessment

A. Observe for uncontrolled bleeding.

B. Assess for signs of shock: tachycardia, restlessness, anxiety.

C. Be alert for symptoms in women with predisposing factors, fetal death, abruptio placenta, etc.

Planning and Analysis

A. Early recognition results in control of bleeding and prevention of shock.

B. Treatment of hypovolemic shock is successful.

C. Source of triggering mechanism is removed.

D. Client's condition is stabilizied.

Implementation

A. Provide emotional support to client and family.

B. Assist with medical management and administration of medications.
   1. Heparin solution prevents clot formation and increases available fibrinogen, coagulation factors, and platelets.
   2. Fresh-frozen plasma and/or platelets may be ordered.

C. Monitor IV therapy as ordered.

D. Administer oxygen at two to three liters/minute.

Evaluation

A. Clotting mechanism returns to normal.

B. No complications (abruptio placenta, fetal death, etc.) have occurred.

C. Circulatory and renal functions monitored.

D. Client's condition is stabilized.

Polyhydramnios

Definition: An excessive amount of amniotic fluid. Normal amount is 500 to 1000 ml.

Characteristics

A. Actual cause is unknown. Occurs frequently in:
   1. Fetal malformations.
   2. Diabetes.
   3. Erythroblastosis.
   4. Multiple pregnancies.
   5. Toxemias.

B. Diagnosis is usually made through clinical observation of the greatly enlarged uterus.

Assessment

A. Observe for greatly enlarged abdomen.

B. Evaluate edema of the lower extremities.

C. Question if general abdominal discomfort is present.

D. Observe for occasional shortness of breath.

E. Assess for presence of diabetes as this condition frequently accompanies it.

Planning and Analysis

A. Relief of discomfort occurs.

B. Medical treatment is implemented.

C. A healthy baby is delivered.

D. Amniocentesis offers temporary relief.

Implementation

A. Monitor condition of uterus.

B. Instruct client to empty bladder so it will not distend.

C. Monitor vital signs.

D. Place client in semi-Fowler's position to assist in breathing if not contraindicated.

E. Give dietary instruction.

Evaluation

A. Discomfort is relieved.

B. Baby is delivered safely.

C. Neonate is examined immediately for any congenital problems.

Fetal Demise

Assessment

A. Assess for cessation of fetal movement.

B. Check for absence of fetal heart rate.

C. Evaluate failure of uterine growth.

D. Assess client's external support system (family, friends, priest, etc.).

E. Test for low urinary estriol.

F. Check for negative pregnancy test—may remain positive for a few weeks due to elevated human chorionic gonadotropin.

Planning and Analysis

A. Safe delivery of dead fetus.

B. Physical condition of mother stabilized.

C. Complications such as disseminated intravascular disease from prolonged retention of the dead fetus do not occur.

D. Emotional stability maintained.

Implementation

A. Provide emotional support to parents—may feel unfulfilled, incomplete and depressed.

B. Guide parents in planning future pregnancies.

C. Do not listen for fetal heart rate or do Leopold's maneuvers.

D. Observe for hemorrhage.

E. Observe for psychological disturbances.

F. Prepare emotionally for delivery process and birth of dead baby.

G. Parents may go through mourning process—encourage them to express feelings; may be angry at staff.

H. Parents may want to see fetus; allow them to do so should they desire.

Evaluation

A. Parents are able to express feelings of guilt, anger, and grief.

B. No signs of complications in the client, i.e., DIC, infection.

C. Emotional and physical condition of client is stabilized.

Pseudocyesis/Pseudopregnancies

Definition: A condition that occurs when all the signs of pregnancy develop without the presence of an embryo.

Assessment

A. Observe for amenorrhea, breast changes, and secretion of colostrum.

B. Check for enlargement of abdomen.

C. Ask for reports of quickening.

D. Assess presence of fetal heart rate or visible fetus on sonogram.

Planning and Analysis

A. Client accepts the fact she is not pregnant.

B. Underlying emotional problem assessed and treated.

Implementation

A. Offer client continued emotional support.

B. Allow client to express her feelings regarding pseudopregnancy.

C. Refer client for continued psychological assistance.

Evaluation

A. Client physically and emotionally accepts that she is not pregnant.

B. Pregnancy symptoms disappear.

C. Client continues with psychological assistance to understand emotional problems.

INTRAPARTUM PERIOD

LABOR AND DELIVERY

Definition: Labor is the process by which the products of conception are expelled from the body. Delivery refers to the actual birth.

Adaptive Processes

Definition: During latter months of pregnancy, the fetus adapts to the maternal uterus enabling it to occupy the smallest space possible. The term *attitude* refers to the posture the fetus assumes in utero; *fetal lie* is the relationship of the long axis of the body to the long axis of the mother.

Presentation

Definition: The part of the fetus that lies closest to the true pelvis.

A. Cephalic: head is presenting part—95–97 percent.
  1. May be vertex, face or brow.
  2. Vertex is most common and most favorable for delivery. Head is sharply flexed in the pelvis with chin near chest.
B. Breech: buttocks or lower extremities are the presenting part.
  1. Types.
    a. Complete or full: buttocks and feet present (baby in squatting position).
    b. Frank: buttocks only present, or legs are extended against anterior trunk with feet touching face.
    c. Incomplete: one or both feet or knees presenting, footling single or double, or knee presentation.
  2. May rotate to cephalic during pregnancy but possibility lessens as gestation nears term.
  3. May be rotated by physician but usually returns to breech position.
C. Transverse lie: long axis of infant lies at right angles to longitudinal axis of mother (necessitates delivery by C-section).

Position

Definition: Relationship of the fetal presenting part to the maternal bony pelvis.

A. Position is determined by locating the presenting part in relationship to the pelvis.
B. Client's pelvis is divided into four imaginary quadrants: right anterior, right posterior, left anterior, and left posterior.
C. Most common positions (abbreviations usually used).
  1. LOA (left occiput anterior): occiput on left side of maternal pelvis and toward front, face down, favorable for delivery.
  2. LOP (left occiput posterior): occiput on left side of maternal pelvis and toward rear or face up.
    a. Usually causes back pain during labor.
    b. May slow the progress of labor.
    c. Usually rotates before delivery to anterior position.
    d. May be rotated in delivery room by physician.
  3. ROA (right occiput anterior): occiput on right of maternal pelvis, toward front, face down, favorable for delivery.
  4. ROP (right occiput posterior): occiput on right side of maternal pelvis, face up. Same problems as LOP.
D. Means of assessing fetal position during labor.
  1. Leopold's maneuver: method of palpating the maternal abdomen to determine information about the fetus such as presentation, engagement, and rough estimate of fetal size.
  2. Vaginal examination.
  3. Rectal examination.

Engagement–Lightening

A. Largest diameter of presenting part has passed into the inlet of the maternal pelvis. Usually takes place two weeks before labor in primiparas, but not until labor in multiparas.
B. May be assessed by Leopold's maneuver or vaginal or rectal examination.

Station

A. Degree to which presenting part has descended into pelvis is determined by the station—the relationship between the presenting part and the ischial spines.
B. Assessed by vaginal or rectal examination.

C. Measured in numerical terms.
   1. At level of spines, 0 station.
   2. Above level of spines, -1, -2, -3.
   3. Below level of spines, $+1$, $+2$, $+3$.
D. Other terms used to denote station.
   1. High: presenting part not engaged.
   2. Floating: presenting part freely movable in inlet of pelvis or may be movable in inlets of pelvis.
   3. Dipping: entering pelvis.
   4. Fixed: no longer movable in inlet but not engaged.
   5. Engaged: biparietal plane passed through pelvic inlet.

Fetal Skull

A. Largest anatomical part of the fetus to pass through the birth canal; usually if the head can pass, the rest of the body can be delivered.
B. Made up of seven bones: two frontal, two parietal, two temporal, and one occipital.
C. Sutures: membranous interspaces between bones.
   1. Sagittal: between two parietal.
   2. Frontal: between two front bones.
   3. Coronal: between frontal and parietal.
   4. Lambdoidals: between posterior margin of parietal and occipital.
D. Fontanels: points where sutures intersect.
   1. Anterior—diamond shaped. Found at the junction of the sagittal and coronal sutures. Becomes ossified sometime after the first year.
   2. Posterior—smaller triangular shaped. Found at the junction of the sagittal and lambdoid sutures. Becomes ossified by the end of the second month after birth.
   3. Other smaller fontanels are also present.
   4. Fontanels allow for fetal skull bones to override as they adapt to the pelvis.
   5. Important points in vaginal or rectal examination to determine position of fetus—posterior or anterior.

The Labor Process

Cause of Labor

A. Alterations in hormonal balance of estrogen and progesterone increase uterine contractibility.
B. Degeneration of the placenta, which no longer provides necessary elements to fetus.

C. Overdistention of uterus creates stimulus-triggering release of oxytocin, which initiates contractions.
D. High levels of prostaglandins near term may stimulate uterine contractions.
E. Hormones secreted by fetus.
F. The type of contraction necessary for true labor may be produced by a combination of several of these physiological occurrences although the actual cause is unknown.

Forces of Labor

A. Muscular contractions primarily of muscles of uterus and secondarily of abdominal muscles.
B. Uterine muscles contract during first stages and bring about effacement and dilatation of the cervix.
C. Abdominal muscles come into play after complete cervical dilatation and help expel the baby—voluntary bearing down effort, urge to push.
D. Contraction of levator ani muscles.

Duration of Labor

A. Varies depending upon individual.
B. Average.
   1. Primipara: up to eighteen hours; some may be shorter, others longer.
   2. Multipara: up to eight hours; some may be shorter, others longer.
C. Length of labor depends on:
   1. Effectiveness of consistent contractions: contractions must overcome resistance of cervix.
   2. Amount of resistance baby must overcome to adapt to the pelvis.
   3. Stretching ability of soft tissue.
   4. Preparation and relaxation of client. Fear and anxiety can retard progress.
D. Important to judge rate of progress: should be regular progression of uterine contraction, progressive effacement and dilatation of the cervix and progressive descent of the presenting part.

Uterine Contractions

A. Characteristics.
   1. Involuntary: cannot be controlled by will of client.
   2. Intermittent: periods of relaxation between contractions. Intervals allow client to rest and

also allow adequate circulation of uterine blood vessels and oxygenation of fetus.

3. Distinguish between true labor (contractions regular, painful, continue with walking) and false labor—Braxton Hicks (regular, painful but go away with walking).
4. Discomfort starts in low back, radiates to abdomen.
5. As labor progresses, intensity increases.

B. Contractions divided into three periods of intensity.
   1. Increment: increasing intensity.
   2. Acme: peak, or full intensity.
   3. Decrement: decreasing intensity.
C. Contractions are monitored by the following:
   1. Place your finger lightly on the fundus of the uterus (the most contractile portion) and relate what you feel in your fingers to seconds and minutes on a clock. Uterus becomes firm, then hardens, and then decreases in hardness.
   2. Electronic monitoring device.
      a. External: less accurate.
      b. Internal: catheter inserted into uterine cavity to measure internal pressures and relay information to a graph.
D. Contractions are monitored for frequency, duration, and intensity.
   1. Frequency: measured by timing contractions from the beginning of one contraction to the beginning of next.
   2. Duration: beginning of contraction to beginning of period of decreasing intensity. Cannot be measured exactly by feeling with the hand.
   3. Intensity: cannot be measured by feeling; must be measured by internal fetal monitoring device. Usually refers to contraction at the beginning of labor. Peaks at about 25 mm Hg. At the end of labor, it may reach 50 to 75 mm Hg.
   4. Contractions may be described as mild, moderate, or intense.
E. Purpose of contractions.
   1. To propel presenting part forward.
   2. To bring about effacement and dilatation of the cervix.

Effacement and Dilatation

A. Effacement: thinning process by which cervical canal is progressively shortened to complete obliteration. Progresses from a structure of 1 to 2 cm long to almost complete obliteration.
B. Dilatation: process by which external os enlarges from a few millimeters to approximately 10 cm.
C. All that remains of the cervix after effacement and dilatation is a paper-thin circular opening about 10 cm in diameter.
D. Primips efface, then dilate; multips efface and dilate at the same time.

Changes in the Uterus

A. Uterus usually becomes differentiated in two distinct portions as labor progresses.
   1. Upper portion: contractile, becomes thicker.
   2. Lower portion: passive, becomes thinner and more expanded.
B. Boundary between the two segments is termed the "physiologic retraction ring."

Signs of Labor

Assessment

A. Assess for premonitory signs: physiologic changes that take place the last several weeks of pregnancy, indicating that labor is near.
B. Observe for lightening: descent of the uterus downward and forward, which takes place as the presenting part descends into the pelvis.
   1. Time in which it takes place varies from a few weeks to a few days before labor. In multigravida, it may occur during labor.
   2. Sensations.
      a. Relief of pressure on diaphragm and breathing is easier.
      b. Increased pelvic pressure leading to leg cramps, frequent micturition, and pressure on rectum.
C. Check presence of Braxton-Hicks contractions.
   1. May become quite regular but do not effectively dilate cervix.
   2. Usually are more pronounced at night.
   3. May play a part in ripening the cervix.
D. Evaluate for decrease in weight: there is usually a decrease in water retention due to hormonal influences.
E. Assess for cervical changes: cervix usually becomes softer, shorter, and somewhat dilated. May be dilated 1 to 2 cm by the time labor begins.
F. Check presence of bloody show.
   1. Tenacious mucus vaginal discharge, usually pinkish or streaked with blood, is expelled from the cervix as it shortens and begins to dilate.

2. Labor usually begins within twenty-four to forty-eight hours.

G. Evaluate rupture of membranes.
1. May break any time before labor or during labor. Occasionally, membranes remain intact and are ruptured by the physician during labor (amniotomy).
2. May gush or trickle.
3. Client usually advised to come to the hospital as labor may begin within twenty-four hours.
4. If labor does not begin spontaneously, it is induced to avoid intrauterine infections.

H. Assess for beginning of true labor.
1. Contractions increase in frequency, intensity and duration.
2. Progressive cervical effacement and dilatation.
3. Progressive descent of presenting part.
4. Presence of bloody show.
5. Contractions increase in intensity with walking.

I. Differentiate true from false labor.
1. Irregular contractions.
2. Contractions may cause discomfort.
3. Usually discomfort is located in abdomen.
4. Labor usually does not intensify.
5. Discomfort may be relieved by walking.
6. Contractions do not bring about appreciable changes in cervix.
7. Sometimes difficult to differentiate false labor from true labor, and client is observed for several hours in the hospital.

Planning and Analysis

A. To provide for the health, comfort, safety, and well-being of the laboring client.
B. Normal progression of labor without complications.
C. Delivery resulting in a healthy neonate and mother.

Implementation

A. Careful monitoring of the client and fetus during the labor and delivery process.
B. Prompt recognition and treatment of complications.
C. Provision of comfort and safety measures during labor and delivery.

D. Supportive assistance to the laboring client or couple to enable them to maintain control during the labor and delivery process.

Evaluation

A. Labor progresses at a normal rate without signs of complications.
B. Delivery is uncomplicated.
C. Delivery of an infant with an Apgar score between 7 and 10 at five minutes.
D. Expressed satisfaction of the client or couple of their performance during labor and delivery and the care they received.

FETAL ASSESSMENT DURING LABOR

Fetal Monitoring

Characteristics

A. Two types of electronic fetal monitoring: external (EFM) and internal (IFM); provide for a continuous data readout of fetal heart rate and uterine contraction pattern.
B. Most common method of obtaining an external recording of the fetal heart rate is with an ultrasound transducer that picks up the motion of the fetal heart valves.
C. External monitoring of uterine contraction is done with a pressure sensitive button placed over the uterine fundus.
D. Heart rate sounds and uterine contractions are translated into electrical impulses reproduced on a printout strip on the fetal monitor.
E. External fetal heart rate tracing does not assess fetal heart rate variability. External uterine contraction monitoring does not quantify the strength of the contractions.
F. Types of external fetal monitors.
1. Abdominal electrodes: elicits fetal and maternal heart rates.
2. Phonotransducer: picks up fetal heart tones.
3. Ultrasonic transducer: picks up fetal heart tones.
4. Tocotransducer: monitors uterine activity.

Assessment

A. Evaluate client's and family's knowledge of rationale for fetal monitoring.

B. Identify client's concerns before procedure is initiated.

C. Assess client's knowledge of procedure.

D. Evaluate position of fetus using Leopold's maneuver.

E. Assess fetal heart rate: normal is 120–160 beats per minute.

F. Assess fetal monitor strip for early and late deceleration.

Planning and Analysis

A. Fetal well-being is monitored throughout the client's labor.

B. Client is well-informed of rationale for monitoring and procedure.

C. Fetal heart rate and uterine activity are clearly displayed on monitor.

Implementation

A. Preparation.
 1. Explain procedure to client.
 2. Plug tocotransducer into monitor inlet.
 3. Turn monitor on and press printout button.
 4. Move stylus to zero. The printout is divided into two parts. The uterine activity waveform is found on the right side.

B. Placement of fetal monitor.
 1. Place tocotransducer over uterine fundus. (Locate fundus using Leopold's maneuvers.)
 2. Position the tocotransducer in place with belt. (Powder belt first to avoid irritating skin.)
 3. When client is free of contractions, tighten belt until stylus on monitor moves to the 50 mm Hg mark on the right side of the printout.
 4. Turn control knob until stylus moves back to the 10 mm Hg mark.
 5. Test tocotransducer by pressing down on transducer. If the baseline recorder moves, tocotransducer is functioning properly.
 6. Record frequency and duration of contractions as required by hospital policy.

C. Monitoring uterine activity.
 1. *Normal fetal heart rate*: 120 to 160 beats/minute; determine baseline.

2. *Early deceleration:* 10 to 20 beat drop in rate usually within normal range of 120 to 160 beats/minute.
 a. Occurs before peak or early contracting phase. Recovery as soon as acme of contraction has passed.
 b. Uniform shape.
 c. Indicate head compression—vagal stimulation results in decreased heart rate.
 d. V-shaped appearance.
 e. Not considered ominous.

3. *Late deceleration:* decrease in fetal heart rate of 10 to 20 beats/minute.
 a. Occurs after peak or late contracting phase.
 b. Uniform shape.
 c. Usually indicates fetal distress.
 d. Likely to appear in any situation where fetal-maternal exchange in placenta is reduced, resulting in hypoxia.

4. *Variable deceleration:* no uniformity in pattern.
 a. Decrease in fetal heart rate occurring any time during contraction phase.
 b. Usually below 120 beats/minute.
 c. May indicate cord compression.
 d. May occur when client pushes.
 e. Must be evaluated carefully—may or may not indicate fetal distress.

5. *Loss of beat-to-beat variation:* baseline is smooth.
 a. May be serious sign of fetal anoxia.
 b. Fetus may be becoming acidotic.
 c. Medication may be affecting fetus.
 d. Neurologic immaturity.

6. *Bradycardia:* any persistent drop of 20 beats below baseline or under 120 beats/minute.
 a. May be indicative of fetal distress.
 b. Congenital heart abnormalities.

7. *Tachycardia:* increase of 10 percent over baseline or over 160 beats/minute.
 a. An ominous sign—requires intervention stat.
 b. Fetal hypoxia; neurologic immaturity.
 c. Maternal fever and/or tachycardia.

Variations in Fetal Heart Rate

Fetal Heart Rate	Possible Etiology	Implementation
Early deceleration 10–20 beat drop. Rate usually within 120–160. Recovery when acme of contraction passes.	Head compression (vagal stimulation).	Often not serious—observed late in labor. Monitor closely. Distinguish from late deceleration.
Late deceleration 10–20 beat decrease in FHR. Occurs after peak contraction.	Hypertonic contractions. Fetal maternal exchange reduced → hypoxia → fetal distress.	Turn client on side to reduce maternal hypotension. Elevate legs. Administer oxygen. D/C oxytocin (as ordered). Increase hydration. Prepare for immediate delivery. (If pattern continues, may result in bradycardia and fetal death.)
Variable deceleration Decrease in FHR. Usually below 120 beats/min.	Cord compression. May or may not result in fetal difficulty.	Mild variable deceleration may not be dangerous—continue to monitor. Change maternal position (knee-chest or Trendelenburg). D/C oxytocin, as ordered. Administer oxygen. Prepare for immediate delivery if continues.
Loss of beat-to-beat variation Smooth baseline. Less than 15 beats/min.	Fetal anoxia (serious sign). Fetal hypoxia and acidosis. Maternal medication. Immature fetus. Fetal malformation.	Monitor that variation does not continue more than 15 minutes. Monitor maternal hypnotics. Decrease stimuli (maternal activity) and recheck rate. Observe for late deceleration pattern.
Bradycardia Drop of 20 beats/min. below baseline (under 120 beats/min.).	Fetal hypoxia. Fetal distress. Congenital heart abnormalities (arrhythmias). Hypothermia (from slow maternal cardiac metabolism).	When preceded by deceleration—fetus is compromised—prepare for immediate delivery. Change maternal position. Administer oxygen.
Tachycardia Increase in FHR over 160 beats/min. for 10 min. period.	Fetal hypoxia. Prematurity—immature ANS. Maternal medication. Maternal fever and/or tachycardia. Maternal anxiety.	Change maternal position. Implement maternal relaxation methods to decrease anxiety. Administer oxygen. Monitor closely to track progress.

STAGES AND PHASES OF LABOR

Definition: Labor is divided into four stages: Stage 1—beginning of true labor to complete cervical dilatation; stage 2—complete dilatation to birth of baby; stage 3—birth to delivery of placenta; and stage 4—first hour after delivery of placenta.

Admission Procedures

A. Check vital signs: temperature, pulse, respirations, and blood pressure.
B. Check fetal heart rate.
C. Determine status of membranes: intact vs. ruptured.
D. Give prep (perineal shave) and enema (if ordered by physician).
E. See that appropriate forms are completed.
F. Determine client's psychological state and readiness for labor: some clients may complain of intense pain in very early labor.
G. Encourage client to void, and check urine for sugar, acetone, and protein.
H. Apply external fetal monitor if ordered.
I. Determine frequency, intensity (mild, moderate, severe), and duration of contractions.
J. Determine amount and character of show.
K. Determine amount of cervical dilatation and effacement.
L. Keep bell cord within easy reach.

Stage 1

Definition: Begins with onset of true labor and ends when cervix is completely dilated at 10 cm.

Assessment

A. Following admission procedures, observe for degree of dilatation.
B. Assess contractions: vary from mild and 5 to 15 minutes apart to intense and close together.
C. Evaluate cervical effacement.
D. Observe presence or increase in bloody show.
E. Assess station.
F. Assess mood of client: comfortable and talkative, or tired and irritable.
G. Assess membrane status: intact or ruptured.

Planning and Analysis

A. Admission procedures are completed.
B. Normal progression of labor to active phase is occurring.
C. Mother will be able to tolerate stage 1 well.
D. Completion of stage 1 is successful.

Implementation
Phase One: Latent Phase

A. Evaluate labor progress.
   1. Begins with onset of regular contractions and ends with dilatation of 3 to 4 cm.
   2. Contractions mild, 5 to 15 minutes apart, lasting 10 to 30 seconds. Averages 6.4 hours.
   3. Station varies -2 to -1.
   4. Show varies from brown to pink—scant amount.

B. Observe for ruptured membranes and take fetal heart rate immediately if membranes rupture.
C. Maintain bed rest if membranes have ruptured. (In some hospitals the client may be allowed out of bed with ruptured membranes if the baby's head is well engaged.)
D. Allow client to walk about if membranes have not ruptured, or provide reading material for client.
E. Auscultate fetal heart rate every 15 minutes.
F. Check blood pressure every 30 minutes or p.r.n.
G. Check vital signs once per shift or more often if needed.
H. Start IV if ordered. Client usually n.p.o.
I. Check for bladder distention.
J. Give periodic vaginal examination to determine progress.
K. Provide support based upon mother's knowledge of the labor process.
L. Reinforce breathing techniques or teach breathing techniques if client has had no classes.
M. Keep family informed of progress.
N. Encourage the presence of client's husband or a significant other person.
O. Reduce stimuli if client wants to rest.

Phase Two: Active Phase

A. Begins with acceleration phase.
   1. Cervix dilates from 3 to 4 to 8 cm.
   2. Fetal descent is progressive.
   3. Contractions three to five minutes apart and lasting 30 to 45 seconds, moderate intensity.
   4. Increase in bloody show.
   5. Station varies from 0 to $+1$.

B. Support client as she becomes tired, less talkative, and shows lack of energy.
C. Instruct client on breathing techniques.
D. Maintain IV fluids.
E. Apply pressure to sacrum during contraction or encourage baby's father to do so.

F. Urge client to stay off back, to avoid supine hypotensive syndrome, and to lie on side.

G. Administer medications as ordered.

   1. Tranquilizers may be given in early labor.

   2. Analgesics are usually not given until labor is well established—4–6 cm dilatation.

H. Assist with anesthesia, if given, and monitor blood pressure and fetal heart rate.

I. Continue support and keep client informed.

J. Once membranes have ruptured (2 to 3 cm dilatation) internal fetal monitor may be applied.

Active Phase – Part Two

A. Deceleration phase is last part of active phase.

   1. Dilatation slows as it progresses from 8 to 10 cm.

   2. Rate of fetal descent increases.

   3. Deceleration should last 3 hours for nulliparas, and one hour for multiparas.

   4. Contractions every 2 to 3 minutes, duration averaging 60 seconds.

   5. Station + 1 to + 2—increased amount of bloody show.

   6. Desire to bear down or defecate.

B. Support client as her attention and feelings become inner-directed; she may feel exhausted and no longer able to cope.

C. Care for symptoms of nausea, vomiting, trembling, burping, and crying.

D. Explain progress to client and encourage her to continue with breathing and relaxing techniques.

E. Discourage bearing down efforts until dilatation is complete.

F. Encourage deep ventilation prior to and after each contraction to avoid hyperventilation.

G. Monitor contractions lightly with fingers as abdomen is sensitive.

H. Accept irritable behavior and aggression and continue supportive care.

I. Help client to push when ready.

J. Observe for signs of imminent delivery and transfer client to delivery room when ready.

Evaluation

A. Admission procedure facilitated and client and family settled in labor facility.

B. Dilatation has progressed to 10 cm.

C. Client has tolerated labor well and is prepared for delivery.

D. No complications observed or diagnosed at this stage.

Stage 2: Process of Expulsion

Definition: Begins with complete dilatation of cervix (10 cm) and ends with delivery of infant.

Mechanism of Labor and Delivery

A. Sequence of movements of presenting part through birth canal. Head usually enters transverse and must rotate LOA or ROA for birth.

B. Engagement: head enters pelvis.

C. Descent: movement that occurs simultaneously with passage of head through pelvis.

D. Flexion: occurs as head descends and meets with resistance. In extreme flexion, the smallest diameter of the head presents.

E. Internal rotation: head usually enters with long diameter conforming to long diameter of inlet (usually transverse position) and must rotate before it can emerge from outlet; head rotates so that smallest diameter presents to conform to pelvis.

F. Extension: follows internal rotation; the head, which is flexed as it passes through birth canal, must extend for birth.

G. External rotation: soon after birth, the head rotates to either mother's right or left side, the fetal position before birth.

H. Expulsion: with delivery of shoulders, rest of body is expelled spontaneously.

Assessment

A. Observe for signs of imminent delivery.

B. Check contractions every two to three minutes; contractions last 60 to 90 seconds.

C. Evaluate vagina and perineum stretching and thinning to allow for passage of baby.

D. Check increase in bloody show.

E. Evaluate urge to push: involuntary bearing down.

F. Observe bulging of perineum.

G. Observe vaginal opening, which distends from a small, narrow opening to a wide, round opening.

H. Observe presenting part as it becomes more visible.

I. Check crowning: widest diameter of baby's head is visible and encircled by vaginal opening.

J. Observe birth of presenting part.

K. Observe rest of body as it is delivered, usually with a gush of fluid.

Planning and Analysis

A. Delivery of the fetus with no complications.

B. Mother comfortable and tolerated delivery well.

Implementation

A. Transfer client carefully from bed to delivery table and place in lithotomy position.

B. Pad stirrups to avoid pressure to popliteal veins and pressure areas. Gently raise both legs simultaneously into stirrups to avoid ligament strain. Adjust stirrups and drape client.

C. Provide client with handles to pull on as she pushes.

D. Cleanse vulva and perineum using sterile technique, commonly referred to as perineal "wash down."

E. Auscultate fetal heart tone every 5 minutes or after each push; transient fetal bradycardia not unusual due to head compression.

F. Check blood pressure and pulse every 15 minutes p.r.n.

G. Administer oxygen if fetal heart tones decrease.

H. Allow baby's father in room, and position him at the head of the delivery table.

I. Catheterize if bladder is distended and prevents descent.

J. Encourage mother and keep her informed of advancement of baby.

K. Encourage mother to take a deep breath before beginning to push with each contraction and to sustain push as long as possible; long pushes are preferable to frequent short pushes.

Evaluation

A. A healthy fetus is delivered.

B. Mother is comfortable and tolerated procedure well.

C. No complications occurred during delivery.

Stage 3

Definition: From birth to expulsion of the placenta, usually 5 to 20 minutes after delivery.

Assessment

A. Observe for signs of placental separation.
   1. The uterus contracts.
   2. The uterus changes from discoid to globular in shape.
   3. A slight gush of blood issues from vagina.
   4. Lengthening of the umbilical cord occurs.
   5. Displacement of the uterus upward occurs.

B. Evaluate placenta after separation.
   1. Schultze (most common): placenta is inverted on itself, and the shiny fetal surface appears; 80 percent separate in center.

2. Duncan: descends sideways, and the maternal surface appears. Separates at edges rather than center.

C. Check to determine placental fragments do not remain in uterus.

D. Continually assess both mother and infant for first critical hour after birth.
   1. Most common cause of death in first hour is hemorrhage—assess vital signs every 15 minutes.
   2. Assess condition of fundus.
   3. Check lochia for color and amount.

Implementation

A. Monitor newborn's status and begin bonding with parents.
   1. Position baby so that mother and baby may have eye-to-eye contact.
   2. Dim lights of birthing room so baby can open eyes fully.

B. Monitor for signs of placental separation.
   1. Uterus rises upward in abdomen; as placenta proceeds downward, umbilical cord lengthens.
   2. Sudden trickle of blood appears.
   3. Uterus changes from discoid to globular shape.

C. Palpate uterus to check for ballooning of uterus caused by uterine relaxation with bleeding into uterine cavity.

D. Splint or support abdominal muscles as mother bears down to assist in delivering placenta.

E. Inspect placental membranes to be sure they are intact after delivery.

F. Palpate fundus of uterus—normal position is at midline and below umbilicus.

Stage 4

Definition: From expulsion of placenta to a period of one to four hours after delivery or until vital signs are stable.

Assessment

A. Continually assess both mother and infant for first critical hour or two after birth.
   1. Assess firmness and position of fundus and that it remains well contracted to ensure that mother has minimal bleeding.
   2. Assess vital signs including blood pressure every 15 minutes.
   3. Assess amount and character of vaginal blood flow.

B. Check that blood pressure returns to prelabor levels and pulse is slightly lower than during labor.

1. Return of B/P is due to increased volume of blood returning to maternal circulation.
2. Lowered B/P and rising pulse may reflect increased blood loss.

COMPLICATIONS OF LABOR AND DELIVERY

Fetal Distress

Assessment

A. Assess fetal heart rate: above 160 or below 120 beats per minute indicates distress.
B. Check for meconium-stained fluid. During hypoxia, bowel peristalsis increases, and meconium is likely to be passed.
C. Assess for fetal hyperactivity.
D. If labor is monitored, check:
  1. Variable deceleration pattern.
  2. Late deceleration pattern.
  3. Fetal pH below 7.2.

Planning and Analysis

A. Relief of fetal distress.
B. Delivery of a healthy baby.

Implementation

A. Discontinue oxytocin if being infused.
B. Turn client to left side; if no improvement, turn to right side. This procedure relieves pressure on umbilical cord during contractions and pressure of uterus on the inferior vena cava.
C. Administer oxygen via mask at 6 to 7 l/minute.
D. Correction of hypotension: elevate legs and increase perfusion of IV fluids.
E. Notify physician.
F. Prepare for emergency cesarean delivery if no improvement.

Evaluation

A. Recognition and diagnosis of fetal distress is made early.
B. Treatment measures relieve fetal distress.
C. Healthy baby is delivered.
D. Mother tolerates delivery well and remains comfortable.

Vena Caval Syndrome (Supine Hypotensive Syndrome)

Definition: Shocklike symptoms that occur when venous return to the heart is impaired by weight of gravid uterus causing partial occlusion of the vena cava.

Assessment

A. Assess for risk factors—multiple pregnancies, obesity, polyhydramnios.
B. Assess shock-like symptoms caused by reduced cardiac output.
  1. Hypotension.
  2. Tachycardia.
  3. Sweating.
  4. Nausea and vomiting.
  5. Air hunger.
C. Assess for fetal distress; caused by reduced flow of blood to placenta from reduced cardiac output.

Implementation

A. Assist mother to turn to left side (use a wedge pillow) to shift weight of fetus off inferior vena cava.
B. Provide oxygen with tight mask if recovery is not immediate after positioning.
C. Monitor fetal heart rate to determine fetal status.

Table 4. COMPLICATIONS AND SIGNS OF DISTRESS IN THE FETUS

Complication	Signs of Distress	Possible Nursing Implementation
Asphyxia	Irregular heart rate Heart rate above 160 or below 120 Passage of meconium in the vertex position	Administer oxygen to the mother—turn on left side Constantly observe and monitor FHT Check for prolapse of the cord Prepare delivery room equipment for possible resuscitation of the baby at birth
Generalized infection	Irregular heart rate Heart rate above 160 or below 120	Administer antibiotics to the mother Keep vaginals to a minimum Follow same interventions as 1, 2, 4 in asphyxia

Premature Rupture of the Membranes

Definition: The spontaneous rupture of membranes prior to the onset of labor irrespective of the gestational age.

Assessment

A. Assess latent period: time from rupture of membranes to onset of labor; interval period is time from rupture of membranes to delivery of fetus.
B. Major maternal risks associated with PROM are ascending uterine infection and precipitation of preterm labor.
   1. Assess time between membrane rupturing and labor began—risk of infection may be directly related to time involved.
   2. Observe for signs of infection: elevated temperature, chills, malaise, WBC.
C. Assess for signs of labor or prolapsed cord.
D. Observe amniotic fluid for foul odor or signs of fetal distress (meconium staining).

Implementation

A. Monitor for signs of contractions.
B. Monitor for fetal heart tones.
C. Alleviate client's fears of "dry birth."
D. Record time, amount, color, and odor of ruptured membranes.
E. Record vital signs, especially temperature, every 4 hours.

Premature Labor and Delivery

Definition: Labor that occurs prior to the end of the thirty-seventh week of gestation.

Characteristics

A. Predisposing factors.
   1. Conditions such as chronic pyelonephritis, cervical incompetence, multiple pregnancies, past history of premature births, sepsis in the fetus, and placental disorders.
   2. Sometimes no specific cause can be identified.
B. Attempts to arrest premature labor are contraindicated when:
   1. Pregnancy is thirty-seven weeks or over.
   2. Ruptured membranes exist; delivery may be delayed if there are no indications of infection to allow fetus to mature.
   3. Maternal disease exists: abruptio placenta, etc.

4. Fetal problems such as Rh isoimmunization become threatening.
C. A drug such as betamethasone (Celestone) may be given to the mother to hasten fetal maturity by stimulating development of lecithin when membranes are ruptured and premature labor cannot be arrested.

Assessment

A. Observe for abrupt change in fetal heart tones or signs of distress.
B. Assess vital signs—blood pressure, pulse, temperature, and respirations.
C. Evaluate for signs of infection, respiratory distress, cardiac status.
D. Check intake and urinary output.
E. Examine urine for glucose and protein.
F. Check for presence of edema.
G. Assess maternal emotional state.

Planning and Analysis

A. Progress of labor will be inhibited to allow for fetal maturity unless contraindicated.
B. Medical treatment is implemented.
C. Client maintains emotional stability during this period.

MEDICAL IMPLICATIONS

- Use of sympathomimetic drugs (Ritodrine, terbutaline) causes an inhibitory effect on uterine smooth muscle and may also cause hypotension, tachycardia and arrhythmias.
- Cardiac monitor and CVP may be used to monitor maternal cardiac function.
- Trendelenburg's or side-lying position minimizes hypotension.
- Magnesium sulfate is used for premature labor.
- Narcotics are usually withheld because of their depressive effect on the infant.
- Drug regimen may be continued on outpatient basis after uterine contractions cease.

Implementation

A. Maintain bed rest.
B. Continuous monitoring of contractions and fetal heart tones.
C. Administer medications according to protocol.

D. Keep client informed and provide support: may be fearful, feel guilty, or be anxious about care of other children at home.

E. Careful observation for signs of complications such as tachycardia.

F. Provide for hygiene and general comfort care.

Evaluation

A. Uterine contractions have ceased and pregnancy continues.

B. No signs of maternal or fetal complications.

C. Delivery of a term infant.

Prolonged Pregnancy

Definition: Pregnancy over forty-two weeks gestation—degeneration of placenta, thus decreased blood flow to fetus.

Characteristics

A. Amniotic fluid decreases and vernix caseosa disappears; infant's skin appears dry and cracked.

B. Infant may lose weight.

C. Chronic hypoxia may occur due to placental dysfunction.

D. Determination of gestational age usually made to ascertain actual duration of pregnancy—estriol studies, sonography.

E. Oxytocin challenge test to determine fetus's ability to tolerate labor.

F. Labor stimulated with oxytocin.

G. Cesarean delivery if induction containdicated.

Assessment

A. Determine actual gestational age.

B. Assess results of oxytocin challenge test to determine fetus's viability.

C. Assess vital signs of client for baseline data before labor is induced.

D. Assess psychological state of client and need for support.

E. Assess external resources of client.

Planning and Analysis

A. Actual gestational age is determined.

B. Placental insufficiency does not exist.

C. Labor is induced successfully.

D. Healthy infant is delivered and mother's condition is stable.

Implementation

A. Support mother during labor process.

B. Prepare for possibility of emergency cesarean section.

C. Monitor FHR continuously—report any late or variable deceleration immediately.

D. Monitor induction of labor if natural labor process occurs.

E. Support family during labor and delivery.

Evaluation

A. No evidence of fetal distress during labor.

B. Healthy infant is delivered vaginally.

C. Mother's condition is stabilized.

Prolapsed Umbilical Cord

Definition: Displacement of the umbilical cord below the presenting part. The cord may protrude through the cervix and into the vaginal canal.

Characteristics

A. Rupture of the membranes before engagement.

B. Abnormal presentations.

C. Premature infant: presenting part does not fill the birth canal, allowing the cord to slip through.

D. Polyhydramnios.

Assessment

A. Observe for presence of cord palpated or seen on vaginal examination.

B. Assess abnormal fetal heart pattern: cord may become compressed and cause fetal hypoxia.

Planning and Analysis

A. Fetal hypoxia is prevented.

B. Healthy baby is delivered.

Implementation

A. Place client in knee-chest or modified Sims' with hips elevated on pillows.

B. Insert fingers of sterile gloved hand into vagina to lift presenting part off umbilical cord.

C. Administer oxygen (5 liters) to mother by mask.

D. Call for assistance.

E. Notify physician.

F. Continuously monitor fetal heart rate.

G. Do not attempt to push in cord.

H. Stay with client and offer support.

I. Prepare for immediate delivery, by cesarean section if necessary.

Evaluation

A. FHR remains stable.

B. A healthy infant is delivered.

Amniotic Fluid Embolism

Definition: The escape of amniotic fluid into the maternal circulation. It is usually fatal to the mother.

Characteristics

A. Amniotic fluid contains debris such as lanugo, vernix, and meconium, which may become deposited in pulmonary arterioles.

B. Usually enters maternal circulation through open venous sinus at placental site.

C. Predisposing factors.

1. Premature rupture of membranes.

2. Tumultuous labor.

Assessment

A. Observe for acute dyspnea.

B. Assess for sudden chest pain.

C. Check for cyanosis.

D. Observe for pulmonary edema.

E. Check vital signs for indications of shock.

F. Assess for uncontrolled hemorrhage.

Planning and Analysis

A. Cardiac and respiratory function is supported.

B. Treatment is implemented.

> MEDICAL IMPLICATIONS
> - Oxygen under pressure.
> - Digitalis for failing cardiac function.
> - Fibrinogen to replace depleted reserves.
> - Heparin to combat fibrinogenemia.
> - Client may be given whole blood.
> - Forceps delivery if cervix is dilated enough to allow for delivery.

Implementation

A. Institute emergency measures to maintain life.

B. If client survives, provide intensive care treatment.

C. Keep family informed and provide emotional support.

Evaluation

A. Support system for client's family is established and maintained as needed.

B. Baby is delivered and is healthy.

Inverted Uterus

Definition: A condition in which the uterus turns inside out, usually during delivery of the placenta.

Assessment

A. Observe for shock, hemorrhage, or severe pain.

B. Check for mild symptoms with incomplete uterine inversion.

Planning and Analysis

A. Uterus is returned to correct position.

B. Maternal mortality from shock is prevented.

C. Medical treatment is implemented.

Implementation

A. Assist with treatment for shock.

B. Monitor for hemorrhage.

C. Monitor vital signs.

D. Assist client while replacement of uterus (if done vaginally) is done.

Evaluation

A. Uterus is replaced.

B. Abnormal bleeding ceases.

C. Vital signs are stable.

Rupture of the Uterus

Definition: The splitting of the uterine wall accompanied by extrusion of all or part of uterine contents into the abdominal cavity. Baby usually dies, and mortality rate in mothers is high due to blood loss.

Assessment

A. Observe for acute abdominal pain and tenderness.

B. Establish that presenting part is no longer felt through cervix.

C. Assess for a feeling in client that something has happened inside her.

D. Evaluate for cessation of labor pains (no contractions).

E. Evaluate for any external bleeding (usually bleeding is internal).

F. Assess for signs of shock: pale appearance, pulse weak and rapid, air hunger, and exhaustion.

Planning and Analysis

A. Maternal and fetal mortality is prevented.

B. Treatment is implemented immediately.

> **MEDICAL IMPLICATIONS**
> - Laparotomy to remove fetus.
> - Hysterectomy, although uterus may be sutured and left in.
> - Blood transfusions.
> - Antibiotics to prevent infection from traumatized tissues.

Implementation

A. Be alert for symptoms since immediate diagnosis is necessary if fetus and mother are to survive.

B. Call for assistance, stay with client, and notify physician.

C. Prepare for emergency surgery.

Evaluation

A. Survival of mother and fetus.

B. Uterus sutured and left in rather than removed.

Prolonged and Difficult Labor

Definition: Dystocia occurs with prolonged and difficult labor and delivery. Labor is considered prolonged when it extends for twenty-four hours or more after the onset of regular contractions.

Characteristics

A. Dysfunctional uterine contractions.
   1. Uterine contractions inefficient; hence, cervical dilatation, effacement, and descent fail to occur.
   2. Contributing factors.
      a. False labor.
      b. Oversedation or excessive anesthesia.
      c. "Unripe" cervix.
      d. Uterine contractions that are hypertonic or hypotonic.
      e. Uterine abnormalities such as fibroids.
      f. Cephalopelvic disproportion (CPD).
      g. Malpositions.
      h. Uterine or other abnormalities.

B. Abnormal presentations and positions.
   1. Occiput posterior position.
      a. Usually prolongs labor because baby must rotate a longer distance (135 degrees or more) to reach symphysis pubis.
      b. May lead to persistent occiput posterior (head does not rotate) or deep transverse arrest (head arrested in transverse position).
      c. Treatment.
         (1) Head usually rotates itself with contraction.
         (2) Rotation may be done by physician manually or with forceps.
   2. Breech: prolongs labor because soft tissue does not aid cervical dilatation as well as the fetal skull.
   3. Face presentation: rare; results in increased prenatal mortality.
      a. Chin must rotate so it lies under symphysis pubis for delivery.
      b. If baby is delivered vaginally, the face is usually edematous and bruised, with marked molding.
      c. Cesarean delivery is indicated if face does not rotate.
   4. Transverse lie.
      a. Long axis of fetus at right angles to long axis of mother.
      b. Spontaneous version may occur. Cesarean delivery is the usual treatment.

C. Cephalopelvic disproportion.
   1. Disproportion between the size of the fetus and the size of the pelvis.
   2. Head is large.
   3. Size of shoulders may also complicate delivery.
   4. Causes.
      a. Multiparity: birth weight may progress with each pregnancy.
      b. Maternal diabetes.
      c. Large baby.
      d. Fetal abnormalities.
         (1) Hydrocephalus.
         (2) Tumors.
         (3) Abnormal development.
   5. Size may be determined by sonography and x-ray.
   6. Treatment.

a. Vaginal delivery if disproportion is not too great. May be fetal injuries: brachial plexus, dislocated shoulder.

b. Cesarean delivery indicated if disproportion too great.

Dystocia

Dystocia may be classified in several ways, and although the divisions are artificial, they are useful in looking at the processes involved.

1. Dysfunction of powers or forces with respect to the utcrus and abdominal muscles.

2. Abnormalities of the passengers—fetus and placenta.

3. Abnormalities of the passages—bony and soft tissue.

4. May be a combination of two or more dysfunctions and abnormalities.

True labor begins but fails to progress. Dystocia may occur during latent or active phase of labor.

It is important to look at the rate of progress as well as the overall length of labor; that is, is the client slowly progressing or is she arrested at one point?

Assessment

A. Observe rate of progress as well as overall length of labor.
1. Latent phase may be considered prolonged.
   a. Parous: labor extends 14 hours or longer.
   b. Nulliparous: labor extends 20 hours or longer.
2. Active phase may be considered prolonged.
   a. Parous: dilatation is slower than 1.5 cm per hour and descent is less than 5 cm/hour.
   b. Nulliparous: dilatation is slower than 1.2 cm per hour and descent is less than 1 cm/hour.
3. Arrested labor—labor fails to progress beyond a certain point.
B. Signs of distress in the mother.
1. Infection.
   a. Elevated temperature.
   b. Elevated pulse.

2. Exhaustion.
   a. Loss of emotional stability.
   b. Lack of cooperation.
3. Dehydration.
   a. Dry tongue and skin.
   b. Concentrated urine.
   c. Acetonuria.
C. Signs of distress in the fetus.
1. Asphyxia.
   a. Irregular heart rate.
   b. Heart rate above 160 or below 120 or decrease of 20 points below baseline.
   c. Passage of meconium in the vertex position.
2. Generalized infection.
   a. Irregular heart rate.
   b. Heart rate above 160 or below 120.

Planning and Analysis

A. Delivery of a healthy baby.
B. Prevention of complications in the mother.
C. Treatment is implemented.

MEDICAL IMPLICATIONS
- Varies with cause.
- Vaginal examination to determine position and station of fetus.
- X-ray pelvimetry or sonography to determine CPD.
- Rest for exhausted client.
- Cautious oxytocic stimulation of labor if malposition, CPD, and other abnormalities are ruled out.
- Cesarean delivery if appropriate.

Implementation

A. Varies with cause. If labor is induced, care of the client with induction of labor.
B. Promote rest: darken room, reduce noise level.
C. Position client for comfort.
D. Give client a back rub.
E. Provide clean linen and gown and allow client to bathe or shower if permissible.
F. Promote oral hygiene.
G. Give client reassurance and support.
H. Explain procedures to client.
I. Let client express feelings and emotions freely.
J. Watch for signs of exhaustion, dehydration, and acidosis.
K. Monitor vital signs.

L. Monitor fetal heart rate.

M. Monitor progress of labor.

N. Watch for signs of excessive bleeding and fetal distress.

O. Administer medications as ordered.

P. Prepare for cesarean section if necessary.

Evaluation

A. Delivery of a healthy baby.

B. No signs of complications in the mother.

Precipitate Delivery

Definition: Rapid or sudden labor of less than three hours duration, from onset of cervical changes to delivery of infant.

Assessment

A. Obtain rapid history by asking focused questions.
   1. "Do you want to push?"
   2. "Have your membranes ruptured?"
   3. "Are you bleeding?"
   4. "Have you had a baby before?"

B. Assess client's ability to understand your directions.

C. Evaluate resources (proximity of physician and/or other assistance).

D. Assess client's psychological state and need for support at this time.

E. Assess signs and symptoms of impending delivery.
   1. Desire to push.
   2. Frequency of strong contractions.
   3. Heavy bloody show.
   4. Membranes ruptured.
   5. Bulging rectum.
   6. Presenting part visible.
   7. Severe anxiety.

F. Observe for above signs continually as labor may progress with unexpected rapidity.

Planning and Analysis

A. Necessary equipment is available.

B. Mother is able to cope with labor without medication and will follow directions.

C. Presentation is vertex occiput anterior so nurse is able to cope with precipitate delivery.

D. Mother's vital signs remain stable.

Implementation

ASSISTING WITH DELIVERY

A. Never leave the client unattended during this time and never hold baby back. Have another employee notify the physician and bring the emergency delivery pack to room.

B. Reassure client that you will remain with her and provide care until the physician arrives.

C. Put on sterile gloves if they are available and if there is time.

D. Break membranes immediately if they have not done so spontaneously.

E. Have client pant rather than push to avoid rapid delivery of the head.

F. With a clean or sterile towel (if available), support baby's head with one hand applying gentle pressure to the head to prevent sudden expulsion and undue stretching of the perineum or brain damage to the infant.

G. If cord is draped around baby's neck, with free hand gently slip it over head.

H. If bulb syringe is available, gently suction baby's mouth and wipe blood and mucus from mouth and nose with towel, if available.

I. Shoulders are usually born spontaneously after external rotation. If shoulders do not deliver spontaneously, ask client to bear down to deliver them.

J. Support the baby's body as it is delivered.

K. All manipulation should be gentle to avoid injury to mother and baby.

CARE AFTER DELIVERY

A. After delivery, hold baby securely over hand and arm with the head in a dependent position to allow fluid and mucus to drain.

B. If baby does not cry spontaneously, gently rub baby's back or the soles of baby's feet.

C. Dry baby to prevent heat loss.

D. Place the baby on the mother's abdomen to provide warmth. The weight on the uterus will help it to contract.

E. Palpate mother's abdomen to make sure uterus is contracting.

F. Watch for signs of placental separation.

G. Support placenta in your hand after it is expelled.

H. Clamp the cord after it stops pulsating if clamp or ties are available. Cord need not be cut; there will be no bleeding from the placental surface.

I. Wrap the baby in a blanket.

J. Put the baby to the mother's breast. This reassures the mother that the baby is all right and helps contract the uterus.

K. Check the uterus after delivery of the placenta. Make sure the uterus is contracting.

L. Keep an accurate record of the time of birth and other pertinent data.

M. If baby is delivered unassisted, in bed, before the nurse arrives (precipitate delivery), the nurse should immediately:
1. Check the baby to make sure breathing is established.
2. Check the mother for excessive bleeding.

N. Comfort mother.

Evaluation

A. Healthy baby with stable fetal heart rate is delivered and placenta follows.

B. Mother's vital signs remain stable.

C. Uterus remains firm and globular.

D. Nurse, mother and baby handle experience with psychological equanimity.

OBSTETRIC MEDICATIONS

Induction of Labor

Definition: To bring about labor through the use of stimulants, such as oxytocin.

Oxytocin Infusion

A. Indications for use.
1. Client overdue (two weeks or more); placental functions reduced.
2. Severe preeclampsia.
3. Diabetes.
4. Premature rupture of membranes (should deliver within twenty-four hours).
5. Uncontrolled bleeding.
6. Rh sensitization: rising titer.

B. Prerequisites for successful induction.
1. Fetal maturity.
2. Cervix amenable for induction; client may be induced for several days consecutively with rest at night to ripen cervix, if it is desirable to deliver fetus due to complications.
3. Normal cephalopelvic proportions.
4. Fetal head engaged.

Assessment

A. Observe for continuous monitoring of contractions and fetal heart rate—danger of ruptured uterus.

B. Evaluate prolonged uterine contractions: over 90 seconds with less than 30-second rest period between. (Safety intervention is to turn off Pitocin.)

C. Assess for change in fetal heart rate pattern indicating fetal distress.

D. Assess for hemorrhage or shock, which may indicate uterine rupture.

E. Check for rigid abdomen, which may indicate abruptio placenta.

F. Assess vital signs: blood pressure for elevations.

G. Evaluate progress of labor.

Planning and Analysis

A. Artificial stimulation of normal labor pattern results in a normal delivery.

B. Healthy, normal baby is delivered.

C. Mother tolerates induction procedure well.

Implementation

A. Maintain client on bed rest and explain procedure.

B. Provide normal care to client in labor.

C. Obtain baseline fetal heart rate and blood pressure; note presence or absence of any contractions.

D. Start IV fluids: usually 50 ml of 5% D/W.

E. Piggyback oxytocin solution into main line: usually 10 units of pitocin in 1000 ml solution. IVAC or Harvard infusion pump may be used to more accurately control drip rate. (Harvard pump may infuse 2.5 units in 50 ml IV fluid.)

F. Begin infusion slowly to test uterine sensitivity to drug: usually begun at rate of 1 mU/minute with dose increased by 2 mU increments every 15 minutes until regular contraction pattern is established.

G. Monitor labor with external monitor.

H. Discontinue oxytocin solution immediately if hypertonic contractions or signs of fetal distress occur and administer 5% D/W solution. Report to physician.

Evaluation

A. Normal labor pattern is established.

B. No complications occur.

C. A healthy baby is delivered.

Analgesia During Labor

Assessment

A. Assess client pain status—individual thresholds vary.

B. Check vital signs and fetal heart rate before and after administration.

C. Evaluate allergies to medication.

D. Check time last pain medication was given if any.

E. Assess progress of labor before and after.

Planning and Analysis

A. Discomfort associated with labor and delivery is relieved.

B. Anesthesia does not harm baby. (Narcotics given to the mother in labor cross placental barrier and affect infant.)

Implementation

A. Never give narcotics until labor is well established in order to avoid retarding progress of labor. Drugs are usually administered between 4 to 6 cm.

B. Do not administer narcotics within two hours of delivery because the infant may be born depressed; drugs are at level of maximum effect two hours after ingestion.

   1. In the uterus, gas exchange takes place through the placenta; therefore, analgesia given in labor does not pose a threat to infant.

   2. After birth, the infants breathe on their own. Analgesics depress the central nervous system and affect the respiratory and other centers.

   3. Some infants do not become fully alert for two to three days after delivery.

C. Continually observe client and keep side rails up.

D. Be familiar with normal dosages and the physiologic effect of preparations used.

E. Record time, type, dosage, and client's response.

F. Use precautions for sedatives that are given early in labor to reduce anxiety.

G. For specific drugs, see appendices 1. and 2.

Evaluation

A. Client reports relief of pain and appears more comfortable and relaxed.

B. Labor continues to progress.

C. Vital signs and fetal heart rate are stable.

Anesthesia During Labor

Characteristics

A. No optimum anesthesia exists.

B. Ranks fourth as the cause of maternal death; other three causes are hemorrhage, infection, and toxemia.

C. History and physical should be obtained before administering anesthesia.

D. Client should be n.p.o. before use.

E. Anesthesia should be administered by trained personnel.

F. Choice of anesthesia in obstetrics is determined by the specific client situation and condition.

GENERAL INHALATION ANESTHETICS

A. Advantages.

   1. May anesthetize client rapidly.

   2. Primary use is for rapid induction for emergency C-Section.

   3. These anesthetics cause uterine relaxation—may be used for manipulation.

   4. Inhalation anesthetics may be preferred in hypovolemic client or if the client's condition prohibits the use of regional anesthetics.

B. Disadvantages.

   1. Client is not awake for delivery.

   2. Brings about respiratory depression of the infant.

   3. May cause emesis and aspiration in the client.

   4. May be flammable.

C. Common types.

   1. Nitrous oxide: danger of aspiration and respiratory depression.

   2. Halothane: potent, used in selected cases only.

   3. Thiopental (Pentothal): IV anesthesia usually used as an adjunct; may depress neonate.

   4. Trichloroethylene—Trilene: often used in self-administration by mask during labor and delivery. Never leave client alone when she is using self-administered anesthesia.

REGIONAL ANALGESIA AND ANESTHESIA

A. Regional analgesia and anesthesia refer to the drugs given to block the nerves carrying sensation from the uterus to the pelvic region.

   1. Some common agents used are: Novocaine, Xylocaine, Pontocaine, and Carbocaine.

2. Vasoconstrictor agents such as epinephrine are commonly used in conjunction with regional anesthetics to:
   a. Slow absorption and prolong the effect of the anesthetic.
   b. Prevent secondary hypotension.
B. Nerve root block is a principle type of regional anesthesia.
   1. General considerations.
      a. Usually relieves pain completely, if administered properly.
      b. Vasodilation below the anesthetic level: may be responsible for a decrease in blood pressure; blood pools in legs.
      c. Does not depress the respiratory center and, therefore, does not harm the client unless hypotension in the client is severe enough to interfere with uterine flow.
      d. May cause postspinal headache.
      e. Contraindicated in a hypovolemic client or in the case of central nervous system disease.
      f. Drug may impede labor if given too early (before 5 to 6 cm dilatation).
      g. Special skill of anesthesiologist required to administer drug.
      h. Infant may need forceps delivery because the client usually cannot push effectively due to anesthesia.
   2. Types.
      a. Caudal (may be continuous).
      b. Lumbar epidural (may be continuous).
      c. Saddle block.
      d. Spinal.
E. Peripheral nerve block is a second principle type of regional anesthesia.
   1. General considerations.
      a. May be done by attending physician—does not require an anesthesiologist.
      b. Local injection of anesthetic to block peripheral nerve endings.
      c. Less effective in relieving pain than nerve root block.
      d. May cause transient bradycardia in fetus, possibly due to rapid absorption of the drug into fetal circulation.
      e. Usually there are no maternal side effects.
      f. Needle guide such as Iowa trumpet usually used.
   2. Types.

a. Paracervical.
b. Pudendal block.

Assessment

A. Observe progress of labor.
B. Check vital signs and fetal heart rate before and after administration of drug (may cause transient fetal bradycardia).
C. Check drug allergies or hypersensitivity.
D. Observe for signs of dizziness, nausea, faintness, and palpitations.
E. Assess level of anesthesia: relief of pain sensation.
F. After delivery, check client for return of sensation to lower body.

Planning and Analysis

A. Relief of sensation of pain is associated with labor and delivery.
B. Mother and baby maintain healthy status after procedure.

Implementation

A. Have client void.
B. Assist client to a knee-chest position over a bolster or onto left side with head flexed and knees drawn up.
C. Monitor blood pressure every three to five minutes until stabilized; then every 30 minutes or p.r.n.
D. Monitor fetal heart rate.
E. If hypotension occurs:
   1. Turn client to left side.
   2. Administer oxygen by mask.
   3. Notify physician.

Evaluation

A. Relief of pain sensation.
B. Client appears relaxed and comfortable.
C. Fetal heart rate remains stable.

OPERATIVE OBSTETRICS

Obstetrical Procedures

Episiotomy

Definition: An incision made into the perineum during delivery to facilitate the birth process.

A. Types of episiotomy.

1. Midline: incision from the posterior margin of the vaginal opening directly back to the anal sphincter.
   a. Healing is less painful.
   b. Incision is easy to repair.
2. Mediolateral: incision made at 45-degree angle to either side of the vaginal opening.
   a. Healing process is quite painful.
   b. Incision is harder to repair.
   c. Blood loss greater.

B. Purposes.
   1. Spare the muscles of perineal floor from undue stretching and tearing (lacerations).
   2. Prevent the prolonged pressure of the baby's head on perineum.
   3. Reduce duration of second stage of labor.
   4. Enlarge vagina for manipulation.

C. Method.
   1. Generally done during contraction, as the baby's head pushes against perineum and stretches it.
   2. Blunt scissors are used.
   3. Client is usually given as anesthetic: regional, local, or inhalation.

Forceps Delivery

Definition: The extraction of a baby from the birth canal by a physician with the use of a specially designed instrument.

A. Types.
   1. Low forceps: presenting part on perineal floor.
   2. Midforceps: presenting part below or at the level of the ischial spine.
   3. High forceps: presenting part not engaged (rarely if ever used today).

B. Indications.
   1. Fetal distress.
   2. Poor progress of fetus through the birth canal.
   3. Failure of the head to rotate.
   4. Maternal disease or exhaustion.
   5. Client unable to push (as with regional anesthesia).

C. Prerequisite conditions for application of forceps.
   1. Fully dilated cervix.
   2. Fetal head engaged in maternal pelvis.
   3. Membranes ruptured.
   4. Absence of cephalopelvic disproportion.
   5. Empty bladder.

6. Fetal heart tones present before and after forceps application.

D. Complications.
   1. Lacerations of the vagina or the cervix; there may be oozing or hemorrhage.
   2. Rupture of the uterus.
   3. Intracranial hemorrhage and brain damage to the fetus.
   4. Facial paralysis of the fetus.

Cesarean Delivery

Definition: A surgical delivery of an infant through an incision cut into the abdominal wall and the uterus.

A. Types.
   1. Classical: vertical incision through the abdominal wall and into the anterior wall of the uterus.
   2. Low segment transverse: transverse incision made into lower uterine segment after abdomen has been opened.
      a. Incision made into part of uterus where there is less uterine activity and blood loss is minimal.
      b. Less incidence of adhesions and intestinal obstruction.
   3. Cesarean hysterectomy: abdomen and uterus are opened, baby and placenta are removed, and then the hysterectomy is performed. The hysterectomy is performed if:
      a. Diseased tissue or fibroids are present.
      b. There is an abnormal pap smear.
      c. The uterus ruptures.
      d. There is uncontrolled hemorrhage or placenta abruptio or uterine atony, etc.

B. Indications.
   1. Fetal distress unrelieved by other measures.
   2. Uterine dysfunction.
   3. Certain cases of placental previa and premature separation of placenta.
   4. Prolapsed cord.
   5. Diabetes or certain cases of toxemia.
   6. Cephalopelvic disproportion.
   7. Malpresentations such as transverse lie.

Assessment

A. Check vital signs: blood pressure, temperature, pulse, respirations.
B. Observe site of incision for bleeding.

C. Assess intake and output (note appearance as well as amount of urine).

D. Assess level of consciousness or return of sensation with regional anesthesia.

E. Check fundus for tone and location.

F. Evaluate lochia for amount and color every 15 minutes for two to three hours.

Planning and Analysis

A. A healthy baby is delivered.

B. Healing in client is promoted.

C. No postsurgical complications in the client observed.

Implementation

POSTOPERATIVE CARE

A. Institute same care as for the postsurgical client.

B. Institute same care as for the postpartum client.

C. Reinforce abdominal dressing as necessary.

D. Assist client to deep breathe, cough, and turn.

E. Change perineal pads as needed.

F. Reassure client that the delivery is over and give information regarding the baby. (If something is wrong with the baby, the physician usually discusses this first with the parents.)

G. If mother is able and desires, show her and let her hold the baby. (Client may be too tired or uncomfortable at this time to do so. Be sensitive to her needs.)

LATER CARE

A. Help ambulate client (usually the first postpartum day).

B. Give stool softener as ordered and needed.

C. Encourage client to talk about delivery and baby; incorporate and accept experience.

D. Reinforce physician's teaching about care at home.
   1. Planned rest periods.
   2. No heavy lifting for four to six weeks.
   3. Signs of infection.
   4. Care of the breast.
   5. Avoidance of constipation.
   6. Nutritious diet.

E. Provide regular postpartum care.

Evaluation

A. Operative obstetrical procedure was successful.

B. Healthy baby was delivered.

C. Mother tolerated procedure well.
   1. Vital signs remained stable.
   2. Healing of surgical procedure.

D. No postsurgical complications in client occurred.

POSTPARTUM PERIOD

PHYSIOLOGY OF THE PUERPERIUM

Definition: The puerperium is the period of four to six weeks following delivery in which the reproductive organs revert from a pregnant to a nonpregnant state.

Uterus

A. Involution: rapid diminution in the size of the uterus as it returns to a nonpregnant state due primarily to a decrease in size of myometrial cells.
B. Lochia: discharge from the uterus that consists of blood from vessels of the placental site and debris from the decidua.
C. Placental site: blood vessels of the placenta become thrombosed or compressed.

Cervix and Vagina

A. Cervix: remains soft and flabby the first few days, and the internal os closes.
B. Vagina: usually smooth walled after delivery. Rugae begin to appear when ovarian function returns and estrogen is produced.

Ovarian Function and Menstruation

A. Ovarian function depends upon the rapidity in which the pituitary function is restored.
B. Menstruation: usually returns in four to six weeks in a nonlactating mother.

Urinary Tract

A. May be edematous and contain areas of submucosal hemorrhage due to trauma.
B. May have urine retention due to loss of elasticity and tone and loss of sensation from trauma, drugs, anesthesia, loss of privacy.
C. Diuresis: mechanism by which excess body fluid is excreted after delivery. Usually begins within the first twelve hours after delivery.
D. Kidney function returns to normal.

Breasts

A. Proliferation of glandular tissue during pregnancy caused by hormonal stimulation.
B. Usually continue to secrete colostrum the first two to three days postpartum.
C. Anterior pituitary: stimulates secretion of prolactin after the placental hormones that inhibited the pituitary are no longer present.
D. In three to four days breasts become firm, distended, tender, and warm (engorged), indicating production of milk.
E. Breast feeding woman: apply warm compress, suckle. Nonbreastfeeding woman: apply cold compress, don't express milk.
F. Milk usually produced with stimulus of sucking infant.
G. Posterior pituitary: discharges oxytocin, alveoli contract and milk flows in response to sucking; "let down reflex."

Blood

A. White blood cells increase during labor and early postpartum period and then return to normal in a few days.
B. Decrease in hemoglobin and red blood cells, and hematocrit usually returns to normal in one week.
C. Elevated fibrinogen levels usually return to normal within one week.

Gastrointestinal Tract

A. Constipation due to stretching, soreness, lack of food, and loss of privacy.
B. Postpartum clients are usually ravenously hungry.

General Assessment

A. Check vital signs every eight hours and p.r.n.: decreased blood pressure, increased pulse, or temperature over 100.4° F indicates abnormality.
B. Observe fundus for consistency and level: massage fundus lightly with fingers if it is relaxed. Immediately after delivery, fundus is 2 cm below umbilicus; twelve hours later it is 1 cm above umbilicus. Fundus gradually descends into pelvic cavity, and by ninth postpartum day should no longer be palpable.
C. Evaluate lochia for amount, color, consistency, and odor. Watch for hemorrhage.
D. Check perineum for redness, discoloration, or swelling.
E. Check episiotomy for healing and drainage.

F. Check breasts for engorgement and cracking of nipples.

G. Assess emotional status of new mother for depression or withdrawal.

H. Assess for problems with flatus, elimination, hemorrhoids and bladder or bowel retention.

I. Observe status of mother-infant relationship.

General Planning and Analysis

A. Involution and healing are promoted.

B. Infection is prevented.

C. Successful lactation is established.

D. Mother-infant relationship is established.

General Implementation

A. Nursing interventions for first critical hour after birth.

B. Routine postpartum continues after first hour.

C. Administer drug to inhibit lactation (if it has not been given immediately postpartum).

D. Administer RhoGAM as ordered within seventy-two hours postpartum to Rh-negative client who is not sensitized.

E. Maintain intake and output until client is voiding a sufficient quantity without difficulty.
   1. Usually the first three voids are measured.
   2. If client fails to void sufficient quantity within 12 to 24 hours, she is usually catheterized.

F. Teach client perineal care and give perineal care until client is able to do so.

G. Encourage ambulation as soon as ordered and as client is able to tolerate it; give assistance the first time.

H. Encourage verbalization of client's feelings about labor, delivery, and baby.

I. Give perineal light as ordered.

J. Give warm sitz baths as ordered.

K. Remind client to return for postpartum checkup.

L. Instruct that sexual relations may be resumed as soon as healing takes place and bleeding stops and client feels comfortable with it.

M. Discuss contraception if client so desires.

N. Provide opportunities to enhance mother-infant relationship—rooming-in, early contact, successful feedings, etc.

General Evaluation

A. Involution takes place within four to six weeks without complications.

B. Lactation is successfully established in breast-feeding mothers.

C. A positive mother-infant relationship is established.

EMOTIONAL ASPECTS OF POSTPARTUM CARE

Parenting

Postpartum Phases as Outlined by Rubin

A. Taking-in phase: first two to three days.
   1. Mother's primary needs are her own: sleep, food.
   2. Mother is usually quite talkative: focus on labor and delivery experience.
   3. Important for nurse to listen and help mother interpret events to make them more meaningful.

B. Taking-hold phase: third postpartum day to two weeks—varies with each individual.
   1. Emphasis on present; mother is impatient and wants to reorganize self.
   2. More in control. Begins to take hold of task of "mothering."
   3. Important time for teaching without making mother feel inadequate—success at this time important in future mother-child relationship.

C. Letting-go phase.
   1. Mother may feel a deep loss over the separation of the baby from part of her body and may grieve over this loss.
   2. Mother may be caught in a dependent-independent role—wanting to feel safe and secure yet wanting to make decisions. Teenage mother needs special consideration because of the conflicts taking place within her as part of adolescence.
   3. Mother may in turn feel resentful and guilty about the baby causing so much work.
   4. May have difficulty adjusting to mothering role.
   5. May feel conflict between the roles of mother and wife.

6. May feel upset and depressed at times—postpartum blues.
7. May be concerned about other children.
8. Important for nurse to encourage vocalization of these feelings and give positive reassurance for task well done.

Assessment

A. Assess maternal and paternal physical and emotional status.
B. Determine what parents know about infant care.
C. Assess parents' own birth—parenting and nurturing.
D. Evaluate impact of parents' cultural background.
E. Assess readiness for parenthood: emotional maturity, pregnancy planned or unplanned, financial status, job status.
F. Assess physical conditions of mother prior to pregnancy, during labor and delivery, and during puerperium.
G. Assess physical conditions of infant at birth, prematurity, congenital defects, etc. (parents may feel guilty, angry, cheated, and so forth).
H. Check for parental career plans.
I. Assess opportunities for early parental-infant interaction.
J. Evaluate parental knowledge of normal growth and development.

Planning and Analysis

A. Successful adaptation to parental role is established.
B. Emotional equilibrium in the mother is stabilized.
C. Physical condition of mother does not impede childcare activities.
D. Mother demonstrates competence in caring for child.

Implementation

A. Promote optimum parent-infant interactions during the early postpartum period (crucial time in parent-infant bonding).
1. Allow periods of time for both mother and father to be alone with infant.
2. Allow parents to hold infant in delivery and recovery rooms, and provide rooming-in and privacy.
B. Based upon assessment of parents, plan nursing care. Be sure to begin at same level as parents.

C. Be alert to parental cues but be careful not to label.
D. Support mother in infant care activities and use these opportunities to promote her self-esteem.
E. Provide a role model for parents.
F. Plan nursing care to reduce maternal fatigue and anxiety so that time with her infant is pleasurable.
G. Explain to parents that it is normal at this time to feel fatigued, tense, insecure, and sometimes depressed.
H. Counsel mother on home care plan.
1. Rest periods to avoid over-fatigue.
2. Time spent away from baby: to be alone, to be with husband, to be with other children, and to resume contact with people.
3. Time for father and baby together.

Evaluation

A. Mother demonstrates increasing levels of competence in carrying out the tasks of newborn care.
B. Mother appears relaxed and secure in her interactions with infant.
C. Couple plan time together.
D. Mother does not appear unduly depressed or anxious.

Breast Feeding

Assessment

A. Assess breasts for tenderness and hardness.
B. Assess for pain, redness, discomfort.
C. Check cracking of nipples.
D. Evaluate maternal nutrition: increased maternal needs of protein, vitamins, and iron during lactation.
E. Check position assumed while nursing and degree of comfort.
F. Evaluate emotional attitude towards nursing: degree of satisfaction, relaxation, tenseness.
G. Assess care given to breast: adequate support, cleansing.

Planning and Analysis

A. Successful lactation is established.
B. Mother adjusts to and finds pleasure in process of breast feeding.
C. Infant is nursing well and growth and development is normal.

Implementation

A. Have mother wash her hands.

B. Put baby to breast as soon as mother's and baby's condition is stable: on the delivery table in some hospitals, or in six to twelve hours in others.

C. Have mother assume comfortable position sitting or lying down.

D. Guide baby to breast; stimulate rooting reflex if necessary—place entire areola in baby's mouth.

E. Gently press breast away from baby's nose.

F. Usually the baby is nursed two to three minutes at each breast the first time, gradually building to ten minutes or so on each side in later feedings.

G. Release suction by inserting a finger into the baby's mouth. The breast will become sore if baby is pulled off it.

H. Burp baby after each breast.

I. Stay with mother each time she nurses until she feels secure or confident with the baby and feedings.

J. Baby should not nurse more than every two hours.

K. Teach mother principles of breast feeding.

   1. Explain to the mother that the baby's stool will be yellow and watery, and it is not uncommon for nursing infants to have three to four stools each day or even one for each feeding.

   2. Dry the breast after feeding and allow it to air occasionally, especially if it is sore.

   3. Use general hygiene and wash the breast once daily; do not use soap as it tends to remove natural oils and increase chances of cracking.

   4. Encourage the mother to eat a well-balanced diet and drink 3000 cc of fluid daily.

   5. Explain to the mother that she may offer sterile water to the baby between feedings, but not formula. (The baby will not be hungry if given formula and will not nurse well.)

   6. Formula may be given at feeding time, or the mother may express milk manually and put it in a bottle if she plans to be away during feeding time.

   7. Breasts may leak between feedings or during coitus. Place a washcloth or pad in brassiere.

   8. Uterine cramping may occur the first few days after delivery while nursing when oxytocin stimulation causes the uterus to contract.

   9. Instruct mother to wear well-fitted brassiere.

L. Instruct mother what to avoid.

   1. Medications or drugs contraindicated unless necessary to save a life—drugs pass to infant through breast milk.

   2. Some foods, such as cabbage or onions, may alter the taste of milk or cause gas in infant.

   3. Birth control pills are usually avoided while nursing as they decrease milk production and are passed to infant in the milk.

Evaluation

A. Infant is gaining weight and appears satisfied between feedings.

B. No pain, redness or hardness in breast.

C. Mother appears relaxed and comfortable while nursing.

D. Mother expresses satisfaction with her ability to breast feed.

COMPLICATIONS OF THE PUERPERIUM

General Assessment

A. Observe for postdelivery hemorrhage (leading cause of maternal death in the world).

B. Check for uterine atony.

C. Assess for lacerations of birth canal.

D. Assess for postdelivery infection (puerperal sepsis).

E. Evaluate for postpartum alterations in mental state, i.e., depression, psychosis, etc.

F. Assess for mastitis.

G. Check for presence of embolism.

General Planning and Analysis

A. Hemorrhage is controlled and blood loss replaced.

B. Shock is prevented.

C. Vital signs remain normal.

D. Health and well-being of the mother are preserved.

E. Normal processes whereby the woman returns to the nonpregnant state are achieved.

General Implementation

A. Postpartum hemorrhage: Identify degree of hemorrhage and implement measures to contain it.

B. Endometritis: Treat inflammation and prevent further complications.

C. Urinary tract infection: Identify presence of infection and initiate treatment.

D. Mastitis: Administer antibiotics, support mother during exacerbation, and perform palliative measures.

E. Subinvolution: Identify condition and initiate treatment.

General Evaluation

A. Specific complication has been treated.

B. Normal process of involution is established.

C. Positive mother-infant relationship is established.

D. Normal reproductive function is maintained.

Postpartum Hemorrhage

Definition: A condition that occurs when 500 ml or more of blood is lost during or after delivery.

Characteristics

A. Uterine atony (exhaustion of muscle) is *primary cause.* Causes for uterine atony include:
  1. Prolonged labor.
  2. Overdistention: multiple pregnancies, polyhydramnios.
  3. Sluggish muscle.
  4. Overmassage of fundus.
  5. Presence of fibroid tumors.
  6. Deep inhalation anesthesia—may inhibit uterine activity.

B. Lacerations of the reproductive tract is a *second cause.*
  1. Lacerations of the cervix or of the high vaginal walls.
  2. Oozing from blood vessels.

C. Retained placental tissue or incomplete separation of the placenta is a *third cause.* (This is the most frequent cause of *late* postpartum hemorrhage.)

D. Hematoma.

E. Late postpartum hemorrhage occurs 12 to 21 days after delivery.

F. Placenta acereta is the abnormal adherence of placenta due to penetration of placental trophoblast into myometrium.
  1. May be partial or complete.

  2. Removal of placenta by hand or hysterectomy if bleeding persists.

Assessment

A. Observe for uterine atony.
  1. Boggy, relaxed uterus.
  2. Dark bleeding.
  3. Passage of clots.

B. Check any lacerations.
  1. Firm fundus.
  2. Oozing of bright red blood.

C. Check for retained placental tissue.
  1. Boggy, relaxed uterus.
  2. Dark bleeding.

D. Evaluate for signs and symptoms of shock.
  1. Air hunger: difficulty in breathing.
  2. Restlessness.
  3. Weak, rapid pulse.
  4. Rapid respirations.
  5. Decrease in blood pressure.

Planning and Analysis

A. Hemorrhage is controlled.

B. Blood loss is replaced.

C. Mother's anxiety is alleviated.

D. Vital signs stabilize and shock is prevented.

Implementation

A. Remain with client.

B. Monitor vital signs every 15 minutes or p.r.n. until stable.

C. Administer intravenous fluids, blood, or volume expanders as ordered.

D. Palpate fundus every 15 minutes or p.r.n. while bleeding continues; then every 2 to 4 hours.

E. Gently massage fundus until firm. Be careful not to overmassage.

F. Administer oxytocin if uterus is boggy.

G. Have physician notified.

H. Weigh pads and linen.

I. Provide warmth for client.

J. Measure intake and output.

K. Explain carefully to client and family to help allay anxiety.

L. Observe for blood reactions and check for clotting defect.

M. Return client to delivery room or to surgery for removal of placental tissue or repair of laceration.

Evaluation

A. Abnormal bleeding ceases; vital signs are stable.
B. Overmassage of uterus does not occur, as this may cause increased bleeding.
C. Lost blood is replaced; fluids and electrolytes regain balance.
D. High anxiety level in mother is alleviated.
E. Lacerations and/or retained placental fragments are treated. No complications occur.

Postdelivery Infection

Definition: An infection in genitalia within 28 days as a consequence of abortion or labor and delivery.

Characteristics

A. Cause.
   1. Organisms that were introduced during labor and delivery.
   2. Bacteria normally present in vaginal tract.
B. Predisposing factors.
   1. Weakened resistance due to prolonged labor and dehydration.
   2. Traumatic delivery.
   3. Excessive vaginal examinations during labor.
   4. Premature rupture of membranes.
   5. Excessive blood loss.
   6. Anemia.
   7. Intrauterine manipulation.
   8. Retained placental fragments.

Assessment

A. Assess for elevated temperature of 100.4°F or 38.0°C for two more consecutive days, not counting first 24 hours.
B. Assess any discomfort in the abdomen and perineum.
C. Evaluate burning on urination and character of urine.
D. Check for foul-smelling lochia or discharge.
E. Assess for pelvic pain.
F. Assess for chills.
G. Check for rapid pulse and assess other vital signs.
H. Evaluate malaise, anorexia.
I. Assess boggy, relaxed, and/or tender uterus.

Planning and Analysis

A. Infection is identified and treated and does not extend upward.
B. Complications (pulmonary embolism, peritonitis, pelvic cellulitis) are prevented.
C. Antibiotic treatment is instituted and symptoms subside.
D. Mother resumes normal feeding schedule and mother-infant relationship is continued.

Implementation

A. Administer IV fluids or blood as ordered.
B. Encourage fluid intake: 3000 to 4000 cc if not contraindicated.
C. Administer medications: broad spectrum IV antibiotics as ordered.
D. Offer warm sitz bath or heat lamp for relief of symptoms.
E. Monitor laboratory studies: blood and urine.
F. Provide high-calorie nutritious diet.
G. Place client in Fowler's or semi-Fowler's position as ordered. Position of client promotes drainage.
H. Provide emotional support to mother, who is usually in isolation and unable to see baby.

Evaluation

A. Complications are avoided; temperature returns to normal range.
B. No malaise or chills are present.
C. Appetite returns.
D. White blood cell count is within normal limits.
E. Fluid and electrolyte balance is maintained.
F. Lochia has no foul odor.
G. General health returns.

Thrombophlebitis

Definition: A vascular occlusion of vessels of the pelvis or lower extremities. Results from infection, circulatory stasis, and increased postdelivery coagulability of blood.

Assessment

A. Assess for discomfort in abdomen and pelvis.
B. Assess for tenderness localized on one side of the pelvis.
C. Assess for femoral symptoms–usually do not appear until the second week or later.
   1. Edema and pain in affected leg.
   2. Chills and fever.

Planning and Analysis

A. Antibiotics reduce and stabilize temperature.
B. Anticoagulants reestablish normal circulation.
C. Bed rest reduces stress on circulatory system.
D. Warm compresses and heat reduce inflammation.

Implementation

A. Provide specific care for extremity.
1. Maintain bed rest; keep bed clothes off leg.
2. Apply warm compresses, as ordered, for fifteen to twenty minutes.
3. Elevate affected leg.
4. Apply bed cradle.
5. Never massage leg and teach client not to do so.
6. Apply antiembolic stocking, and teach client its proper use.
B. Provide diversion.
C. Administer medications as ordered.
D. Teach client to administer heparin.
E. Teach client to watch for signs of excessive bleeding.
F. Allow client to express fears and concerns.
G. Watch for signs of pulmonary embolism.

Evaluation

A. No tenderness or redness in affected area.
B. No edema in leg.
C. Leg and toes feel warm to touch.
D. No fever or chills.
E. No abnormal bleeding.

Urinary Tract Infection

Definition: Postdelivery urinary tract infections are usually caused by the coliform bacteria and generally occur soon after vaginal delivery.

Characteristics

A. Edema and hyperemia of bladder due to stretching and trauma in labor and delivery.
B. Temporary loss of bladder tone; pressure and injury may result in bladder being less sensitive to fullness.
C. Overdistention and residual urine or inability to void may occur.
D. Trauma to urethra may cause difficulty in voiding.

Assessment

A. Assess for suprapubic or perineal discomfort.
B. Check for frequent urination, burning, dysuria.
C. Check for hematuria.
D. Assess for elevated temperature.
E. Assess for pyelitis–pain in flank.
F. Perform urine cultures and chemical tests to determine presence and number of bacteria.
G. Evaluate microscopic examination for detailed identification of the organism (especially important in chronic infections).
H. Note that a colony count of over 100,000/ml is most important lab finding and designates infection.

Implementation

A. Observe client closely postpartum for full bladder or residual urine.
1. Palpate bladder for distention.
2. Palpate fundus: full bladder displaces fundus upward and to the sides.
B. Institute measures to help client void.
C. Insert catheter, as ordered, using sterile technique.
D. Force fluids to 3000 cc per day.
E. Administer drugs as ordered. (Most common are NegGram, Mandelamine, and Furadantin.) May give systemic antibiotics.
F. Obtain urine specimens for microscopic examination.
G. Provide emotional support to client: allow her to express feelings about her illness and the baby.

Evaluation

A. No organisms found in microscopic examination.
B. No fever, chills, malaise.
C. No pain or burning on urination.
D. Client able to void on own.

Mastitis

Definition: An infection in breast tissue usually caused by the staphylococcus organism. It occurs in about one percent of women who have recently delivered.

Characteristics

A. Infected hands of client or attendants.
B. Bacteria normally present in lactiferous glands.

C. Fissure in nipples.

D. Bruising of breast tissue.

E. Stasis of milk or overdistention may injure tissue, but does not cause infection in itself.

F. Infected baby.

Assessment

A. Assess for chills.

B. Assess for elevated temperature: 103°F or 39.5°C or above.

C. Check for elevated pulse rate.

D. Evaluate breast lobe which may appear hard, red, painful, and evidence localized tenderness.

Planning and Analysis

A. Cause identified immediately and treated to prevent breast abscess.

B. Antibiotic therapy is instituted.

C. Discomfort is decreased and symptoms diminish.

D. Normal lactation pattern is reinstituted.

Implementation

A. Provide support for breast. Make sure client wears snug-fitting, supportive brassiere.

B. Administer antibiotics as ordered.

C. Apply ice or heat to breast.

D. Teach client to empty breast every four hours if nursing is to be discontinued.

E. Wash hands before touching client's breast.

F. Teach client careful handwashing and care of the breast.

Evaluation

A. No redness, tenderness or pain in breast, and client responds to treatment.

B. No breast abscesses develop.

C. Symptoms of infection (chills, elevated temperature, increased pulse) subside.

D. Normal breast feeding pattern is reestablished.

Subinvolution

Definition: Failure of the uterus to revert to normal postpartum state, caused by retained placental tissue or fetal membranes, endometritis, or uterine tumors.

Assessment

A. Assess for enlarged, boggy, and tender uterus.

B. Assess for profuse red lochia or hemorrhage.

C. Check for pelvic discomfort and backache.

Planning and Analysis

A. Normal involution of the uterus is established.

B. Profound hemorrhage is avoided or treated immediately.

C. Client is instructed to note symptoms and is able to differentiate between normal bleeding and frank bleeding.

Implementation

A. Monitor ergonovine (0.2 mg every four hours for three days) to cause contractions.

B. Administer antibiotics to prevent infection as ordered.

C. Assist physician in manual replacement of malposition.

D. Explain condition and treatment to client.

Evaluation

A. Uterus decreases in size and descends into the pelvis.

B. Bleeding is controlled and loss of blood minimized.

C. Client's anxiety is allayed.

D. Infection is prevented.

NEWBORN

Delivery Room

Universal Precautions: All newborns must be handled with gloves until after first bath.

Assessment: Delivery Room

A. Assess respiratory status, especially tachypnea (earliest sign of a problem), nasal flaring, retractions, expiratory grunt.
B. Apgar scoring, one and five minutes (see Table 5); based on the scoring method developed by Virginia Apgar.
C. Assess for obvious congenital malformation.
D. Check umbilical cord: two arteries and one vein.
E. Look for meconium staining: skin, nails.
F. Evaluate abnormal cry or no cry.
G. Assess any injuries caused by birth trauma, i.e. dislocated shoulder, edema of scalp, lacerations.
H. Assess neurological status: reflexes, tremors, and twitching.
I. Check for anal and nasal patency.

Assessment: Nursery

A. Observe for jaundice: check general skin color, blanching, sclera of the eyes.
B. Check for respiratory difficulty: mucus, flaring of nostrils, grunting, etc.
C. Note tremors, twitching, muscle tone, reflexes, and irritability.
D. Take baby's temperature each shift.
E. Check baby's weight daily.
F. Note amount voided and number of stools.
G. Check for signs of infection on the skin and cord: redness, drainage, odor, and bleeding.
H. Assess formula or breast milk intake each feeding.
I. Check sleep patterns.

J. Evaluate mother's and infant's response to each other.

Planning and Analysis

A. Body temperature is maintained.
B. Respirations and cardiovascular functions are stable.
C. Infection and injury are prevented.
D. Nutrition is maintained and growth promoted.
E. Positive mother-infant relationship is promoted.

Implementation: Delivery Room

A. Wipe off mucus from baby and wrap in warm blanket.
B. Place in heated crib or give to mother and/or father to hold (mother may be too tired to receive baby at this time).
C. Avoid excessive exposure as body temperature is variable.
D. Place infant on side or modified Trendelenburg's to facilitate drainage of mucus or blood.
E. Suction mucus as needed with bulb or suction catheter attached to mucus trap.
F. Provide oxygen as needed.
G. Apply 1 percent silver nitrate or broad spectrum antibiotic, erythromycin, to eyes.
H. Clamp cord if physician has not done so.
I. Identify baby with bands.

Implementation: Nursery

A. Check axillary temperature.
B. Weigh and measure: total length and head circumference.
C. Place in heated crib.
D. Check respiratory rates every hour for two to three hours and p.r.n.
E. Check for nasal flaring, retractions, expiratory grunt, breath sounds.

Table 5. APGAR SCORING

Sign	0	1	2
Heart tone	Absent	Slow (less than 100)	Over 100
Respiratory effort	Absent	Slow, irregular	Good crying
Muscle tone	Flaccid	Some flexion of extremities	Active motion
Reflex irritability	No response	Cry	Vigorous cry
Color	Blue, pale	Body pink, extremities blue	Completely pink

F. Check apical pulse every hour for two to three hours; watch for above 180 or below 100.

G. Keep bulb syringe available and suction as needed.

H. Administer vitamin K as ordered.

I. Bathe and dress baby when infant's temperature is stable.

J. Place in an open crib when infant's temperature is stable.

K. Administer feeding as ordered; usually sterile water is given within four to six hours.

L. Assess baby for congenital defects, tremors, color, acrocyanosis. (Acrocyanosis is normal for one to two hours after birth and when infant is cold, because of sluggish peripheral circulation.)

M. Apply alcohol to cord daily p.r.n.

N. Provide circumcision care.
   1. Observe for bleeding.
   2. Change petroleum gauze as necessary.
   3. Keep area clean to prevent infection.

O. Arrange appointment for phenylketonuria (PKU) test to be done within two weeks of birth.

P. Teach mother how to hold and burp the baby.

Q. Use proper hand washing between handling of babies to prevent spreading infection.

R. Isolate babies with known or suspected infections.

S. Be sure that the mother understands the doctor's orders regarding care of the infant.

T. Ensure mother plans follow-up visits to the physician.

Evaluation

A. Normal body temperature is maintained and infant shows no signs of cold stress.

B. Respirations are between 40 to 60; heart rate is 120 to 160 at rest.

C. No signs of infection or other complications.

D. Weight stabilizes, and infant takes adequate nutrition.

E. Normal cry, sleep patterns, and reflexes present.

F. Infant's skin color shows signs of adequate circulation, except for possible mild acrocyanosis or mottling on chilling.

G. Mother appears relaxed with baby, and is able to comfort baby. Mother-infant bonding continues.

Schedules of Newborn Feeding

A. First feeding.

1. May be breast fed on the delivery table.

2. Feed in first hour of life.

3. Latest to start feeding is 2 to 3 hours (when normal low blood sugar occurs).

4. Sterile water, a few swallows to ½ oz.

5. Discontinue water and give full strength formula or breast milk for first feeding.

6. Glucose water no longer recommended—aspiration pneumonia.

B. Subsequent feeding.

1. Routine schedule: 2- to 4-hour feedings.

2. Self-demand: baby is fed according to needs, when hungry, usually every 3 to 6 hours. (Breast fed may be 1½ to 2 hours.)

Calories and Fluid Needs

A. Fluid: 105 ml/kg of body weight in twenty-four hours. More fluids should be given in hot weather or when the baby has an elevated temperature.

B. Caloric needs: approximately 115 kca/kg.

General Assessment

A. Assess respiratory status.

1. Infant's respiratory system must function immediately after loss of placental function; adequate maturation at birth is necessary.

2. From 20 to 30 cc of fluid are present in the lungs at birth.
   a. Approximately one-third is removed as a result of compression of the chest during delivery.
   b. The remainder is carried off through pulmonary circulation and by the lymph system.

3. Surfactant is a phospholipid found in the lungs.
   a. It reduces surface tension in alveoli and keeps them from collapsing.
   b. Surfactant is necessary to maintain lung expansion and to prevent respiratory distress syndrome.

4. Normal respiration is about 30 to 50.
   a. Over 60 or below 30 indicates a problem.
   b. Tachypnea is earliest symptom of many neonatal problems (respirations above 60).

c. Respiration may be slightly elevated during crying episodes or shortly afterward. (Always count for one full minute.)

B. Assess circulatory status.

1. Ductus arteriosus, ductus venosus, and foramen ovale should close (may not be complete for one or two days).

2. Peripheral circulation may be sluggish; there may be mottling, acrocyanosis.

3. Pulse may be variable (normal 120–160).

   a. It may be as high as 170 with crying or below 120 when resting.

   b. Always take apical pulse for one full minute.

4. Anemia is common in early months because of the decrease in erythropoiesis and breakdown of red blood cells. Baby may need an iron-supplemented formula.

5. Plethora (red coloring to skin) especially visible when baby cries; may be present due to increase in red blood cells.

6. Physiologic jaundice: normal level less than 1 mg per 100 ml blood.

   a. Jaundice visible in skin, sclera.

   b. Does not become visible until the second or third day after birth.

   c. Caused by impairment in the removal of bilirubin—deficiency in the production of glucuronide transferase, which is needed to convert indirect insoluble bilirubin to direct water soluble bilirubin which is excreted.

   d. Jaundice begins to decrease by the sixth or seventh day.

   e. Should be watched carefully although usually does not require treatment.

   f. Usual treatment is phototherapy (13 mg/ 100 ml blood; lower in premature infants). If the indirect bilirubin continues to go up, a cause other than physiologic jaundice is searched for.

   g. Infant may be on force fluids between feeding to aid in excretion of bilirubin as it is broken down.

7. Transitory deficiency in the ability of the blood to clot.

   a. Bacteria in the intestines are necessary for the production of vitamin K.

   b. Bacteria are not present in the intestines during the first few days after birth.

   c. Vitamin K IM usually given after birth to aid in blood coagulation.

C. Assess ability of newborn to maintain body heat.

1. Baby suffers loss of heat primarily from head because of being wet and coolness of delivery room.

   a. Put knit cap on head, dry off, and place immediately in a warmer.

   b. Wrap in warm blanket and give infant to mother.

2. Means of heat production in the newborn.

   a. Increasing metabolism.

   b. Shivering—poor in newborn.

   c. Metabolism of brown fat—less mature infants have less brown fat.

3. Effects of chilling—cold stress.

   a. Increased consumption of oxygen.

   b. Use of glucose stored as glycogen.

   c. May become hypoglycemic.

   d. May develop metabolic acidosis—products of incomplete metabolism accumulate with fatty acids from breakdown of brown fat.

4. The baby may have a decrease in the production of surfactant.

   a. Glucose, pO_2, and proper pulmonary circulation are necessary for the production of surfactant.

   b. Decrease in surfactant may lead to respiratory distress.

5. Temperature may be taken by rectum or axilla (latter method is usual).

D. Assess newborn's weight.

1. Infants usually lose between 5 to 10 percent of their body weight the first few days, because of low fluid intake and loss of excess fluid from tissue.

2. Usually regain weight lost within seven to fourteen days.

E. Assess head size and shape.

1. Head or face may be asymmetrical due to birth trauma.

2. Molding of head may be present (elongation of head as it passes through birth canal to accommodate pelvis); usually disappears in about a week.

3. Caput succedaneum: diffuse swelling of soft tissues of scalp, caused by an arrest in circulation in those tissues present over the cervix as it dilates.

4. Cephalohematoma: extravasation of blood beneath periosteum of one of the cranial bones because of a ruptured blood vessel during the trauma of labor and delivery.
5. Anterior and posterior fontanel.
   a. Should be open.
   b. Should neither bulge (may indicate intracranial pressure) nor be depressed (may indicate dehydration).
6. Ears well formed and cartilage present.

E. Assess gastrointestinal system.
   1. Salivary glands immature.
   2. May have Epstein's pearls: white raised areas on palate caused by an accumulation of epithelial cells.
   3. May have transient circumoral cyanosis.
   4. Sucking pads: fatty tissue deposits in each cheek that aid in sucking. They usually disappear when no longer needed.
   5. Infant stools.
      a. Meconium plug: thick gray-white mucus passed before meconium.
      b. Meconium: sticky, black, tarry looking stools, consisting of mucus, digestive secretions, vernix caseosa, and lanugo; usually passed during the first twenty-four hours after birth.
      c. Transitional stool: second to fifth day; greenish-yellow color and loose (partly meconium and partly milk).
      d. Breast-fed baby's stools: soft, nonfoul-smelling, and more frequent.
      e. Bottle-fed baby's stools: formed, foul-smelling.
      f. Observe for color, frequency, and consistency.
   6. Regurgitation following feeding is common. It may be reduced by frequent burping during feedings.

F. Assess genitourinary system.
   1. Urinary functions.
      a. Observe ability to concentrate urine and check to see if specific gravity elevated.
      b. Uric acid crystals (pink or reddish spots) may appear on diaper due to high uric acid secretion.
   2. Female genitalia.
      a. May have heavy coating of vernix between labia.
      b. Usually has mucus discharge. Mucus may be blood-tinged due to elevated hormonal levels in mother.
   3. Male genitalia.
      a. Size of penis and scrotom vary.
      b. Testicles should be descended or in inguinal canal.
      c. Circumcision: surgical removal of foreskin of penis by physician.
         (1) Usually performed by the second or third day.
         (2) Observe for bleeding from postoperative site.

G. Assess skin.
   1. Should be pinkish color; may appear dry.
   2. Acrocyanosis (cyanosis of extremities) may be present for the first hour or two after birth. Presistent blueness may indicate complications such as heart disease.
   3. Lanugo and vernix caseosa may be present.
   4. Petechiae may be present because of the trauma of birth.
   5. Milia (secretions of sebaceous materials in obstructed sebaceous glands) may be present and will disappear.
   6. Erythema toxicum neonatorum (small harmless eruptions on the skin); transient in nature.
   7. Hemangiomas may be present on nape of neck or upper eyelids.
   8. Mongolian spots (bluish pigmented areas) present on the buttocks of babies of Oriental, Negro, or Mediterranean heritage.
   9. Mottling may occur if the infant is chilled.

H. Assess for possible effects of maternal hormones.
   1. Maternal hormones may cause enlargement of breast in both male and female infants, and "witches" milk, a milk-like substance, may be excreted from the breasts.
   2. Vaginal bleeding in female infant.
   3. Hypertrophy of labia or scrotum.

I. Assess neurological system.
   1. Reflexes present at birth.
   2. Muscle tone.
      a. Fist usually kept clenched.
      b. Baby should offer resistance when change in position is attempted.
      c. Head should be supported when baby is lifted.
      d. Muscles should not be limp.
   3. Cry.
      a. Cry should be loud and vigorous.
      b. Baby should cry when hungry or uncomfortable.

4. Hunger.
   a. Usually becomes fretful and restless at three- to four-hour intervals.
   b. May suck fingers or anything placed near mouth.
5. Sleep.
   a. Sleeps about twenty out of twenty-four hours.
   b. Often stirs and stretches while sleeping.
J. Assess functioning of senses.
  1. Eyes.
   a. Eyelids may be edematous or have purulent discharge from the chemical irritation of silver nitrate.
   b. Light perception is present.
   c. Eye movement is uncoordinated.
   d. Usual color of eyes is blue-gray.
   e. May have subconjunctival hemorrhages, which disappear in a week or two.
   f. May gaze at or follow bright objects.
  2. Nose.
   a. Newborn breathes through nose.
   b. Sense of smell is present.
  3. Ears: hearing is present at birth.
  4. Taste is present at birth.
  5. Touch is present at birth. Responds to stimuli and discomfort.
K. Immunity factors.
  1. May receive from the mother some passive immunity to infectious diseases, such as measles, mumps, and diphtheria.
  2. Capacity to develop own antibodies is slow during first few months.
  3. Has little resistance to infection.

General Implementation

A. Maintain body temperature.
  1. Place infant in heated incubator or crib with radiant heat.
  2. Wipe off fluid, mucus, and excessive vernix.
  3. Avoid excessive exposure.
  4. Wrap infant in warm blankets.
  5. Transfer to the nursery after parents have seen and held infant.
B. Maintain respiration.
  1. Place infant on side, in modified Trendelenburg's position, to prevent cerebral edema and to facilitate drainage of mucus and blood.
  2. Suction mucus as needed with bulb or suction catheter attached to mucus trap.
  3. Provide oxygen as needed.
C. Prevent infection and injury.

1. Eye care.
   a. To prevent eye infection from gonorrhea.
   b. Usually one percent silver nitrate: two drops in conjunctival sacs; flush eyes with water after about two minutes.
   c. Most common treatment: broad-spectrum antibiotic ointment applied to eyes.
2. Cord care—use sterile scissors and clamp.
3. Never handle newborn baby without wearing gloves until after first bath—observe universal precautions.

Newborn with AIDS

A. Don gloves and gown to protect self from contamination.
B. Wait until newborn's temperature is stable in the nursery to provide care.
C. Wash infant carefully with Neutrogena soap.
D. Administer cord care with alcohol.
E. Wrap infant in clean blanket.
F. Dispose of gloves and gown in plastic bag.
G. Teach principles of care to mother of HIV baby.
  1. Breast feeding is discouraged when mother tests positive for HIV.
  2. Circumcisions are not done on infants with HIV positive mothers until infant's status is determined.
  3. Immunizations with live vaccine (oral polio, MMR) should not be done until child's status is confirmed. If child is infected, live vaccine will not be given. Inactivated Polio Vaccine (IPV) will be administered.
  4. Excellent hygiene procedures should be carried out in the home.
  5. Inform the care giver exposed to infant's body fluids of the potential for infection transmission.
  6. Teach the importance of good handwashing techniques.

General Evaluation

A. Newborn functions independently out of womb; all systems appear normal.
  1. Maintains respirations.
  2. Maintains body temperature.
B. Newborn appears alert, cries, and scores normal on Apgar scale.
C. Infection does not develop in newborn.
D. No birth trauma is evident in newborn.
E. Vital signs remain stable.

SUMMARY CHART OF NEWBORN ASSESSMENT

ASSESSMENT	NORMAL	ABNORMAL
SKIN ASSESSMENT		
Note skin **color** and **lesions**	Pink	Cyanosis, pallor, beefy red
	Mongolian spots	Petechiae, ecchymoses, or purpuric spots: signs of possible hematologic disorder
	Capillary hemangiomas on face or neck	Cafe au lait spots (patches of brown discoloration): possible sign of congenital neurological disorder
		Raised capillary hemangiomas on areas other than face or neck
	Localized edema in presenting part	Edema of peritoneal wall
	Cheesy white vernix	Poor skin turgor: indicates dehydration
	Desquamation (peeling off)	Yellow discolored vernix (meconium stained)
	Milia (small white pustules over nose and chin)	Impetigo neonatorum (small pustules with surrounding red areas)
	Jaundice after 24 hours; gone by second week	Jaundice at birth or within 12 hours
		Dermal sinuses (opening to brain)
		Holes along spinal column
		Low hairline posteriorly: possible chromosomal abnormality
		Sparse or spotty hair: congenital goiter or chromosomal abnormality
Note color of **nails**	Pink	Yellowing of nail beds (meconium stained)
Note **skin tone**	Strong, tremulous	Flaccid, convulsions
		Muscular twitching, hypertonicity
HEAD AND NECK ASSESSMENT		
Note **shape of head**	Fontanels: anterior open until 18 months; posterior closed shortly after birth	Depressed, tense, bulging, or absent fontanels: indicates hydrocephalus or dehydration
		Cephalohematoma that crosses the midline
		Microcephaly and macrocephaly

ASSESSMENT	NORMAL	ABNORMAL
Assess **eyes**	Slight edema of lids	Purulent discharge
		Lateral upward slope of eye with an inner epicanthal fold in infants not of Oriental descent
		Exophthalmos (bulging of eyeball): may be congenital anomaly, sign of congenital glaucoma or thyroid abnormality
		Enophthalmos (recession of eyeball): may indicate damage to brain or cervical spine
	Pupils equal and reactive to light by three weeks of age	Constricted pupil, unilateral dilated fixed pupil, nystagmus (rhythmic nonpurposeful movement of eyeball): continuous strabismus
	Intermittent strabismus (occasional crossing of eyes)	
	Conjunctival or sclera hemorrhages	Haziness of cornea
	Symmetrical light reflex (light reflects off each eye in the same quadrant): sign of conjugate gaze	Absence of red reflex; asymmetrical light reflex
Note **placement of ears,** shape and position		Low set ears: may indicate chromosomal or renal system abnormality
Assess **nose**	Discharge, sneezing	Thick, bloody nasal discharge
Assess **mouth**	Sucking, rooting reflexes	Cleft lip, palate
	Retention cysts (pears)	Flat, white nonremovable spots (thrush)
	Occasional vomiting	Frequent vomiting: may indicate pyloric stenosis
		Vomitus with bile: fecal vomiting
		Profuse salivation: may indicate tracheoesophageal fistula
Assess **neck**	Tonic neck reflex (Fencer's position)	Distended neck veins
		Fractured clavicle
		Unusually short neck
		Excess posterior cervical skin
		Resistance to neck flexion
Assess **cry**	Lusty cry	Weak, groaning cry: possible neurological abnormality
		High-pitched cry; hoarse or crowing inspirations; cat-like cry: possible neurological or chromosomal abnormality

ASSESSMENT	NORMAL	ABNORMAL
CHEST AND LUNG ASSESSMENT		
Assess the **chest**	Circular Enlargement of breasts Milky discharge from breasts	Depressed sternum Retractions, asymmetry of chest movements: indicates respiratory distress and possible pneumothorax
Assess the **lungs**	Abdominal respirations Respiration rate: 30 to 50 Respiration movement irregular in rate and depth Resonant chest (hollow sound on percussion)	Thoracic breathing, unequal motion of chest, rapid grasping or grunting respirations, flaring nares Deep sighing respirations Grunt on expiration: possible respiratory distress Hyper-resonance of chest or decreased resonance
HEART ASSESSMENT		
Assess the **rate, rhythm,** and **murmurs** of the heart	Rate: 100 to 160 at birth; stabilizes at 120 to 140 Regular rhythm Murmurs: significance cannot usually be determined in newborn	Heart rate above 200 or less than 100 Irregular rhythm Dextrocardia, enlarged heart
ABDOMEN AND GASTROINTESTINAL TRACT ASSESSMENT		
Assess the **abdomen**	Prominent	Distention of abdominal veins: possible portal vein obstruction
Assess the **gastrointestinal tract**	Bowel sounds present Liver 2 to 3 cm below right costal margin Spleen tip palpable May be able to palpate kidneys Bladder percussed 1 to 4 cm above symphysis pubis Umbilical cord with one vein and two arteries Soft granulation tissue at umbilicus	Visible peristaltic waves Increased pitch or frequency: intestinal obstruction Decreased sounds: paralytic ileus Distention of abdomen Enlarged liver or spleen Midline suprapubic mass: may indicate Hirschsprung's disease Enlarged kidney Distended bladder; presence of any masses One artery present in umbilical cord: may indicate other anomalies Wet umbilical stump or fetid odor from stump

ASSESSMENT	NORMAL	ABNORMAL
GENITOURINARY TRACT ASSESSMENT		
Assess the **genitalia**	Edema and bruising after delivery Unusually large clitoris in females a short time after birth Vaginal mucoid or bloody discharge may be present in the first week	Inguinal hernia
Urethra orifice	Urethra opens on ventral surface of penile shaft	Hypospadias (urethra opens on the inferior surface of the penis) Epispadias (urethra opens on the dorsal surface of the penis) Ulceration of urethral orifice
Testes	Testes in scrotal sac or inguinal canal	Hydroceles in males
SPINE AND EXTREMITIES ASSESSMENT		
Assess the **spine**	Straight spine	Spina bifida, pilonidal sinus; scoliosis
Assess **extremities**		Asymmetry of movement
	Soft click with thigh rotation	Sharp click with thigh rotation: indicates possible congenital hip Uneven major gluteal folds: indicates possible congenital hip Polydactyly (extra digits on a hand or foot); syndactyly (webbing or fusion of fingers or toes)
Assess **anus and rectum**	Patent anus	Closed anus: no meconium

HIGH RISK INFANTS

Premature Infant

Definition: An infant born before the end of the thirty-seventh week regardless of birth weight.

Characteristics

A. Maternal factors: diabetes, toxemia, chronic disease, chronic poor nutrition, premature rupture of membranes, placenta previa, abruptio placenta, incompetent cervix, other premature births, age, multiple pregnancies, etc.
B. Fetal factors: congenital anomalies, infection, other diseases.
C. Socioeconomic factors: low socioeconomic status, poor nutrition, unmarried, under seventeen years of age.
D. Other: cause unknown; accounts for large percentage of premature births.
E. Incidence: 8 percent of all live births.
   1. Factors associated with prematurity make it the leading cause of death in neonates.
   2. Primarily due to respiratory distress syndrome, infection, and intracranial hemorrhage.

Assessment

A. Assess digestive system.
   1. Gag and suck reflexes weak and poorly developed.
   2. Suck and swallow reflexes uncoordinated.
   3. Small stomach capacity.
   4. Poor ability to tolerate fats.
   5. Immature enzyme system.
B. Assess central nervous system and muscle tone.
   1. Poor muscle tone: muscles appear limp; baby assumes frog-like position when placed on abdomen.
   2. Weak, feeble cry.
   3. Weak reflexes.
   4. Heat regulation unstable.
      a. Body temperature below normal, small muscle mass, absent sweat or shiver responses.
      b. Large body surface in proportion to body weight.
      c. Lack of subcutaneous fat.
      d. Poor capillary response to environmental changes.

   5. Susceptibility to brain damage from high levels of bilirubin.
C. Assess respiratory system.
   1. Insufficient production of surfactant.
   2. Immaturity of alveoli.
   3. Immaturity of musculature and rib cage.
   4. Prone to respiratory disease.
D. Assess integumentary system.
   1. Skin thin and capillaries easily seen.
   2. Little subcutaneous fat.
   3. Lanugo prominent: hair on head is fine and fuzzy.
   4. Vernix may cover body if born between 31 and 33 wccks.
E. Assess immune system: resistance to infection decreased.
   1. Lack of passive immunity from mother (occurs late pregnancy).
   2. Inability to produce own antibodies—immature system.
   3. Skin is thin and offers little protection from disease-causing organisms.
F. Assess hepatic system: liver immature.
   1. Poor glycogen stores—increased susceptibility to hypoglycemia.
   2. Inability to conjugate bilirubin—susceptible to hyperbilirubinemia.
   3. Decreased ability to produce clotting factors.
   4. Decreased ability to produce immune factors.
G. Assess circulatory system.
   1. Capillary fragility increases susceptibility to hemorrhage, especially intracranial.
   2. Prone to anemia—poor iron stores.
H. Assess renal system.
   1. Renal function immature—poor ability to concentrate urine.
   2. Fluid and electrolyte balance precarious.
   3. Easily dehydrated.

Planning and Analysis

A. Needs of family are met.
   1. Separation is kept to a minimum.
   2. Information on baby's progress is given.
   3. Feelings and concerns are expressed.
   4. Instruction is provided.
B. Needs of infant are met.
   1. Baby is kept warm.
   2. Oxygen and humidity are administered.
   3. Nutrition and hydration status is maintained.
   4. Infection is prevented.

424

5. Circulatory status is maintained.
6. Normal development and feelings of trust are promoted.

Implementation

A. Provide for family's needs to be met.
   1. Allow parents to visit baby frequently; as soon as possible, involve parents in infant care to promote parent-to-infant attachment.
   2. Answer questions openly, provide up-to-date information on baby's progress.
   3. Allow parents to talk freely about infant, give support as needed, and help parents to accept reality of situation.
   4. Explain specialized care to parents. Have them report to pediatrician any of the following symptoms: diarrhea, vomiting, lack of appetite, or elevated temperature.
   5. Allow mother to feel confident in caring for infant before discharge. Explain to mother infant's special needs.
B. Provide immediate care to infant.
   1. Give immediate attention in delivery room and transport to nursery to maintain heat.
      a. Maintain skin temperature at about 36°C or 97.6°F in isolette or heated crib.
      b. Gradually wean infant from heated environment and watch temperature closely until stable.
      c. Warming infant too quickly may cause apneic spells.
   2. Administer humidity (distilled water) usually between 40 to 70 percent as ordered.
C. Evaluate respiratory status.
   1. Check respiratory rate–every hour and p.r.n.
   2. Observe for the following signs of respiratory distress:
      a. Color of skin.
      b. Flaring of nares.
      c. Grunting retractions.
   3. Auscultate breath sounds with stethoscope.
   4. Analyze oxygen concentration one to two hours or as necessary to prevent retrolental fibroplasia and to ensure adequate oxygenation.
   5. Observe for periods of apnea and stimulate by gently rubbing chest or tapping foot.
   6. Percuss, vibrate and suction as ordered to remove mucus.
D. Reposition every two hours to promote aeration of all lobes of lung and facilitate drainage.

E. Monitor blood gases and electrolytes frequently; IV regulated by infusion pump to prevent circulatory overload.
F. Initiate feedings as ordered (usually begin with sterile water or breast milk); progress to dilute formula or breast milk to full strength as tolerated.
G. Give gavage feeding if respirations are about 60 breaths per minute.
   1. Use premie nipple if bottle feeding.
   2. Infants often require alternate feedings of gavage and bottle feeding.
H. Maintain intake and output including stool and weigh daily.
I. Organize care to conserve energy with rest periods after each feeding.
J. Measure head circumference and length at least once a week.
K. Maintain aseptic technique and strict isolation techniques with infected babies.
L. Prevent skin breakdown: change position, careful cleansing and handling.
M. Observe for signs of infection: vomiting, jaundice, lack of appetite and lethargy.
N. Check heart rate by apical pulse for a full minute every one to two hours.
O. Frequently check for bleeding from umbilical catheter.
   1. Apply pressure to puncture site as necessary to prevent bleeding.
   2. Administer vitamin K as ordered after birth to prevent hemorrhage.
   3. Frequently check monitors if monitored electronically.
P. Gently stroke and talk to baby when giving care.
Q. Hang colorful mobiles or other nonharmful objects in crib.
R. Hold baby during feeding as soon as condition permits.
S. Encourage parents to hold, cuddle, feed, and diaper baby as soon as baby's condition permits.

Evaluation

A. Parents visit baby frequently, are interested and involved in the baby's care, and touch and gently stroke baby.
B. Parents ask questions and are able to express fears, concerns, and any feelings of guilt.
C. Infant's skin temperature remains between 36.1° to 36.5° C.

D. Blood gases are within normal limits, and there are no signs of respiratory distress, i.e., nasal flaring, grunting, poor color.

E. Infant is gaining weight, and there are no signs of dehydration or hypoglycemia.

F. Infant is urinating and passing stool.

G. No signs of infection are present.

H. Respirations and apical pulse are within normal limits.

I. No signs of abnormal bleeding.

Respiratory Distress Syndrome

Definition: A group of clinical symptoms signifying that the infant is experiencing problems with the respiratory system—also called hyaline membrane disease.

Characteristics

A. Symptoms are the result of a decrease in the amount of surfactant in the infant's lungs caused by one of the following conditions.
   1. Prematurity: immaturity of lungs and inability to produce surfactant.
   2. Hypoxia and acidosis.
   3. Hypothermia.
   4. High concentration of oxygen.

B. Respiratory distress syndrome is the most common cause of death in infants.

Assessment

A. Assess for increased respirations: greater than 60/min.

B. Assess for retractions: sternal and intercostal.

C. Check for presence of cyanosis and expiratory grunting.

D. Assess for increased apical pulse.

E. Evaluate nasal flaring and chin lag.

F. Evaluate for lack of activity or movement.

G. Assess for inability to take in sufficient oxygen leading to low oxygen and hypoxemia.

H. Assess for hypercarbia due to elevated levels of carbon dioxide.

I. Check for respiratory acidosis due to retention of carbon dioxide owing to inadequate pulmonary ventilation.

J. Evaluate for decreased body temperature.

K. Check for metabolic acidosis due to increased production of lactic acid.

L. Evaluate x-ray examination which may reveal:
   1. Atelectasis: collapsed portions of lung.
   2. Reticulogranular pattern bilaterally.
   3. Air bronchograms.

Planning and Analysis

A. Early diagnosis is made which is critical to survival rate.

B. The degree of respiratory distress is determined.

C. Measures are taken to relieve respiratory distress.

D. Hypoxemia is prevented.

E. Respiratory acidosis or alkalosis is prevented.

F. Emergency equipment is available.

Implementation

A. Prevent cold stress: infant is usually placed in isolette or open crib with overhead radiant warmer. Skin temperature is maintained with probe at 97.6°F or 36°C—thermoneutral environment.

B. Provide for nutrition and hydration: usually give IV glucose fluids during acute periods, then gradually increase feedings as tolerated.

C. Do careful monitoring of blood gases and electrolytes, color, and activity.

D. Administer oxygen to maintain pa O_2 50 to 70 mm Hg warmed and humidified. Monitor and record. Adjust concentration based on ABG's. Administer via hood, nasal prongs, endotracheal tubes, or bag and mask. Oxygen may be given at atmosphere or increased airway pressure.

E. Administer continuous positive pressure applied to lungs during spontaneous breathing. CPAP may be used.

F. Apply intermittent positive pressure to lungs during expiratory cycle. PEEP may be used.

G. Check and change nasal prongs; frequently analyze oxygen concentration.

H. Loosely tape endotracheal tube and check frequently for correct placement and connection at adapter site.

I. Suction infant with endotracheal tube:
   1. Disconnect from respirator at site of adapter.
   2. Instill a few minims to 0.5 ml of sterile normal saline into tube to loosen secretions.
   3. Suction no longer than five seconds using sterile catheter.
   4. Ventilate infant as needed during procedure.
   5. Reconnect tube to respirator, being sure it is in place and adapter is secure.
   6. Auscultate chest for breath sounds.

J. Gently handle infant with as little disturbance as possible.
K. Provide postural drainage and percussion if ordered.
L. Keep parents informed of infant's progress.
M. Allow parents to visit infant as much as possible and express their feelings about infant's illness.
N. Gently stroke and talk with infant while giving care.

Evaluation

A. Early recognition is made so early treatment is instituted.
B. Respiratory status is maintained (no signs of distress, such as grunting, retractions, or nasal flaring are exhibited).
C. Acid-base balance is maintained.
D. Body temperature is stabilized through specific measures to maintain warmth.
E. Blood gases are within normal limits.
F. Nutritional and metabolic status is maintained through IV feedings.
G. Monitoring of blood values, vital signs, and technical equipment allows close observation of infant's condition.
H. Infant is in restful environment and has psychosocial needs met.
I. Parents of ill infant are supported.

Small for Gestational Age

Definition: Refers to infants who are significantly undersize for gestational age. Also called intrauterine growth retardation (IUGR).

Characteristics

A. Postmature infants.
B. Defective embryonic development.
C. Placental insufficiency.
D. Associated factors: diabetes, toxemia, maternal infection, maternal malnutrition, cigarette smoking, multiple gestation.
E. Infant appearance.
  1. Little subcutaneous tissue.
  2. Loose, dry, scaling skin.
  3. Appears thin and wasted; old for size.
  4. May be meconium staining of skin, nails.
  5. Sparse hair on head.

6. Active, alert, seems hungry.
7. Cord dries more rapidly than normal infants.

Assessment

A. Assess for hypoglycemia or poor glucose control: nervousness, cyanosis, apnea, temperature instability, weak cry.
B. Assess for hypothermia: lethargy, poor feeding pattern, cold to touch, slow respiration.
C. Assess for asphyxia: may have been deprived while in utero or aspirated amniotic fluid. Infant may require resuscitation at birth.
D. Assess for polycythemia: usually asymptomatic but may have tachypnea, retractions.

Planning and Analysis

A. Any congenital anomalies are identified and appropriate treatment begun.
B. Normal body temperature is maintained.
C. Hypoglycemia identified and normal blood glucose levels are maintained.
D. Adequate growth and development are promoted.

Implementation

A. Provide care similar to premature infant until the infant is stabilized.
B. Protect from cold stress: keep warm, usually in isolette.
C. Perform tests for glucose levels.
D. Weigh daily and maintain intake and output.

Evaluation

A. Environmental heat is provided to maintain infant's temperature at 36.5°C or 97.7°F.
B. Glucose control remains stable and there are no signs of hypoglycemia.
C. Measures are taken to treat polycythemia.
D. Infant has steady weight gain and accurate daily weights are recorded.
E. Parents of infant are supported.

Postmature Infants

Definition: Refers to infants of over forty-two weeks gestation.

Characteristics

A. Placental function decreased.
B. Nutritional and oxygen needs are not met.

C. Infants exposed to chronic hypoxia.

D. Easily stressed during labor.

E. Increased morbidity and mortality due to above factors.

Assessment

A. Assess that vernix and lanugo are no longer present.

B. Assess skin: appears dry and wrinkled.

C. Check fingernails and toenails: usually long and may be meconium stained.

D. Assess size: may be SGA due to nutritional deficiency and chronic hypoxia.

E. Observe for hypoglycemia.

F. Observe for signs of birth injury: dislocated shoulder, fractured pelvis, facial paralysis, and CNS injury.

Planning and Analysis

A. Meconium aspiration as a complication is prevented by adequate suctioning before infant's first breath.

B. Infant's physiologic processes are stabilized, especially the respiratory system.

C. Nutritional and oxygen needs are met.

D. Measures to promote warmth begun and body temperature is maintained.

E. Possible complications such as asphyxia neonatorum and polycythemia are identified early and treatment instituted.

Implementation

A. Similar to care given to premature infants if premature characteristics are observed.
1. Immediate attention in the delivery room.
2. Heated crib or isolette to prevent cold stress.
3. Evaluate respiratory rate consistently.
4. Observe for signs of respiratory distress—administer oxygen and humidification if necessary.
5. Monitor blood gases and electrolytes.
6. Check need for IV feedings.
7. Maintain intake and output records.
8. Observe for signs of infection; monitor administration of antibiotics.
9. Prevent skin breakdown.

B. Symptomatic depending upon condition at birth. Care for as SGA in those infants who are underweight for gestational age.

Evaluation

A. Signs of hypoglycemia are identified and treatment begun.

B. Oral feeding or IV glucose shortly after birth prevents hypoglycemia.

C. Respirations and apical pulses are within normal range and respiratory distress avoided.

D. No signs of birth injuries or their complications.

E. Parents' anxiety is alleviated and concerns talked through.

Hyperbilirubinemia

Definition: An abnormal elevation of bilirubin in the newborn (above 13 to 15 mg/100 ml) in full term infant.

Characteristics

A. Functional immaturity of the liver: usually appears after twenty-four hours and disappears after ten days; physiologic jaundice.

B. Bacterial infections.

C. ABO and Rh incompatibilities: usually show up in the first twenty-four hours and may be severe.

D. Enclosed bleeding, such as hematoma, from trauma of delivery.

E. Pregnanediol hormone, present in mother's breast milk, may contribute to jaundice. (It inhibits conjugation of bilirubin by glucuronyl transferase.)

Assessment

A. Observe for jaundice which progresses from head to extremities.
1. Physiologic jaundice occurs three to five days after birth.
2. When levels reach above 12 mg/100 ml in full term infants and 15 mg/100 ml in premature infants jaundice may be termed pathological.

B. Observe for pallor.

C. Evaluate activity level: infant may be lethargic and feed poorly.

D. Assess if urine is concentrated and stools are light in color.

E. Assess progress of condition: if untreated, infant may progress from muscular rigidity or flaccidity to increased lethargy, high-pitched cry, respiratory distress, decreased Moro's reflex and spasms.

F. Evaluate blood tests.
1. Hemoglobin.

2. Bilirubin: important to measure amount of indirect bilirubin in blood, since unbound bilirubin is free to deposit in body tissues, such as skin, cardiac muscle, brain, and kidney. Unconjugated bilirubin deposited in the brain determines the extent of kernicterus.

Planning and Analysis

A. Infant's skin is observed and increase in jaundice is recognized.
B. Any changes in urine are identified.
C. Fluid balance is maintained.
D. The amount of unconjugated indirect bilirubin in the serum is reduced via phototherapy.
E. No side effects of phototherapy are noted.

Implementation

A. Observe infant for signs of increased jaundice.
B. Observe for and prevent acidosis/hypoxia and hypoglycemia, which decrease binding of bilirubin to albumin and contribute to jaundice.
C. Maintain adequate hydration and offer fluids between feedings as ordered.
D. Maintain skin temperature at 97.6°F; avoid cold stress.
E. Prevent infection.
F. Provide phototherapy: fluorescent light breaks down bilirubin into water soluble products.
   1. Do not clothe infant.
   2. Cover infant's eyes to prevent retinal damage.
   3. Change baby's position every two hours to ensure adequate exposure.
   4. Remove infant from light and remove eye patches during feedings; dress to keep infant warm.
   5. Carefully examine eyes for signs of irritation from eye patches.
   6. Keep an accurate record of hours spent under fluorescent lights.
G. Meet infant's emotional needs: cuddle, talk to infant, etc.
H. Reinforce physician's teaching to parents and allow parents to express concerns and feelings.
I. Monitor exchange transfusion: considered when bilirubin reaches high levels (20 mg/ml in full term infant; lower levels in premature infants).
   1. Exchange transfusion is usually performed in operating or delivery room.
   2. Infant is usually placed in radiant warmer and restrained.
   3. Resuscitative equipment and oxygen should be available.
   4. Blood should be no more than twenty-four hours old and warmed.
   5. Stomach contents are aspirated to prevent vomiting.
   6. Baseline vital signs are obtained and checked every fifteen to thirty minutes.
   7. Transfusion is usually given via umbilical catheter.
   8. Exchange usually done by alternately withdrawing and adding blood. Maximum 500 ml Rh-negative blood is given.
   9. Exchange usually takes forty-five to sixty minutes.
J. Administer care after transfusion.
   1. Observe for bleeding from the umbilical cord.
   2. Observe vital signs frequently.
   3. Maintain warmth.
   4. Administer oxygen if needed.
   5. Observe for signs of hypoglycemia, sepsis, cardiac arrest, or irregularities.
   6. Handle infant.
   7. Resume feedings after four to six hours.
   8. Keep umbilical cord moist in case other transfusions are indicated.

Evaluation

A. Decrease in the level of serum bilirubin occurs either due to phototherapy or exchange transfusions.
B. Complications in the infant from high levels of bilirubin do not occur (especially kernicterus).
C. Nutrition and hydration status are maintained.
D. Parent's anxiety is alleviated when they understand the condition and result of treatment program.
E. Emotional needs of infant are met during period of hospitalization.

Hemolytic Disease (Erythroblastosis Fetalis)

Definition: The destruction of red blood cells that results from an antigen-antibody reaction and is characterized by hemolytic anemia or hyperbilirubinemia.

Characteristics

A. Rh incompatibility: Rh antigens from the baby's blood enter the maternal bloodstream. The mother's blood does not contain Rh factor, so she produces anti-Rh antibodies. These antibodies are harmless to the mother but attach to the erythrocytes in the fetus and cause hemolysis. Exchange of fetal and maternal blood takes place primarily when the placenta separates at birth.

1. RhoGAM, $Rh_0(D)$ human immune globulin, should be given during first 72 hours after delivery if Rh-negative mother delivers Rh-positive fetus but remains unsensitized.
2. Sensitization rare with first pregnancy.
3. Diagnosis of Rh incompatibility.
   a. Begins in pregnancy, with discoveries of antibodies in an Rh-negative mother's blood by means of indirect Coombs' test.
   b. Titration is used to determine the extent to which antibodies are present.
   c. Spectrophotometric analysis of amniotic fluid for bilirubin determines the severity of the disease—the higher the bilirubin content, the more severe the disease.
   d. Testing of cord blood—direct Coombs' test—determines the presence of maternal antibodies attached to baby's cells.

B. ABO incompatibility—usually less severe.

Assessment

A. Assess for anemia which is caused by destruction of red blood cells.
B. Assess for jaundice which develops rapidly after birth, before 24 hours.
C. Evaluate for edema—usually seen in stillborn infants or those who die shortly after birth; most likely due to cardiac failure.

Planning and Analysis

A. Continued destruction of red blood cells is reversed and treatment reverses hyperbilirubinemia.
B. Anemia is relieved.
C. Brain damage from high levels of unconjugated bilirubin is prevented.
D. Complete recovery is expected if kernicterus does not occur.

Implementation

A. Administer immunization against hemolytic disease with Rho-GAM as ordered. (Now given at 28 weeks and postpartum.)
B. Monitor exchange transfusion after birth or intrauterine transfusion.
C. Follow interventions listed under hyperbilirubinemia.

Evaluation

A. Decrease in high levels of serum bilirubin.
B. No evidence of brain damage or other complications from high levels of bilirubin.
C. Complete recovery occurs.
D. Mother of infant is reassured that infant is fine and will suffer no untoward effects from condition.

Sepsis in the Neonate

Definition: Generalized infection resulting from the presence of pathogenic bacteria in the bloodstream.

Predisposing Factors

A. Prolonged rupture of membranes, over twenty-four hours.
B. Long difficult labor or prolonged resuscitation after birth.
C. Maternal infection.
D. Aspiration of amniotic fluids or vaginal secretions during birth.
E. Aspiration of formula after birth.
F. Infection within nursery or among nursery personnel (nosocomial).
G. Usually appears within the first forty-eight hours after birth but may begin prenatally or post-delivery.
H. May quickly lead to septicemia or meningitis if not treated promptly.

Assessment

A. General assessment is important as symptoms may be vague.
B. Assess feeding, which may be poor, and sucking reflex.
C. Check for presence of diarrhea.
D. Assess for periods of apnea or irregular respirations.
E. Check for jaundice.
F. Assess for low-grade fever or subnormal temperature.
G. Evaluate activity level for lethargy.
H. Assess for irritability.

I. Diagnosis is made from aspiration of gastric contents, which are examined for polymorphonuclear cells, or cultures taken of blood, urine, spinal fluids, throat, skin lesions, and the umbilical area.

Planning and Analysis

A. Identification of infectious process made.
B. Infectious process is treated.
C. Infant status is viable.
D. Mother of infant and family reassured.

Implementation

A. Administer antibiotics and observe carefully for toxicity because of liver and kidney immaturity.
B. Maintain warmth—usually in an isolette.
C. Administer oxygen as necessary.
D. Administer IV fluids if ordered; otherwise, give fluids as ordered to maintain hydration, electrolytes, and calories.
E. Maintain isolation and proper hand washing techniques.
F. Check respiratory apical pulse frequently.
G. Stimulate if apnea is present by gently rubbing chest or foot.
H. Maintain intake and output.
I. Check temperature.
J. Weigh daily.
K. Observe for signs of jaundice.
L. Keep parents informed of infant's progress.
M. Allow parents to visit infant as much as possible.
N. Talk and gently stroke infant while giving care.

Evaluation

A. Infant's temperature is within the normal range.
B. Infant is taking adequate nutrition.
C. Respirations are regular and within normal limits.
D. Infant is active and calm (not irritable).

Infants of Diabetic Mothers

Characteristics

A. May be delivered early to prevent intrauterine death; usually delivered after thirty-six weeks.
B. Often delivered by cesarean section.
C. Children with diabetic mothers have a higher incidence of congenital anomalies than the general population.

D. High incidence of hypoglycemia, respiratory distress, hypocalcemia, and hyperbilirubinemia.

Assessment

A. Assess for excessive size and weight due to excess fat and glycogen in tissues.
  1. High blood sugar levels in mother cross the placenta and enter the baby's bloodstream, elevating blood sugar levels.
  2. High blood sugar stimulates infant's metabolic system to store glycogen and fat and increase the production of insulin.
B. Assess appearance of infant—may be puffy in face and cheeks.
C. Observe for signs of hypoglycemia—twitching, difficulty feeding, lethargy, apnea, seizures, and cyanosis.
D. Observe for signs of respiratory distress—tachypnea, cyanosis, retractions, grunting, nasal flaring.
E. Hyperbilirubinemia.

Planning and Analysis

A. Hypoglycemia prevented.
B. Normal growth and development promoted.
C. Respiratory status is maintained.
D. No untoward complications occur.

Implementation

A. Administer care similar to premature infant.
B. Feed glucose as necessary: infant may need IV therapy depending upon condition.
C. Be aware that any infant of a diabetic mother will be started on hypoglycemia protocol regardless of weight.

Evaluation

A. No signs of hypoglycemia. Evaluate two blood glucose levels within normal range.
B. No signs of respiratory distress.

Hypoglycemia

Definition: Abnormal low level of sugar in the blood.

Characteristics

A. Placental dysfunction.
B. Diabetes in mother.

C. Cold stress.

D. Renal disease, cardiac disease, preeclampsia, or chronic infection in the mother.

E. Small for gestational age infants.

F. Postterm infant.

G. Asphyxia at birth.

H. Infection in infant or any condition that stresses the metabolic rate and increases the need for glucose.

Assessment

A. Assess for presence of cyanosis.

B. Assess for increased respiratory rate.

C. Check any twitching, nervousness or tremors.

D. Evaluate for lethargy and poor muscle tone.

E. Assess unstable temperature.

F. Assess for shrill or intermittent cry.

G. Check for any feeding problems.

H. Evaluate apneic periods closely.

I. Evaluate blood sugar values: normal is 45 to 100/100 ml of blood; usually around 60 to 75/100 ml.
  1. Term infant: 30/40 mg/100 ml blood.
  2. Preterm: 20 mg/100 ml blood.

J. Monitor screening that is done with special testing sticks, with laboratory studies as a follow-up.

Planning and Analysis

A. Normal blood glucose level is maintained.

B. Respiratory status is maintained.

C. Infection is prevented.

D. Normal growth and development are maintained.

Implementation

A. Prevent low blood glucose through early feedings.

B. Administer glucose orally or IV, depending on baby's condition.

C. Perform close monitoring of blood sugar values every one to two hours.

D. Give care as for other high risk infants.

Evaluation

A. Blood glucose level remains within normal limits.

B. Cold stress is avoided and respiratory status is normal.

C. Complications do not occur.

D. Infant begins to put on weight and responses are within normal limits.

Infant Born to Mother with Drug Addiction

Characteristics

A. There is a direct relationship between the duration of addiction, dosage, and the severity of symptoms.

B. Heroin addicted mother: infant may appear normal at birth with a low birth weight.
  1. Withdrawal within 12–24 hours—may last 5–7 days.
  2. Infant appears less ill than when mother is taking methadone.
  3. Heroin causes early maturity of the liver.

C. Mother on methadone.
  1. Withdrawal 1–2 days to 1 week or more; most evident 48–72 hours and may last 6 days to 8 weeks.
  2. Infant may appear to be very ill.
  3. May develop jaundice due to prematurity.

D. Mother addicted to cocaine, a stimulant.
  1. Infant evidences decreased interactive behavior, feeding problems, irregular sleep patterns, diarrhea.
  2. 7 out of 1000 mothers will have infants with major deformities—especially of the kidneys.

Assessment

A. Assess for irritability, tremors, hyperactivity, and hypertonicity.

B. Assess for respiratory distress and ventilatory capacity.

C. Observe for the following signs:
  1. Vomiting.
  2. High-pitched cry.
  3. Sneezing.
  4. Fever.
  5. Diarrhea.
  6. Excessive sweating.
  7. Poor feeding.
  8. Extreme sucking of fists.

D. Assess for convulsions, which are rare.

Planning and Analysis

A. Withdrawal symptoms do not lead to complications.

B. Withdrawal symptoms are of reduced severity.

C. Respiratory status is maintained.

D. Feeding schedule resumes and infant tolerates food well.

E. Gastrointestinal tract functions normally.

Implementation

A. Monitor respiratory and cardiac rates every thirty minutes and p.r.n.

B. Take temperature every four to eight hours and p.r.n.

C. Maintain warmth and swaddle infant in blanket.

D. Reduce external stimuli and handle infant infrequently.
E. Hold infant firmly and close to body during feedings and when giving care.
F. Pad sides of crib to protect infant from injury.
G. Administer small, frequent feedings as ordered.
H. Suction if necessary.
I. Provide careful skin care: cleanse buttocks and anal area carefully.
J. Measure intake and output.
K. Keep mother informed of infant's progress.
L. Promote mother's interest in infant.
M. Administer medications as ordered, usually paragoric or phenobarbital.

Evaluation
A. Irritability gradually decreases.
B. Temperature remains stable.
C. No signs of skin rash.
D. Infant is maintaining adequate nutrition and weight gain.
E. No signs of injury or complications.

Fetal Alcohol Syndrome
Characteristics
A. Maternal alcohol abuse throughout pregnancy results in fetal alcohol syndrome.
 1. Most serious cause of teratogenesis.
 2. In affected infants, growth is retarded; they are microcephalic with severe mental retardation.
B. Lesser amount of alcohol ingested throughout pregnancy results in less severe symptoms.
 1. Prenatal and/or postnatal growth retardation.
 2. Developmental delay.
 3. May not be diagnosed until early childhood.

Assessment
A. Monitor for respiratory distress and apnea.
B. Observe for cyanosis.
C. Observe for seizures.
D. Check for major brain dysfunction symptoms.

Implementation
A. Position on side to facilitate drainage of secretions.
 1. Keep resuscitation equipment at bedside.
 2. Have suction available, especially following feeding.

B. Administer small feedings and burp well.
C. Support family and assist to accept anomalies.

INFERTILITY

Definition: The inability to conceive after one year of regular intercourse with no contraceptive measures, or the inability to deliver a live fetus after three consecutive conceptions.

Characteristics
A. General statistics indicate that two-thirds of couples achieve pregnancy within six months and 80 percent within one year.
B. Approximately 40–50 percent of all infertility is attributed to the female.
 1. Following investigation and treatment, 50–70 percent achieve pregnancy.
 2. Of the 30–50 percent who do not achieve pregnancy, 10 percent have no pathologic basis for infertility.

Assessment
A. Causes of infertility.
 1. Female.
  a. Functional: hormonal dysfunction causing insufficient gonadotropin secretions.
  b. Anatomic: ovarian factors, uterine abnormalities, tubal, peritoneal, and cervical factors.
  c. Chronic infections.
  d. Psychological problems.
  e. Immunologic reaction to partner's sperm.
 2. Male.
  a. Semen disorders—volume, motility, or density; abnormal or immature sperm.
  b. Systemic disease such as diabetes.
  c. Genital infection.
  d. Disorders of the testes.
  e. Structural abnormalities.
  f. Genetic defects.
  g. Immunologic disorders.
  h. Chemicals, drugs, and environmental factors.
  i. Psychological problems.
  j. Sexual problems.

B. Tests for infertility.
   1. Female.
      a. Complete physical exam and health history.
      b. Basal body temperature graph.
      c. Endometrial biopsy.
      d. Progesterone blood levels.
      e. Tests to determine structural integrity of the tubes, ovaries, and uterus.
      f. Male-female interaction studies.
   2. Male.
      a. Detailed history and physical examination.
      b. Semen analysis (most conclusive).
      c. Other laboratory tests: gonadotropin assay, serum testosterone levels, and urine 17-ketosteroid levels.
      d. Testicular biopsy.
C. Treatment.
   1. Female.
      a. Identification of underlying abnormality or dysfunction and correction.
      b. Hormone therapy.
      c. Surgical restoration.
      d. Drug therapy.
   2. Male.
      a. Correction of anatomic dysfunctions or infections.
      b. Counseling for sexual dysfunctions (education, counseling, or therapy).
      c. Proper nutrition with vitamin supplements.
      d. Hormone supplements: testosterone or chorionic gonadotropin.

Implementation

A. Education of couple.
   1. Information about diagnostic and treatment techniques.
   2. Information about reproductive and sexual function and factors that may interfere with fertility.
B. Provide emotional support.
   1. Encourage couple to discuss frustration, anger, etc., and express feelings.
   2. Suggest couple join groups to share concerns with other couples.
C. Explore alternatives such as adoption.
D. Provide information and preparation for surgery, if necessary.

Influences on Parenthood

A. Tendency toward smaller families.
B. Career-oriented women who limit family size or who do not want children.
C. Early sexual experimentation, necessitating sexual education, contraceptive information.
D. Tendency toward postponement of children.
   1. Until education is completed.
   2. For economic factors.
E. High divorce rates.
F. Alternate family designs.
   1. Single parenthood.
   2. Communal family.

FAMILY PLANNING

General Concepts

A. General concepts.
   1. Dealing with individuals with particular ideas regarding contraception.
   2. No perfect method of birth control.
   3. Method must be suited to individual.
   4. Individuals involved must be thoroughly counseled on all available methods and how they work, including advantages and disadvantages.
   5. Once a method is chosen both parties should be thoroughly instructed in its use.
   6. Individuals involved must be motivated to succeed.
B. Effectiveness depends upon:
   1. Method chosen.
   2. Degree to which couple follows prescribed regimen.
   3. Thorough understanding of method.
   4. Motivation on part of individuals concerned.

Role of Nurse in Family Planning

A. Education of client in various methods available, their effectiveness, and their side effects.
B. Help clients explore their feelings regarding birth control and what they find acceptable and not acceptable.
C. Create open relaxed atmosphere allowing clients to express concerns and feelings about birth control.
D. Thorough explanation of how method works.
E. Instruction of client in possible complications and side effects.

CONTRACEPTIVE METHODS

Natural Contraceptive Methods

A. Periodic abstinence: 75% effective.
  1. Based on three principles:
    a. Ovulation usually occurs fourteen days before period begins.
    b. An ovum may be fertilized twelve to twenty-four hours after release from ovary.
    c. Sperm usually survives only 24 hours in the uterine environment.
    d. If coitus is avoided during the fertile period, pregnancy should not occur.
  2. Cervical mucus: couple avoids intercourse during peak 72-hour period of cycle, when mucus becomes clear, stringy, stretchable, and slippery.
B. Coitus interruptus: 60% effective.
  1. Requires withdrawal of penis before ejaculation.
  2. Pre-ejaculatory fluid may contain sperm.
C. Lactation—unreliable.
  1. Breast-feeding has contraceptive effect.
  2. Prolactin's inhibition of luteinizing hormone which maintains menstruation.

Mechanical Methods

A. Condom: 95–98% effect with proper application.
  1. Acts as mechanical barrier by collecting sperm and not allowing contact with vaginal area.
  2. Prevents spread of disease.
B. Diaphragm: 80% effective; with proper use, 98%.
  1. Functions by blocking external os and closing access to cervical canal by sperm. It is a mechanical barrier.
  2. Must be used in conjunction with vaginal cream or jelly to be effective.
C. Contraceptive sponge: 80–90% effective.
  1. Inserted deep into vagina, sponge releases spermicide.
  2. Decreases risk of STDs.
  3. May be risk of developing toxic shock syndrome.
D. Cervical cap: 80–90% effective.
  1. Rubber cap with spermicide placed over cervical opening.
  2. May decrease risk of STD.
E. Intrauterine devices: 95% effective.
  1. Methods of action—not completely clear.
    a. More rapid transport of ovum through tube reaching endometrium before it is "ready" for implantation.
    b. IUD may cause substances to accumulate in uterus and interfere with implantation.
    c. IUD may stimulate production of cellular exudate, which interferes with the ability of sperm to migrate to fallopian tubes.
  2. Usually made of soft plastic or nickel-chromium alloy.
  3. Complications: perforation of uterus; infection: increased incidence of PID; spotting between periods; heavy menstrual flow or prolonged flow; and cramping during menstruation.

Chemical Methods

A. Oral contraceptives: 96–98% effective.
  1. Contraceptive effect occurs by:
    a. Artificially raising the blood levels of estrogen and/or progesterone, thereby preventing the release of FSH and LH. Without FSH the follicle does not mature and ovulation fails to take place.
    b. Endometrial changes.
    c. Alteration in cervical mucus, making it hostile to sperm.
    d. Altered tubal function.
  2. Types of birth control pills.
    a. Combined: contains both estrogen and progesterone.
    b. Sequential (mimics normal hormonal cycle): estrogen given alone for 15 to 16 days, followed by combination of estrogen and progestin for the next five days.
  3. Minor side effects, which usually diminish within a few months: breast fullness and tenderness; edema, weight gain; nausea and vomiting; chloasma; and breakthrough bleeding.
  4. More serious side effects: thrombophlebitis; pulmonary embolism; hypertension.
B. Chemical agent: Nonoxynol-9 or octoxynol-9
  1. Agent acts by killing or paralyzing sperm—may kill STD agents.
  2. Agent acts as a vehicle for spermicide as well as a mechanical barrier through which sperm cannot swim.
  3. Available forms are foams, creams, jellies or suppositories.

Operative Sterilization Procedures

A. Vasectomy.
  1. Surgical procedure with local anesthesia on outpatient basis.
    a. Incision made over ductus deferens on each side of scrotum; sperm ducts isolated and severed.
    b. Ends ligated, lumen coagulated, clipped or polyethylene tubing used with a stopcock for

potential reversal.

c. Absorbable sutures used to close the skin.

2. Client instruction for care.

a. Apply ice with pain or swelling.

b. Use scrotal support for one week.

c. Inform client that it takes 4–6 weeks and 3–36 ejaculations to clear sperm from ductus.

d. Sperm samples (2 or 3) should be checked for sperm count.

e. Client rechecked at 6 and 12 months to insure fertility has not been restored by recanalization.

3. Possible side effects of procedure.

a. Hematoma, sperm granulomas, and spontaneous reanastomosis.

b. For those who wish to reverse process, 65 percent are successful.

B. Tubal ligation most common method; (removal of uterus and ovaries is permanent method of sterilization).

1. Accomplished by abdominal or vaginal procedures; most common method is transection of fallopian tubes.

a. Tubes are isolated, then crushed, ligated, or plugged (newer reversible procedure).

b. The postpartal and mini-laparotomy procedures require hospitalization.

c. A newer procedure, laparoscopic sterilization requires an incision at the umbilicus, the tube coagulated, and may be transected.

2. Complications of procedure include bowel perforation, infection, hemorrhage, and adverse anesthesia effects.

a. Reversal of tubal ligations results in overall pregnancy rate of 15 percent.

b. Three-quarters of these pregnancies result in live births and 10 percent are tubal pregnancies.

THERAPEUTIC ABORTIONS

General Considerations

A. Legality.

1. Abortion is now legal in all states as the result of a Supreme Court decision in January 1973.

2. It is regulated in the following manner. First trimester—decision between client and physician; second trimester—decision between client and physician (state may regulate who performs the abortion and where it can be done); third trimester—states may regulate and prohibit abortion except to preserve the health or life of the mother.

B. Indications.

1. Medical: psychiatric conditions or diseases such as chronic hypertension, nephritis, severe diabetes, cancer, or acute infection such as rubella; possible genetic defects in the infant or severe erythroblastosis fetalis.

2. Nonmedical: socioeconomic reasons, unmarried, financial burden, too young to care for infant.

C. Preparation of the individual.

1. Advise client of available sources of abortion.

2. Inform client as to what to expect from the abortion procedure.

3. Provide emotional support during decision-making period.

4. Maintain an open, nonjudgmental atmosphere in which the individual may express concerns or guilt.

5. Encourage and support the individual once the decision is made and after surgery.

6. Give information about contraceptives.

D. Complications and effects.

1. Abortion should be performed before the twelfth week, if possible, because complications and risks are lower during this time.

2. Complications.

a. Infection.

b. Bleeding.

c. Sterility.

d. Uterine perforation.

Techniques

A. First trimester.

1. Dilatation and curettage (D & C).

a. Cervical canal is dilated with instruments of increasingly large diameter.

b. Fetus and accessory structure is removed with forceps.

c. Endometrium is scraped with curette to assure that all products of conception are removed.

d. Process usually takes fifteen to twenty minutes.

2. Vacuum aspirator.

a. Hose-linked curette is inserted into dilated cervix.

b. Hose is attached to suction.

c. The vacuum aspirator lessens the chance of uterine perforation, reduces blood loss, and reduces the time of the procedure.

B. Second trimester abortion.
1. Hysterotomy.
   a. Incision is made through abdominal wall into uterus.
   b. Procedure is usually performed between the fourteenth and sixteenth week in pregnancy.
   c. Products of conception are removed with forceps.
   d. Uterine cavity is curetted.
   e. Tubal ligation may be done at same time.
   f. Client usually requires several days of hospitalization.
   g. Operation requires general or spinal anesthesia.
2. Intraamniotic injection or amniocentesis abortion.
   a. Performed after the fourteenth to sixteenth week of pregnancy.
   b. From 50 to 200 ml of amniotic fluid are removed from the amniotic cavity and replaced with hypertonic of 20 to 50 percent saline instilled through gravity drip over a period of forty-five to sixty minutes.
   c. Increased osmotic pressure of the amniotic fluid causes the death of the fetus.
   d. Uterine contractions usually begin in about twelve hours and the products of conception are expelled in twenty-four to thirty hours.
   e. Oxytocic drugs may be given if contractions do not begin.
   f. Complications.
      (1) Infusion of hypertonic saline solution into uterus.
      (2) Infection.
      (3) Disseminated intravascular coagulation disease may develop during procedure.
      (4) Hemorrhage.
3. Prostaglandins.
   a. These hormone-like acids cause abortion by stimulating the uterus to contract.
   b. They may be administered IV into the uterine cavity through the cervical canal, into the posterior fornix of the vagina, or after twelve weeks into the amniotic cavity. The

IV method is least effective and has many possible side effects.

Abortion Procedure

Assessment
A. Observe for excessive bleeding.
B. Assess for symptoms of infection.
C. Assess for hypernatremia in saline abortions.
D. Check for nausea and vomiting.

Implementation
A. Administer preoperative medications.
B. Ensure that client understands the procedure.
C. Offer emotional support and let client express feelings.
D. Monitor IV.
E. Check vital signs pre- and postoperatively.
F. Administer pain medications as ordered.
G. Instruct client to watch for signs of excessive bleeding (more than a normal menstrual period) and infection (elevated temperature, foul-smelling discharge, persistent abdominal pain).
H. Administer oxytocic drug as ordered.
I. Administer RhoGAM as ordered for an Rh-negative client.
J. Offer fluids as tolerated, after vital signs are stable and client is alert and responsive.

PRENATAL DIAGNOSIS

Genetic Amniocentesis

Indications
A. Advanced maternal age—over 35, or suspected abnormality.
   1. Previous child with chromosomal abnormality.
   2. Parent carrying chromosomal abnormality.
   3. Mother carrying X-linked disease.
   4. Parents carrying inborn error of metabolism.
   5. Both parents carrying autosomal recessive disease.
B. Test provides clearest chromosome profile, but is usually done at 16 weeks—may be done as early as 12 weeks.

Procedure
A. Amniotic fluid obtained via transabdominal or suprapubic amniocentesis.
   1. Complications rare (less than 1 percent).
   2. Rh-negative women would receive Rh-immune

globulin after amniocentesis, if not already sensitized.

B. Performed at about 16 weeks; takes 2 to 4 weeks for results.

C. Positive test indicates fetus has genetic disorder.

Chorionic Villus Sampling (CVS)

Indications

A. Diagnostic capability similar to amniocentesis; may replace it for prenatal diagnosis in the future.

B. Advantage is that diagnostic information available before end of first trimester of pregnancy, between 8 and 12 weeks.

Procedure

A. A transcervical approach used to aspirate chorionic villi from the placenta through endocervix.

B. Syringe contents (villi) inspected microscopically and prepared for culture.

C. Results are available in 1 to 2 weeks.

Alpha Feto-Protein (AFP)

A. Principle screening procedure for detection of neural tube defect (spina bifida, hydrocephalus; incidence is 1-2/1000 births in U.S.).

    1. Recently researchers have matched AFP levels to other problems.

    2. Low levels detect Down's syndrome; high levels risk of premature delivery, toxemia, low birth weight, etc.

B. Multi-purpose test done at 15 weeks.

C. Mother's blood is analyzed for amount of AFP that liver normally re-releases at a known and increasing amount as pregnancy proceeds.

D. Procedure allows families to choose whether to have a child with an identified birth defect.

Appendix 1. COMMON DRUGS IN OBSTETRICS AND GYNECOLOGY

Name of Drug and Action	Uses and Side Effects	Nursing Implications
Oxytocin, Syntocinon, Pitocin Classification: oxytocic Produces rhythmic contractions of uterine musculature Dosage: varies with method and purpose of administration. IV: 5–10 USP units in 500 or 1,000 ml 5% dextrose in saline solution infused at rate 0.5–0.75 ml/min. Calibrated pump 2.5 USP units in 50 ml 5% D/W. Start at 1 mic/min and increase as necessary	Used to induce labor, constrict uterus, and decrease hemorrhage after delivery and postabortion Stimulates contractile tissue in lactating breast to eject milk Side effects: water intoxication, allergic reactions, death due to uterine rupture, pelvic hematomas, bradycardia Excessive contractions more frequent than every 2 1/2 minutes or lasting longer than 40-60 seconds.	Observe for signs of sensitivity and overdose Monitor strength and duration of uterine contractions Check FHT every 15 minutes and p.r.n. Take pulse and blood pressure every hour Contractions of 90 seconds with no resting period stop infusion immediately and notify physician
Methergine Classification: oxytocic Produces constrictive effects on smooth muscle of uterus (more prolonged constrictive effects as compared to rhythmic effects of oxytocin); also has generalized vasoconstrictive effect Usual IM dose 0.2 mg; may be repeated in 2–4 hrs; usual oral dose 0.2 mg 3–4 × a day for 2 days	Used primarily after delivery to produce firm uterine contractions and decrease uterine bleeding May be used to prevent postabortal hemorrhage Side effects include nausea, vomiting, dizziness, increased blood pressure, dyspnea, and chest pain	Check blood pressure and pulse before administration of medication, and check vital signs frequently after administration Injectable form deteriorates rapidly when exposed to lights and heat; do not use if discoloration occurs

Name of Drug and Action	Uses and Side Effects	Nursing Implications
Apresoline (hydralazine hydrochloride) Classification—antihypertensive Dosage: p.o. 12.5 mg b.i.d., increased incrementally to maximum 100 mg b.i.d.	Decreases peripheral resistance and peripheral vasodilatation Side effects: flushing, headache, nausea, vomiting, tachycardia, palpitations, lupus syndrome and leukopenia	Monitor blood pressure and pulse rate. Observe for orthostatic hypotension, tachycardia, palpitations, headache, dizziness, nausea, vomiting Give drug with meals to increase absorption.
Magnesium sulfate Depressive effects on central nervous system, and smooth, skeletal, and cardiac muscle Produces peripheral vasodilation Given IV in preeclampsia and eclampsia; dosage varies Usual dosage: initial dosage 4 gm in 250 cc 5% D/W at 5 cc/30 sec (approximately 20 min) or in continuous infusion	Used to prevent convulsions in preeclampsia and eclampsia. Also counteracts uterine tetany after large doses of oxytocin Side effects: *Maternal:* extreme thirst, hypotension, flaccidity, circulatory collapse, depression of CNS and cardiac system. *Fetal:* crosses placenta, lethargy, hypotonia Antidote: Calcium Gluconate. Keep available at bedside	Observe carefully for signs of magnesium toxicity: extreme thirst, feeling hot all over; loss of patellar reflex Monitor respirations (greater than 12/min), BP (hypotension), and P closely in order to assess effect of drug. Never leave client alone Patellar reflex should be checked continuously Check urine output continuously (greater than 30 cc/hr)
Vasodilan (isoxsuprine) Classification: vasodilator, pure beta drug, B_2 receptor stimulant; sympathomimetic Relaxing effects on circulatory and uterine smooth muscle IV 50 mg in 500 ml infusion by calibrated pump 0.1 mg/min. Increase rate q. 10 min until 1.5 mg/min max. IM dosage 10–20 mg q. 2–3 hrs. Usual oral maintenance dose 10–20 mg; tablets 3–4 times daily. Continue for 24 hours until contractions stop or side effects indicate need to stop infusion	Treatment of premature labor or during labor when contractions are unusually frequent and not coordinated; most effective when given in early latent phase of labor; rarely stops active labor Side effects: nausea, vomiting, dizziness, transient hypotension and tachycardia Doses greater than 10 mg may cause hypotension Antagonist: propranolol 0.25 mg to 1 mg IV bolus × three doses	Take blood pressure and pulse frequently; may be on continuous monitoring Observe for signs of tachycardia (pulse > 140) and hypotension (BP < 90/60) Maintain bed rest Trendelenburg's or side-lying position Monitor uterine activity and FHT
Ritodrine (improved analog of isoxsuprine)	Hydrate woman prior to infusion with IV solution of 1000 cc normal saline Continuous monitoring (Swan-Ganz) of mother and infant important as mother-infant deaths have occurred	Same as above
Terbutaline, B_2 receptor stimulant; sympathomimetic	Treatment of premature labor and requires hospitalization Side effects: tachycardia, palpitations, sweating, tremors, restlessness, lethargy, drowsiness, headache, nausea, vomiting	Same as above

Appendix 2. DRUGS ADVERSELY AFFECTING THE HUMAN FETUS

Drugs	Adverse Effect	Comments
Analgesics		
Heroin and morphine	Respiratory depression; neonatal death; addiction	Near term Fairly well documented
Salicylates	Neonatal bleeding; coagulation defects	Near term
Anesthetics		
Mepivacaine	Fetal bradycardia; neonatal depression	Near term More studies needed
Antibacterials		
Chloramphenicol	"Gray syndrome" and death	Near term Fairly well documented
Nitrofurantoin	Hemolysis	Near term More studies needed
Novobiocin	Hyperbilirubinemia	Near term More studies needed
Streptomycin	8th nerve damage; hearing loss; multiple skeletal anomalies	Throughout pregnancy Debatable, more studies needed
Sulfonamides (long acting)	Hyperbilirubinemia and kernicterus	Near term Fairly well documented
Tetracyclines	Inhibition of bone growth; discoloration of teeth	2nd and 3rd trimesters Fairly well documented
Anticarcinogens		
Amethopterin	Cleft palate; abortion	1st trimester Fairly well documented
Aminopterin	Cleft palate; abortion	1st trimester Known teratogen
Cyclophosphamide	Severe stunting; fetal death; extremity defects	1st trimester More studies needed
Anticoagulants		
Warfarin	Fetal death; hemorrhage	Throughout pregnancy More studies needed
Antidiabetics		
Chlorpropamide	Prolonged neonatal hypoglycemia	Throughout pregnancy More evidence needed before implication
Tolbutamide	Congenital anomalies	Throughout pregnancy One reported case only; evidence lacking
Antimalarials		
Quinine	Deafness	More studies needed
Antimitotic Agents		
Podophyllum	Fetal resorption; multiple deformities	More studies needed
Antithyroid Agents		
Methimazole	Goiter and mental retardation	From 14th week on Fairly well documented
Potassium iodide	Goiter and mental retardation	From 14th week on Fairly well documented

440

Appendix 2. DRUGS ADVERSELY AFFECTING THE HUMAN FETUS (continued)

Drugs	Adverse Effect	Comments
Antithyroid Agents (continued)		
Prophylthiouracil	Goiter and mental retardation	From 14th week on Fairly well documented
Radioactive iodine	Congenital hypothyroidism	From 14th week on Fairly well documented
Depressants		
Phenobarbital	Neonatal bleeding; increased rate of neonatal drug metabolism	In excessive amounts
Reserpine	Nasal block	Near term One report only More studies needed
Thalidomide	Phocomelia; hearing defect	28th–42nd day Known teratogen
Diuretics		
Ammonium chloride	Acidosis	
Thiazides (Hydrochlorothiazide) (Chlorothiazide) (Methyclothiazide)	Thrombocytopenia; neonatal death	Latter part of pregnancy One report only; evidence lacking
Stimulants		
Dextroamphetamine	Transposition of great vessels	One report only More evidence needed
Phenmetrazine	Skeletal and visceral anomalies	4th–12th week One report only More evidence needed
Sex Steroids		
Androgens, estrogens and oral progestogens	Masculinization and labial fusion (early in pregnancy); clitoris enlargement (later in pregnancy)	Fairly well documented
Miscellaneous		
Acetophenetidin	Methemoglobinemia	More studies needed
Cholinesterase inhibitors	Transient muscular weakness	Throughout pregnancy More studies needed
Hexamethonium bromide	Neonatal ileus and death	Throughout pregnancy More studies needed
Iophenoxic acid	Elevation of serum protein-bound iodine	
Isonicotinic acid hydrazide (INH)	Retarded psychomotor activity	More studies needed
Lysergic acid diethylamide (LSD)	Chromosomal damage; stunted offspring	1st trimester More studies needed
Nicotine and smoking	Small babies	Throughout pregnancy More studies needed
Vitamin A	Congenital anomalies; cleft palate; eye damage, syndactyly	Throughout pregnancy In large doses only
Vitamin D	Excessive blood calcium; mental retardation	Throughout pregnancy In large doses only
Vitamin K analogues	Hyperbilirubinemia; kernicterus	Near term; In large doses
Cocaine	Decreased interactive behavior; feeding problems; possible deformities	Addiction throughout pregnancy

6

PEDIATRIC
NURSING

This chapter presents an overview of the basic principles of pediatric nursing and is organized by system and according to the nursing process. In addition to a thorough exploration of each illness or disease, this chapter describes therapeutic approaches for each phase of child development. An understanding of pediatric concepts enables the nurse to deal more effectively with the psychological implications of illness and hospitalization for the child and the child's family.

The appendices feature useful tables on immunization, dental development, and pediatric assessment. These appendices are an excellent reference source for the student who is reviewing pediatrics.

GENERAL ASSESSMENT OF THE CHILD

GENERAL PRINCIPLES

A. Maturational ability of the child to cooperate with the examiner is of major importance to adequate physical assessment.
B. When planning physical assessment of the child, the following points should be considered:
1. Establish a relationship with the child prior to the examination.
   a. Determine child's maturational level.
   b. Allow the child an opportunity to become more accustomed to the examiner.
2. Explain in terms appropriate to the child's level of understanding the extent and purpose of the examination.
3. Realize that the physical examination may be a stressful experience for the child, who is helpless and depends on others for protection.
4. Limit the physical examination to what is essential in determining an adequate nursing diagnosis.
5. Proceed from the least to the most intrusive procedures.
6. Allow active participation of the child whenever possible.

Assessment of the Infant

A. Accomplish as much of the examination as possible while the infant is sleeping or resting undisturbed.
B. Assess general condition.
1. Symmetry and location of body parts.
2. Color and condition of the skin.
3. State of restlessness and sleeplessness.
4. Adjustment to feeding regimen.
5. Quality of cry.
C. Congenital anomaly assessment.
1. Assess the neurological system.
   a. Reflexes: absent or asymmetrical (see Neurological section).
   b. Head circumference: microcephaly, hydrocephaly.
      (1) 35 cm at birth.
      (2) 40 cm at 3 months.
      (3) 45 cm at 9 months.
      (4) At birth, the head size is 2 cm larger than the chest. Equals or exceeds chest until 2 years of age.
   c. Fontanels: closed, bulging.
      (1) Anterior measures 3.5 cm × 3.5 cm and closes by 18 months.
      (2) Posterior measures 1 cm × 1 cm and closes at 2 months.
   d. Eyes: cataracts, lid folds, spots on iris.
2. Assess the respiratory system.
   a. Breath sounds: signs of aspiration, asymmetry of lung expansion, retractions, grunting.
   b. Apnea.
3. Assess the cardiovascular system.
   a. Color: cyanosis.
   b. Rate and rhythm: murmurs, tachycardia, bradycardia.
   c. Energy level: cannot suck for fifteen minutes without exhaustion or cyanosis.
4. Assess the gastrointestinal tract.
   a. History of polyhydramnios.
   b. Patency: mucus, spitting, cyanosis, cannot pass nasogastric tube to stomach.
   c. Mouth: palate or lip not intact.
   d. Anus: not patent.
5. Assess the genitourinary system.
   a. Umbilical vessels: missing, normal two arteries and one vein.
   b. Urine: abnormal stream.
   c. Masses: abdominal (Wilms' tumor).
   d. Boys: undescended testicles, hernia, urethra no opening at the end of the penis.
   e. Girls: labial adhesions.
6. Assess the skeletal system.
   a. Fractured clavicle.
   b. Dislocated hip: asymmetric major gluteal folds, hip click.
   c. Legs and feet: clubbing, without straight tibial line.
   d. Spine: curved, inflexible, open.
D. Assess for common problems.
1. Ear infections.

a. Assess for increased temperature.

b. Check for irritability.

c. Determine if infant pulls or rubs ear.

d. Determine if change in eating habits has occurred recently.

2. Respiratory infections.

a. Assess duration and severity of symptoms.

b. Look for wheezing, barking cough, anxiety, restlessness, use of accessory muscles.

c. If throat is sore, check for white patches on tonsils.

3. Rashes.

a. Assess onset, duration, and location.

b. Provide accurate description of rash.

c. Determine if infant recently ingested new food or was exposed to animals.

4. Contact dermatitis.

a. Assess if history of allergies. ·

b. Evaluate diaper area rash: use of soap, lotions, powders.

c. Determine method of cleaning cloth diapers.

5. Hernias.

a. For inguinal, assess for lump in groin, with or without pain.

b. For umbilical, determine if lump can be pushed back without difficulty or pain.

6. Scalp: cradle cap.

a. Assess for scaling or crusted areas.

b. Determine method of washing hair.

c. Evaluate lotions or balms applied to hair.

7. Birth marks.

a. Assess for change in size, color, or shape.

b. Look for any bleeding or irritation.

8. Eye symmetry.

a. Assess frequency of problem with eye alignment.

b. Determine if the eyes wander at any particular time of day.

c. Determine if light reflex is symmetrical in both eyes.

E. Utilize screening procedures for assessment.

1. Developmental landmarks—DDST (Denver Developmental Screening Test).

2. Vision.

3. Hearing.

4. Growth charts: head circumference, weight, length.

F. Provide guidance in the following areas:

1. Growth and development changes.

2. Anxiety toward strangers.

3. Separation anxiety.

4. Transitional objects.

5. Prevention of accidents.

Assessment of the Toddler and the Preschool Child

A. General considerations.

1. Remember that separation anxiety is most acute at toddler age and body integrity fears most acute at preschool age.

2. Involve the parent in examination as much as possible.

3. Restrain child as much as necessary to protect the child from injury.

4. Give careful explanation of each portion of the exam.

5. Allow the child to handle the equipment and try out on doll.

6. Take into account child's need for autonomy.

7. Do not disparage imaginary friends.

8. Allow for rituals and routines.

B. Assess for common problems.

1. Feeding and eating.

a. Review food intake for last 48 hours.

b. Assess types of food ingested.

c. Ensure adequate source of vitamins and minerals.

2. Temper tantrums.

a. Assess frequency and duration.

b. Determine precipitating event.

c. Evaluate response of caretaker.

3. Toilet training.

a. Check ability to ambulate (indicates neuromuscular maturity).

b. Determine if child is bothered by wet diapers.

c. Evaluate child's interest in toileting.

4. Respiratory infections.

a. Assess duration and severity of symptoms.

b. Look for wheezing, barking cough, anxiety, restlessness, use of accessory muscles.

c. If throat is sore, check for white patches on tonsils.

5. Communicable diseases.

a. Assess onset of symptoms.

b. Evaluate progression of disease.

c. Determine treatment of symptoms.

    d. Look for complications.

  6. Gastrointestinal infections.

    a. Assess onset and duration.

    b. Evaluate intake and output.

    c. Check for signs of dehydration.

C. Utilize screening procedures for assessment.

  1. Developmental landmarks: DDST (Denver Developmental Screening Test).

  2. Vision.

  3. Hearing.

  4. Growth charts: head circumference, weight, length.

Assessment of the School-Age Child

A. General considerations.

  1. Modesty important, heightened concern for privacy.

  2. Explain all procedures clearly.

  3. Direct questions to child.

B. Assess for common problems.

  1. School.

    a. Assess for signs of school phobias, i.e., vomiting, procrastination.

    b. Determine child's attitude toward school.

  2. Nervous habits.

    a. Assess onset and duration of such habits as stuttering, twitching.

    b. Determine precipitating event.

    c. Evaluate anxiety of child and parent over problem.

  3. Accident trauma.

    a. Gain understanding of accident.

    b. Determine ways accident can be avoided.

    c. Assess if physical limitations may have caused accident.

  4. Respiratory infections.

    a. Assess duration and severity of symptoms.

    b. Look for wheezing, barking cough, anxiety, restlessness, use of accessory muscles.

    c. If throat is sore, check for white patches on tonsils.

  5. Gastrointestinal infections.

    a. Assess onset and duration.

    b. Evaluate intake and output.

    c. Check for signs of dehydration.

C. Utilize screening procedures for assessment.

  1. Snellen vision testing.

  2. Sweep check audiometry.

  3. Height and weight measurement.

  4. Inspection of skin and teeth.

Assessment of the Adolescent

A. General considerations.

  1. Examine child alone if he or she wishes (privacy is important).

  2. Note signs of puberty.

  3. Ascertain feelings about body image.

B. Assess for common problems.

  1. Acne.

    a. Evaluate existing skin care program.

    b. Assess child's personal hygiene.

  2. Dysmenorrhea.

    a. Evaluate degree of pain, i.e., absences from school.

    b. Determine use of analgesics.

    c. Assess amount of exercise.

  3. Obesity.

    a. Determine eating patterns.

    b. Evaluate family concern for problem.

    c. Assess amount of exercise.

C. Utilize screening procedures for assessment.

  1. Snellen vision testing.

  2. Sweep check audiometry.

  3. Height and weight measurement.

  4. Inspection of skin and teeth.

D. Provide guidance in the following areas.

  1. Hazards of cigarette smoking and alcohol.

  2. Transmission and symptoms of venereal disease.

  3. Sex education.

  4. Accident prevention, particularly automobile.

  5. Principles of nutrition.

PSYCHOSOCIAL ADJUSTMENT

Psychological Assessment of the Infant

A. Assess psychological implications of hospitalization on child.
   1. Separation from the mother.
   2. Decrease in sensory stimuli.
   3. Breakdown in mother-infant relationship due to:
      a. Maternal guilt.
      b. Hostile, cold hospital environment.
      c. Mother's feelings of inadequancy in the mothering role.
      d. Subordination of the parents by the staff.
B. Assess behavior of infants in response to illness.
   1. Indication of discomfort or pain.
      a. Cries frequently.
      b. Displays excessive irritability.
      c. Appears lethargic or prostrate.
      d. Has high temperature.
      e. Has decreased appetite.
   2. Positive reaction behaviors.
      a. Cries loudly.
      b. Appears fussy and irritable.
      c. Rejects everyone except mother.
   3. Negative reaction behaviors.
      a. Withdraws from everyone.
      b. Cries monotonously.
      c. Appears completely passive.

Implementation

A. Nursing actions help prevent the detrimental effects of hospitalization.
B. Hold a prehospitalization nursing interview with the parents and give a tour of the pediatric unit.
   1. Parents should meet the staff, have procedures and regulations explained to them, and be told the rationale behind the rules.
   2. They should be encouraged to visit frequently and/or to room in if possible.
C. Counsel the parents regarding the infant's illness, and elicit their understanding of the disease and its course of action. Correct any misconceptions, and if appropriate, reassure them that they are not the cause of the illness.
D. Encourage the parents to participate in the infant's care if they show an interest in doing so.
   1. Teach the parents procedures they are capable of doing.
   2. Show respect for their superior knowledge of infant's likes, dislikes, and habits.
E. Nurse's role for the absent mother.
   1. Limit the number of people handling the infant in the beginning.
   2. Allow one person to become familiar with the infant and gradually introduce others.
   3. Provide closeness and warmth (cuddling).
   4. Avoid isolating the infant from sensory stimulation.
   5. Provide stimulation for the infant during feeding.
   6. Hang brightly colored mobiles within the infant's sight.
   7. Encourage play activities.

Psychological Assessment of the Toddler and Preschooler

A. Assess psychological implications of hospitalization.
   1. Hospitalization is a very threatening experience to the child because of the total number of new experiences involved.
   2. Because of the threat involved, hospitalization has the potential for disrupting the toddler's new sense of identity and independence.
   3. Separation anxiety—the child mourns the absence of the mother through protest, despair, and denial.
   4. The child fears the loss of "body integrity." The child also has no realistic perception of how the body functions and may overreact to a simple procedure. Some toddlers believe that drawing blood will leave a hole and that the rest of their blood will leak out.
   5. The child resents the disruption of normal rituals and routines. Toddlers are often very rigid about certain procedures, which allows them a sense of security and control over otherwise frightening circumstances.
   6. Loss of mobility is frustrating to the child.

7. Regression—the toddler frequently abandons the most recently acquired behaviors and reverts to safer, less mature patterns.

B. Assess behavior of toddlers-preschoolers in response to illness.

1. Indications of discomfort or pain.
   a. Cries frequently.
   b. Displays excessive irritability.
   c. Appears lethargic.
   d. Has high temperature.
   e. Changes eating pattern.
   f. Verbalizes discomfort.
2. Positive reaction behaviors.
   a. Shows aggressive behavior.
   b. Appears occasionally withdrawn.
   c. Fantasizes about illness and procedures.
   d. Shows regressive behavior.
3. Negative reaction behaviors.
   a. Appears completely passive or excessively aggressive.
   b. Displays excessive regressive behavior.
   c. Withdraws from everyone.

C. Evaluate separation anxiety syndrome.

1. Protest is the first stage.
   a. Characteristics: cries loudly, throws tantrums.
   b. Nursing behaviors: stay close to the child to provide warmth and support.
2. Despair is the second stage.
   a. Characteristics: in periods of longer hospitalization, the child withdraws and shows no interest in eating, playing, etc.
   b. Nursing behaviors: recognize the syndrome and establish a relationship with the child—attempt to engage and involve the child in an activity.
3. Denial is the final stage.
   a. Characteristics: exhibits behavior that is often mistaken for happy adjustment; ignores mother and may regress.
   b. Nursing behaviors: reassure the mother, build a relationship with the child, and provide warmth and support to the child during long hospitalization.

Implementation

A. Introduce the child to hospital surroundings, preferably prior to hospitalization.

B. Explain in simple terms all the procedures; elaborate on them if child shows inclination.

Table 1. MANAGING BEHAVIOR THROUGH PLAY

Nursing Goals	Nursing Interventions
To bathe child	Give tub toys such as boats, cups, bottles, syringes without needles Give child something he can wash, such as a doll or a car
To administer soaks	Give child something to look at, such as a viewmaster or kaleidoscope Read a story or have child tell you one Set a timer so that child has the concept of time For hand and foot soaking, give child something to hold down or count
To encourage mobility	Extend environment through use of "fantasy trips," decoration of bed and surrounding area, or imaginative movement Move bed outdoors or to a playroom or a different room Have other children come to visit restricted child Use Atari or video games for older children
To ambulate	Give child something to pull or push or ride on Set reasonable distance goal for child to reach Take to visit another child or place Have a parade with hats, horns, etc. Have child walk for a reward, such as a visit to a sibling or the cafeteria
To encourage deep breathing	Give child bubbles, balloons, or surgical gloves to blow Have child blow through straws to race cotton balls Have child play kazoos or harmonicas Give child straws to suck up pieces of paper or cotton balls

Table 1. MANAGING BEHAVIOR THROUGH PLAY (continued)

Nursing Goals	Nursing Interventions
To encourage coughing	Put squeaky toy on child's abdomen so toy makes a noise when the child coughs Have child squeeze a pillow or stuffed animal
To maintain NPO status	Arrange special activities during meal time, such as a walk or visit to a special place
To encourage child to eat	Sit child with other children who are eating Serve food in small portions on a small plate Use a game or story to encourage eating Have child prepare foods that he likes
To restrict fluids	Give child a choice of fluids and time when he wants to drink them
To encourage child to drink	Give small amounts of liquid over a period of time Use a special decorated cup Let child use syringe instead of straw or cup Give popsicles, jello, or slushes Sit child with other children and have a tea party
To administer medication	Give child a choice of methods to take medication: whole, cut up, with water or apple juice Let older child give medication to himself Have special decorated cup for medications Give rewards (stars, stickers) for taking medication

C. Encourage rooming-in or frequent visits of parents once the child is hospitalized.
D. Suggest that the mother leave an object closely connected with her for the child to "care for" until she can return. This procedure assures the child that his or her mother will return.
E. Encourage the parents to be honest about when they are going and coming, i.e., do not tell the child they will stay all night and then leave when the child is asleep.
F. Have the family pictures pasted to the crib.
G. Use puppet play to explain procedures and to gain an understanding of the child's perception of hospitalization. Use puppets to work out child's anxiety, anger, and frustration.
H. During developmental history, elicit exact routines and rituals that the child uses; attempt to modify hospital routine to continue these rituals.
I. Provide stretchers, wheelchairs, and carts for immobilized children.
J. Do not punish the child for regression, and explain the reasons for its occurrence to the parents.

Problem Behaviors

A. Depressed behavior.
 1. Encourage child to express himself through play.
 2. Talk through a doll or stuffed animal for younger children.
 3. Determine child's level of understanding and clarify misconceptions.
 4. Don't avoid child; continue to interact and support.
 5. Structure child's day.
B. Aggressive behavior.
 1. Channel energy positively: older children may enjoy competitive activities; younger children can release tension through pounding boards, large motor activity, or clay projects.
 2. Set limits.
 3. Praise for jobs well done.
 4. Help child gain a sense of mastery.
C. Passive behavior.
 1. Structure the child's day.
 2. Give simple choices.
 3. Encourage self-care.
 4. Spend more time with the child and attempt to stimulate interest.
D. Regressed behavior.
 1. Regression is acceptable to a point because it allows child a brief return to a less mature and demanding time.
 2. Support independence, mastery of tasks, and self-care.
 3. Give alternatives to regressive behavior.
 4. Do not reprimand or shame regressive behavior.

Psychosocial Assessment of the School-age Child

A. Assess psychological implications of hospitalization.
   1. The school-age child wants to understand why things are happening.
   2. There is a heightened concern for privacy.
   3. The child is modest and fears disgrace.
   4. Hospitalization means an interruption in the child's busy school life, and the child fears that he or she will be replaced or forgotten by peer group.
   5. Absence from peer group means a disruption of close friendships.
B. Assess behavior of school-age children in response to illness.
   1. Indications of discomfort or pain.
      a. Expresses that something is wrong. ("I feel sick.")
      b. Cries easily.
      c. Tells adult he or she is ill so adult can do something about it.
   2. Positive reaction behaviors.
      a. Shows anger.
      b. Feels guilty.
      c. Fantasizes and is fearful.
      d. Displays increased activity in response to anxiety.
      e. Reacts to immobility by becoming depressed or angry or by crying.
      f. Cries or aggressively resists treatment.
      g. Needs parents and authority.
   3. Negative reaction behaviors.
      a. Is excessively guilty and angry and is unable to express feelings.
      b. Experiences night terrors.
      c. Displays excessive hyperactivity.
      d. Will not talk about experience.
      e. Is regressive and completely withdrawn.
      f. Shows excessive dependency.
      g. Has insomnia.

Implementation

A. Teach the child about his or her illness; take the opportunity to explain the functioning of the body.
B. Explain all procedures completely; allow the child to see special rooms (e.g., intensive care, cardiac cath. lab) prior to being sent there for treatments.
C. Provide opportunities for the child to socialize with peer group at meals and through team tournaments of cards, chess, and checkers.
D. Allow telephone privileges for calls to home and friends.
E. Provide outlets, such as a dart board and a boxing bag, for anger and frustration.
F. Give the child the opportunity to make choices and use independence.
G. Protect child's privacy.
H. Continue child's schooling by providing tutors.
I. Provide child with the opportunity to master developmental tasks of age group.

Psychosocial Assessment of the Adolescent

A. Assess psychological implications of illness.
   1. Disruption of social system and peer group.
   2. Alteration of body image.
   3. Fear of loss of independence.
   4. Alteration in plans for future.
   5. Interruption in development of heterosexual relationships.
   6. Loss of privacy.
   7. The degree to which the young adult is affected is dependent on:
      a. Whether the illness is chronic or acute.
      b. Whether the prognosis necessitates a change in the client's future aspirations.
      c. How many changes must be accepted.
B. Assess behavior of adolescents in response to illness.
   1. Indications of discomfort or pain.
      a. Realizes something is wrong and seeks help.
      b. Shows high anxiety level.
      c. Verbalizes discomfort.
   2. Positive reaction behaviors.
      a. Shows resistance to accepting illness.
      b. Rebels against authority.
      c. Demands control and independence.
      d. Is fearful.
      e. Temporarily withdraws from social scene.
      f. Verbalizes how illness has affected him or her.
   3. Negative reaction behaviors.
      a. Holds in feelings about illness.
      b. Tries to manipulate staff.
      c. Becomes completely dependent.
      d. Denies illness.

Implementation

A. Adolescents should be in rooms with their peers.

B. Allow telephone privileges, with some limit setting.

C. Encourage the feeling of self-worth by allowing as much independence as possible.

D. Allow heterosexual relationship to develop within reason.

E. Provide for privacy.

F. Assist client in identifying role models.

G. Realistically discuss problems of the illness with the client.

H. Always provide information honestly.

I. Encourage the adolescent, if possible, to accept some responsibility on the hospital unit.

Table 2. ASSESSMENT OF VITAL SIGNS

Age	Range of Normal Pulse	Average Pulse	Average Blood Pressure	Average Respiration
Newborn	110–160	120	80/45	30–50
1 year	80–160	115	96/65	20–40
2 years	80–130	110	99/65	20–30
4 years	80–120	100	99/65	20–25
6 years	75–115	100	100/56	20–25
8 years	70–110	90	105/56	15–20
10 years	70–110	90	110/58	15–20

Table 3. PEDIATRIC PHYSICAL ASSESSMENT

ASSESSMENT	NORMAL	ABNORMAL
MEASUREMENTS		
Measure **height** and **weight** and plot on a standardized growth chart	Height/weight proportional Sequential measurements: pattern follows normal growth curves	Height/weight below third percentile Sudden drop in percentile range of height and/or weight: possible sign of disease process or congenital problem
Assess **temperature** (axillary until six years of age)	Axillary 97°F; 36.4°C Elevations following eating or playing not unusual	Temperature of 104° to 105°F: corresponds roughly with 101° to 102°F in an adult Large daily temperature variations Hypothermia: usually result of chilling
Measure **circumference of head and chest** Examine or check circumferences when child is less than two years old Compare measurements with standardized charts	Head at birth: about 2 cm greater than chest During first year: equalization of head and chest After two years: rapid growth of chest; slight increases in size of head	Increase in head circumference greater than 2.5 cm per month: sign of hydrocephalus

ASSESSMENT	NORMAL	ABNORMAL
VITAL SIGNS		
Assess **pulse** apically	Birth to one year: 120 to 140 One year: 80 to 160 Two years: 80 to 130 Three years: 80 to 120 Over three years: 70 to 115	Pulse over 180 after first month of life: cardiac or respiratory condition Inability to palpate femoral pulses: possible coarctation of the aorta
Assess **respirations**	Birth: 30 to 50 Six years: 20 to 25 Puberty: 14 to 16 (Young children have abnormally high respiration rate with even slight excitement)	Consistent tachypnea: usually a sign of respiratory disease Respiratory rate over 100: lower respiratory tract obstruction Slow rate: may be sign of CNS depression
Assess **blood pressure**	Birth: 60 to 90 mm Hg systolic 20 to 60 mm Hg diastolic Rise in both pressures: 2 to 3 mm Hg per year of age Adult level reached at puberty	Elevated blood pressure in upper extremities: coarctation of aorta Narrowed pulse pressure (normal or elevated diastolic with lowered systolic; less than 30 mm Hg difference between systolic and diastolic readings): possible sign of aortic or subaortic stenosis or hypothyroidism Widened pulse pressure: possible sign of hyperthyroidism
APPEARANCE		
Observe **general appearance**	Alert, well-nourished comfortable, responsive	Lethargic, uncomfortable, malnourished, gross anomalies, dull
Listen to **voice and cry**	Strong, lusty cry	Weak cry, low- or high-pitched cry: may indicate neurological problem or chromosomal abnormality
	Facial expression animated No indications of pain	Expressionless, unresponsive Doubling over, rubbing a body part, general fretfulness
	No odor	Musty odor: sign of phenylketonuria, diphtheria Odor of maple syrup: may be maple syrup urine disease Odor of sweaty feet: one type of acidemia Fishy odor: may be metabolic disorder Acetone odor: acidosis, particularly diabetic ketoacidosis

ASSESSMENT	NORMAL	ABNORMAL
SKIN ASSESSMENT		
Assess **pigmentation**	Usually even Pigmented nevi common Large, flat, black and blue areas over sacrum, buttocks (mongolian spots)	Multiple cafe au lait spots: possible neurofibromatosis Cyanosis Jaundice Pallor
Assess **lesions**	Usually none Adolescence: acne	Erythematous lesions Multiple macules, papules, or vesicles Petechiae and ecchymoses: may indicate coagulation disorder Hives Subcutaneous nodules: may indicate juvenile rheumatoid arthritis
Note **consistency of skin**	Good turgor Smooth and firm	Poor turgor Dryness Edema Lack or excess of subcutaneous fat: sign of malnutrition or excess nutrition
Assess **nails**	Nail beds: normally pigmented Good nail growth	Cyanosis Pallor Capillary pulsations Pitting of the nails: possible sign of fungal disease or psoriasis Broad nail beds: possible sign of Down's syndrome or other chromosomal abnormality
Assess **hair** (consistency appropriate to ethnic group)	No excessive breaking	Dry, coarse, brittle hair: possible sign of hypothyroidism Alopecia (loss of hair): may be psychosomatic or due to drug therapy Unusual hairiness in places other than scalp, eyebrows, and lashes: may indicate hypothyroidism, vitamin A poisoning, chronic infections, reaction to Dilantin therapy Tufts of hair over spine or sacrum: may indicate site of spina bifida occulta or spina bifida Absence of the start of pubic hair during adolescence: possible hypothyroidism, hypopituitarism, gonadal deficiency, or Addison's disease

ASSESSMENT	NORMAL	ABNORMAL
Assess **lymph nodes**	Nontender, movable, discrete nodes up to 3 mm in diameter in occipital, postauricular, parotid, submaxillary, sublingual, axillary, and epitrochlear nodes Up to 1 mm in diameter inguinal and cervical nodes	Tender or enlarged nodes: may be sign of systemic infection
HEAD AND NECK ASSESSMENT		
Assess **scalp**	Usually without lesions	Ringworm, lice
Assess frontal and maxillary **sinuses**	Nontender	Tenderness: indicative of inflammatory process
Assess **face**	Symmetrical movement	Signs of facial paralysis Twitching: could be due to psychosomatic causes
Evaluate the **eyes**		
Gross screening of vision with Snellen chart	With younger child, ability to follow movement and to see objects placed a few feet away	Inability to follow movement or to see objects placed a few feet away
Sclerae	Completely white	Yellow sclera: sign of jaundice Blue sclera: may be normal or indicative of osteogenesis imperfecta
Placement in eye socket	Normally placed	Exophthalmos (protrusion of eyeball) Enophthalmos (deeply placed eyeball)
Iris	At rest: upper and lower margins of iris visible between the lids	Setting sun sign (iris appears to be beneath lower lid): if marked, may be sign of increased intracranial pressure
Movement	In newborn, intermittent strabismus	Fixed strabismus or intermittent strabismus continuing after six months of age: indication of muscle paralysis or weakness Nystagmus (constant motion of eye): characteristic of cerebellar lesions and brain tumors
Eyelids	Fully covers eye Fully raised on opening	Ptosis of eyelid: may be an early sign of a neurological disorder Sty
Conjunctiva	Clear	Inflammation Conjunctivitis Hemorrhage Stimson's lines (small red transverse lines on conjunctiva)
Cornea	Clear	Opacity: sign of ulceration Inflammation Redness

ASSESSMENT	NORMAL	ABNORMAL
Discharge	Tears	Purulent discharges: note amount, color, consistency
Pupils	Round, regular Clear, equal Brisk reaction to light Accommodation reflex (pupil contraction as object is brought near the eye)	Sluggish or asymmetrical reaction to light: indicates intracranial disease Lack of accommodation reflex
Lens	Clear	Opacities (cataracts)
Evaluate the **ears**		
Sinuses	None present	Small holes or pits anterior to ear: may be superficial but could indicate the presence of a sinus leading into brain
Position	Top of ear above level of eye	Top of ear below level of eye: congenital defects
Discharge	None	Discharge: note color, odor, and amount
Hearing	In infant: turning to sound In older child: response to whispered command	Diminished hearing in one or both ears
Assess the **nose**	No secretions	Secretions: note characteristics Any unusual shape or flaring of nostrils
	Breathing through nose	Breathing through mouth
Assess the **mouth**		Circumoral pallor: possible sign of cyanotic heart disease, scarlet fever, rheumatic fever, hypoglycemia; also seen in other febrile diseases Asymmetry of lips: seen in nerve paralysis
	Intact palate	Cleft palate
	Teeth in good condition In older child, presence of permanent teeth	Delayed appearance of deciduous teeth: may indicate cretinism, rickets, congenital syphilis, or Down's syndrome; may be normal Poor tooth formation: may be seen with systemic diseases Green or black teeth: seen after iron ingestion or death of tooth Stained teeth: may be seen after prolonged use of tetracyclines
Assess the **gums**	Retention cysts in newborn	Inflammation, abnormal color, drooling, pus, tenderness Black line along gums: may indicate lead poisoning
Assess the **tongue**	Moves freely	Tremors on protrusion: may indicate chorea, hyperthyroidism White spots (thrush) Tongue-tie

ASSESSMENT	NORMAL	ABNORMAL
Assess the **throat**	Tonsils normally enlarged in childhood	White membrane over tonsils White pus on sacs, erythema
Assess the **larynx**	Normal vocal tones	Hoarseness or stridor: possible respiratory tract obstruction
Assess the **neck**	Short in infancy Lengthens at two to three years Trachea slightly right midline	Trachea deviated to left or right: may indicate shift with atelectasis
Thyroid	Not enlarged	Enlarged: may be due to hyperactive thyroid, malignancy, goiter
Motion	Full lateral and upward/downward motion	Limited movement with pain: may indicate meningeal irritation, lymph node enlargement, rheumatoid arthritis, or other diseases
LUNGS AND THORAX ASSESSMENT		
Assess the **lungs**	Normally clear breath sounds bilaterally	Presence of rhonchi, rales or wheezes Diminished breath sounds heard over parts of lung
	No retractions	Mild or severe intercostal or sternal retractions
	Symmetry of diaphragmatic movement	Asymmetry of movement
Assess the **sputum**	None or small amount of clear sputum in morning	Thick, tenacious sputum with foul odor Blood-tinged or green sputum
Assess the **breasts**	Slightly enlarged in infancy Generally slightly asymmetrical at puberty	Discharge or growth in male
HEART ASSESSMENT		
Assess **heart sounds**	S_1, S_2, S_3	S_4: indicates congestive heart failure
Assess **femoral pulses**	Strong	Weak
Note **edema**	None present	Edema: note location (initially periorbital) and duration
Note **clubbing** of fingers	None present	Clubbing: note location and duration
Note **murmurs**		Murmur grade three or higher
Note **cyanosis**	None normally present	Circumoral or peripheral cyanosis: indicates respiratory or cardiac disease Abnormal pulse rate for age

ASSESSMENT	NORMAL	ABNORMAL
ABDOMEN ASSESSMENT		
Assess **skin condition**	Soft	Hard, rigid, tender
Assess for **peristaltic motion**	Not visible	Visible peristalsis: may indicate pyloric stenosis
Assess **shape**	Slightly protuberant in standing adolescent	Large protruding abdomen: may indicate pancreatic fibrosis, hypokalemia, rickets, hypothyroidism, bowel destruction, constipation
		Inguinal hernias, unilateral or bilateral: observe for reducibility
	Umbilical protrusion	Umbilical hernia
GENITOURINARY TRACT ASSESSMENT		
Assess **female genitalia**		
Discharge	Mucoid	Foul or copious discharge; any bleeding prior to puberty
Assess **male genitalia**		
Presence of urethral orifice	Orifice on distal end of penis	Hypospadias or epispadias (urethral orifice along inferior or dorsal surface)
Urethral opening	Normal size	Stenosis of urethral opening
Foreskin	Covers glans completely	Foreskin incompletely formed ventrally when hypospadias present
Placement of testes	Descended testes	Undescended testes
		Enlarged scrotum
Assess **urine output**	Full, steady stream of urine	Urine with pus, blood, or odor
		Excessive urination or nocturia: possible sign of diabetes
Check **anus and rectum**	No masses or fissures present	Hemorrhoids, fissures, prolapse, pinworms
		Dark ring around rectal mucosa: may be sign of lead poisoning
MUSCULOSKELETAL ASSESSMENT		
Assess **extremities**	Coloration of fingers and toes consistent with rest of body	Cyanosis: can indicate hypothermia, respiratory, or cardiac disease
		Clubbing of fingers and toes: indicates cardiac or repiratory disease
	Quick capillary refill on blanching	Sluggish blood return on blanching: indicates poor circulation
	Temperature same as rest of body	Temperature variation between extremities and rest of body: indicates neurological or vascular anomalies

ASSESSMENT	NORMAL	ABNORMAL
	Presence of pedal pulses	Absence of pedal pulses indicates circulatory difficulties
	No pain or tenderness	Presence of localized or generalized pain
	Straight legs after two years of age	Any bowing after two years of age: may be hereditary or indicate rickets
	Broad-based gait until four years of age; feet straight ahead afterwards	Scissoring gait: indicates spastic cerebral palsy
		Persistence of broad-based gait after four years of age: possible abnormalities of legs and feet or balance disturbance
		Any limp or ataxia
Assess **spine**	No dimples	Presence of dimple or tufts of hair: possible spina bifida
	Flexible	Limited flexion: indicates central nervous system infections
		Hyperextension (opisthotonos): indicates brainstem irritation, hemorrhage, or intracranial infection
	No lateral curvature or excessive anterior posterior curvature	Presence of lordosis, kyphosis, or scoliosis
Assess **joints**	Full range of motion without pain, edema, or tenderness	Pain, edema, or tenderness: indicates tissue injury
Assess **muscles**	Good tone and purposeful movement	Decreased or increased tone
	Ability to perform motor skills approximate to development level	Spasm or tremors: may indicate cerebral palsy
		Atrophy or contractures
NEUROLOGICAL ASSESSMENT		
Refer to adult section on neurological assessment for complete overview		
Assess **fine motor movements**	Presence of fine motor activity approximate to age	Continued presence of primitive reflexes after fading of reflex should normally occur: may indicate brain damage
Assess presence of **reflexes**	Positive Babinski until age two	Any asymmetry of movement

NEUROLOGICAL SYSTEM

The central nervous system (brain and spinal cord), the peripheral nervous system (cranial and spinal nerves), and the automatic nervous system comprise the neurological system; together these provide control functions for the entire body.

System Assessment

A. Assess for increased intracranial pressure.
   1. Shrill, high-pitched, cry.
   2. Bulging, tense fontanels.
   3. Sunset sign.
   4. Lethargy.
   5. Increasing head circumference.
   6. Projectile vomiting.
B. Assess motor function.
   1. Symmetry of movements.
   2. Muscle tone.
   3. Tremors or twitching.
   4. Seizure activity.
C. Assess eye movement and pupillary response.
D. Assess for presence or absence of reflexes.
E. Assess for signs of infection.
F. Assess level of consciousness.
G. Assess for signs of meningeal irritation.
H. Assess sensory function.
I. Assess any seizure activity.

Diagnostic Procedures

Pneumoencephalogram

A. A procedure in which air is injected into the subarachnoid space to visualize the ventricular system.
B. Nursing responsibilities prior to procedure.
   1. Ensure child is n.p.o. six to eight hours before procedure.
   2. Explain to child and/or parents exactly what is going to be done.
   3. Child may be premedicated to produce maximum relaxation and cooperation.
   4. Obtain base line data on level of consciousness.
C. Nursing responsibilities following procedure.

   1. Observe for any changes in level of consciousness.
   2. Observe neurological signs and vital signs every 15 minutes until stable.
   3. Encourage fluid intake.
   4. Keep flat and promote rest.
   5. Observe for signs of headache, nausea, vomiting, and elevated temperature.

Myelogram

A. Visualization of the spinal subarachnoid space to define it and to evaluate lesions involving neural elements.
B. Nursing responsibilities prior to procedure.
   1. Ensure child is n.p.o. six to eight hours before procedure.
   2. Maintain base line record of vital signs and neurological status.
   3. Administer sedative as ordered.
C. Nursing responsibilities following procedure.
   1. Frequently observe neurological signs and vital signs and compare to base line.
   2. Check for adequate voiding.
   3. Keep flat for 24 hours and promote rest.
   4. Watch for signs of infection.
   5. Slightly elevate head if some contrast media is retained.

Angiogram

A. Radiopaque substance is injected into cerebral vasculature or its extracranial sources to evaluate vascular anomalies, lesions, or tumors.
B. Nursing responsibilities prior to procedure.
   1. Shave and prep area where puncture is to be made.
   2. Ensure child has no solid food for six to eight hours prior to procedure.
   3. Keep base line record of neurological and vital signs.
   4. Frequently a sedative is administered to relax child.
C. Nursing responsibilities following procedure.
   1. Observe for changes in level of consciousness, transient hemiplegia, seizures, sensory or motor deterioration, or elevation of blood pressure with widening pulse pressure.
   2. Apply cold compress to injection site.
   3. Keep child flat and promote rest.
   4. Encourage fluid intake.
   5. Check extremity for adequate peripheral pulses, color, temperature.

Table 4. NEWBORN REFLEXES

Reflex	Response	Stimulus	Duration
Babinski's Sign	Toes, especially the great toe, hyperextend.	Stroke lateral side of the sole of the foot from heel to base of toes.	Present at birth; disappears between twelve to eighteen months.
Neck Righting Reflex	Shoulder, arms, and legs of opposite side will flex to follow head in turn.	Turn infant's head to left or right.	Evolving at four months; involuntary movement disappears at nine to twelve months.
Palmar Grasp	Grasps and holds adult finger; automatic reflex of full-term newborns.	Place finger in infant's palm.	Present at birth; disappears at four months.
Asymmetrical Tonic Neck Reflex	Assumes fencer's position: arm extends on side to which head is turned; opposite arm is flexed.	Turn infant's head to one side.	Present at birth; disappears at four months.
Moro's Reflex (Startle Reflex)	Body stiffens; legs are drawn up; arms are brought up, out, and then in front in an embracing position.	Make a loud noise .	Present at birth; disappears at four months.
Reciprocal Kicking (Stepping)	Steps alternately from one foot to the other.	Hold infant upright with feet touching a firm surface.	Evolving at birth; disappears at nine months.
Rooting Reflex	Turns head to side which has been stimulated.	Brush infant's cheek with fingertips.	Present at birth; rooting while awake disappears at three to four months; rooting while asleep at seven to eight months.
Sucking Reflex	Makes sucking movements.	Touch infant's lips with any object.	Present at birth; involuntary sucking disappears at nine months.

Lumbar Puncture

A. Withdrawal of cerebral spinal fluid by insertion of a hollow needle between lumbar vertebrae into subarachnoid space to identify intracranial pressure, signs of infection, or hemorrhage.

B. Nursing responsibilities prior to procedure.
   1. Maintain base line record of vital signs.
   2. Explain to the parents and child exactly what will happen.

C. Nursing responsibilities during procedure.
  1. Place child on side in knee-chest position with head flexed on chest.
  2. Help child remain steady in this position and reassure child throughout procedure.
D. Nursing responsibilities following procedure.
  1. Keep child flat in bed.
  2. Encourage fluid intake.
  3. If headache occurs when sitting up, return child to flat position and give analgesic.
  4. Observe neurological status for signs of deterioration.

System Planning and Analysis

A. Signs of increased intracranial pressure have been identified.
B. Casefinding of abnormal motor functioning completed.
C. Seizure activity is prevented and controlled.
D. Any abnormal neurological signs have been observed.
E. Infection is prevented.
F. Adequate nutrition is promoted.
G. Client's family is supported during diagnosis and treatment.
H. Child receives emotional support from staff.

System Implementation

For Infants

A. Take daily head circumferences, and graph results.
B. Observe for changes in the fontanels.
C. Note activity level.
D. Observe for the continuous presence of sunset sign.
E. Observe for presence of all newborn reflexes. Note the symmetry of movement and the presence of hypertonia or hypotonia.

For Children

A. Note activity level and watch for changes in activity.
B. Control and prevent seizure activity. (For specific actions, refer to Epilepsy.)
C. Carefully position child to prevent aspiration if vomiting is an actual or potential problem.
D. Check pupillary responses every shift. Note presence of nystagmus or strabismus or abnormal responses.
E. Assess vital signs every four hours or more frequently if unstable.
F. Report intake and output for every 24-hour period.
G. Evaluate the nutritional status of the child if vomiting is present.
H. Provide sterile field for any treatment that involves an area with open entry to the nervous system.
I. Evaluate level of consciousness (see neurological system, Medical-Surgical nursing).
J. Assess child for presence of meningeal irritation.
  1. Kernig's sign: Extension of leg causes spasm of the hamstring, pain, and resistance when child is in supine position with thigh and knee flexed to right angle.
  2. Brudzinski's sign: Flexion of head causes flexion of knees and both thighs at the hips.
K. Support the family through accurate reports of the child's condition and by allowing the family to participate in the child's care as much as possible.
L. Explain all procedures in truthful manner to the child. Allow time for questions.

System Evaluation

A. Normal head growth.
  1. Increase of approximately 2.5 cm per month.
  2. Decrease or increase in growth may be indicative of neurological disorder.
B. Fontanels normotensive.
  1. Normal for fontanels to become tense during vigorous crying.
  2. Should always be soft when child is quiet or asleep.
C. No persistent sunset sign.
  1. May be transitory in newborn period.
  2. If persistent, evaluate for other signs of increased intracranial pressure.
D. Normal activity level for age.
  1. Increasing lethargy and drowsiness may be indicative of increased intracranial pressure.
  2. Restlessness can be early indication of increasing pressure.

E. Normal reflex pattern.
1. Reevaluate any abnormal patterns when child fully alert.
2. Drowsiness can slow or diminish reflexes.
3. Continued abnormalities of response may be the first sign of neurological disorder.
F. Pupils equal and reactive to light.
1. Intermittent strabismus normal up to six months.
2. Any nystagmus or abnormal pupillary response should be further evaluated.
G. Normal respiratory pattern.
1. Abnormal changes indicative of increased intracranial pressure.
2. Respiration rate, depth, and rhythm are the most sensitive index of increasing intracranial pressure.
H. Normal pulse and blood pressure for age.
1. Slowed pulse is associated with increased intracranial pressure.
2. Increasing blood pressure with enlarging pulse pressure is a sign of increasing intracranial pressure.
I. Balanced intake and output.
1. Overhydration can increase cerebral edema.
2. Diminished output may indicate inappropriate secretion of antidiuretic hormone due to hypothalamus dysfunction.
J. Normal nutritional status.
K. No evidence of infection.
L. No sign of meningeal irritation.
M. Family supported by appropriate resource persons.

NEUROLOGICAL DISORDERS

Head Injury

Definition: Any trauma to the scalp, skull, meninges, or brain caused by mechanical force.

Characteristics

A. Accidental head injury is the major single cause of death in the pediatric age group. Approximately 200,000 children are admitted every year for evaluation and treatment of head injury.
B. Causes.
1. Falls are most frequent under one year; 75 percent result in some type of head injury.
   a. More boys than girls are injured by falls.
   b. Highest incidence is in 8–9 age group.
2. Auto accidents are the second most frequent cause.
C. Types of injuries.
1. Most head injuries are caused by physical forces that impact on the head through acceleration and deceleration.
   a. Acceleration: slower moving contents of cranium strike bony prominences or dura (coup).
   b. Deceleration: moving head strikes fixed object and brain rebounds, striking opposite side of cranium (contrecoup).
2. Concussion is most common: violent jarring of the brain within the skull; temporary loss of consciousness; seizure activity.
3. Contusion and laceration: the bruising of the brain and tearing of cerebral tissue.
4. Closed head injuries: skull is intact.
5. Open head injuries include deep scalp lacerations that require suturing.
6. Fractures: the majority of fractures are linear; other types are depressed, compound, and comminuted. A child's skull can withstand a great amount of force before it fractures.
D. Complications.
1. Epidural hemorrhage: usually the result of skull fracture. Blood accumulates between dura and skull and forms a hematoma.
   a. Signs of intracranial compression occur within a few minutes or hours after the injury.
   b. Clinical signs include headache, vomiting, hemiparesis, and loss of consciousness.
2. Subdural hemorrhage: bleeding between dura and cerebrum. (Common in infants due to birth trauma.)
   a. Most common clinical signs are seizures, vomiting, and irritability.
   b. May be evidence of increased intracranial pressure.
3. Subarachnoid and intracerebral hemorrhages may also occur from head injury.
4. Cerebral edema (diffuse brain swelling) leads to signs of increased intracranial pressure but no focal signs.

Assessment

A. Assess for level of consciousness; changes appear earlier than changes in vital signs.

B. Check for nausea and vomiting.

C. Observe for pupillary changes: epsilateral dilated pupil.

D. Monitor changes in vital signs, reflecting increased intracranial pressure or shock.

E. Observe for seizure activity and describe fully if noted.

F. Observe for changes in position and movement: nuchal rigidity; opisthotonos.

G. Check for headache. (If child is too young to verbalize, he may be fussy and irritable.)

H. Observe for vasomotor or sensory losses.

I. Assess for rhinorrhea and otorrhea (infrequent in children).
   1. Bleeding from ear suggests basal skull fracture.
   2. Drainage from nose should be tested with Dextrostix; if glucose present, it is evidence of cerebrospinal damage.

J. Observe child for any unusual behavior: make interpretation of this behavior in terms of child's normal behavior.

K. Identify any overt scalp or skull trauma.

Implementation

A. Monitor for complications: determine neurological status. (See previous section.)
   1. Check for signs of increased intracranial pressure.
      a. Level of consciousness: alert and easily aroused or lethargic; in a stupor or coma.
      b. Restless, irritable, crying behavior.
      c. Vital signs: changes in respiratory rate, increased blood pressure, pulse pressure, decreased pulse.
   2. Avoid actions that might increase intracranial pressure.
      a. Sudden changes in position.
      b. Bowel straining.
      c. Confused, noisy environment.

B. Monitor vital signs. Report changes immediately.

C. Maintain adequate respiratory exchange. Increased carbon dioxide levels increase cerebral edema.

D. Protect from injury by using safety measures.
   1. Maintain bedrest.
   2. Keep padded siderails up.

E. Position head to promote fluid drainage, promoting venous return from brain: 15–30 degrees with head straight.

F. Monitor and protect child if seizure activity.
   1. Observe and record type of seizure.
   2. Note behavior that preceded seizure.

G. Prevent infection if there is drainage from auditory canal or nose.
   1. Place dry, sterile cotton loosely at orifice.
   2. If drainage from nose is positive for glucose, do not suction nares (risk of secondary infection).
   3. Maintain strict asepsis.

H. Provide adequate nutrition and hydration.
   1. Provide clear liquids as ordered.
   2. Measure intake and output accurately.
   3. Monitor IV if in place.

Hydrocephalus

Definition: A condition in which the normal circulation of the spinal fluid is interrupted, resulting in pressure on the brain, deformity, and the progressive enlargement of the head.

Assessment

A. Assess for gradual enlargement of the head (more than 2.5 cm per month).

B. Check for separation of skull sutures.

C. Assess that sclera is visible above the iris (sunset sign).

D. Check for hyperactive reflexes.

E. Evaluate presence of irritability, failure to thrive, and high-pitched cry.

F. Assess for presence of projectile vomiting.

Implementation

A. Actions depend on the cause of increased pressure.
   1. Removal of part of choroid plexus to decrease production of cerebral spinal fluid.
   2. Shunting of the fluid out of the brain to the heart or to the peritoneal cavity.

B. Preoperative care.
   1. Prevent pressure sores on head by changing child's position, placing child's head on sheepskin, or by holding the infant.
   2. Provide good head support when the child is sitting.
   3. Promote optimal nutritional status.

C. Postoperative care.
   1. Observe for shunt malfunction: watch for progressive increase in head circumference and signs of increased intracranial pressure.

2. Observe for infection: increased temperature, rapid pulse, irritability.

3. Position child flat on unoperated side.

4. Prevent postoperative complications: turn every four hours, evaluate lung sounds, and assess for signs of infection.

5. Protect the operative site: avoid pressure on the site; ensure sterile dressing changes.

Spina Bifida

Definition: The failure of the posterior portion of the lamina of the bony spine to form, which causes an opening in the spinal column.

Assessment

A. Spina bifida occulta type.
   1. Involves a bony defect only and does not involve the spinal cord or the meninges.
   2. Requires no treatment.
B. Meningocele type.
   1. The meninges of the spinal cord extend through the opening in the spine.
   2. Usually causes no paralysis.
   3. Treatment involves removal of sac.
C. Meningomyelocele type.
   1. The cord and the meninges extend through the defect in the spine.
   2. This defect causes neuromuscular involvement, which can vary from flaccidity and lack of bowel and bladder innervation to weakness of lower extremities.
   3. Assess for presence of hydrocephalus.
   4. Check urological involvement.
      a. Frequent bladder infections.
      b. Potential for progressive renal damage.
      c. Ileal conduit surgery is frequently required.
      d. Credé method of managing urinary retention involves systematic "milking" of the bladder at periodic intervals.
   5. Assess for orthopedic involvement.

Implementation

A. Actions dependent on the severity of the condition.
B. Neurological interventions.
   1. Observe for signs of hydrocephalus as it is a frequent complication.
   2. Measure head circumference daily.

3. Observe for signs of increased intracranial pressure.
C. Urological interventions.
   1. If child is catheterized, use sterile technique.
   2. Keep a careful record of intake and output.
   3. Teach parents Credé method if treatment is ordered.
   4. Observe for signs of urinary tract infection.
      a. Increased temperature.
      b. Foul-smelling urine.
      c. Cloudy urine with possible mucus.
D. Orthopedic interventions.
   1. Provide opportunities for the child to exercise and develop unaffected areas.
   2. Prevent contractures through proper positioning.
      a. Provide foot brace to prevent footdrop.
      b. Provide support for legs to prevent external rotation of the hips.
   3. Implement range-of-motion exercises.

Epilepsy

Definition: A series of seizures that result from focal or diffuse discharges in cortical neurons—symptoms of abnormal brain function.

Etiology

A. Seizure disorders are idiopathic—cause unknown or acquired—result of brain injury caused by trauma, hypoxia, infection, toxins, or other factors.
B. Seizures more common during first 2 years than any other period.
C. Most common cause by age group.
   1. Young infants—birth injury, hemorrhage, anoxia, and congenital defects of the brain.
   2. Late infancy and early childhood—infections frequent cause; infrequent in middle childhood.
   3. Children older than 3 years—idiopathic epilepsy most common.

Assessment

A. Simple partial seizure.
   1. Localized (confined to a specific area) motor symptoms, accompanied by autonomic or somatosensory symptoms.
   2. Manifestations.
      a. Aversive seizure—most common motor seizure in children. Eye(s) turn away from

focus side.

    b. Sylvan seizures—most common during sleep. Tonic-clonic movements involving face.

    c. Jacksonian march—rare in children. Sequential clonic movements.

3. Complex partial (psychomotor) seizure.

    a. Area of brain most involved in temporal lobe (thus, this type of seizure is called psychomotor).

    b. Most common in children from 3 years to adolescence.

    c. Characterized by complex sensory phenomena, a period of altered behavior and amnesia (child is not aware of behavior).

    d. May perform such mannerisms as lip smacking, chewing, picking at clothes, etc.

    e. May appear dazed, but only loses consciousness for a few seconds.

B. Generalized Seizures.

1. Tonic-clonic seizures, traditionally known as "grand mal."

    a. May begin with an aura, then a tonic phase (lasting 10–20 seconds): stiffening or rigidity of muscles, particularly arms and legs; eyes roll up; followed by loss of consciousness; may be apneic and become cyanotic.

    b. Clonic phase follows (lasts about 30 seconds, but may last as long as 30 minutes): hyperventilation with rhythmic jerking of all extremities; may foam at the mouth and become incontinent; full recovery may take several hours.

    c. Status epilepticus—a series of seizures that run together and do not allow the child to regain consciousness between attacks.

        (1) A neurological emergency with generalized tonic-clonic seizures.

        (2) State can lead to exhaustion and death.

2. Absence seizures, formerly "petit mal."

    a. Brief duration, often just 5–10 seconds, brief loss of consciousness; almost no change in muscle tone.

    b. May occur 20–30 times/day.

    c. Common in children; may appear to be "day dreaming," or inattentive.

3. Myoclonic seizure.

    a. Characterized by a brief, generalized jerking or stiffening of the extremities.

    b. Seizure may throw person to the floor; no loss of consciousness.

4. Atonic or akinetic seizures, also called "drop attacks."

    a. Onset between 2 and 5 years of age.

    b. Characterized by sudden, brief loss of muscle tone.

    c. Person may fall to ground, momentary loss of consciousness.

5. Infantile spasms.

    a. Most common between 3–12 months of age; more common in males; usually low intelligence.

    b. Characterized by sudden, brief, symmetrical contractions; head flexed, legs drawn up, arms extended.

    c. May experience numerous attacks during the day without postictal drowsiness.

Implementation

A. Prevent injury during seizure.

1. Remove any objects that may cause harm.

2. Remain with child during seizure and provide privacy if possible.

3. Do not force jaws open during seizure.

4. Do not restrict limbs or restrain.

5. Loosen restrictive clothing.

6. Check that airway is open. Do not initiate artificial ventilation during a tonic-clonic seizure.

7. Following seizure, turn head to side to prevent aspiration and allow secretions to drain.

B. Observe and document seizure pattern.

1. Note time, level of consciousness, and presence of aura before seizure.

2. Record type, character, progression of movements.

3. Note duration of seizure and child's condition throughout.

4. Observe and record postictal state.

C. Administer and monitor medications—complete control achieved 50–70% of epileptic children.

1. Drugs prescribed for partial or generalized seizures: carbamazepine (Tegretol), phenytoin (Dilantin), and mephenytoin.

2. Drug of choice for absences is ethosuximide.

D. Administer postseizure procedures—speed of recovery.

1. Reduce stimuli—noise, lights, conversation.

    a. Place sources of light behind client.

    b. Keep away from fluorescent lights.

2. Remain with child after consciousness returns.

a. Speak and move slowly.

b. Use simple phrases—give child time to respond.

3. Encourage rest following a seizure (child will be exhausted) and maintain privacy.

Cerebral Palsy

Definition: This term is used to describe a group of neuromuscular disorders caused by malfunctions of the motor centers and pathways of the brain.

Assessment

A. Etiology is anoxia to the brain. Infections of the CNS are also a major factor.

B. Assess for abnormal movements.

1. Spasticity.
   a. Voluntary muscles lose normal smooth movements and respond with difficulty to both active and passive movement.
   b. Increased deep tendon reflexes, scissoring.
   c. Contractures of antigravity muscles.
   d. Persistence of primitive reflexes.
   e. Lack of normal postural control.

2. Athetoid (dyskinetic).
   a. Involuntary muscle action with smooth, writhing movement of extremities.
   b. Reflexes usually normal.

3. Ataxia: lack of coordination and possibly hypotonia.

C. Assess for seizures which occur in many children with cerebral palsy.

D. Check for vision disturbance which occurs in 20 percent of these children.

E. Assess mental functioning; at least 50 percent function at a subnormal level. Many cerebral palsy children are diagnosed as mentally retarded due to slow motor skills or aphasia.

Implementation

A. Each child requires an individualized program according to the particular manifestations of the disease and the child's capacities.

B. Major focus of interventions.

1. To develop motor control.
2. To develop communication skills.
3. To provide adequate nutrition.
4. To prevent orthopedic complications.

Poliomyelitis

Definition: An acute viral infection that affects the spinal cord and brain stem; may lead to paralysis or death.

Characteristics

A. A contagious disease caused by three viruses: type 1, 2, and 3.

B. Incubation period is usually 7–14 days with range of 5–35 days.

C. Communicable: throat holds virus for about one week; feces 4–6 weeks.

D. Manifests in three forms: abortive, nonparalytic (most common), and paralytic.

E. Recent statistics indicate that parents are very susceptable to contracting polio if infants receive live vaccine when the parents have never been immunized.

Assessment

A. Assess symptoms of different types.

1. Abortive: fever, sore throat, headache, anorexia, vomiting, abdominal pain. May last few hours to days.

2. Nonparalytic: same as above but more severe with stiff neck, back, and legs.

3. Paralytic (spinal and bulbar types): similar course as nonparalytic; apparent recovery followed by paralysis.

Implementation

A. Preventive: education of public about oral trivalent polio immunization.

B. Maintain complete bedrest during acute period.

C. Provide respiratory ventilation if respiratory paralysis occurs.

D. Assist with physiotherapy (most important factor in recovery) following acute stage.

E. Evaluate for potential complications.

Meningitis

Definition: An acute inflammation of the meninges.

Assessment

A. Assess cause: usually bacterial or viral agents.

B. Assess disease by culturing CSF.

C. Assess for symptoms of nuchal-spinal rigidity: headache, irritability, nausea, vomiting, fever.

D. Assess for positive Kernig's and Brudzinski's signs.

Implementation

A. Isolate child until the causative agent is identified.

B. Administer medications on time.

C. Promote hydration: prevent dehydration and over-hydration (causes an increase in cerebral edema).

D. Monitor neurological signs.

E. Maintain bedrest and position child comfortably; most children prefer a side-lying or flat position; sitting up increases pain.

F. Observe for signs of subdural effusion (collection of fluid in the subdural space).
   1. Increasing intracranial pressure.
   2. Irritability.

G. Maintain patent airway; administer oxygen if ordered. May be prone to respiratory arrest.

Reye's Syndrome

Definition: Acute encephalopathy with fatty degeneration resulting in marked cerebral edema and enlargement of the liver with marked fatty infiltration.

Characteristics

A. Children from two months to adolescence contact illness; ages 6 and 11 years most often affected.

B. Usually follows a viral infection, especially varicella and influenza B.

C. Aspirin is now contraindicated with influenza—Tylenol medication of choice.

D. Incidence of Reye's decreased dramatically since change from aspirin to Tylenol.

Assessment

A. Assess for prodromal symptoms: malaise, cough, rhinorrhea, sore throat.

B. Assess level of consciousness.

C. Evaluate temperature changes.

D. Evaluate clinical stages of the syndrome.
   1. Stage 1: vomiting, lethargy and drowsiness.
   2. Stage 2: CNS changes, disorientation, delirium, aggressiveness and combativeness, central neurologic hyperventilation, hyperactive reflexes and stupor.
   3. Stage 3: comatose, hyperventilation, decorticate posturing.
   4. Stage 4: increasing comatose state, loss of ocular reflexes, fixed, dilated pupils.
   5. Stage 5: seizures, loss of deep tendon reflexes, flaccidity and respiratory arrest.

E. Evaluate lab findings.
   1. Associated with liver dysfunction; SGOT, SGPT, LDH are all elevated, dependent clotting factors, decreased prothrombin time, bilirubin and alkaline phosphate unchanged.
   2. Associated with renal dysfunction: reduced blood sugar levels to below 50 mg/100 ml, reduced insulin levels and decreased glucagon response.

F. Assess fluid and electrolyte balance; intake and output.

Implementation

A. Monitor for signs of increased intracranial pressure; most important intervention, may result in death.
   1. Major effort is toward recognizing and reducing cerebral edema, as this may lead to death.
   2. Monitor IV mannitol or glycerol when administered to reduce blood osmolarity, thus reducing cerebral edema.

B. Prepare for tracheal intubation and controlled ventilation (to decrease carbon dioxide level).

C. Monitor vital signs frequently and decrease temperature as needed.

D. Monitor closely for signs of seizure activity and utilize seizure precautions.

E. Provide nursing care appropriate for semi-conscious and unconscious client as neurological status alters.
   1. Maintain head elevation at 30 degrees.
   2. Monitor reflexes as indicative of clinical stage of syndrome.

F. Provide adequate fluid balance.
   1. Ensure adequate urinary output of at least 1 ml/1 kg/hr.
   2. Provide and monitor intravenous fluids.
   3. Observe closely for cerebral edema or dehydration.

G. Provide low protein diet.

H. Provide respiratory care; suctioning, ventilation and oxygen as ordered.

I. Provide emotional and supportive care for client and family.

CARDIOVASCULAR SYSTEM

The heart is the center of the cardiovascular system, which, by contracting rhythmically, pumps blood through the body to nourish all of the body tissues and cells. This is one of the most essential body systems because failure to function results in death of the client.

System Assessment

A. Assess feeding capability.
1. Unable to complete feeding without long rest periods.
2. Poor sucking reflex.
B. Evaluate for retarded growth and failure to thrive.
C. Assess for respiratory difficulties.
1. Dyspnea.
2. Tachypnea.
3. Frequent respiratory infections (generally seen in acyanotic defects).
4. Orthopnea.
5. Retractions and/or grunting.
D. Observe for flaccid position of limbs.
E. Check for signs of congestive heart failure.
F. Check for tachycardia or bradycardia.
G. Evaluate for presence of murmurs.
H. Evaluate for decreased arterial blood saturation (seen in cyanotic defects).
1. Polycythemia.
2. Cyanosis.
3. Clubbing of the fingers and toes.
4. Cerebral changes, i.e., fainting, confusion.
I. Observe for signs of congestive heart failure.
1. Tachycardia.
2. Dyspnea.
3. Tachypnea.
4. Hemoptysis.
5. Costal retractions.
6. Fluid retention (weight gain).
7. Rales, wheezing, or ronchi.

Diagnostic Procedures

Cardiac Catheterization

A. A procedure in which a catheter is passed into the heart and its major vessels for examination of blood flow, pressures in all chambers and vessels, and oxygen content and saturation. The catheter may be passed through the arterial system into the left side of the heart or through the venous system into the right side of the heart.
B. Nursing responsibilities before procedure.
1. Prepare parents and child for procedure by showing equipment, procedures, table.
2. Establish vital sign base line.
3. Promote good physical condition prior to test.
C. Nursing responsibilities during procedure.
1. Carefully observe vital signs.
2. Observe for cyanosis or pallor, bradycardia, and apnea.
3. Assist in restraining and comforting the child.
D. Nursing responsibilities following procedure.
1. Check for peripheral pulses, distal to the site in the extremity used for catheter.
2. Take and record vital signs every fifteen minutes; observe for subnormal temperature.
3. Observe for thrombosis: warmth of extremities, weak arterial pulses, cyanosis, blanching of extremity, skin color.
4. Check for progressive return to normal.
5. Observe for hypotension (internal bleeding) and signs of infection.
6. Check incision site for bleeding.
7. Observe for reactions to dye used in procedure.

Echocardiography

A. A noninvasive cardiac procedure that reflects mechanical cardiac activity. Usually used to diagnose valvular and other structural anomalies.
B. Nursing responsibilities.
1. Before procedure, assure child that procedure is painless, and prepare child for procedure to help ensure cooperation.
2. After procedure, provide general reassurance (no specific care is indicated).

Phonocardiogram

A. A graphic recording of the occurrence, timing, and duration of the sounds of the heart.
B. Nursing responsibilities.

1. Before procedure, explain equipment to child.
2. Take precautions to eliminate any extraneous noises during procedure.

System Implementation

Congenital Heart Disease

A. Organize care and feedings to provide sufficient periods of rest.
B. Feed the child by nipple or nasogastric tube. Formula should contain appropriate caloric concentration and fluid volume.
C. Monitor regular analysis of oxygen concentration in isolette to ensure appropriate levels.
D. Position infant in the knee-chest position. The toddler assumes the squatting position by himself.
E. Note laboratory values for oxygen saturation and signs of polycythemia. Oxygen saturation of arterial blood that is less than 92 percent is considered a sign of cyanotic heart disease. Hematocrit higher than 52 percent may be a sign of polycythemia or dehydration.
F. Obtain vital signs every four hours or more frequently if warranted.
G. Check for signs of impending heart failure.
   1. Increase in weight.
   2. Increased pulse.
   3. Presence of adventitious breath sounds.
   4. Increase in cyanosis.
H. Monitor daily weights for changes that may indicate alterations in the infant's fluid status.

Congestive Heart Failure

A. Infant signs and symptoms: increased respiratory rate and infections; enlarged liver and spleen, generally no edema, may see periorbital edema; babies do not have distended jugular veins (they do not have necks).
B. Promote rest for child with heart failure.
   1. Provide outlets such as drawing, doll play, and reading for child with restricted activity.
   2. Organize care to promote child's rest periods.
C. Supervise diet.
   1. Provide small, frequent feedings.
   2. Failure to thrive often present, so meals should be high calorie, attractive, and foods child will eat.
D. Monitor medication administration.

1. Digoxin.
   a. Monitor vital signs every hour during digitalization. If pulse under 90–100, notify physician.
   b. Observe for digoxin toxicity; nausea, vomiting and diarrhea (seen most often in children); anorexia, dizziness and headaches, arrhythmias, and muscle weakness.
2. Diuretics—important part of treatment.
   a. Observe for electrolyte abnormalities.
   b. Weigh child daily.
   c. Common diuretics: lasix, diuril (depletes potassium), and aldactone (preserves potassium).
E. Monitor for signs of complications (other than medications).
   1. Dehydration—important to keep child hydrated.
   2. Increased respiratory effort; children usually able to monitor own oxygen expenditure.
      a. Tachycardia, retractions, grunting cyanosis.
      b. Do not take child to high altitudes (above 5000 feet)—hypoxemia may occur.
   3. Cardiovascular collapse—pallor, cyanosis, hypotonia.
F. Prepare family for home care of infant or child.
   1. Encourage family to participate in care.
      a. Administration of medications.
      b. Signs of medication toxicity.
      c. Techniques for conserving children's energy.
      d. How to contact others for help and guidance.
   2. Support family relationships.
      a. Reinforce positive coping mechanisms.
      b. Assist family to express feelings and fears.
      c. Support as normal a life as possible for child.

System Evaluation

A. Parents are prepared to take infant home when they can demonstrate:
   1. How to feed baby—provide adequate calories without excessive strain.
   2. How to administer medications—know signs of toxicity.
   3. When to call physician—recognize signs of complications.
B. Vital signs do not deteriorate or improve.
   1. Child's activity level is appropriate for condition.
   2. There are no clinical signs of a worsening condition.

Table 5. FETAL TO INFANT CIRCULATION

	Fetal Circulation	Infant Circulation	Acyanotic Congenital Defects
Ductus venosus	Oxygenized blood from umbilical vein to inferior vena cava; shunts blood past portal circulation	Becomes nonfunctional	Ventral-septal defect Acyanotic: blood from left to right side
Foramen ovale	Opening between right and left atria; shunts blood past lungs	Functional closure by 3 months	Atrial septal defect: patent foramen ovale and ostium defect
Ductus arteriosus	Connects aorta and pulmonary artery; shunts blood past lungs	Contracts and becomes occluded by 4 months	Patent ductus arteriosus: normal closing fails to occur
Aorta	Receives mixed blood from heart and pulmonary arteries	Carries oxygenated blood from left ventricle	Coarctation of aorta; aortic stenosis
Pulmonary artery	Carries some mixed blood to lungs	Carries oxygenated blood to lungs	Pulmonic stenosis: narrowing of pulmonic valve
Ventricles	Ejecting chambers of the heart; pump blood	Ejecting chamber of the heart	Ventricular septal defect: oxygenated blood passes from left to right ventricle
Umbilical vein	Carries oxygenated blood from placenta to fetus	Obliterated at birth	
Umbilical arteries	Two arteries; carry oxygenated (venous) blood from fetus to placenta	Obliterated at birth	
Inferior vena cava	Carries oxygenated blood from umbilical vein and ductus venosus and mixed blood from body	Carries unoxygenated blood	

CONGENITAL HEART CONDITIONS

Fetal Circulation

A. Major structures of fetal circulation.
  1. Ductus venosus: a structure that shunts blood past the portal circulation.
  2. Foramen ovale: an opening between the right and left atria of the heart that shunts blood past the lungs.
  3. Ductus arteriosus: a structure between the aorta and the pulmonary artery that shunts blood past the lungs.
B. Changes in circulation at birth.
  1. The umbilical arteries and vein and the ductus venosus become nonfunctional.
  2. The lungs expand, reducing resistance, and greater amounts of blood enter the pulmonary circulation.
  3. More blood in the pulmonary circulation increases the return of blood to the left atrium, which initiates the closure of the flap of tissue covering the foramen ovale.
  4. The ductus arteriosus contracts and the blood flow decreases; eventually, the duct closes.
C. Two major clues to presence of heart disease.
  1. Congestive heart failure.
    a. Begins before one year of age in majority of infants.
    b. Most infants are less than six months old.
  2. Cyanosis.

Table 6. CONGENITAL HEART DEFECTS

Cyanotic Type of Defect	Acyanotic Type of Defect
Conditions that allow unoxygenated blood into the systemic circulation or conditions that result in obstructive pulmonary blood flow.	Conditions that interfere with normal blood flow through the heart either by slowing it down, or by shunting blood back to the right side of the heart.
A. Signs and symptoms. 1. Retarded growth and failure to thrive 2. Lack of energy 3. Frequent infections 4. Polycythemia 5. Clubbing of fingers and toes 6. Squatting 7. Cerebral abscess B. Diseases in the cyanotic category. 1. Tetralogy of Fallot 2. Complete transposition of the great vessels 3. Truncus arteriosus 4. Tricuspid atresia	A. Signs and symptoms. 1. Audible murmur 2. Discrepancies in pulse pressure in the upper and lower extremities 3. Tendency to develop respiratory infections 4. May develop heart failure with little stress B. Diseases in the acyanotic category. 1. Patent ductus arteriosus 2. Atrial septal defect 3. Ventricular septal defect 4. Coarctation of the aorta 5. Pulmonic stenosis 6. Aortic stenosis

CYANOTIC TYPE OF DEFECTS

Definition: Conditions that allow unoxygenated blood into the systemic circulation even though cyanosis is not clinically evident.

Tetralogy of Fallot

Definition: A cardiac malformation with anatomic abnormalities caused by the underdevelopment of the right ventricular infundibulum.

Characteristics

A. Ventricular septal defect.
B. Dextroposition of aorta so that it overrides the defect.
C. Hypertrophy of the right ventricle.
D. Stenosis of the pulmonary artery.
E. Hemodynamics: a right to left shunt arises in this anomaly due to the position of the aorta and the hypertrophied right ventricle; thus, partially unoxygenated blood is sent back to the systemic circulation.

F. Cyanosis not immediately evident in the newborn due to patent ductus arteriosus.

Assessment

A. Observe for signs already mentioned for cyanotic conditions.
B. Assess for hypoxic episodes with potential for seizure activity.
C. Assess pulse rate.
D. Evaluate fatigue with exercise.
E. Observe for dyspnea and tachypnea.
F. Observe for signs of polycythemia (can lead to clotting problems and cerebral vascular diseases).

Implementation

A. Provide appropriate nursing interventions discussed under general implementation section.
B. Provide postoperative care for child having Blalock-Taussig or Potts procedure (increases blood flow to the lungs).
C. Provide postoperative care for corrective treatment of pulmonary stenosis and ventricular septal defect.

Complete Transposition of the Great Vessels

Definition: In this condition the aorta arises from the right ventricle and the pulmonary artery arises from the left ventricle, which is not compatible with survival unless there is a large defect present in the ventricular or atrial septum.

Characteristics

A. Aorta is anterior to pulmonary artery.
B. Pulmonary artery ascends parallel to aorta rather than crosses it.
C. Ventricular septal defect.
D. Atrial septal defect.
E. Patent ductus arteriosus.

Assessment

A. Evaluate for development of subvalvular pulmonic stenosis, decreased pulmonary blood flow, hypoxia, and polycythemia.
B. Observe for profound cyanosis.
C. Assess for signs of heart failure.

Implementation

A. Provide appropriate nursing interventions as listed under general implementation section.
B. Provide postoperative care for palliative surgery (creation or enlargement of a large septal defect, allowing for greater mix of oxygenated and unoxygenated blood).
C. Provide postoperative care for palliative surgery (creation of a patent ductus arteriosus or pulmonary artery banding to decrease blood flow through lungs).
D. Provide postoperative care for corrective Mustard procedure.
   1. Removal of the atrial septum with creation of a new septum.
   2. The systemic venous return is directed into the pulmonary artery from the left ventricle, and the pulmonary venous return is directed into the aorta.

Truncus Arteriosus

Definition: A single arterial trunk arising from both ventricles that supplies the systemic, pulmonary, and coronary circulations. A ventricular septal defect and a single, defective, semilunar valve also exist.

Assessment

A. Assess for mottled skin and ashen color.
B. Evaluate for other cyanotic symptoms.
C. Determine if systolic murmur is present.

Implementation

A. Provide nursing care as outlined in general intervention section.
B. Provide postoperative care for palliative treatment (banding of both pulmonary arteries as they arise from the truncus arteriosus).

Tricuspid Atresia

Definition: Complete closure of the tricuspid valve and hypoplastic right ventricle, frequently accompanied by ventricular and atrial septal defect.

Assessment

A. Evaluate for a right-to-left shunt through the atrial septal defect. Blood mixes with pulmonary venous blood and enters the left ventricle. From the left ventricle, some blood is shunted to the right ventricle and then to the pulmonary artery. The rest passes into the aorta.

B. Assess for symptoms of cyanotic conditions.

C. Observe for cyanosis at birth.

Implementation

A. Provide nursing care as outlined in general intervention section.

B. Provide postoperative care for palliative surgery designed to increase pulmonary blood flow.

ACYANOTIC TYPE OF DEFECTS

Definition: Conditions that interfere with normal blood flow through the heart, either by interference with the normal flow or by defects that allow blood to be shunted from the left to the right side of the heart.

Patent Ductus Arteriosus

Definition: A patent ductus is present when normal closing after birth fails to occur. The potential for difficulty with this defect is dependent on the amount of blood passing through the defect.

Assessment

A. Assess for machinery-type murmur over pulmonary artery.

B. Check for low diastolic blood pressure and for widened pulse pressure.

C. Evaluate for poor feeding habits.

D. Check for distress and frequent respiratory infections.

E. Palpate for bounding peripheral pulses.

Implementation

A. Provide appropriate nursing care as listed under general implementation.

B. Provide postoperative care for surgical ligation of ductus, which is usually done at two or three years of age.

Atrial Septal Defect

Definition: Involves two types of defects that occur during the development of the atrioventricular canal.

Characteristics

A. Patent foramen ovale.

  1. In 20 percent of all births, a slit-like opening remains in the atrial septum.

  2. This defect is usually a functional murmur and requires no surgical intervention.

B. Ostium defects.

  1. A high defect, ostium secundum, in which the foramen ovale fails to close.

    a. Frequently asymptomatic.

    b. Murmur in area of pulmonary artery.

    c. Usually well tolerated in childhood.

  2. A low defect, ostium primum, in which there is inadequate development of endocardial cushions. The atrial septum allows a flow of blood from the left high pressure chamber to the right atrial chamber.

    a. Usually accompanied by mitral insufficiency.

    b. Frequently asymptomatic if there are no other abnormalities.

Assessment

A. Assess for widely fixed and split S_2 heart sound.

B. Auscultate for ejection systolic murmur.

C. Monitor for signs of congestive heart failure (usually not present in infants and children).

Implementation

A. Provide symptomatic care (usually not a nursing care problem).

B. If severe pulmonary hypertension occurs, provide appropriate respiratory care, i.e., oxygen, maintain bed in semi-Fowler's position, etc.

C. Provide postoperative care following closure of defect.

Ventricular Septal Defect

Definition: The majority of defects occur in the membranous septum, and severity is related to the size of the defect and amount of pulmonary blood flow.

Assessment

A. Signs and symptoms depend on size of shunting. Usually children with large defects present with symptomatology.

  1. Assess for cardiac enlargement.

  2. Assess for pulmonary engorgement.

3. Assess for dyspnea.

4. Assess for frequent respiratory infections.

5. Evaluate loud systolic murmur.

B. Assess for signs of congestive heart failure.

C. Assess for tendency to tire easily.

D. Assess for frequent respiratory infections.

E. Assess for poor weight gain.

F. Assess for blowing pansystolic murmur.

Implementation

A. Usually no nursing care needs for child with small defects.

B. Provide symptomatic nursing care for child with large defects as shunting of blood can produce pulmonary dysfunction.

C. Provide preoperative and postoperative care for repair of VSD using a patch.

Pulmonic Stenosis

Definition: Narrowing of the pulmonic valve.

Assessment

A. Assess for increase in right ventricular pressure.

B. Evaluate for a decrease in exercise tolerance, evidence of tiring easily, and dyspnea.

C. Assess for right ventricular hypertrophy.

D. Be aware that some children may be asymptomatic.

E. Assess for signs of congestive heart failure.

F. Assess for cyanosis.

Implementation

A. Provide symptomatic nursing care. Clients with mild or moderate stenosis may not need care.

B. Monitor drug and oxygen therapy if needed.

C. Provide preoperative nursing and monitor postop problems: arrhythmias and conduction problems.

Aortic Stenosis

Definition: The narrowing or the stricture of the aortic valve.

Assessment

A. Be aware that many infants are asymptomatic.

B. Assess for left ventricular hypertrophy, which will occur with resistance to blood flow from the left ventricle.

C. Assess for chest pain during exercise. Be aware that in rare conditions sudden death may occur after exercise because of inadequate blood flow to the heart muscle.

D. Evaluate child's exercise tolerance.

E. Observe for episodes of syncope or vertigo.

Implementation

A. Teach children to evaluate their exercise tolerance and to not exceed their limit.

B. Provide preoperative and postoperative care for surgical intervention.

Coarctation of Aorta

Definition: The constriction of the lumen of the aorta.

Assessment

A. Assess for high blood pressure and bounding pulses–areas of the body that receive blood from vessels proximal to the constriction may result in these conditions.

B. Evaluate for a diminished blood supply in areas of the body distal to the defect.

C. Infant diagnosis: Assess for discrepancies in pulses and blood pressure between upper and lower extremities and left-right sides.

D. Older child diagnosis: Assess for increased cerebral flow: headache, dizziness, epistaxis, fainting.

E. Evaluate for possible complications (in untreated cases): intracranial hemorrhage, stroke, hypertension, or congestive heart failure.

F. Assess for leg pain on exertion.

Implementation

A. Provide symptomatic nursing care as necessary.

B. Monitor blood pressure and neurological signs in nonsurgical clients.

C. Provide preoperative and postoperative nursing care.

D. Observe for postsurgical signs of gastrointestinal disturbance and systemic hypertension.

ACQUIRED CARDIAC DISEASE

Rheumatic Fever

Definition: A systemic inflammatory (collagen) disease that usually follows a group A beta-hemolytic streptococcus infection.

Assessment

A. Utilize Jones criteria for diagnosis (there is no single clinical pattern).
B. Two major criteria, or one major and two minor criteria, are necessary for a diagnosis.
   1. Major criteria.
      a. Assess for carditis.
      b. Check for polyarthritis.
      c. Evaluate if chorea is present.
      d. Assess for erythema marginatum.
      e. Ascertain if subcutaneous nodules are present.
   2. Minor criteria.
      a. Assess for fever.
      b. Check for arthralgia.
      c. Determine if child has had rheumatic fever or rheumatic heart disease.
      d. Evaluate for elevated erythrocyte sedimentation rate.
      e. Check for positive C-reaction protein.
      f. Determine if P-R interval is prolonged.
C. Evaluate supporting evidence.
   1. Recent scarlet fever.
   2. Positive throat culture for group A streptococci.
   3. Increased streptococcal antibodies.

Implementation

A. Provide antibiotic therapy against any remaining streptococci.
B. Administer aspirin for joint symptoms.
C. Ensure sufficient bed rest.
D. Prevent further infection.
E. Instruct on use of long-term antibacterial prophylaxis.

Subacute Bacterial Endocarditis

Definition: An infectious disease involving abnormal heart tissue, particularly rheumatic lesions or congenital defects.

Assessment

A. Look for insidious onset of symptoms.
B. Assess for fever.
C. Check for lethargic behavior and general malaise.
D. Assess for anorexia.
E. Evaluate for splenomegaly.
F. Assess for retinal hemorrhages.

Implementation

A. Provide large doses of antibiotic therapy, usually penicillin.
B. Ensure adequate bed rest.
C. Monitor erythrocyte sedimentation rate and increased leukocytes.
D. Repeat blood cultures as ordered.

CARDIAC SURGERY

Assessment

A. Preoperative.
   1. Determine if child is physically prepared for surgery.
   2. Determine if child is psychologically prepared for surgery.
   3. Assess readiness of child to learn postoperative procedures.
   4. Observe for signs of infection.
   5. Check that all laboratory tests are completed.
B. Postoperative.
   1. Observe for patency of the airway.
   2. Evaluate vital signs and blood pressure.
   3. Ensure environment provides opportunity for rest.
   4. Evaluate child's hydration and nutrition status.
   5. Monitor cardiac rate and rhythm.
   6. Evaluate chest tube drainage.
   7. Observe for postoperative complications.

Implementation

A. Preoperative.
   1. Evaluate laboratory values for presence of infection.
   2. Discuss with the parents of the child the extent of preparation that the child has received.
   3. Plan with the parents the approach and timing of preoperative teaching.

4. Utilize dolls or models to explain the surgery and postoperative treatment.
5. Conduct a tour of the intensive care unit for the parents and the child and introduce the child to the staff.
6. Teach the child how to cough and deep breathe using blow bottles or other devices.

B. Postoperative.
1. Maintain adequate pulmonary function.
   a. Maintain patent airway.
   b. Instruct child to deep breathe and cough. Monitor use of IPPB.
   c. Maintain ventilator if required by child.
   d. Suction if necessary.
   e. Administer oxygen as ordered.
   f. Check rate and depth of respirations.
2. Maintain adequate circulatory functioning.
   a. Check vital signs.
   b. Monitor rate of IV replacement fluids.
   c. Replace blood when required.
   d. Maintain hourly intake and output records.
3. Monitor chest tube drainage and patency.
4. Provide for rest through organized care.
5. Establish adequate hydration and nutrition.
6. Observe for complications of cardiac surgery.
   a. Pneumothorax.
   b. Hemothorax.
   c. Shock.
   d. Cardiac failure.
   e. Heart block.
   f. Cardiac tamponade.
   g. Hemorrhage.
   h. Hemolytic anemia.
   i. Postcardiotomy syndrome: sudden fever, carditis, and pleurisy.
   j. Postperfusion syndrome (three to twelve weeks after surgery): fever, malaise, and splenomegaly.
   k. Embolism, air or clot.
7. Observe for late complications.
   a. Respiratory: pneumonia.
   b. Infection: incision area.
   c. Congestive heart failure.
   d. Postpericardiotomy Syndrome (assess for symptoms of fever, pericardial friction rub, and pleural effusion).
   e. Postperfusion Syndrome (assess for fever, hepatosplenomegaly, leukocytosis, malaise, and maculopapular rash).

RESPIRATORY SYSTEM

The respiratory system accomplishes pulmonary ventilation through the process of inspiration and expiration. The act of breathing involves a complex chemical and osmotic process in which oxygen is taken into the lungs and carbon dioxide, the end product, is given off.

System Assessment

A. Assess vital signs.
B. Assess rate and rhythm of respirations.
C. Evaluate use of accessory muscles for respiration.
D. Assess presence of cyanosis.
E. Check clubbing of the fingers and toes.
F. Auscultate lungs for rales, rhonchi, wheezes, or diminished breath sounds.
G. Assess presence of pain on respiration.
H. Evaluate cough: productive or nonproductive; color or consistency of sputum.
I. Assess signs of dehydration (poor output, dry mucous membranes, sunken fontanel, poor skin turgor).
J. Check signs of restlessness.
K. Assess need for oxygen administration.
   1. Gasping and/or irregular respirations.
   2. Bradycardia.
   3. Flaring nostrils.
   4. Tachycardia.
   5. Cyanosis.
   6. Increased blood pressure followed by decreased blood pressure.

System Planning and Analysis

A. Client's energy is conserved.
B. Fluid balance is maintained.
C. Temperature is controlled.
D. Air is humidified.
E. Adequate oxygen supply is maintained.
F. Isolation procedures maintained providing infection control.
G. Clinical manifestations are continually monitored for potential complications.

System Implementation

A. Ensure adequate rest and provide a stress-free environment.
B. Organize nursing care to give adequate rest periods.
C. Maintain IV and/or oral fluid levels.
D. Administer antipyretic medication, such as Tylenol or aspirin, tepid sponge baths, or cooling mattress.
E. Provide cool mist tent for humidifying the air. (Keep child dry by changing bedclothes frequently.)
F. Administer oxygen as ordered. (No smoking allowed in room in which oxygen is running.)
G. Provide postural drainage (coughing, deep breathing, and cupping or clapping) to aid in the removal of secretions.
H. Administer antibiotic therapy if bacterial infection occurs.

Conditions Necessary for Avoiding Respiratory Distress

A. Functioning respiratory center in the brain.
B. Intact nerve cells to regulate respiratory muscles.
C. Patent airway for exchange of gases.
D. Alveoli that are able to expand and contract.
E. Adequate pulmonary capillary bed to allow exchange of gases.
F. Adequate supply of oxygen.
G. Functioning cardiovascular system.

System Evaluation

A. Adequate rest is provided for child.
　1. Evaluate environmental conditions if child appears exhausted.
　　a. Noise level.
　　b. Lighting.
　　c. Frequency of interruptions by medical personnel.
　　d. Feeding schedule.
　2. Evaluate child's medical status for exhaustion.
　　a. Respiratory efforts increased.
　　b. Increasing restlessness due to decreasing oxygenation.
B. Adequate hydration is provided for child.
　1. Assess for the following conditions:
　　a. Moist mucous membranes.
　　b. Good skin turgor.
　　c. Adequate output.
　　d. Normal fontanel.
　2. If fluid intake appears to be inadequate, institute the following procedures.
　　a. Increase oral intake.
　　b. Discuss intravenous volume with physician.
C. Normal temperature is maintained.
　1. Monitor treatments to decrease temperature.
　2. Alter treatments as temperature changes.
　3. Ensure mist tent provides cool, visible mist.
D. Adequate oxygenation is maintained.
E. Successful respiratory therapy is provided.
　1. Ensure productive cough.
　2. Auscultate for improvement of breath sounds.
F. Decreased symptoms of bacterial infection.
G. General improvement in respiratory status occurs.
　1. Check for normal rate and rhythm.
　2. Ensure decreased use of accessory muscles for breathing.
　3. Ensure decreased abnormal breath sounds.
　4. Check for decrease in cyanosis.

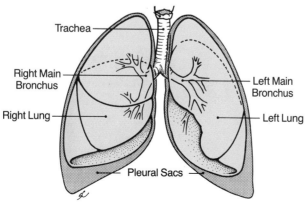

Table 7. SYMPTOM DIFFERENTIATION BETWEEN HIGH AND LOW OBSTRUCTION

High Obstruction (Inspiration Problems)	Low Obstruction (Expiration Problems)
1. Toxicity	1. Toxicity
2. Fatigue	2. Fatigue
3. Air hunger	3. Air hunger
4. Increasing dyspnea	4. Increasingly severe dyspnea
5. Severe sternal retractions	5. Intercostal retractions (mild chest wall)
6. Prolonged inspiratory phase	6. Prolonged expiratory phase
7. Respiratory rate: 45–50 per minute	7. Respiratory rate: 100–110 per minute
8. Cardiac rate: 140–160 per minute	8. Cardiac rate: 180–200 per minute
9. Tracheostomy at cardiac rate over 160	9. No tracheostomy necessary
10. Barking cough	10. Harsh cough
11. Marked inspiratory stridor with hoarseness	11. Expiratory wheeze and grunt
	12. Moist rales
	13. Flaring alae nasi

LOW OBSTRUCTIVE RESPIRATORY CONDITIONS

Bronchitis

Definition: An infection of the major bronchi.

Assessment

A. Assess for hacking and moderately productive cough.
B. Examine for rhonchi and rales.
C. Assess for acute respiratory distress with acute bronchitis.

Implementation

A. Perform postural drainage.
1. Focus on timing—never after meals.
2. Complete according to client's tolerance.
B. Administer humidified air.
C. Increase and monitor fluid intake.
D. Instruct child how to cough and deep breathe deeply.
E. Administer expectorant as ordered.

Bronchiolitis

Definition: Thick production of mucus that causes occlusion of the bronchiole tubes and small bronchi. It occurs most frequently in infants and young children and is usually preceded by an upper respiratory infection.

Assessment

A. Assess for abrupt onset of accelerated respiratory rate and intercostal retractions with prolonged expiratory phase.
B. Check for tachycardia.
C. Check for cyanosis.
D. Evaluate for harsh cough with expiratory wheeze and grunt.

Implementation

A. Conserve child's energy.
B. Administer cool, moist oxygen.
C. Place in semi-Fowler's position to facilitate breathing. Some children may prefer being on their abdomen.
D. Maintain adequate hydration.
E. Observe for signs of dehydration.
1. Sunken fontanel.
2. Poor skin turgor.
3. Decreased and concentrated urinary output.

Types of Pneumonia

Definition: Inflammation of the alveoli caused by bacteria, virus, mycoplasma organisms, aspiration, or inhalation.

Pneumococcal Pneumonia

Assessment

A. Note that symptoms appear suddenly.
B. Assess for high fever.
C. Evaluate if respiratory rate is increased and retractions are present.
D. Assess for increased pulse rate.
E. Check for cough with expectoration.
F. Assess for signs of dehydration.

Implementation

A. Supervise antibiotic therapy.
B. Conserve child's energy.
C. Reduce body temperature with antipyretic medication, cool water mattress, or sponge baths.
D. Maintain isolation for protection.
E. Monitor fluid balance.
F. Measure intake and output.

Staphylococcal Pneumonia

Assessment

A. Note that onset of the disease is rapid.
B. Assess for high fever, cough, and respiratory distress.
C. Check for possible severe dyspnea and cyanosis.
D. Assess for tension pneumothorax or empyema (caused by lesions on the periphery of the lungs that eroded into the pleural space).

Implementation

A. Maintain strict isolation.
B. Supervise administration of medications (frequently methicillin) and watch for side effects (hematuria and proteinuria).
C. Give oxygen therapy.
D. Monitor patency of chest tubes and drainage when inserted.
E. Monitor fluid balance.
F. Maintain accurate intake and output records.

Viral Pneumonia

Assessment

A. Note that illness usually follows an upper respiratory infection.
B. Assess for low-grade fever, nonproductive cough, and tachypnea.
C. Evaluate breath sounds for rales and diminished air exchange.

Implementation

A. Administer therapy similar to that for bacterial pneumonia.
   1. Humidified oxygen.
   2. Chest physiotherapy.
B. Observe for signs of complications.

   1. Atelectasis.
   2. Bronchiectasis.

Asthma

Definition: A pulmonary disorder in which physical or chemical irritants cause the release of histamine and other substances resulting in edema of the bronchial walls, excess secretion of mucus by the bronchial glands, and constriction of the bronchi.

Assessment

A. Check conditions that led to asthmatic attack: exposure to certain foods, infections, vigorous activity, or emotional excitement.
B. Assess for spasms of bronchiolar musculature.
C. Observe for thick, tenacious mucus that accumulates and causes obstruction of air passages.
D. Look for obstructive emphysema caused by trapping of air.
E. Assess for wheezing and rales.
F. Assess for continual cough.
G. Check for distended neck veins.
H. Assess for cyanosis.
I. Evaluate psychological state of child who may be anxious and upset.
J. Constantly monitor symptoms, which may become rapidly worse resulting in acute respiratory failure with cyanosis and acidosis.

Implementation

A. Suspected allergen is identified and removed.
B. Supervise medication administration.
   1. Epinephrine: acts to reduce congestion and edema.
   2. Ephedrine sulfate: reduces congestion and edema.
   3. Aminophylline: bronchodilator.
C. Ensure removal and control of secretions.
   1. Encourage large fluid intake: liquefies secretions and maintains electrolyte balance.
   2. Place in mist tent.
   3. Perform chest physical therapy and postural drainage with lower airway congestion.
D. Provide emotional support for parents and child to reduce anxiety.
E. Educate child to live optimally with chronic problem.

HIGH OBSTRUCTIVE RESPIRATORY CONDITIONS

Laryngotracheobronchitis

Definition: Viral croup is a syndrome caused by a variety of inflammatory conditions of the upper airway. Viral croup is the most common, and bacterial croup is the most serious.

Assessment

A. Ascertain if rhinitis and cough have preceded croup for several days.

B. Assess for gradual onset, then barking cough and inspiratory stridor—usually for 3 to 7 days.

C. Look for symptoms in children less than three years old.

D. Assess for mild elevation in temperature (below 102° F).

E. Observe for hypoxemia which results in anxiety and restlessness.

F. Assess for cyanosis, a late sign, which may indicate complete airway obstruction.

Implementation

A. Plan for home treatment if no inspiratory stridor.
   1. Instruct parents in signs of airway obstruction.
      a. Tachypnea.
      b. Cyanosis.
      c. Increased anxiety.
   2. Instruct parents in using the shower for warm mist therapy. (Cool mist is preferable but usually not available at home.)

B. Provide hospital care for acute onset with inspiratory stridor.
   1. Monitor vital signs every 1–2 hours; check temperature every 2 hours while in cool mist tent.
   2. Check respiratory status every 1–2 hours, depending upon severity of distress.
   3. Monitor accompanying signs and symptoms.
      a. RR (respiratory rate).
      b. GFR (grunting, flaring, retracting).
      c. Stridor.
      d. Color.
      e. Auscultation of breath sounds.
      f. Restlessness.
      g. Use of accessory muscles.
   4. Obtain baseline ABG/CBC.
   5. Place in cool mist oxygen tent every 4–6 hours, depending on severity of distress.

6. Monitor hydration status.
   a. If RR>60 and NPO, start intravenous fluids; if RR<60 and will take fluids, give clear liquids only as tolerated.
   b. Monitor urinary output, specific gravity, and skin turgor.
   c. Maintain patency of IV.

7. Place on cardio-respiratory monitor if signs of hypoxia or respiratory failure.

Epiglottitis

Definition: An acute viral or bacterial infection of the epiglottis. Usually caused by Hemophilus influenza type B or pneumococci streptococci.

Assessment

A. Observe that illness occurs most frequently in young children, 3–7 years of age.

B. Ascertain if illness was preceded by an upper respiratory infection.

C. Assess for rapid onset with inspiratory stridor and retractions, cough, muffled voice.

D. Assess for high temperature (100°–104°F).

E. Assess for respiratory distress.

F. Evaluate difficulty in swallowing as manifested by excessive drooling and refusal to take liquids.

Implementation

A. Prepare for lateral neck films STAT to confirm diagnosis. Keep child in upright position. Supine position may cause occlusion of the airway and respiratory arrest.

B. Never use restraints; never use a tongue blade.

C. Do not elicit a gag reflex—may cause further spasm of epiglottis.

D. Prepare child for OR if elective intubation is to be done.

E. Maintain tracheostomy set/intubation tray at bedside.

F. Provide cool oxygen mist at all times.

G. Monitor vital signs with respiratory status every 1 hour with continuous close observation.
   1. Monitor respiratory rate, grunting, retracting, stridor, color, restlessness.
   2. Auscultate breath sounds; evaluate use of accessory muscles.

H. Monitor hydration status. Keep child NPO.
   1. Start IV. Check urinary output, specific gravity, skin turgor, tears.

2. Maintain patency of IV.
I. Monitor temperature every 2 hours—give Tylenol for temperature > 100°F as ordered.
J. Place on cardiorespiratory monitor.
K. Isolate for 24 hours after start of antibiotic therapy.
L. Prepare for intubation.
  1. Maintain child in upright position.
  2. Administer humidified oxygen—assist with CPAP or mechanical ventilation as necessary.
  3. Check every 1 hour to maintain tube patency.
  4. Restrain child *well* to prevent accidental extubation (remains intubated 12–48 hours).
M. Monitor signs prior to extubation.
  1. Ability to swallow.
  2. Resolution of sepsis.
  3. Temperature within normal limits for 12 hours.
  4. Resolution of swelling.
  5. NPO 4 hours prior to extubation.

Tonsillitis and Adenoiditis

Definition: Infection and inflammation of the palatine tonsils and adenoids. Primary causes are Group A beta-hemolytic streptococcus and viruses.

Assessment

A. Assess for tonsillitis.
  1. Observe for fever, sore throat, and anorexia.
  2. Assess for general malaise and difficulty in swallowing.
B. Assess for adenoiditis.
  1. Evaluate for stertorous breathing.
  2. Assess for pain in ear and recurring otitis media.
C. Evaluate if indications for surgery are present.
  1. Surgery is performed only when absolutely necessary because tonsils are thought to have important protective immunologic functions.
  2. Assess for repeated episodes of tonsillitis, which indicates infection.
  3. Assess for difficulty in swallowing, which indicates enlargement of tonsils or adenoids.
  4. Observe for interference with breathing.
  5. Evaluate for blocked eustachian tube. (Chronic otitis media).

Implementation

PREOPERATIVE INTERVENTIONS

A. Take samples for blood tests (CBC, Hgb, Hct, bleeding and clotting time), serologic tests, and throat culture.
B. Obtain complete health history, including history of allergies.
C. Provide emotional support for the child.
  1. Separation from family.
  2. Hospitalization procedure.
  3. Physical layout of surgery room.
  4. Induction of anesthesia.
  5. Recovery room procedure.
  6. Postoperative pain.
  7. Postoperative activity level (play therapy useful).
D. Provide routine preoperative care.

POSTOPERATIVE INTERVENTIONS

A. Maintain in prone or Sims' position until fully awake to facilitate drainage of secretions and prevent aspiration. Then change to semi-Fowler's.
B. Avoid suctioning and coughing to prevent hemorrhage.
C. Observe for signs of shock.
  1. Restlessness.
  2. Alterations in vital signs (increased pulse, decreased blood pressure, increased respiration).
  3. Frequent swallowing.
  4. Excessive thirst.
  5. Vomiting of blood.
  6. Pallor.
D. Maintain calm, quiet environment to prevent anxiety, which can lead to shock.
E. Provide ice collar.
F. Force fluids.
  1. Encourage cold fluids, popsicles, ice chips.
  2. Avoid use of citrus juices, mild, hot liquids.
  3. Do not use straws.
G. Administer Tylenol for pain as ordered.

ASSOCIATED CONDITIONS

Cystic Fibrosis

Definition: Cystic fibrosis is a genetic disorder in which the mucus-producing glands, particularly those of the lungs and pancreas, are abnormal. They produce thick and viscous mucus. Abnormal mucus production in the pancreas leads to pancreatic insufficiency and, in the lungs, to emphysematous changes.

Assessment

A. Assess weight gain because infants with high-caloric intake do not gain weight.
B. Evaluate for recurrent, severe respiratory infections caused by thick mucous and bronchial plugs, which can cause atelectasis.
C. Assess for mild diarrhea with greasy, malodorous stools caused by malabsorption of fats and proteins.
D. Evaluate diagnostic tests, including the sweat test for sodium content and trypsin test. (Trypsin is absent in cystic fibrosis.)

Implementation

A. Provide adequate nutritional maintenance.
 1. Pancreatic enzymes, Viokase and Cotazym, prior to meals.
 2. Water-soluble vitamins.
 3. Fat-soluble vitamins A, D, and E in water-miscible form.
 4. Diet high in calories and protein and low in fat.
 5. Sodium balance.
B. Provide adequate respiratory maintenance. Major objective is to keep lungs clear of mucus.
 1. IPPB mucomist.
 2. Mist tent at night to liquefy secretions.
 3. Postural drainage t.i.d. following IPPB.
 4. Breathing exercises. (Children tend to breathe shallowly.)
C. Administer antibiotics as ordered to prevent infection.
D. Provide parental education.
 1. Information about the disease and its long-term effects.
 2. Genetic counseling.
 3. Resource centers such as National Foundation for Cystic Fibrosis and local organizations.
 4. Care of the child at home.
  a. Normal family routine.
  b. Children are irritable, frightened, and insecure.
  c. Children need attention, discipline, and reassurance.

Otitis Media

Definition: A common complication of an acute respiratory infection that occurs when edema of the upper respiratory structures trap the infection in the middle ear.

Assessment

A. Assess for high fever.
B. Observe for pulling or rubbing of one or both ears.
C. Observe for irritability and restlessness.

Implementation

A. Supervise use of antibiotics, usually ampicillin, penicillin, or, if chronic, Keflin.
B. Supervise use of decongestant to open the eustachian tubes.
C. Administer analgesic for pain as ordered.
D. Advise parents that during the course of the infection the child will usually have a conductive hearing loss.
E. Conserve child's energy by providing sedentary activities.
F. Maintain adequate diet and fluid intake.

Sudden Infant Death Syndrome (SIDS)

Definition: The sudden, unexplainable death of an infant during sleep.

Characteristics

A. Most frequent cause of death after neonatal period.
B. Peak incidence from 2 to 4 months of age. No danger first month; rare after 6 months.
C. Higher incidence in winter, June and July, and in low-income groups.
D. On autopsy, inflammation of upper respiratory tract is found.
E. Maternal factors: SIDS more common in unwed mothers, younger mothers, multiparous mothers with shorter between-pregnancy intervals, cigarette-smoking mothers, and mothers who do not fully utilize health care facilities or use them later in pregnancy.
F. Infant factors: SIDS more common in prematures and small-for-gestational-age infants; infant's growth after birth is slower than average.
G. Sleep: most deaths are unobserved; death during sleep is common although not universal.

H. Feeding: bottle-feeding more prevalent in SIDS, but breast-fed infants are not immune.
I. Familial recurrence: greater than normal population, but only 1–2 percent risk. No evidence of genetic link.
J. Specificity: occurrence rate of SIDS parallels the rate for general infant mortality.
K. Etiology unknown and controversial. Theories involve carbon dioxide, sensitivity, massive virus, allergic reaction, and poor response to stimulus.

Assessment

1. Assess age of infant and remaining epidemiologic findings.
2. Assess for prematurity/low birth weight infant.
3. Check for respiratory pauses, sleep apnea.
4. Check for gastroesophageal reflux/apnea associated with regurgitation after feeding, or tiring during feeding.
5. Assess for past history of oxygen administration.
6. Assess for history of allergic response.

Implementation

A. Apneic episode discovered: infant responds when stimulated (near-miss SIDS). Instruct parents in care.
   1. Shake/stimulate infant. If no response, immediately begin CPR.
   2. Take infant to physician or nearest emergency room.
      a. Record accurate history from parents: time of discovery of infant, color of infant, skin temperature, spontaneous respirations after stimulation.
      b. Ask relevant questions: Was CPR begun? How long after? How long was it continued? Did infant respond? Did there appear to be regurgitation of formula when infant was discovered? When did infant last eat?
   3. Assist physician to do complete neurological, developmental, and physical exam of infant, including labwork.
   4. Teach parents CPR.
   5. Instruct parents about care of a child on a home monitor.
   6. Give parents phone numbers for respite care and support groups.
   7. Suggest to parents that infant join sleep study program (polygraph monitoring of near-miss SIDS infants).
B. Infant dies; upon autopsy, SIDS is diagnosed.
   1. Support parents through loss and grieving process. Reassure parents that they did everything right for the child. Emphasize *blamelessness* of parents and siblings.
   2. Inform parents of result of autopsy as soon as possible so grieving process may begin.
   3. Refer parents to National Foundation for SIDS.
   4. If other infants in home, suggest they be tested for possible sleep apnea.

Kawasaki Disease

Definition: A children's disease, most frequently seen in boys under two of Asian ancestry. It responds like a viral disease of lymph nodes, but has an unknown cause.

Assessment

A. Assess for age, sex, and ancestry to determine if child fits usual profile.
B. Assess for viral symptoms: fever, rash, swollen hands and feet, redness of the eyes, swollen lymph glands in the neck, inflammation of mouth, lips, and throat.
C. Assess for potential heart involvement (aneurysm, blocked coronary artery leading to a heart attack, myocarditis or pericarditis; arrhythmias can also occur).

Treatment

A. Since cause is unknown, no specific treatment is ordered.
B. Monitor aspirin to reduce fever, pain, and inflammation; intravenous gamma globulin may prevent coronary artery disease if given early.

GASTROINTESTINAL SYSTEM

The primary function of the alimentary tract is to provide the body with a continual supply of nutrients, fluids, and electrolytes for tissue nourishment. This system has three components: a tract for ingestion and movement of food and fluids; secretion of digestive juices for breaking down the nutrients; and absorption mechanisms for the utilization of foods, water, and electrolytes for continued growth and repair of body tissues.

System Assessment

A. Assess for obstruction.
   1. Absent or abnormal stools.
   2. Presence of vomiting.
   3. Distended abdomen.
   4. Hyperactive bowel sounds above level of obstruction.
B. Assess for infection.
   1. Diarrhea.
   2. Vomiting.
   3. Increased pulse, respirations.
   4. Elevated temperature.
C. Assess hydration status.
   1. Signs of dehydration.
   2. Change in daily weight.
D. Assess nutritional status.
   1. Failure to gain weight.
   2. Abnormal stools.

Diagnostic Procedures

Barium Enema

A. A procedure in which a barium mixture is placed in the large intestine via a rectal catheter for x-ray visualization of the entire large intestine.
B. Nursing responsibilities prior to procedure.
   1. Cleanse the bowel through enemas.
   2. Restrict diet (clear fluids for 24 hours).

C. Nursing responsibilities following procedure.
   1. Avoid impaction from barium.
      a. Provide child with large fluid intake.
      b. Administer laxative or cleansing enemas.
   2. Advise parents and child that stools will be white for 24 to 72 hours following procedure.

System Implementation

A. Interventions for possible obstruction in infants.
   1. Check on passage of meconium during first three days.
   2. Attempt to pass a nasogastric tube into stomach and aspirate contents as ordered.
   3. Evaluate for excessive mucus and choking.
   4. Observe for presence of cyanosis and choking on first feeding.
   5. Check for projectile vomiting following feedings.
   6. Check for presence of abdominal distention.
   7. Document evidence of abdominal pain.
   8. Evaluate for absent or abnormal stooling cycle.
B. Interventions for possible infection.
   1. Evaluate vital signs.
   2. Check for presence of watery stools.
   3. Evaluate laboratory results of stool culture.
   4. Evaluate vomiting pattern.
   5. Isolate child until the causative organism is identified.
   6. Provide meticulous skin care.
   7. Be aware that taking temperature with rectal thermometer is contraindicated if diarrhea is present.
C. Interventions for maintaining hydration.
   1. Check for signs of dehydration.
      a. Dry mucous membranes.
      b. Sunken fontanels (infant).
      c. Poor skin turgor.
      d. Decrease in output.
      e. Increase in urine specific gravity.
      f. Sunken eyeballs.
      g. Increased pulse.
      h. Increased irritability.
   2. Monitor intravenous fluid administration.
   3. Monitor daily weights.
   4. Check specific gravity of urine.
D. Interventions for maintaining nutritional status.
   1. Compare child's growth with standardized growth chart.
   2. Evaluate food intake and meal pattern.
   3. Record stooling pattern and reaction to feed-

ings. (If fatty, bulky stools, assess for malabsorption problem.)

4. Determine child's likes and dislikes and orient diet accordingly.

5. Allow bottle if child regresses and is comforted by sucking.

6. Allow between-meal snacks that are both nutritious and fun (popsicles, fruit bars).

System Evaluation

A. Early identification of obstruction.
   1. Meconium passes in the first few days after birth.
      a. If not, assess the child for abdominal distention.
      b. If more than 20 cc of gastric contents is aspirated through nasogastric tube, assess for lower intestinal obstruction.
   2. No symptoms of esophageal atresia present.
      a. Excessive drooling, choking, and cyanosis may indicate esophageal atresia.
      b. Inability to pass nasogastric tube at birth indicates esophageal atresia.
   3. Absence of projectile vomiting.
      a. If not, evaluate infant's diet. (Overfeeding can cause projectile vomiting.)
      b. If vomiting occurs, evaluate for signs of infection or increased intracranial pressure.
      c. If these conditions are not present, vomiting may be a sign of an obstruction.
   4. Presence of slightly protuberant abdomen, which is normal. If abdomen is distended or excessively hard, evaluate for possible obstruction.
   5. Normal crying pattern.
      a. It is abnormal for an infant to have abdominal pain, but it is necessary to distinguish this from colic.
      b. If the child has very harsh intermittent crying or continual crying, evaluate the stool cycle for normal stools that follow the normal infant stool cycle. Ribbon-shaped stools, bulky, foul-smelling stools, or other abnormalities can be signs of a gastrointestinal abnormality.

B. Absence of infection.
   1. No vomiting and/or diarrhea present.
   2. No vital sign changes.
      a. Increased temperature and pulse are signs of infection.
      b. If significant dehydration has occurred, respirations will be rapid.

C. Normal hydration status maintained.

D. Normal nutrition maintained.
   1. Child remains in the same percentile range for height and weight according to growth and development chart.
   2. Growth appears normal for age.
   3. Skin and hair appear healthy.

GASTROINTESTINAL DISORDERS

Poisoning

Definition: Ingestion of toxic substances which may result in death or severe illness.

A. The most common age group affected is 2-year-olds because of their exploration of the environment through tasting.

B. The major cause of poisoning is improper storage of toxic agents.
   1. Legislation has mandated child-proof tops on prescription drugs, but many children can still remove the tops.
   2. Some new forms of drugs, such as transdermal patches or lozenges, are packaged so that they present a danger.

C. General principles of care for poisoning.
   1. Identify the toxic substance and retrieve the poison.
   2. Notify the local poison control and inform them of the toxic substance.
   3. Reverse the effect of the poison.
      a. Induce vomiting with syrup of ipecac or apomorphine.
         (1) Families of small children should keep this substance in the house in case of accidental poisoning.
         (2) Dose is 15 ml for children and 30 ml for young adults; follow with tap water.
         (3) Child should vomit within 30 minutes— important to bring up the syrup of ipecac to avoid cardiac complications.
      b. Activated charcoal may be used to carry toxic substance out of the body.
   4. Vomiting is contraindicated with some substances.
      a. If child or person is in a coma, in shock, convulsing, or exhibits no gag reflex.

b. If person has ingested low viscosity hydrocarbons or corrosive substances (acid or alkaloid).

Pyloric Stenosis

Definition: The pyloric canal, which is at the distal end of the stomach and connects with the duodenum, is greatly narrowed. This narrowing is believed to be caused by a combination of muscular hypertrophy, spasms, and edema of the mucous membrane.

Assessment

A. Assess for vomiting in newborn. Vomiting usually begins after two weeks and before two months of age.
   1. Progressively increases in frequency and force.
   2. Projectile vomitus may contain mucus and blood.
B. Check for constant hunger, fussiness, and frequent crying.
C. Evaluate stools for decrease in size and number, and assess for constipation.
D. Observe for peristaltic waves: frequently noted passing from left to right during or immediately following a feeding.
E. Assess for later symptoms, which may include malnutrition, dehydration, electrolyte imbalance, and alkalosis.

Implementation

A. Monitor infant for metabolic alkalosis from vomiting.
B. Provide preoperative care.
   1. Ensure accurate regulation of IV to prevent dehydration.
   2. Accurately record intake and output.
   3. Observe feeding behavior for definitive diagnosis.
   4. Support mother and infant.
C. Maintain proper insertion and observation of gastric tube.
   1. Measure length of tube externally on infant from bridge of nose to ear to stomach.
   2. Check position of the tube. Infant should show no sign of respiratory difficulty with external end of tube occluded.
   3. Aspirate gastric contents. Insert 2–5 cc air through tube and listen for "whooshing" sound with stethoscope.
   4. No gagging, redness, or coughing should be observed.

D. Perform nursing care following surgery. Follow standard postoperative procedures for Fredet-Ramstedt intervention.
   1. Maintain patent airway.
   2. Observe for shock.
   3. Keep a careful record of feeding behavior to assist physician in determining progress of feedings.
   4. Begin feedings four to six hours after surgery to prevent adhesion formation.
   5. After anesthesia has worn off, place in semi-Fowler's position.
   6. Do not handle infant excessively after feeding.

Esophageal Atresia with Tracheoesophageal Fistula (TEA)

Definition: Failure of the esophagus to be continuous from the pharynx to the stomach. TEA is an abnormal connection between the trachea and the esophagus.

Characteristics

A. Anomaly occurs during embryonic development. Cause is unknown.
B. There are several different types of esophageal atresia.
   1. The most simple type involves the narrowing of the esophagus.
   2. The second type involves the upper and lower segments of the esophagus that are not attached to each other, creating two blind pouches.
   3. Other types involve fistulas between the upper and/or lower segments of the esophagus and trachea.
C. Fistulas may be present when the esophagus is patent, when it is narrowed, or when it is not joined to its distal portion.
D. Infants at risk for TEA: premature infants and those with polyhydramnios.

Assessment

A. Assess infant status. Early recognition of the defect is imperative to prevent aspiration.
B. Assess for excessive amounts of mucus with much drooling.
C. Assess for coughing, choking, and cyanosis when fed.

D. Check to see if food is expelled through the nose immediately following feeding.
   1. Assess severe coughing and choking.
   2. Assess struggling with resulting cyanosis.
E. Evaluate frequent respiratory problems.
F. Check for abdominal distention caused by inspired air going into the stomach.

Implementation

A. Maintain patent airway; observe for signs of respiratory distress.
B. Prevent aspiration pneumonia.
   1. Discontinue oral fluids immediately.
   2. Position infant at least 30 degrees for head elevation to decrease potential of aspiration. Infant seat works well for positioning.
   3. Change position every two hours.
   4. Suction accumulated secretions frequently.
C. Initiate and monitor IV fluids as ordered to prevent dehydration.
D. Prepare for gastrostomy tube insertion (decompresses stomach and prevents aspiration of gastric contents from fistula).
   1. Administer gastrostomy tube feedings.
   2. Observe for patency of all tubes. Do not clamp gastrostomy tube.
   3. Use gentle suctioning of the upper pouch to minimize aspiration of saliva.
   4. Monitor the gastrostomy tube in place until total repair is performed.
E. Postoperative care
   1. Maintain patent airway.
      a. Suction secretions as necessary.
      b. Position for comfortable ventilation.
      c. Administer oxygen as needed.
      d. Maintain care of chest tubes.
   2. Prevent infection.
      a. Provide meticulous care of operative site.
      b. Observe for signs of inflammation or infection.
   3. Maintain fluid and electrolyte balance.
      a. Monitor IV fluids; record intake and output.
      b. Record weight daily.
      c. Measure specific gravity of urine.
   4. Maintain infant in Isolette or radiant warmer with nebulized humidity.
   5. Provide adequate nutrition.
      a. Administer gastrostomy feedings (usually after third postoperative day).
      b. Continue until infant tolerates oral feedings, 10–14 days postoperatively (based on condition of child and degree of healing).
      c. Monitor gradual increase in feedings and elevation of gastrostomy tube.
         (1) Feed slowly to allow for swallowing and to provide infant rest.
         (2) Position upright to prevent aspiration.
         (3) Burp frequently.
   6. Meet sucking needs by providing a pacifier (if approved by physician).
   7. Prepare parents for discharge.
      a. Teach techniques parents will need for home care: tube feedings, suctioning, etc.
      b. Educate parents to look for signs of complications such as esophageal constriction: difficulty in swallowing, choking, breathing difficulties.

Intussusception

Definition: A segment of the bowel telescopes into the portion of bowel immediately distal to it. Probably results from hyperactive peristalsis in the proximal portion of the bowel, with inactive peristalsis in the distal segment. Usually occurs at the junction of the ileum with the colon. Common in children with cystic fibrosis and celiac disease.

Assessment

A. Assess for sudden onset. Condition occurs most often when the child is between four and six months old.
B. Evaluate for vomiting, abdominal pain and distention, and infrequent stools with blood and mucus (appears like currant jelly).
C. Note child's behavior; if child frequently pulls knees to chest, this is an indication of pain.
D. Assess level of hydration.

Implementation

A. Prepare child for barium enema x-ray, which frequently reduces the bowel.
B. Observe and monitor for recurrence of symptoms. Surgery may need to be performed for bowel reduction.
C. Observe and maintain IV fluid and electrolyte replacement.
D. Perform nasogastric suction to deflate the stomach to prevent vomiting.

E. Gradually reintroduce fluids and foods.

F. Maintain care of operative site following surgery.

Diarrhea (Severe)

Definition: Diarrhea is seen when there is a disturbance of the intestinal tract that alters motility and absorption and accelerates the excretion of intestinal contents (three to thirty stools per day). Fluids and electrolytes that are normally absorbed are excreted, causing electrolyte imbalances. Most infectious diarrheas in this country are caused by a virus. Diarrhea can be a separate disease, or it may be a symptom of another disease.

Assessment

A. Assess for increased rate of peristalsis carrying intestinal contents (include base-bicarbonates) along.
   1. Blood, pus, or mucus in stools, which are often green in color.
   2. Increase in frequency of stools of watery consistency.
B. Assess for signs of dehydration.
   1. Mucous membranes become dried and cracked.
   2. Skin dries and loses its normal elasticity.
   3. Fontanels are depressed, and eyes appear sunken.
   4. The urine decreases greatly in amount and becomes dark in color (concentrated).
   5. Acidosis is a common result.

Implementation

A. Provide a period of rest for the gastrointestinal tract—usually ordered for twenty-four to forty-eight hours.
B. Monitor diet as it progresses from water to carbohydrates, proteins, fats, fruits, and vegetables as tolerated.
C. Maintain strict isolation until causal organism or other factors are determined.
D. Dispose of stools and diapers in proper containers.
E. Maintain careful ongoing assessment of dehydration level and acidosis.
F. Complete accurate recording of the number and consistency of stools.
G. Prevent dehydration and electrolyte imbalance.
   1. Maintain strict observation of intake and output.

   2. Supervise IV therapy if ordered.
   3. Monitor electrolyte laboratory results.
H. Maintain excellent skin care to prevent excoriation caused by alkaline stools.

Hirschsprung's Disease (Megacolon)

Definition: A disease caused by the congenital absence of parasympathetic nerve ganglion cells in the distal bowel. As a result, this portion of the bowel is unable to transmit regular peristaltic waves, which are coordinated with the proximal portion of the bowel. When a stool reaches the diseased area, it is not transmitted on down the colon, but accumulates in the segment just proximal to this area, forming a functional obstruction. The bowel above the obstructed portion eventually becomes hypertrophied in its attempts to transmit the stool.

Assessment

A. Assess for failure to pass meconium in newborn.
B. Assess for symptoms of bile-stained vomiting and reluctance to feed.
C. Evaluate for signs of intestinal obstruction.
D. Evaluate for signs of constipation and abdominal distention.
E. Assess for foul odor of breath and stool.
F. Note that in older child symptoms of constipation, offensive odor, and ribbon-like stools may be present.

MEDICAL IMPLICATIONS
A. In mild cases, treatment is enemas, stool softeners, and low-residue diet.
B. The first stage of treatment is usually a transverse or sigmoid colostomy.
C. The child is then brought back to optimal health and nutritional status.
D. The final procedure consists of dissection and removal of the nonfunctional bowel and anastomosis.
E. Final treatment is closure of temporary colostomy.

Implementation

A. Prior to diagnosis, observe carefully for all gastrointestinal manifestations of the disease and report them accurately.
B. Prior to the colostomy procedure.
   1. Cleanse bowel.

a. Stool softeners.
b. Liquid diet.
c. Colonic irrigation—saline.
2. Prepare parents for the procedure.
   a. Clarify the surgical technique.
   b. Describe stoma.
   c. Prepare for care of the child with a colostomy.
   d. Give parents the opportunity to express their feelings about the procedure.
C. Postoperative care.
1. Maintain optimal nutrition.
2. Closely observe stools for reestablishment of normal elimination pattern.
3. Maintain skin care of colostomy and anal areas.

Cleft Lip

Definition: A birth defect that involves a fissure resulting from incomplete merging of embryonic processes that normally form the face or jaws. The condition is usually considered hereditary but may be familial.

Assessment

A. Assess for adequate nutrition.
B. Assess vital signs for base line data.
C. Assess respiratory status.

Implementation

A. Preoperative care for surgical repair.
1. Use soft or regular nipple with crosscut.
2. Place nipple on opposite side from cleft.
3. Bubble frequently.
B. Postoperative care.
1. Observe for respiratory distress and swelling of tongue, nostrils, and mouth.
2. Avoid circumstances that will cause crying.
3. Watch for hemorrhage.
4. Use elbow restraints and provide supervised rest periods to exercise arms.
5. Feed with rubber-tipped medicine dropper on unoperated side for three weeks.
6. After feeding, clean suture line with half-strength hydrogen peroxide.
7. Prevent crust formation on suture line.
8. Lay infant on unoperated side or back with support; goal is to prevent rubbing suture site on the sheet.

Cleft Palate

Definition: A birth defect in which the palates—opening between the nose and the roof of the mouth—fail to close properly. It is usually considered hereditary. Types include clefted soft palate, clefted hard palate, and a cleft that infrequently involves the nose.

Assessment

A. Assess for difficulty in sucking.
B. Assess for increase in upper respiratory infections.
C. Evaluate mother-child relationship—i.e., mother feels frustrated and baby is fussy.

MEDICAL IMPLICATIONS

A. Surgical repairs: some surgeons prefer to wait until the palate has had the opportunity to grow; others prefer to operate prior to the onset of speech.
B. Repair in stages: may be required with extensive defects.
C. Surgical repair usually needs to be followed by treatment from an orthodontist, a speech therapist, and a plastic surgeon.

Implementation

A. Preoperative care.
1. Observe for respiratory infections.
2. Ensure that child is sitting up when fed.
3. Provide frequent mouth care.
4. Introduce the method of postoperative feeding; for example, have the child drink from a cup.
5. Practice arm restraints on the child, so that child becomes familiar with them.
6. Prepare parents and give them support.
B. Postoperative care.
1. Immediate postoperative period.
   a. Place child on abdomen to prevent aspiration of mucus or blood.
   b. Observe for signs of airway obstruction, and have suction apparatus at the bedside.
   c. Observe for shock or hemorrhage.
   d. Utilize elbow restraints but release frequently.
   e. Irrigate suture line frequently.
   f. Provide a mist tent.
2. Second postoperative day prior to discharge.
   a. Start introducing fluids by paper cup; avoid straws and glasses.
   b. Advance diet as tolerated.
   c. Irrigate sutures following feedings.

Celiac Disease (Gluten-Induced Enteropathy)

Definition: A chronic disease of intestinal malabsorption precipitated by ingestion of gluten or protein portions of wheat or rye flour.

Characteristics

A. A major cause of malabsorption in children, second only to cystic fibrosis.
B. Highest incidence occurs in caucasians.
C. Major problem is an intolerance to gluten, a protein found in most grains.
D. Basic defect is believed to be an inborn error of metabolism or an autoimmune response.
E. Primary physiological effect is inadequate fat absorption; as disease progresses it affects absorption of all ingested elements.
F. Long-term effects can be anemia, poor blood coagulation and osteoporosis.

Assessment

A. Assess age disease occurs: usually when child begins to ingest grains. It may begin as early as six months and continue until fifth year.
B. Assess for diarrhea or loose stools: bulky, foul smelling, pale, and frothy.
C. Check for failure to gain weight after a bout of diarrhea.
D. Check for abdominal distention.
E. Assess for anorexia.
F. Evaluate behavioral changes: irritability and restlessness.
G. Assess for celiac crisis.
   1. Vomiting and diarrhea.
   2. Acidosis and dehydration.
   3. May be precipitated by respiratory infection.
   4. Excessive perspiration.
   5. Cold extremities.

Implementation

A. Monitor appropriate diet.
   1. Wheat and rye gluten as well as barley and oats are eliminated.
   2. Low fat.
   3. Slow feedings, small amounts at a time.
   4. Strict intake and output.
   5. Strict calorie control.
   6. Supplemental vitamins and iron.

B. Instruct parents to recognize impending celiac crisis.
   1. Teach primary symptoms of crisis.
   2. Institute medical intervention to correct dehydration and metabolic acidosis.
C. Give parental support.
   1. Teach diet.
   2. Provide for follow-up by public health nurse for continued teaching and assistance.
   3. Explain prognosis: clinical symptoms decrease with increasing age.
D. Prevent infection.

Obesity

Definition: A condition resulting from an excess of caloric intake over caloric output from over-eating.

Characteristics

A. The impact of childhood obesity becomes most obvious at adolescence when body image and peer approval become important.
B. Occasionally, obesity is a sign that the child is missing other satisfaction.
C. Sometimes food is the only source of pleasure a child can find.
D. Eating can relieve anxiety for some children.
E. The child is often the victim of nagging and begins to associate overweight with feelings of worthlessness.
F. Usually, a strong familial tendency toward obesity exists.

Assessment

A. Assess height and weight according to standard growth and development scale.
B. Identify possible genetic factors related to the child.
C. Evaluate eating patterns and habits.
D. Assess length of time child has been obese.
E. Evaluate child's and family's feelings and attitudes about obesity.

Implementation

A. Provide a balanced diet with limited calories.
B. Set up a routine of daily exercise; frequently, groups for after-school exercise programs can be organized by school nurses.
C. Help the young person work through underlying problems causing or caused by obesity.

D. Provide family counseling.
   1. Examine the eating patterns of the family. Some cultures have a high proportion of starches; others associate large meals with prosperity.
   2. Suggest the use of positive reinforcement for the adolescent rather than shaming the child.
   3. Have family support child by removing high calorie food from their meals.

Ulcerative Colitis

Definition: An inflammatory disease of the colon and the rectum in which the mucous membrane becomes hyperemic, bleeds easily, and tends to ulcerate. The etiology is unknown; however, the incidence is highest in young adults and middle-age groups.

Assessment

A. Assess for diarrhea.
B. Check for weight loss.
C. Assess for rectal bleeding.
D. Evaluate for abdominal pain, nausea, and vomiting.
E. Assess for presence of anemia.
F. Assess for fever and dehydration.
G. Evaluate personality and attachments; children with the disease tend to be passive, pessimistic, fearful, and strongly, though ambivalently, attached to a parent.

Implementation

A. Control inflammation.
   1. Supervise medication regime.
   2. Provide adequate hydration with intravenous therapy and oral fluids as indicated.
B. Provide rest to intestinal tract.
   1. Observe for amount of bowel activity and symptoms of bleeding and hyperactive peristalsis.
   2. Administer tranquilizers, and observe for side effects.
C. Monitor diet therapy.
   1. Provide a high-fiber, bland, high-protein diet.
   2. Institute vitamin therapy.
   3. Avoid cold foods because they increase gastric motility.
   4. Arrange for attractive environment with opportunities for socialization at mealtimes.

   5. Avoid sharp cheeses, highly spiced foods, smoked or salted meats, fried foods, raw fruits, and vegetables.
D. Provide counseling activities.
   1. Educate child about diet, medication, and symptoms of bleeding.
   2. Observe for signs of psychological problems; initiate referral if necessary.

Imperforate Anus

Definition: A congenital abnormality in the formation of the anorectal canal or in the location of the anus resulting in the rectum ending blindly. A fistula or a severe narrowing of the anal canal.

Assessment

A. Assess patency of anal opening with small finger or soft catheter if the following symptoms are present.
   1. No meconium stool within 24 hours.
   2. Green-tinged urine.
   3. Progressive abdominal distention.
B. Assess for presence of other anomalies if imperforate anus is present.
C. Observe for signs of distress.

Implementation

A. Withhold feedings when anomaly is diagnosed.
B. Check vital signs frequently.
C. Maintain temperature by using Isolette or radiant warmer.
D. Administer postoperative care.
   1. Prevent infection of operative site.
   2. Provide colostomy care if colostomy is performed and prevent skin breakdown.
   3. Check for return of peritalsis so that oral feedings may be started.
E. Provide supportive care to parents before and after surgery.

PARASITIC WORMS

Definition: Worms affect not only the gastrointestinal system but also are found in the lungs, heart, and other body systems. As parasites, they feed off the host which leads to a variety of symptoms.

Roundworms

Characteristics

A. Eggs are laid by the worm in the gastrointestinal tract of any host animal and passed out in feces.

B. After the worms have been ingested, egg batches are laid.

C. Larvae in the host invade lymphatics and venules of the mesentery and migrate to the liver, the lungs, and the heart.

D. Larvae from lungs reach the host's epiglottis and are swallowed; once in the gastrointestinal tract, the cycle is repeated—larvae mature and mate, and the female lays eggs.

Assessment

A. Assess for atypical pneumonia.

B. Assess for gastrointestinal symptoms: nausea, vomiting, anorexia, and weight loss.

C. Determine if insomnia is present.

D. Evaluate for signs of irritability.

E. Assess for presence of intestinal obstruction.

Implementation

A. Prevent infection through the use of a sanitary toilet.

B. Provide hygiene education of the family.

C. Dispose of infected stools carefully.

D. Administer piperazine citrate.

Pinworms (Enterobiasis)

Characteristics

A. Most common parasite infection in U.S., especially in warm climates.

B. Eggs ingested or inhaled.

C. Eggs mature in cecum, then migrate to anus.

D. Worms exit at night and lay eggs on host's skin.

Assessment

A. Assess for acute or subacute appendicitis.

B. Evaluate for eczematous areas of skin.

C. Determine if irritability is present.

D. Ascertain loss of weight and anorexia.

E. Determine if child suffers from insomnia.

F. Diagnose condition by tape test: place transparent adhesive tape over anus and examine tape for evidence of worms.

Implementation

A. During treatment, maintain meticulous cleansing of skin, particularly anal region, hands and nails.

B. Ensure that bed linens and clothing are boiled.

C. Use ointment to relieve itching.

D. Teach careful hygiene as a preventative measure.

E. Instruct all infected persons living communally that they must be treated simultaneously.

F. Drugs available: piperazine citrate; pyrantel pamoate; drug of choice is mebendazole.

Giardiasis

Definition: The most common intestinal parasitic pathogen in the U.S., this condition is caused by the protozoan, *Giardia lambia*.

Characteristics

A. Very common in children in day-care centers (estimates are 9–38%).

B. Major mode of transmission is person-to-person; water (especially mountain lakes and streams), food and animals.

C. Adults may be asymptomatic, but children usually manifest symptoms.

Assessment

A. Infants and young children.
   1. Diarrhea.
   2. Vomiting and anorexia.
   3. Failure to thrive.

B. Children over 5 years of age.
   1. Abdominal cramps.
   2. Loose stools—may be intermittent.
   3. Stools may be watery, pale and smelly.

C. Assess condition through stool specimens—may need six or more over several weeks.

Implementation

A. The most important nursing measure is to teach prevention—meticulous sanitary practices during diaper changes and cleaning of children.
   1. Inform parents of importance of handwashing.
   2. Drink water that is purified, especially when out in the open.

B. Administer drugs available for treatment: quinacrine, furazolidone (drug of choice), and metronidazole.
   1. If cost is a factor, quinacrine is usually given; administer with or after meals and crush tablets into jam or syrup.
   2. Quinacrine has most side effects: nausea and vomiting.

RENAL SYSTEM

The genitourinary system—the kidneys and their drainage channels—is essential for the maintenance of life. This system is responsible for excreting the end products of metabolism as well as regulating water and electrolyte concentrations of body fluids.

System Assessment

A. Assess fluid and electrolyte balance.
   1. Assess degree of edema.
   2. Assess distribution of edema.
   3. Monitor daily weights.
B. Assess normal renal functioning.
   1. Assess intake and output.
   2. Check for signs of diuresis.
   3. Measure specific gravity.
C. Check presence of infectious process.
   1. Inspect urine for cloudy appearance.
   2. Use hemastix to note presence of red blood cells.

Diagnostic Procedures

Cystoscopy

A. Direct visualization of bladder and urethra done under general anesthesia.
B. Nursing responsibilities.
   1. Prior to procedure—child is n.p.o. 6–8 hours.
   2. Following procedure—check I & O, observe for urinary retention and hematuria.

Intravenous Pyelogram (IVP)

A. A radiographic study of kidneys, bladder and other structures via contrast media injection.
B. Nursing responsibilities.
   1. Prior to IVP—child n.p.o. 6–8 hours; bowels cleaned with cathartic; have child void.
   2. Following procedure—evaluate for dye reaction; assess child's alertness and gag reflex; check for signs of perforation (intense pain in stomach).

System Implementation

A. Monitor laboratory results of serum electrolytes. (Refer to Medical-Surgical chapter for major electrolyte disorders.)
B. Monitor edema formation through daily weights and abdominal circumferences.
   1. Measure abdominal girth at umbilicus.
   2. If ascites present, evaluate for respiratory embarrassment from pressure on the diaphragm.
   3. Place child in semi-Fowler's position if massive edema is present.
C. Provide excellent skin care.
   1. Bathe body surfaces frequently.
   2. Turn and position client frequently to prevent skin breakdown.
   3. Support edematous areas such as the scrotum.
D. Monitor IV solutions for appropriate electrolytes depending on the disorder.
E. Measure intake and output for renal shutdown or for signs of diuresis following the initiation of medical intervention.
   1. Normal output:

Age	24-hour Period
6 months to 2 years	540–600 cc
2 to 5 years	500–780 cc
5 to 8 years	600–1200 cc
8 to 14 years	1000–1500 cc
14 years to adult	1400 cc

   2. Always evaluate output in relation to input and insensible water losses.
F. Utilize Hemastix and Clinitest for each voiding. Check presence of blood, protein, and ketones.
G. Describe the appearance of urine: dark, light, cloudy, pink, mucus present.
H. Evaluate the specific gravity of the urine.
I. Monitor vital signs every four hours or more frequently if warranted.
J. Administer antihypertensive medications.
K. Evaluate for rapid respirations associated with acidosis.
L. Isolate children who have an increased susceptibility to infection.
M. Control infection if present with appropriate medications.
N. Collect urine specimens from children suspected of having urinary tract infections.
O. Record symptoms of urinary tract infection: burning on urination; cloudy, foul-smelling urine; increased temperature.
P. Provide diet appropriate for condition. If there is a high-protein loss in urine, a large protein intake is important.
   1. Restrict foods rich in potassium and sodium as ordered.

2. Allow parents to bring in appropriate foods from home.
3. Sit with child during meals and talk about subjects other than food.
4. Provide nutritious snacks between meals.

Q. Provide appropriate diet for degree of renal dysfunction.
   1. Glomerulonephritis: low sodium, regular diet.
      a. Evidence of renal failure: restrict protein and potassium.
      b. Edema, hypertension or congestive heart failure: restrict fluids.
   2. Nephrosis: low sodium, high potassium. Fluids may be restricted if severe edema is present.

System Evaluation

A. Electrolytes remain in balance.
B. Edema diminishes or is absent.
C. Skin remains intact; no sign of breakdown.
D. IVs are appropriate for disorder.
E. Intake and output remains within normal limits for age.
   1. Any significant drop in output could be a sign of renal failure.
   2. Serious sign if output drops below 200 to 300 cc/24 hours (8 to 12 cc/hour) in the younger child.
   3. Serious sign if output drops below 500 cc/24 hours (20 cc/per hour) in the older child.
   4. For severe renal disease, it is imperative that the child be catheterized for accurate assessment of output.
F. Urine remains clear and yellow with no ketones, protein, blood, or sugar.
G. Specific gravity corresponds to clinical findings.
   1. Morning specimen usually concentrated around 1.020 to 1.030.
   2. Diluted urine around 1.001 may be found in normal infants or in children going through diuresis.
H. Blood pressure remains normal for age.
   1. If upward trend, child should be evaluated for other renal problems.
   2. No side effects occur from medications.
I. Respirations normal range for age.
J. Children with increased susceptibility to infection are isolated.
K. No symptoms of urinary tract infections are present.
L. Diet appropriate for child's age and condition is maintained.

RENAL DISORDERS

Acute Glomerulonephritis

Definition: Acute glomerulonephritis is believed to be an antigen-antibody reaction usually secondary to an infection from group A beta-hemolytic streptococci originating elsewhere in the body.

Assessment

A. Assess renal system.
   1. Protein and blood cells present in urine.
   2. Oliguria and occasional anuria.
   3. Mild edema—facial and extremities.
   4. Tea-colored urine.
B. Assess cardiovascular system.
   1. Possible hypertension and slowed pulse.
   2. Possible congestive heart failure or circulatory congestion.
C. Assess for preceding tonsillitis and fever.
D. Assess for anorexia and fatigue.

Implementation

A. Maintain bed rest during acute stage.
B. Monitor antibiotic treatment if there are positive bacterial cultures.
C. Monitor diet and fluid intake.
   1. Elevated BUN and oliguria—restrict protein moderately (acute renal failure—restrict protein severely).
   2. Liberal carbohydrates for energy.
   3. Restrict sodium if edema present.
D. Give antihypertensive drugs, e.g., reserpine, magnesium sulfate, as ordered.
E. Prevent fluid overload—replace fluid loss only.
   1. Weigh daily.
   2. Measure intake and output.
F. Prevent complications.
   1. Observe for signs of cerebral edema: headache, dizziness, vomiting.
   2. Monitor for renal failure: nausea, vomiting, oliguria.
   3. Prevent skin breakdown.

The Nephrotic Syndrome

Definition: A symptom complex with multiple and varied pathological manifestations and causes, the etiology of which is unknown. Usually occurs at two-and-a-half years of age.

Assessment

A. Assess for generalized edema.
  1. Periorbital edema.
  2. Abdominal edema.
  3. Respiratory difficulty with pleural effusion.
  4. Diarrhea, vomiting, and malabsorption from edema of gastrointestinal tract.
B. Assess for marked proteinuria.
C. Assess for malnutrition.
D. Assess for potential hypertension.

Implementation

A. Isolate the child to prevent infection due to increased susceptibility.
B. Monitor edema.
  1. Meticulous skin care.
  2. Daily weights.
  3. Change body position.
  4. Accurate intake and output.
  5. Diuretics.
C. Monitor use of steroids. Prednisone, which reduces edema and proteinuria, is drug of choice.
  1. Produces diuresis in ten to twelve days.
  2. Tapered dosage.
  3. Prepare child and family for side effects:
    a. Cushing's syndrome.
    b. Weight gain.
    c. Acne.
    d. Hirsutism.
D. Provide appropriate diet.
  1. High protein.
  2. Possibly low sodium—500 mg/day.
  3. High calorie diet.

URINARY DISORDERS

Hypospadias

Definition: Malposition of the urethral opening behind the glans penis, along the ventral surface. Epispadias is a condition in which the urethra is located on the upper surface of the penis.

Assessment

A. Assess severity of malposition.
B. Assess location of urethral opening on penis.
C. Assess ability to void in normal elevated position.
D. Check for presence of fistulas, chordee.

E. Assess child's understanding of procedure (word for penis, urine).
F. Evaluate parents' understanding of surgery and fears.

Implementation

A. Pre-operative care.
  1. Use drawings or dolls to reinforce physician's explanation.
  2. Prepare child for presence of urinary catheter(s).
  3. Prepare child for the possibility of post-op bladder spasms.
  4. Prepare child for nursing and medical personnel looking at his bandages frequently.
B. Post-operative care.
  1. Maintain adequate hydration.
    a. Measure urine specific gravity.
    b. Encourage fluid as needed.
  2. Expect a Foley catheter that may be sutured in place; urine should be rose-colored immediately post-op, gradually becoming clear.
  3. If it is a first stage repair, expect a supra-pubic catheter for urinary diversion and a Foley catheter.
  4. Tape catheters in place securely. (Do not adjust position or remove catheter.)
  5. Administer analgesics as ordered.
  6. Remove Foley and clamp supra-pubic intermittently to allow child to void through the meatus.
  7. After Foley is removed, note presence of fistula (should not be present).
  8. Chart when the child voids through the meatus; report to physician:
    a. Character of flow, presence of spray, dribbling, leaking, pain.
    b. Expect pain on the first voids; should decrease in subsequent voids.

Cryptorchidism (Undescended Testis)

Definition: The absence of one or both testes from the scrotum.

Assessment

A. Assess for presence of testis in scrotal sac.
B. Assess for presence of accompanying hernia (present in 50 percent of clients).
C. Evaluate normal development of secondary sex characteristics.

Implementation

A. Support child and family during surgery. Orchiopexy usually performed before age 5.
B. Provide postoperative care: maintain traction which anchors testis to scrotum (5-7 days); prevent contamination of incision.

Urinary Tract Infections

Definition: Urinary tract infection is a term that refers to a wide variety of conditions affecting the urinary tract in which the common denominator is the presence of microorganisms.

Characteristics

A. Escherichia coli most frequent organism.
B. The most important factor influencing ascending infection is obstruction of free urine flow.
   1. Free flow, large urine output, and pH are antibacterial defenses.
   2. If defenses break down, the result may be an invasion of the tract by bacteria.
C. More common in girls than in boys.

Assessment

A. Perform urine cultures and chemical tests to determine presence and number of bacteria.
B. Evaluate microscopic examination for detailed identification of the organism (especially important in chronic infections).
C. Note that a colony count of over 100,000/ml is most important lab finding and designates infection.

Implementation

A. Force fluids to amount appropriate for age.
B. Administer urinary antiseptics as ordered.
   1. Common drugs—NegGram, Mandelamine, Furadantin.
   2. Monitor side effects: nausea, vomiting, diarrhea, rash pruritus, urticaria.
C. Monitor administration of systemic antibiotics as ordered.
   1. Specific for causative bacteria (given one to two weeks).
   2. Common drugs: streptomycin, kanamycin, neomycin, gentamicin.
   3. Monitor side effects: vertigo, nausea, vomiting, rash.
D. Teach mother and remind staff to wipe child front to back.
E. If stool in diaper, clean immediately.

DISORDERS OF THE BLOOD AND LYMPH SYSTEM

The circulatory system, a continuous circuit, is the mechanical conveyor of the body constituent called blood. Blood, composed of cells and plasma, circulates through the body and is the means by which oxygen and nutrients are transported to the tissues. The lymph system collects lymph from the tissues and carries it to the blood.

Blood Transfusions

Assessment

A. Identify type of therapy to be administered.
   1. Whole blood.
   2. Packed red blood cells.
   3. Platelets.
B. Check that type and crossmatch is correct before administering blood.
C. Assess base line vital signs.

Implementation

A. Check identification of child with blood slip and Identaband before administering blood.
B. Obtain base line vital signs.
C. Ensure that proper IV tubing is used for blood administration.
D. Monitor blood flow and vital signs frequently.
E. Never give medications in blood, and never hang blood with dextrose and water.
F. Observe for transfusion reaction: backache, generalized discomfort, chilly sensations, distention of neck veins, tachycardia, tachypnea, and fall in blood pressure.
G. Observe for allergic reactions: wheezing, laryngeal edema, hives, itching and rash, and flushed appearance.
H. If either reaction occurs, close off transfusion, assess symptoms, and call physician.

I. Never use blood that is discolored or cloudy or that has been unrefrigerated for more than twenty minutes.

Sickle Cell Anemia

Definition: An hereditary disorder in which red blood cells sickle when under low oxygen tension. Usually confined to Blacks, it is considered to be inherited as an autosomal recessive disorder.

Assessment

A. Assess major symptoms.
   1. Severe chronic anemia— pallor.
   2. Periodic crises with abdominal and joint pain.
   3. Lethargy and listlessness.
   4. Irritability.
   5. High fever.
   6. Enlarged spleen from increased activity.
   7. Jaundice from excessive blood cell destruction.
   8. Widening of the marrow spaces of the bones.
   9. Gallstones.
B. Assess periods of crisis.
   1. Thrombotic crises.
      a. Most frequent type.
      b. Caused by occlusion of the small blood vessels producing distal ischemia and infarction.
      c. Beginning of crises may be characterized by the swelling of the hands and feet or decreased appetite, irritability, or fever.
      d. May experience pain and swelling in abdomen.
   2. Sequestration crises.
      a. Occurs usually in children under five.
      b. Caused by pooling of blood in spleen.
      c. Enlargement of spleen and circulatory collapse.

Implementation

A. Alleviate pain with analgesics.
B. Prevent dehydration with intravenous infusion, if necessary, and increased fluid intake.
C. Keep child warm.
D. Offer parents genetic counseling.
E. Counsel the family on physiology and prognosis of disease.
F. During sequestration crises, supervise blood transfusions.

Thalassemias

Definition: An inherited group of hemolytic anemias caused by too few hemoglobin polypeptide chains. A chronic condition.

Assessment

A. Assess for skin breakdown, especially leg ulcers.
B. Observe for jaundice; serum bilirubin elevated.
C. Check for intolerance of fatty foods and abdominal discomfort.
D. Check blood studies, fetal hemoglobin as high as 90%.

Implementation

A. Supportive: rest, decreased activity, heat lamp to open wounds, excellent skin care.
B. Administer packed red cells or chelating agents (DTPA) as ordered.
C. Prepare for splenectomy if transfused cells are rapidly destroyed by spleen.

Hemophilia

Definition: A sex-linked disorder in which certain factors necessary for coagulation of the blood are missing. Transmission of sex-linked traits are passed from unaffected carrier females to affected males.

Characteristics

A. Hemophilia A—Factor VIII deficiency: treated with cryoprecipitate or fresh-frozen plasma.
B. Hemophilia B—Factor IX deficiency (Christmas disease): treated with cryoprecipitate or fresh-frozen plasma.
C. Hemophilia C—Factor XI deficiency: treated with fresh-frozen plasma.

Assessment

A. Assess for type A or B.
   1. Possible bleeding tendency in neonatal period because factors are not passed through the placenta.
   2. Excessive bruising.
   3. Large hematomas from minor trauma.
   4. Persistent bleeding from minor injuries.
   5. Hemarthrosis with joint pain, swelling, and limited movement.
   6. Possible progressive degenerative changes with osteoporosis, muscle atrophy, and fixed joints.

B. Assess for type C.
   1. Usually appears as a mild bleeding disorder.
   2. Autosomal dominant trait with both sexes affected.

Implementation

A. Prevent bleeding.
   1. Protect child from environment by padding crib and playpen.
   2. Supervise child carefully when child is learning to walk.
B. Observe for signs of blood transfusion reaction.
C. Observe for signs of volume overload with plasma administration.
D. Treatment if bleeding occurs:
   1. Apply cold compresses and pressure.
   2. Hemarthrosis (effusion of blood into joint).
      a. Immobilize joint initially.
      b. Initiate passive range of motion within forty-eight hours to prevent stiffness.
   3. Immobilize site of bleeding.

Anemia

Definition: A deficit of red blood cells or hemoglobin caused by impairment of red blood cell production or increased erythrocyte destruction.

Assessment

A. Assess for early changes in behavior: listlessness, fatigue, sluggishness and anorexia.
B. Assess for late symptoms: pallor, weakness, tachycardia.
C. Determine if nutritional deficiency is present: iron, folic acid, vitamin B_6 or B_{12}.
D. Evaluate tests for impairment of red blood cell production: red cell, aplastic, or hemolytic anemia or leukemia. Refer to page 282.

Implementation

A. Prevent infection by maintaining nutritious diet with vitamin supplements, excellent hygiene, adequate rest, and avoidance of exposure to infections.
B. Monitor blood transfusions and observe for signs of transfusion reactions.
C. Administer iron injections by special method (Z-track) and take special precautions.

Infectious Mononucleosis

Definition: An infectious disease, believed to be viral in origin, that causes an increase in the mononuclear elements of the blood.

Assessment

A. Evaluate length of incubation period: around eleven days.
B. Assess for specific symptoms:
   1. Malaise.
   2. Sore throat with pharyngitis.
   3. Prolonged fever.
   4. Enlargement of the lymph nodes.
   5. Splenomegaly.
   6. Skin rashes.

Implementation

A. Provide symptomatic and supportive measures.
   1. Initially bed rest is indicated.
   2. Increase in activity should be gradual.
   3. Salicylates are given for fever, chills, and muscle pain.
B. Administer antibiotics.

MUSCULOSKELETAL SYSTEM

The musculoskeletal system comprises the bones, joints, and muscles. In order to effectively assess and treat disorders associated with this system, it is necessary to consider the effects of the blood vessels, skin, nerves, and tendons.

System Assessment

A. Assess length and shape of the extremities.
B. Assess movement, gait, and balance.
C. Evaluate strength of muscles.
D. Assess for presence of pain or tenderness in the extremities.
E. Check adequacy of circulation.
F. Assess that traction is intact.
G. Assess that cast is intact and appropriate for condition.

System Planning and Analysis

A. Abnormality of the musculoskeletal structure is identified.
B. Abnormal movements are prevented.
C. Limitation of movement is prevented.
D. Pain is controlled.
E. Adequate circulation is maintained.
F. Alignment is maintained through traction.
G. Healing is promoted through proper casting and cast care.

System Implementation

A. Identify abnormality of musculoskeletal structure.
   1. Evaluate newborn for congenital abnormality of the musculoskeletal system.
   2. Check for adequate range of motion in all extremities.
   3. Check for normal hip sockets in newborn.
   4. Check for spinal curvature (usually seen in the school-age child).
B. Prevent abnormal movement.
   1. Limit movement if developing abnormal patterns.
   2. Establish program of teaching ambulation with a physical therapist.
C. Prevent limitation of movement.
   1. Position body parts in proper alignment.
   2. Complete appropriate active and passive range of motion.
D. Control pain.
   1. Schedule painful procedures around analgesic schedule.
   2. Implement measures to reduce pain, i.e., massage, heat and/or cold compresses, relaxation techniques, etc.
E. Promote adequate circulation.
   1. Remove any restrictive garments or bandages.
   2. Check circulation of extremities at frequent intervals.
      a. Capillary filling.
      b. Temperature.
      c. Color.
      d. Peripheral pulses.
      e. Edema.
F. Promote alignment through traction.
   1. Check the vascular status of the extremity.
   2. Check the neurological status of the extremity.
      a. Level of sensation.

      b. Motion.
   3. Observe traction for intactness in both skeletal and skin traction.
   4. Check the traction equipment.
      a. Check the ropes for fraying.
      b. Make sure ropes are in the center of the pulley.
      c. Check the weights for correct number of pounds and to see if they are hanging free.
G. Promote healing through proper casting and cast care.
   1. Check the vascular status of the extremity.
   2. Examine the cast for signs of bleeding. If bleeding is present, draw a circle around the site, indicating time and date.
   3. Examine the cast for any pressure areas.
   4. Pull stockinette over cast edges and secure with tape (prevents cast crumbs from falling down cast).
   5. Keep the cast clean and dry.
   6. If appropriate, keep the level of the cast above the heart to prevent edema formation.

System Evaluation

A. Structure is within normal limits.
B. Movement is normal.
C. Joints can be put through full range of motion.
D. Pain is diminished.
E. Circulation to extremities is normal.
F. Traction is intact; vascular status normal.
G. Casting is appropriate; vascular status normal.
   1. No signs of continued bleeding.
   2. No signs of pressure areas under the cast.

MUSCULOSKELETAL DISORDERS

Legg-Perthes Disease

Definition: A self-limiting disease in which aseptic necrosis of the femoral head produces hip deformation and dysfunction.

Characteristics
A. Usually affects children 3–12 years of age and males 4–8 years of age; usually unilateral.
B. Four stages.
   1. Septic necrosis or infarction of the femoral capital epiphysis—the avascular stage.
   2. Capital bone absorption—the revascularization stage.

498

3. New bone formation, calcification or ossification—the reparative stage.
4. Gradual reformation of the head of the femur—the regenerative stage.

Assessment

A. Assess for pain in hip or knee; most evident on rising or at end of the day.
B. Assess for limp or joint dysfunction on the affected side—may be intermittent.
C. Assess for stiffness and tenderness over hip capsule.

Implementation

A. Goal of treatment is to keep head of the femur contained in the acetabulum.
   1. Initial therapy is rest to reduce inflammation and restore motion.
      a. Active motion is encouraged during this phase.
      b. Traction may be applied to stretch tight adductor muscles.
   2. Containment accomplished by several measures.
      a. Nonweight-bearing devices such as abduction brace, leg cast or leather harness sling that prevents weight-bearing on affected limb.
      b. Weight-bearing appliances such as abduction-ambulation brace or cast.
   3. Conservative treatment continued for 2–4 years.
   4. Disease is self-limiting, but early treatment is essential to avoid permanent damage.
B. Most care is out-patient so nursing emphasis is on teaching.
   1. Teach family use of corrective device selected for therapy.
   2. Stress importance of compliance for resolution of disease.

Congenital Dislocation of the HIP

Definition: The malrotation of the hip at birth; cause is usually unknown.

Assessment

A. Check for unequal major gluteal folds.
B. Assess for presence of a hip "click" on abduction.
C. Assess for femur that may appear shortened.

Implementation

A. Complete casefinding and referral.
B. Teach parents how to apply splint and maintain splint in alignment.
C. Protect skin under the splint.
D. Bring environment to child: surround with age-appropriate toys.
E. Maintain hip in flexion and abduction.
F. Continue double diapering.
G. Monitor Bryant's traction.

Osteomyelitis

Definition: Infection usually of the long bones caused most frequently by Staphylococcus aureus. Occurs most frequently in boys between five and fourteen years old.

Assessment

A. Assess for abrupt onset.
B. Check for fever, malaise, and pain.
C. Assess for localized tenderness in the bone at the metaphysis.
D. Evaluate for swelling and redness over affected bone.

Implementation

A. Control infection.
   1. Supervision of antibacterial therapy.
   2. Careful handling of drainage.
B. Control pain.
   1. Immobilization of affected limb.
   2. Analgesics.
C. Monitor occupational activities during immobilization.
   1. Painting and crafts.
   2. Passive games.
   3. Interaction with peers.

Juvenile Rheumatoid Arthritis

Definition: This is a systemic collagen disorder with multiple manifestations, arthritis being the most characteristic. Etiology is unknown.

Assessment

A. Assess for inflammation of joints.
B. Assess for edema and congestion of synovial tissues. (As the disease progresses, synovial material

fills the joint spore, causing narrowing, fibrous an-
kylosis, and bony fusion.)

C. Assess for premature closure or accelerated epi-
physeal growth.

D. Assess joint involvement.
1. Arthritis may start slowly with gradual development of joint stiffness, swelling, and loss
of motion.
2. Most frequently affects knees, ankles, feet,
wrists, and fingers—although any joint may be
involved.
3. Affected joints are swollen, warm, painful, and
stiff.
4. Young children appear irritable and anxious,
guarding their joints.
5. Weakness and atrophy of muscles appear
around affected joints.
6. Chronically affected joints may become de-
formed, dislocated, or fused.

E. Assess systemic involvement.
1. Frequent.
2. Irritability, anorexia, and malaise.
3. Fever.
4. Intermittent macular rash is occasionally
seen.
5. Hepatosplenomegaly and generalized lymphadenopathy in 20 percent of the clients.
6. Anemia is common with active cases of the disease.
7. Inflammation of eye: redness, pain, photophobia, decreased visual acuity, and nonreactive
pupil.

Implementation

A. Supervise medication administration.
1. Salicylates given in large doses.
2. Signs of toxicity and side effects.
   a. Ringing in the ear.
   b. Gastric irritation. (Give drug with milk or
   antacids.)
   c. Headaches.
   d. Disturbances of mental state.
   e. Hyperventilation and drowsiness.
3. Gold salts.
   a. Usually given in weekly injections.
   b. Side effects.
      (1) Dermatitis.
      (2) Stomatitis.
      (3) Nephritis with hematuria or albumi-
      nuria.

(4) Thrombocytopenia.
(5) Bone marrow depression.
c. Weekly blood and urine tests.
4. Steroids.
   a. Side effects and toxicity.
      (1) Masked infection.
      (2) Hypertension.
      (3) Vascular disorders.
      (4) Mental disturbances.
      (5) Edema and weight gain.
      (6) Increased appetite.
      (7) Peptic ulcer.
   b. Regular observation of vital signs.
   c. Careful supervision during initiation and
   tapering off of drug.

B. Maintain joint mobility.
1. Exercise joints.
2. Provide night splints.
3. Educate parents in how child should perform
exercises and impress upon them the child's
need for physical therapy and night splints.

C. Prevent eye damage—encourage parents to report
any signs of eye problems in the child immediately
to the physician.

D. Counsel family.
1. Explain physiology and unpredictable nature
of the disease to the parents and the child.
2. Provide emotional support to the parents for
dealing with a chronically ill child or adolescent.
3. Encourage independence in the child.
4. Encourage mastery of developmental tasks appropriate to the age group of the child.

Muscular Dystrophy

Definition: Gradual degeneration of muscle fibers
with progressive weakness of the skeletal muscles.

Characteristics

A. Duchenne's muscular dystrophy is the most common type and the most severe.

B. Genetic pattern is an X-linked recessive; 30–50
percent have no family history.

C. Usual age this disease appears is 2–6 years; rare
in infancy or at birth.

D. Death usually occurs from pneumonia 10–15
years after diagnosis.

Assessment

A. Assess for delay in motor development: clumsiness, walking on toes, waddling gait.

B. Assess for abnormal fatigue when walking or running.

C. Check for presence of Gower's maneuver: climbing up on legs from supine position.

D. Assess for progressive muscle weakness: axial and proximal before distal.

Implementation

A. Provide support so that child can maintain independence as long as possible.
  1. Assist parents to develop physical therapy program.
  2. Support use of wheelchair when necessary to maintain mobility.

B. Counsel parents to prevent respiratory infection.
  1. Teach deep breathing exercises.
  2. Maintain adequate diet to promote healthy status.

C. Counsel parents to monitor child's weight to promote mobility and health.

D. Assist parents to obtain emotional support to deal with child more adequately at home.
  1. Identify community resources that will support family.
  2. Counsel family to deal with chronic illness with eventual death of the child.

Fracture

Definition: A break in the continuity of bone that occurs when the resistance of the bone against the stress exerted yields to the force.

Characteristics

A. Fractures are a common injury in children.

B. A child's bone can be bent 45 degrees before breaking; thus, it is much more flexible than adult bones.

C. Common types.
  1. Greenstick.
    a. A crack; the bending of a bone with incomplete fracture. Only affects one side of the periosteum.
    b. Common in skull fractures or in young children when bones are pliable.
  2. Comminuted.
    a. Bone completely broken in a transverse, spiral, or oblique direction.
    b. Bone broken into several fragments.
  3. Open, or compound: bone is exposed to air through a break in the skin.
  4. Closed, or simple: skin remains intact.
  5. Compression: fractured bone has been compressed by other bones.
  6. Complete: bone is broken with a disruption of both sides of the periosteum.
  7. Impacted: one part of fractured bone is driven into another.
  8. Depressed fracture: bone or fragments of bone are driven inward.

D. Healing process.
  1. Occurs over several weeks.
  2. New bone tissue occurs in region of break.
  3. Repair is initiated by migration of blood vessels and connective tissue from periosteum in break area.
  4. Dense fibrous tissue fills in the break and forms a callus (temporary union).
  5. Cells deposit cartilage between broken surfaces.
  6. Cartilage is slowly replaced by mineralized bone tissue, which completes repair.

Assessment

A. Observe for signs of a fracture.
  1. Cardinal signs.
    a. Pain or tenderness over involved area.
    b. Loss of function of the extremity.
    c. Deformity.
      (1) Overriding.
      (2) Angulation: limb in an unnatural position.
  2. Crepitation: sound of grating bone fragments.
  3. Ecchymosis or erythema.
  4. Edema.
  5. Muscle spasm.

B. Assess emotional status of child admitted for a suspected fracture.
  1. Degree of anxiety present.
  2. Readiness for treatment.

C. Evaluate type of treatment.
  1. Traction.
  2. Reduction (restoring bone to proper alignment).
    a. Closed reduction.
      (1) Manual manipulation.

(2) Usually done under anesthesia to reduce pain and relax muscles, thereby preventing complications.

(3) Cast is usually applied following closed reduction.

b. Open reduction.

(1) Surgical intervention.

(2) Usually treated with internal fixation devices (screws, plates, wires, etc.).

(3) Cast application.

Implementation

A. Provide emergency care of fractures.

1. Immobilize affected extremity to prevent further damage to soft tissue or nerve.

2. If compound fracture is evident, do not attempt to reduce it.

a. Apply splint.

b. Cover open wound with sterile dressing.

3. Splinting.

a. External support is applied around a fracture to immobilize the broken ends.

b. Materials used: wood, plastic (air splints), magazines.

c. Function of splinting is to prevent additional trauma, reduce pain, decrease muscle spasm, limit movement, and prevent complications, such as fat emboli in long bone fracture.

B. Monitor traction for fracture treatment.

1. Skeletal traction.

a. Mechanical, applied to bone using pins (Steinmann), wires (Kirschner), or tongs (Crutchfield).

b. Most often used in fractures of femur, tibia, and humerus.

c. Balanced suspension traction.

(1) Thomas' splint with Pearson attachment is used in conjunction with skin or skeletal traction (particularly with skeletal traction for fractured femur).

(2) Balanced suspension traction is produced by a counterforce other than the child.

2. Skin traction.

a. Applied by use of elastic bandages, moleskin strips, or adhesive.

b. Used most often in alignment or lengthening.

c. Most common types.

(1) Russell traction.

(2) Buck's extension.

(3) Cervical traction, for temporary immobilization.

(4) Pelvic traction.

3. Alignment through proper care of traction.

a. Ensure that weights hang freely and do not touch the floor.

b. Ensure that pulleys are not obstructed.

c. Check that ropes in the pulley move freely.

d. Secure knot in rope to prevent slipping.

e. Maintain proper body alignment (up in bed, in direct line with traction) and proper countertraction.

f. Do not remove or lift weights without specific order. (Exceptions are pelvic and cervical traction that clients can remove at intervals.)

g. Cover sharp edges on traction apparatus with hollowed out rubber balls to prevent injury to personnel.

C. Promote fracture healing through proper cast care.

1. After application of cast, allow 24 to 48 hours for drying. For synthetic cast, allow 30 minutes for drying.

2. Do not handle cast during drying process as indentations from fingermarks can cause skin breakdown under cast.

3. Keep extremity elevated to prevent edema.

4. Provide for smooth edges surrounding cast.

5. Observe casted extremity for signs of circulatory impairment.

6. Keep cast dry; it can break down when water comes in contact with plaster. Synthetic cast can be cleaned—does not break down as easily.

7. Utilize isometric exercises to prevent muscle atrophy and to strengthen the muscle. Isometrics prevent joint from being mobilized.

8. Position client with pillows to prevent strain on unaffected areas.

9. Turn frequently to prevent skin breakdown.

Scoliosis

Definition: Scoliosis is a lateral curvature of the spine and may be "C-shaped" or "S-shaped." The "S-shaped" curve has a secondary or compensatory curve.

Characteristics

A. Age of onset—the younger the child the greater the chances for deformity.

1. Deformity increases during growth periods.
2. Usually not noticed until adolescence.
3. Affects more girls than boys.

B. Size of curve—curves between 20–45° usually treated non-surgically. Curves more than 45° warrant surgical intervention.

C. Pattern of curve—when the primary curve is thoracic, there is a greater likelihood that deformity will occur.

D. Types.
1. Kyphosis: flexion deformity usually at thoracic spine.
2. Lordosis: fixed extension deformity usually occurring to compensate for other abnormalities.
3. Scoliosis: lateral curvature of the spine.
   a. Nonstructural: caused by changes outside the spine; treated with exercises.
   b. Structural: the spine itself has rotated, treated by bracing, exercise, insertion of the Harrington rod or Lugue procedure.

MEDICAL IMPLICATIONS

Non-surgical correction of curvature.
1. Exercise.
2. Plastic braces (orthoses).
3. Milwaukee Brace (usually when curve is 20–24°).
4. Halo Traction.
5. Casting.

Surgical correction options.
1. Considerations: any patient with a curve of 45° is considered to be a candidate for surgery—after growth stops, a lateral curve can continue to progress at about 1° a year.
2. Spinal fusion: prevents progression of scoliosis and is done by inserting bone chips to achieve fusion of the vertebrae.
3. Harrington Rod Instrumentation: straightens the spine; acts as a splint to allow solid fusion of bony parts. Steel rods are placed along the spine and attached by wires at the cephalo and caudal ends of the spine.
4. Dwyer Instrumentation: anterior spinal fusion and instrumentation; used as first part of two-part surgery with Harrington Rod Instrumentation (posterior).
5. Lugue Segmental Spinal Instrumentation: rigid internal fixation of the spine; a method of internal segmental spinal instrumentation by wiring each vertebra to steel rods.

Assessment

A. Assess for subjective symptoms—fatigue, dyspnea, backache.

B. Question client about ability to breathe and when client usually has difficulty breathing.

C. Assess physical status—expose back and check for deviations.
1. Difference in shoulder height, elbow level, and height of iliac crests.
2. The infolding of one flank and flattening of another.

D. Assess range of motion of the spine.

E. Observe for deviations of the hips, rib cage, shoulders, and iliac crest.

F. Assess for mild pain and/or discomfort.

Implementation

A. Instruct on use of Milwaukee brace.
1. Teach adolescent to wear the brace correctly and remove it only to bathe or as prescribed by the physician.
2. Explain necessity for good skin care where brace touches.
3. Assist adolescent to understand the need for the brace, and help the client deal with the altered body image.

B. Provide care when child undergoes surgery.
1. Harrington Rod.
   a. Decortication of the bone over the laminas and spinous processes.
   b. Bone grafts from iliac crest are inserted to achieve fusion of the vertebrae.
   c. Rods are inserted along the vertebrae and attached by Harrington hooks and wires to achieve tension along the spine.
   d. Casting is required postoperatively to protect the spinal fusion and to add stability.
2. Lugue procedure.
   a. Placement of wire loops under the lamina at each vertebral level.
   b. Steel rods aligned along the curvatures of the spine are fixated to the spine by the wires.

C. Operative nursing management.
1. Preoperative care.
   a. Evaluate child's level of understanding regarding condition and development progression.
   b. Check preop labwork to assure all values are within normal limits.

c. Assist child with pulmonary function tests. Teach child to do tri-flows, cough and deep breathe. Explain the importance of doing this postoperatively.

d. Evaluate child's and parents' understanding of surgical procedure. Explain to their level of understanding. Discuss postoperative course with child and parents to help them know what to expect. Answer questions they may have.

e. Visit the ICU with family and child to familiarize them with the surroundings.

2. Postoperative care.

a. Check vital signs every 15 minutes until stable, then every hour.

b. Watch for signs and symptoms of hypovolemia, tachycardia, BP. (Blood loss in the OR is considerable.)

c. Assess respiratory function—BS, RR, chest excursion, color, GFR (grunting, flaring, retractions); check ABG's. (Continual assessment of respiration function with vital signs is essential; pneumothorax or punctured lung is a risk after surgery.)

d. Maintain strict I & O; monitor urine output after one hour. Urine output must be adequate; if low, may indicate hypovolemia.

e. Check specific gravity to assess hydration status.

f. Start tri-flows as soon as awake after 1 hour. Encourage to cough and deep breathe between use of tri-flows.

g. Check CMS (color, movement, sensation) of lower extremities and feet q̄ 1 hr. × 8 hrs., q̄ 2 hr. × 24 hrs., then q̄ 4 hr.

h. Turn after 1 or 2 hours by logrolling only. Maintain alignment of spine.

i. Medicate child prior to turning or doing procedures (per orders).

(1) It is important to keep child comfortable, but watch for signs of respiratory depression with large doses of narcotics.

(2) Observe vital sign changes as indicative of pain.

j. Maintain NPO until child has positive bowel sounds, is passing flatus or has had a stool.

k. Start diet with ice chips only. (Paralytic ileus is a common side effect.)

l. Check skin and dressing every two hours to assess for skin breakdown and bleeding.

m. Instruct child to flex feet to improve circulation and maintain muscle tone.

D. Rehabilitation

1. Harrington Rod.

a. Most children are casted after recovery from surgery; they can get up 1–2 weeks after the cast has been applied.

b. Cast stays on 6 months.

c. Once cast is removed, a Milwaukee brace or thoracolumbar support is worn approximately 3 months—only removed at night.

2. Lugue procedure.

a. After the wound is healed (approximately 3–5 days), child may sit at the side of the bed.

b. Progresses to ambulation. No postop immobilization is required.

Congenital Clubfoot (Talipes Equinovarus)

Definition: Congenital deformity in which the foot has a club-like appearance: inner area of foot is turned up, anterior half of foot is adducted, and foot is in plantar flexion.

Assessment

A. Assess whether foot deformity is accompanied by other problems such as neurological defects or spina bifida.

B. Assess general health status of infant in preparation for treatment.

C. Determine aspects of treatment: occurs in three stages and includes exercises, manipulation, casting, and splinting.

Implementation

A. Assist in passive exercises (manipulation) of the foot following a demonstration by physician: hold position to count of 10 and continue for 10 minutes several times a day.

B. Provide cast care (change frequently).

C. Assist in care if infant is put in Denis Browne Splint (flexible horizontal bar attached to footplates).

D. Instruct parents in cast and/or splint care.

INTEGUMENTARY SYSTEM

The integumentary system comprises the skin, including the epidermis and the dermis, as well as all the derivatives of the epidermis, such as hair, nails, and various glands. It forms a barrier against the external environment and participates in many vital body functions.

System Assessment

A. Identify the type of abnormal lesions.
1. Macule: a small, flat, colored lesion.
2. Papule: a small, solid, elevated lesion.
3. Vesicle: an elevated lesion filled with fluid.
4. Nodules: larger solid forms of papules.
5. Petechia: pinpoint hemorrhage in the skin.
6. Tumors: an abnormal mass.
7. Hives: an eruption of itching wheals.
B. Observe distribution of lesions and any other symptoms that occur simultaneously.
C. Assess the pigmentation of the skin.
D. Assess the color of the skin: jaundice, cyanosis, pallor, or cherry red coloring.
E. Observe for abnormal texture: edema or poor skin turgor.

System Planning and Analysis

A. Plan for treating skin lesions is devised.
B. Skin lesions diminish.
C. Abnormal changes in skin lesions are noted.
D. Underlying causes of abnormal coloring are identified.
E. Abnormal texture is corrected.
F. Secondary infection is prevented.
G. Allergic responses are prevented.

System Implementation

A. Identify and treat cause of skin disorder.
1. Record the size, shape, and distribution of skin lesions.
2. Note all other concurrent symptoms.
3. Evaluate child's recent history, particularly medications, new foods, and exposure to communicable diseases.
4. Isolate possible allergen and remove from environment.
B. Assist in reducing pruritus.
1. Apply lotion (i.e., calamine lotion) to reduce itching.
2. Administer antihistamine if ordered.
3. Apply topical medication if ordered.
C. Note abnormal change in skin lesions.
1. Describe accurately the placement, size, shape, and distinguishing characteristics of all lesions.
2. Evaluate for changes on a routine basis.
3. Teach family to notify physician if any skin lesions such as birthmarks or moles change shape or color or start to bleed.
D. Observe and record any abnormal coloring.
1. Describe cyanosis if present. Include location and under what conditions (i.e., during feeding) it occurred.
2. Check the child for other signs of cardiac or respiratory disease or chilling.
3. Evaluate child's laboratory values if pallor is present to determine presence of anemia. Ask for a 24-hour accounting of diet.
4. Monitor jaundice for change.
E. Correct any abnormal texture.
1. For poor skin turgor:
a. Increase the fluid intake.
b. Monitor intake and output.
c. Monitor specific gravity.
2. For edema:
a. Establish and treat the underlying cause.
b. Give meticulous skin care.
c. Monitor intake and output.
F. Prevent secondary infections.
1. Encourage the child not to scratch the lesions.
2. Pin sleeves of the infant's undershirt over hands.
3. Keep child's hands and nails clean with the nails trimmed.
4. Keep infant clean and dry. Change diapers frequently.
G. Prevent allergic responses.
1. Assist in obtaining an accurate environmental history including exposure to common household allergens, food, and medications.
2. Educate the family on changes in the environment that are necessary.

System Evaluation

A. Skin lesions diminished.
B. Symptoms of lesions decreased.
C. Changes in lesions noted accurately.
D. Abnormal coloring diminished.
E. Skin texture normal.
F. No presence of secondary infection.
G. Decrease in allergic response.

SKIN DISORDERS

Impetigo

Definition: A skin infection caused by streptococcus, staphylococcus, or pneumococcus.

Assessment

A. Assess for multiple macular-papular rash seen at various stages of healing.
B. Check rupture of papules, which produce serous exudate and form a crust.
C. Assess location: usually found on head and neck.

Implementation

A. For newborn, monitor local and systemic antibiotic therapy.
B. For older child and adult, administer frequent cleansing with soap and remove crusts.
C. Cut nails to avoid scratching.
D. Provide isolation protection for newborn.

Eczema

Definition: An atopic dermatitis generally seen in children with allergic tendencies.

Assessment

A. Assess for erythema, papules, vesicles.
B. Check drainage if crusting is present.
C. Assess for intense itching.
D. Look for symptoms in children four months to four years.
E. Assess when symptoms appear: often commences with the introduction of new foods, particularly eggs and cow's milk and the cessation of breast feeding.

Implementation

A. Eliminate foods which exacerbate problem.
B. Remove dust-carrying objects in environment (stuffed animals).
C. Eliminate all strong soaps.
D. Provide symptomatic treatment of lesions: frequent soaks with Burow's solution or normal saline.
E. Prevent scratching.

Acne (see page 270)

Burns

Assessment

A. Assess for first-degree or superficial: involves only reddening of the skin.
B. Assess for second-degree or partial thickness: skin blisters, regeneration of epithelium without grafting.
C. Assess for third-degree or full thickness: destruction of most of the epidermal tissue; unable to regenerate without graft.
D. Assess type of treatment appropriate to degree of burn.
 1. First aid.
  a. Provide comfort and prevent chilling.
  b. Wash area with cool, sterile solution or water if no sterile solution is available.
  c. Cover with a sterile cloth to prevent liquid contamination.
  d. Do not apply greasy substances until burn is evaluated.
  e. Wash surrounding area thoroughly with mild detergent.
 2. Exposed method: No dressing is used so that hard eschar forms, protecting wound from infection. This method is excellent for areas difficult to bandage effectively. Requires reverse isolation and is difficult for a child.
 3. Closed method: Sterile occlusive dressing is applied frequently, usually with topical medications. Debridement occurs every time the dressing is changed, preventing a large loss of blood at one time, as when eschar is removed.
 4. Silvadene has broad antimicrobial activity. Inhibits bacteria resistant to other antimicrobials.

5. Sulfamylon therapy: This treatment is effective against many gram negative and positive organisms, but it may cause acid-base derangements and is painful when applied.
E. Assess for complications associated with burns.
1. Fluid and electrolyte imbalances.
   a. In deeper wounds, edema appears around the wound from damage to capillaries.
   b. There is a loss of fluid at the burn area.
   c. On the second day, there is a large loss of potassium.
   d. Objective of fluid therapy is to maintain adequate tissue perfusion.
2. Circulatory changes.
   a. Drop in cardiac output, initially.
   b. Decrease in blood volume from loss of plasma protein into extravascular and extracellular spaces.
   c. Moderate amount of hemolysis of red blood cells.
3. Pulmonary changes— inhalation injury.
   a. Pulmonary edema.
   b. Obstruction of the air passages from edema of the face, neck, trachea, and larynx.
   c. Restriction of lung mobility from eschar on chest wall.
4. Renal changes.
   a. Renal insufficiency caused by reaction to hypovolemic shock.
   b. Decreased blood supply to kidneys results in decreased renal perfusion.
   c. In burns of 15 to 20 percent of the body surface, there is a decreased urinary output that must be avoided or reversed.
   d. Urinary tract infections are frequent.
5. Gastrointestinal changes.
   a. Acute gastric dilation.
   b. Paralytic ileus.
   c. Curling's ulcer—producing "coffee ground" aspirant.
   d. Hemorrhagic gastritis—bleeding from congested capillaries in gastric mucosa.
F. Assess ability to cope with lifelong disfigurement.
1. Psychological problems associated with disfigurement.
2. Problems encountered with long-term plastic surgery.
3. Distortion of self-image and lowering of self-esteem due to disfigurement.

Implementation
A. Prevent infection.
1. Provide sterile technique and environment.
2. Observe for signs of infection, increased temperature and pulse.
3. Provide prophylactic measures: tetanus and antibiotics.
B. Prevent pulmonary complications.
1. Establish and observe for adequate airway.
2. Suction p.r.n.
3. Provide humidified oxygen p.r.n.
4. Teach coughing and deep breathing.
5. Provide frequent position changes.
C. Establish adequate circulatory volume.
1. Observe for signs of hypovolemia, e.g., thirst, vomiting, increased pulse, decreased blood pressure, and decreased urinary output.
2. Observe for signs of circulatory overload, particularly around the second to fifth day, when fluid in extracellular tissues returns to circulation. There is danger of congestive heart failure.
3. Monitor intravenous fluid therapy.
4. Monitor intake and output.
D. Prevent contractures.
1. Keep body parts in alignment.
2. Elevate burned extremities.
3. Provide active and/or passive range of motion to all joints.
E. Provide adequate nutrition.
1. Give twice the normal amount of calories.
2. Give three to four times the normal requirement for protein.
3. Provide small, frequent and attractive meals.
4. Encourage child, who is frequently anorexic, to eat.
F. Design activities for the burned child while child is hospitalized.
1. Actively involve the child, e.g., acting out part of a story verbally.
2. Provide television, books, and games.
3. Allow the child to associate with friends.
G. Counsel parents.
1. Parents and child have difficulty dealing with disfigurement and need assistance.
2. Parents frequently feel guilty, although they are usually not at fault and need assistance working out these feelings.

ENDOCRINE SYSTEM

The endocrine system consists of a series of glands that function individually or conjointly to integrate and control innumerable metabolic activities of the body. These glands automatically regulate various body processes by releasing chemical signals called hormones.

System Assessment

A. Assess for any growth imbalance.
 1. Excessive growth.
  a. Pituitary or hypothalamic disorders.
  b. Excess adrenal, ovarian, or testicular hormone.
 2. Retarded growth.
  a. Endocrine and metabolic disorders; difficult to distinguish from dwarfism.
  b. Hypothyroidism.
B. Assess for obesity.
 1. Sudden onset suggests hypothalamic lesion (rare).
 2. Cushing's syndrome (with characteristic buffalo hump).
C. Assess for abnormal skin pigmentation.
D. Assess for abnormal hirsutism.
 1. Normal variations in body occur on nonendocrine basis.
 2. First sign of neoplastic disease.
 3. Indicates change in adrenal status.
E. Assess for appetite changes.
 1. Polyphagia is a common sign of uncontrolled diabetes.
 2. Indicates thyrotoxicosis.
 3. Nausea and weight loss may indicate Addisonian crisis or diabetic acidosis.
F. Assess for presence of polyuria and polydipsia.
 1. Symptoms usually of nonendocrine etiology.
 2. If sudden onset, suggest diabetes mellitus or insipidus.
 3. May be present with hyperparathyroidism or hyperaldosteronism.
G. Assess any noticeable mental changes.

 1. Though often subtle, may be indicative of underlying endocrine disorder.
  a. Nervousness and excitability may indicate hyperthyroidism.
  b. Mental confusion may indicate hypopituitarism, Addison's disease, or myxedema.
 2. Mental deterioration is observed in untreated hypoparathyroidism and hypothyroidism.
 3. Mental retardation is present in some endocrine gland disorders.

System Planning and Analysis

A. Endocrine gland imbalance is identified early.
B. Imbalance is corrected.
C. Maintenance of vital functions is preserved.
 1. Growth and development normal.
 2. Reproduction glands normal.
 3. Fluid, electrolyte, and acid-base balance maintained.
 4. Energy metabolism preserved.
D. Hormone regulation is maintained; deficit or excess in production is corrected.

System Implementation

A. Give medications on schedule to maintain accurate blood level.
B. Instruct the child and parent on signs and symptoms and side effects of medications.
C. Instruct the child and parent on methods to decrease infection.
D. Provide appropriate nutrition.

System Evaluation

A. No hyperplasia of the endocrine glands is found.
B. Imbalances in hormone production (either deficits or excesses) are corrected by replacement hormones, surgery, etc.
C. Side effects of replacement hormones are minimal, and child functions well.
D. Vital functions directed by endocrine glands are preserved.
E. Side effects of hormone imbalance diminish after treatment.

THYROID GLAND DISORDERS

Cretinism (Hormone Hypofunction)

Definition: Cretinism is a condition caused by severe hypofunction of the thyroid gland in the fetus, in utero, or soon after birth.

Assessment

A. Assess for severe retardation of physical development, resulting in grotesque appearance, sexual retardation.
B. Evaluate severe mental retardation, apathy.
C. Assess for dry skin; coarse, dry, brittle hair.
D. Evaluate constipation.
E. Assess teething pattern (usually slow).
F. Assess for poor appetite.
G. Examine tongue (usually large).
H. Check for pot belly with umbilical hernia.
I. Assess for sensitivity to cold.
J. Examine skin (usually yellow).

Implementation

A. Evaluate laboratory values to confirm diagnosis.
   1. T_4 under 3 μg/100 ml.
   2. Elevated serum cholesterol.
   3. Low radioactive iodine uptake.
B. Monitor administration of drugs.
   1. Desiccated thyroid.
   2. Synthroid drug of choice.
   3. Cytomel used when rapid response is needed.

PITUITARY GLAND DISORDERS

Giantism (Hormone Hyperfunction)

Definition: Hypersecretion of growth hormone by the anterior pituitary, which occurs in childhood prior to closure of the epiphyses of the long bones.

Assessment

A. Assess for symmetrical overgrowth of the long bones.
B. Assess for increased height in early adulthood (eight to nine feet).
C. Evaluate deterioration of mental and physical processes, which may occur in early adulthood.

Implementation

A. Care for client as irradiation of pituitary program is instituted.
B. Administer care for hypophysectomy.

Dwarfism (Hormone Hypofunction)

Definition: Hyposecretion of growth hormone by the anterior pituitary. Growth is symmetrical but decreased.

Assessment

A. Assess for retarded physical growth.
B. Assess for premature body-aging processes.
C. Examine pale, dry, smooth skin.
D. Assess for poor development of secondary sex characteristics and external genitalia.
E. Assess for slow intellectual development.

Implementation

A. Monitor administration of human growth hormone injections (HGH) if the imbalance is diagnosed and treated in early stage.
B. Support family and refer to social services if condition has not been arrested.

DISORDER OF THE PANCREAS

Insulin Dependent Diabetes: Type I

Definition: A disorder characterized by metabolic conditions that interfere with the production, availability, or effectiveness of insulin.

Characteristics

A. Pathology.
   1. Interference with the utilization of sugar.
   2. Impaired transportation of glucose across cellular membranes and impaired utilization within the cell.
   3. Increased glycogenesis.
   4. Diuresis from hyperglycemia, resulting in glucosuria and excessive losses of electrolytes and water.
   5. Increased oxidation of fats and proteins, leading to proteinuria and acidosis.
B. Prognosis: degenerative changes associated with diabetes mellitus begin in young adults who have had the disease for ten to twenty years.

Table 8. TYPE I, INSULIN DEPENDENT (IDDM)

Etiology	Hereditary predisposition Environmental Acquired
Causes	Insulin deficiency
Other terms	Juvenile, Ketosis-prone, insulin dependent
Age of onset	Usually under 35 but can be at any age
Clinical manifestations	+ + Polyuria + + Polydipsia* + Blurred vision + + Fatigue, weakness + Vaginitis + Peripheral neuropathy Weight loss Anorexia, nausea, vomiting Muscle cramps
Nutritional state	Poorly nourished
Treatment	ADA diet and insulin
Common complications	Insulin reaction, Ketoacidosis

Note:
+ Present
+ + Significantly present
 * Polyphagia is not always present

1. Arteriosclerosis with hypertension.
2. Retinal changes and cataracts.
3. Nephropathy.

Assessment

A. Assess for rapid onset.
B. Assess for loss of weight.
C. Check for symptoms of increased thirst and appetite, polydipsia, polyphagia, polyuria, and nocturia.
D. Assess for presence of ketoacidosis, an acute, life-threatening condition.
   1. Drowsiness.
   2. Dryness of skin.
   3. Flushed cheeks.
   4. Acetone breath.
   5. Hyperpnea.
   6. Nausea, vomiting, and abdominal pains.

Implementation

A. Monitor administration of insulin. (Oral hypoglycemic agents generally do not produce satisfactory results because they require some pancreatic function to be effective.)
   1. Side effects: hypoglycemia with hunger, irritability, nervousness, headaches, and slurred speech.
   2. Types of treatment (see table in Medical-Surgical chapter).
B. Monitor diet.
   1. Diet should be adequate for normal growth and development and regulated according to diabetic needs.
   2. The type of diet prescribed is influenced by the philosophy of the physician.
   3. Diets vary from free diets to strict dietary control.

510

C. Provide family and client education.
   1. Signs and symptoms of disease, including acidosis and hypoglycemia.
   2. Instruction in insulin injection, sterile technique, and urine testing.
   3. Diet control as prescribed by the physician.
   4. Prevention of infections through adequate skin and foot care.
   5. Knowledge of the effects of increased physical activity and stress on food needs.
   6. Client's responsibility for administering insulin and managing diet.
   7. Normal activity and life style appropriate.
D. Provide special counseling because of adolescent's heightened sensitivity to being different and their frequently unusual dietary habits.

PEDIATRIC ONCOLOGY

The signs and symptoms of pediatric malignancy may be subtle and not easily recognized. In addition, the causal factors associated with cancer in children are not clearly defined. Current treatment focuses on chemotherapy, radiation therapy, a combination of the two, and surgical intervention. The specialty area of pediatric oncology is becoming more prominent as the incidence goes up and the etiology remains a mystery.

CHEMOTHERAPY

Characteristics

A. Chemotherapeutic agents work on dividing cells.
B. Tumor's location and cell type affect choice of drugs.
C. Most antineoplastic drugs are metabolized in the liver and excreted by the kidneys so they must be in functioning order to prevent toxicity.

Assessment

A. Assess if more than one chemotherapeutic agent is being administered.
B. Identify potential side effects of medications.
   1. G.I. disturbance.
   2. Loss of hair.
C. Assess for fluid and electrolyte imbalances associated with drug therapy.
D. Assess for adequate urine output.
E. Monitor laboratory values.
F. Assess oral cavity for irritation and bleeding gums.

Implementation

A. Establish base line data.
   1. Nutritional status.
   2. Oral condition.
   3. Skin condition.
   4. Degree of mobility.
   5. Psychological status.
   6. Neurological condition.

B. Observe for side effects of cell breakdown.
   1. BUN on rise.
   2. Stone formation in urinary tract.
C. Maintain chemotherapy flow sheet.
D. Observe for side effects on rapidly dividing cells.
   1. Gastrointestinal mucosa: diarrhea, nausea, vomiting.
      a. Administer antiemetics.
      b. Provide mouth care with hydrogen peroxide every four hours. Do not use toothbrush or glycerin.
      c. Administer anesthetic spray to mouth prior to meals.
      d. Provide frequent cold, high-calorie beverages.
   2. Hair follicles: loss of hair.
      a. Prepare client for loss, i.e., suggest wig, scarf.
      b. Reassure client that hair will grow back in six weeks.
      c. Apply tourniquet around scalp during chemotherapy and in two to three hours following chemotherapy to lessen amount of hair lost.
E. Monitor administration of common drugs.
   1. Prednisone, an immunosuppressive agent.
      a. Monitor side effects, which may include ravenous appetite, change in fat distribution, retention of fluid, hirsutism, occasional hypertension, and psychological disturbance.
      b. Monitor serum blood sugar levels.
      c. Monitor tapering of medication.
   2. 6-Mercaptopurine: interrupts the synthesis of purines essential to the structure and function of nucleic acids.
      a. Monitor side effects: very little toxicity in children but the kidneys must excrete increased amount of uric acid.
      b. Observe kidney function and possible increase in fluid intake.
   3. Methotrexate: folic acid antagonist that suppresses the growth of abnormal cells enough to permit regeneration of normal cells.
      a. Monitor side effects: ulceration of oral mucosa and nausea, vomiting, diarrhea, and abdominal pain.
      b. Observe for ulcerations. Discontinue drug temporarily at the appearance of ulcers.
      c. Observe renal function, e.g., drug is excreted through kidneys.

4. Cytoxan: alkylating agent that suppresses cellular proliferation; it has greater effect on abnormal than normal cells.
   a. Monitor side effects: hemorrhagic cystitis.
   b. Provide large quantities of fluids preceding and immediately following drug administration to prevent side effects.
5. Vincristine: alkylating agent used to induce remissions rapidly.
   a. Monitor side effects: insomnia, severe constipation, and peripheral neuritis or palsies.
   b. Once disease is in remission, maintain client on another less toxic drug as ordered.

RADIATION

Characteristics

A. Radiation affects all cells but is particularly lethal to rapidly developing cells.
B. Radiation can be utilized in conjunction with chemotherapy.
C. Radiation may be used to eradicate tumors or to relieve pressure.

Assessment

A. Assess for easy fatigability.
B. Assess fluid and electrolyte imbalances due to vomiting, diarrhea, and urinary frequency associated with radiation therapy.
C. Monitor hemoglobin and hematocrit.
D. Assess skin condition in radiated area.
E. Assess for dental caries and gum disease.
F. Assess condition of hair.

Implementation

A. Treat radiation sickness.
   1. Monitor symptoms: nausea, vomiting, malaise.
   2. Offer frequent high-calorie feedings (milkshakes with extra protein and vitamins).
   3. Make food trays attractive and palatable.
B. Observe side effects of cell breakdown: BUN on rise, accumulation of uric acid, and stone formation in urinary tract.
C. Treat side effects of cell breakdown.
   1. Increase fluid intake.
   2. Monitor intake and output.

D. Treat skin breakdown.
   1. Check client regularly for any redness or irritation at radiation site.
   2. Notify physician immediately.
   3. Apply lotion to area following termination of radiation therapy.
   4. Avoid any irritation to area from clothing, soap, or weather extremes.
E. Treat bone marrow depression.
   1. Watch lab values carefully.
   2. Isolate client because of susceptibility (low leukocytes).
   3. Avoid injections (low platelets).
   4. Administer antibiotics.

MALIGNANT DISEASES

Wilms' Tumor (Nephroblastoma)

Definition: A cancerous unilateral tumor of the kidney. The most common type of renal cancer in children.

Assessment

A. Complete routine assessment on child's abdomen. Assess for presence of a mass.
B. Assess for presence of fever or abdominal pains.
C. Assess for adequate kidney function.

Implementation

A. Avoid palpation of the tumor as it may spread.
B. Provide support for the family. (Counsel family that prognosis is good if surgery is done early.)
C. Observe carefully intake and output.
D. Observe for toxic reactions to chemotherapy, such as mouth lesions.
E. If x-ray therapy is given, provide good skin care.

Leukemia

Definition: A potentially fatal malignant disease caused by the proliferation of leukocytes and their precursors. Average life expectancy was three to four years, but new medications have extended life expectancy. Types include acute lymphocytic leukemia which is responsible for about 80 percent of all childhood cases, and chronic myelocytic leukemia which affects young adults.

Assessment

A. Assess for early manifestations.
1. Bone and abdominal pain.
2. Fever.
3. Bruising.
4. Lethargy and pallor.
5. Lymph node enlargement.
B. Assess for late manifestations.
1. Oral and rectal ulcers.
2. Hemorrhage.
3. Infection.

> MEDICAL IMPLICATIONS
>
> A. Clinical course.
> 1. Untreated: rapid deterioration and death.
> 2. Treated: with chemotherapy, 90 percent of those treated experience at least an initial remission.
> B. Initial remission usually occurs following the commencement of chemotherapy.
> C. Chemotherapy is usually continual for three years of remission and then stopped.
> D. Drugs most commonly used for initiations and maintenance of remissions:
> 1. Prednisone.
> 2. Mercaptopurine.
> 3. Methotrexate.
> 4. Cytoxan.
> 5. Vincristine.
> E. Methotrexate usually administered soon after start of remission to prevent central nervous system involvement.

Implementation

A. Prevent infection.
1. Avoid contact with communicable diseases.
2. Do not give regular immunizations.
3. Provide oral hygiene.
4. Change intravenous tubing daily.
5. If resistance very low, reverse isolation.
B. Prevent hemorrhage.
1. Watch platelet count.
2. Avoid all unnecessary intramuscular and intravenous injections.
3. Avoid aspirin, alcohol, spicy foods.
4. Use electric razor to shave legs and face.
C. Prevent uric acid build up—treat hyperuricemia (due to increased cellular proliferation and the breakdown of leukemia cells).

1. Increase fluids; observe pH of urine.
2. If ordered, administer allopurinol.
D. Promote healthy nutrition.
1. Administer antiemetic one-half hour before meals.
2. Use anesthetic mouthwash before meals.
3. Avoid toothbrushes.
4. Offer cold liquids high in calories.
E. Observe for side effects and signs of the toxicity of chemotherapy.
F. Counsel parents and siblings.
1. During periods of remission, encourage normal activity.
2. Assist in psychological preparation for death.
3. Refer to parents' group.
4. Provide for continuing follow-up of family following death.

Hodgkin's Disease

Definition: A malignancy of the lymph system characterized by a large, primitive, reticulum-like, malignant cell. Prognosis is guarded.

Assessment

A. Assess age. Symptoms usually peak between fifteen to twenty-nine years of age.
B. Evaluate enlarged painless lymph nodes, i.e., nodes are firm and movable.
C. Assess for frequent infections.
D. Assess for stage of disease.
1. Stage I: Disease is restricted to single anatomic site or is localized in a group of lymph nodes; asymptomatic.
2. Stage II(a): Two or three adjacent lymph nodes in the area on the same side of the diaphragm are affected.
3. Stage II(b): Symptoms appear.
4. Stage III: Disease is widely disseminated into the lymph areas and organs.

Implementation

A. Provide symptomatic relief of the side effects of radiation and chemotherapy.
1. Radiation is used for stages I, II, and III in an effort to eradicate the disease.
2. Radiation and chemotherapy used in combination is treatment of choice.

B. Counsel client.
  1. Assist the family and the adolescent client to accept the process of treatment.
  2. Encourage independence where possible.
C. Observe for pressure from enlargement of the lymph glands on vital organs, particularly for respiratory problems from the compression of the airway.

Brain Tumors

Definition: Two-thirds of brain tumors arise in the infratentorial region of the brain. The most common types are cerebellar astrocytoma, medulloblastoma, and brain stem glioma.

Characteristics

A. Seventy-five percent of childhood brain tumors are impossible to remove or are so situated as to cause damage if completely removed.
B. Tumors occur most frequently in the five-to-seven age group.
C. Location: most tumors occur in the posterior fossa.
D. Types most frequently seen in children:
  1. Astrocytoma.
    a. Located in the cerebellum.
    b. Insidious onset and slowly progressive course.
    c. Surgical removal usually possible.
  2. Medulloblastoma.
    a. Located in the cerebellum.
    b. Highly malignant.
    c. Prognosis poor.
  3. Ependymoma.
    a. Usually, a ventricular blockage, which leads to signs of increased intracranial pressure.
    b. Treated with incomplete internal compression and radiation therapy.
  4. Brain stem gliomas.
    a. Seventy-five percent of childhood brain tumors.
    b. Develops slowly with initial symptoms of cranial nerve palsies.
  5. Neuroblastoma
    a. A malignant, solid tumor primarily occurring in infants and young children.
    b. The tumor generally arises in the adrenal gland, but may originate in any part of the sympathetic chain.

c. Growth is by extension and invasion; prognosis is guarded.
d. Chemotherapy (Vincristine and cyclophosphamide) can be successful, especially under one year of age.

Assessment

A. Assess for increased intracranial pressure.
  1. Vomiting without nausea.
  2. Headache.
  3. Diplopia.
B. Check any enlargement of the head in children under four years old.
C. Assess any mental change: lethargy, irritability, drowsiness, and stupor.

Implementation

A. Control and relieve symptoms.
B. Institute seizure precautions.
C. Administer postoperative care.
  1. Maintain child flat in bed on unaffected side.
  2. Log roll for change of position.
  3. Control fever with hypothermia mattress.
  4. Frequently observe vital signs until stable.
  5. Reinforce a wet dressing with sterile gauze.
  6. Notify physician of increased wetness of dressing (possible cerebral spinal fluid leakage).
D. Educate and counsel family.
  1. Counsel family and child through the stages of acceptance of the disease.
  2. Instruct on the use of medications and dosage.
  3. Alert them to signs of increased intracranial pressure.
  4. Suggest the use of a wig, a hat, or a scarf to cover the child's shaved head.
  5. Encourage return of the independence of the child.
E. Monitor radiation therapy.
  1. Prepare parents for toxic effects of treatment (see section on radiation side effects).
  2. Treat side effects as they arise.

BONE TUMORS

Osteogenic Sarcoma

Definition: A malignant tumor originating from osteoblasts (bone-forming cells). Occurs twice as frequently in boys as in girls.

Assessment

A. Assess for tumor. Usually located at the end of the long bones (metaphysis). Most frequently seen at the distal end of the femur or the proximal end of the tibia.
B. Assess for pain at site, swelling, and limitation of movement.
C. Evaluate lungs which is a common site of metastasis.

Implementation

A. Provide care for amputation followed by chemotherapy.
B. Administer and monitor frequently used drugs.
   1. Vincristine.
   2. Cytoxan.
   3. Actinomycin D.

Ewing's Sarcoma

Definition: A malignant tumor of the bone originating from myeloblasts with early metastases to lung, lymph nodes, and other bones.

Assessment

A. Assess for tumor. Usually located on the shaft of the long bones. Femur, tibia, and humerus are common sites.
B. Assess for pain at site.
C. Assess for swollen area with tenderness.
D. Check elevation in temperature.

Implementation

A. Monitor for side effects of radiation.
B. Provide postoperative amputation care, which sometimes follows radiation therapy.
C. Administer chemotherapy to treat tumor and prevent metastases.
   1. Vincristine.
   2. Cytoxan.
   3. Actinomycin D.
C. Treat the side effects of chemotherapy and radiation.
D. Encourage inclusion of child in discussions of treatment, options, risks, and prognosis.
E. Listen to parents, child, and siblings as they work through denial, anger, acceptance; allow them their grieving process.
F. Promote age-appropriate activities and group discussions with peers.
G. Assist parents in avoiding overprotection.

SPECIAL TOPICS IN PEDIATRIC NURSING

Special topics in pediatric nursing include a broad category of subjects relevant to pediatrics but which do not fit in the system format. This section encompasses venereal diseases, the mentally retarded child, accidents, the battered child syndrome, and, finally, death and children.

THE MENTALLY RETARDED CHILD

General Concepts of Mental Retardation

A. The child is treated according to developmental age rather than chronological age.
B. The child needs as much stimulation and love as a normal child.
C. Retarded children are frequently more susceptible to infections and disease.
D. Behavioral modification frequently works well with these children.
E. Help support parents' reaction to the birth of a mentally retarded child.
   1. Birth presents a threat to the parents' marital relationship and family dynamics.
   2. Stages of reactions.
      a. Denial: initial reaction of defense, which protects the parents from admitting that this child, this extension of themselves, is not normal.
      b. Self-awareness: recognition of difference between their child and other children.
      c. Recognition of problem: active search for information on their child's problem and for professional advice.
F. Developmental delay may be first indication of mental retardation. (Almost 75 percent have no physical abnormality.)
G. Diagnosis is difficult and should be done by skilled team to ensure no child is mislabeled.

516

Down's Syndrome

Etiology

A. Caused by the presence of an extra chromosome or the translocation of a chromosome in the genetic chain.

B. The chromosome is usually number 21.

Assessment

A. Assess facial characteristics: almond-shaped eyes, round face, protruding tongue, flattened posterior and anterior surfaces of the skull, epicanthus, and flat nose.

B. Assess musculoskeletal system: muscles are flaccid and joints are loose.

C. Assess extremities: broad hands, abnormal palmar crease, incurved fifth finger, first and second toe widely spaced.

D. Assess mental capacity: ranges from slightly incapacitated (educable) to severely retarded.

Implementation

A. Refer parents for genetic counseling.

B. Following discharge from hospital, provide follow-up for the family for counseling and child guidance.

C. Refer to the community health agency for follow-up.

D. Alert the parents to the child's increased susceptibility to infections and the need for extra precautions to prevent illness.

E. Assist the parents in developing a program for the child by identifying for them signs of neurological development in the child that indicates readiness for developmental tasks such as sitting, self-feeding, and crawling.

Phenylketonuria

Definition: A genetically transmitted condition in which an infant fails to metabolize the amino acid phenylalanine normally. High levels of this amino acid in the blood can cause mental retardation.

Assessment

A. Assess results of PKU tests: most states have mandatory PKU testing before discharging the infant from the hospital.

B. Assess any arrested brain development by four months of age and suspect PKU.

C. Observe for signs.
1. Lethargy.
2. Anorexia.
3. Anemia.
4. Skin rashes.
5. Diarrhea.

Implementation

A. Monitor restriction of phenylalanine in the diet, e.g., Lofenalac formula.

B. Restrict foods high in protein, e.g., meat, poultry, fish, eggs, nuts, legumes, and milk products.

C. Provide nutrition referrals and follow-up.

D. Educate the parents about the disease.

E. Provide continued counseling throughout childhood for the prevention of emotional problems that can arise from diet restriction.

F. Screen future children born to the same parents.

G. Provide genetic counseling.

Table 9. LEVEL OF MENTAL RETARDATION

Type I	Type II	IQ	Description
Mild	Educable	50–75	Can develop social and sensorimotor skills. Can be self-supporting.
Moderate	Trainable	35–50	Can communicate. Minimal learning ability. Poor social interaction skills, but can be independent with supervision.
Severe	Trainable	20–35	Poor communicative, social, and sensorimotor skills. Needs supervision and can benefit from habit training.
Profound	Custodial	Below 20	Minimal capacity to function. Needs constant supervision.

ACCIDENTS

Definition: Unexpected events that lead to recognizable injury or metabolic changes.

General Categories of Accidents

A. Incidence: Accidents are the leading cause of death from the age of one year through twenty-four years.
B. Most common types of fatal accidents by age.
  1. Infant under twelve months.
    a. Aspiration.
    b. Motor vehicle.
  2. From one to four years.
    a. Motor vehicle.
    b. Fires or burns.
  3. From five to nineteen years.
    a. Motor vehicle.
    b. Drowning.

Prevention of Accidents

A. Control of agent when possible.
  1. Education of parents as to what substances are hazardous and how to "safety-proof" a home.
  2. Safe storage of poisons.
  3. Safety caps on prescriptions.
  4. Use of special car seats and seat belts.
B. Recognition of risk.
  1. Provide accident prevention education appropriate to the age of the child.
  2. For children with a history of accidents, take special care to make the environment safe.
C. Control of the environment; during crisis periods in families, suggest help for child care and supervision.

Treatment of Poisoning at Home

A. At a well-child visit, give parent the telephone number of the local poison control center.
B. Suggest keeping ipecac syrup with the poison control telephone number wrapped around it.
C. Instructions to the family.
  1. When poisoning occurs, telephone the control number. Be sure to know the brand name of the poison and the approximate amount ingested.
  2. Institute the program suggested by poison control.

  3. If no telephone number is available, call a physician and take the child to the emergency room; bring the bottle of poison and have a neighbor or a friend drive.
D. Diagnostic information the physician will need.
  1. What infant ingested.
  2. The amount ingested.
  3. Odor on breath.
  4. Pupil changes.
  5. Presence of abdominal pain, nausea, or vomiting.
  6. Convulsions.

PSYCHOSOCIAL DISORDERS

Attention Deficit Disorder

Definition: A developmental disorder that involves a group of behavioral symptoms such as hyperactivity, hyperkinesis, or over-activity. Also called minimal brain damage, minor cerebral dysfunction.

Assessment

A. Identify child with this disorder by assessing presence of diagnostic criteria (modified from American Psychiatric Association DSM-III).
  1. Inattention—child demonstrates three or more of the following.
    a. Does not complete things.
    b. Does not appear to listen.
    c. Demonstrates difficulty in concentrating.
    d. Easily distractable.
    e. Cannot stick to a play activity.
  2. Impulsivity—child demonstrates three or more of the following.
    a. Often acts before thinking.
    b. Moves rapidly from one activity to another.
    c. Cannot organize work effectively.
    d. Requires close supervision.
    e. Interrupts in class.
    f. Cannot wait to take turns; has difficulty in group activities.
  3. Hyperactivity—child demonstrates two or more of the following.
    a. Runs around, jumps, and climbs constantly.
    b. Cannot sit still or stay seated for very long.
    c. Moves around during sleep.
    d. Seems to be always active.

4. Onset before the age of seven.
5. Duration of at least 6 months.
6. Cause is not identified as schizophrenia, affective disorder, or mental retardation.

B. Observe for additional traits.
1. Negativistic.
2. Emotional lability.
3. Easily frustrated.
4. Nonlocalizing neurological signs, learning disabilities, and abnormal EEG may or may not be present.

Implementation

A. Coordinate treatment plan with physician, family, and educational counselor.
B. Provide safe environment with minimal stimulation.
1. Decrease number of stimuli; reduce extraneous stimuli.
2. Set limits on behavior.
3. Structure activities.
4. Provide for energy outlets: allow large muscle movements.
5. Provide for quiet area and time.
C. Establish primary relationship, if possible, with short contact times.
D. May establish behavior modification program; encourage positive behavior. Assist to build self-esteem, which is usually low.
E. Assist client to establish own controls and behavior.
F. Coordinate diet: limit sugar, additives, and artificial colors.
G. Administer medication if ordered: Ritalin, a mild nervous-system stimulant, is extremely controversial at the present time.

Failure to Thrive

Definition: A syndrome characterized by an infant's failure to grow and develop with or without characteristic posturing or "body language." Etiology is nonspecific. May be organic or nonorganic.

Assessment

A. Assess history of infant: feeding problems, vomiting, sleep disturbance, irritability, sucking ability, aversion to formula, and irregularity in daily activities.

B. Assess general physical-physiological status to assist in ruling out organic cause of disorder.
C. Assess normal nutritional intake to help to determine if cause is related to deficient intake, malabsorption, or poor assimilation.
1. Assess number of calories, quality of calories, and feeding patterns.
2. Check weight daily and observe reaction to nutritional program.
D. Assess nature of mother-child relationship.
1. Relationship patterns.
2. Ability of mother to perceive infant's needs.

Implementation

A. Priority—provide sufficient nutrients so that infant will grow.
1. Develop a structured feeding routine.
2. Weigh daily to assess weight gain.
B. Provide nuturing to infant.
1. Ensure a warm, loving environment through holding, cuddling, and physical contact.
2. Limit number of persons interacting with infant; primary nursing preferred.
3. Spend time talking to infant and building a trusting relationship.
4. Maintain as much eye-to-eye contact as possible.
C. Provide a positive, quiet, nonstimulating environment to promote psychosocial growth.
D. Assist mother to develop a positive relationship with infant.
1. Do not be judgmental in evaluating mother-infant relationship. Accept mother of infant.
2. Support mother as she attempts to cope with situation.
3. Encourage mother to express feelings.
4. Include mother in plan of care.
5. Evaluate continuing mother-infant relationship.
E. Document feeding behaviors and evaluate infant progress.
F. Coordinate referral services from family when infant discharged.

Battered Child Syndrome

Definition: Any nonaccidental physical abuse resulting from an absence of reasonable standards of care by the parents or the child's caretaker.

Epidemiology

A. Incidence.
  1. Six out of 1,000 children born become battered children.
  2. In the hospital emergency room, it is estimated that 10 percent of the injuries seen in children under five are actually caused by parents or are the result of negligence.
B. Victims.
  1. One-third of the victims are less than six months old.
  2. One-third are six months to three years old.
  3. One-third are over three years old.
  4. Premature infants have a three times greater risk of becoming battered children than full-term infants.
  5. Stepchildren have an increased risk.
C. Environment.
  1. The abused child usually has characteristics that make him or her demanding.
  2. The abuse usually occurs on the same day as a crisis or stressful event.
  3. The abuse usually occurs in anger after the parent is provoked.

Clinical Indications of Abuse

A. History of the problem.
  1. The cause given for the condition is implausible, e.g., punishment is inappropriate for the age of the child.
  2. There are discrepancies in the history from neighbors or various members of the family.
  3. There is a delay in seeking medical help for the child.
B. Physical examination and indications for diagnosis.
  1. Bruises, welts, and scars in multiple stages of healing.
  2. Fingermark pattern of bruises.
  3. Bite, rope, or choke marks.
  4. Cigarette and/or hot water burns.
  5. Eye damage, subdural hematoma, failure to thrive, and/or intraabdominal injuries.
  6. Radiographic findings of multiple bone injuries at different stages of healing.
  7. Passive, noncommunicative, and/or withdrawn child.

Characteristics of Abusive Parents

A. Parents were usually abused as children.
B. Abusers are unable to utilize outside help (neighbors, friends, or professionals) when angry at their child.
C. Abusers usually are isolated people.
D. Spouse of abuser frequently does not know how to prevent the occurrence or recurrence of the abuse.
E. Abusive parents frequently have unreasonable expectations of their children—they expect a baby to meet their needs.
F. Personality characteristics.
  1. Dependent personality.
  2. Low self-esteem and poor self-image.
  3. Immature personality.
  4. Low impulse control and inability to handle feelings.

Legal Responsibility

A. Both nurse and doctor are legally responsible to report a suspected battered child to the proper authorities.
B. The designated community authorities are responsible to determine placement of the abused child.

Lead Poisoning

Definition: An environmental disease caused by the ingestion of lead-based materials, such as paint. Death results in 25 percent of the cases of lead encephalopathy, and there are many neurologic residual problems in survivors.

Assessment

A. Assess age of child: usually twelve months to thirty-six months old.
B. Assess gastrointestinal symptoms.
  1. Unexplained, repeated vomiting.
  2. Vague chronic abdominal pain.
C. Assess central nervous system symptoms.
  1. Irritability.
  2. Drowsiness.
  3. Ataxia.
  4. Convulsive seizures.

Implementation

A. Institute preventive measures.
  1. Inspection of buildings twenty-five years old or older.

2. Areas painted with lead paint should be covered with plywood or linoleum.
3. Education of parents.

B. Treat condition.
1. Acute: gastric lavage followed by magnesium sulfate.
2. Chronic: medications that aid in removal of lead calcium disodium edetate (EDTA) dimercaprol (BAL).
   a. Prepare child for painful, frequent injections.
   b. Inject slowly.
   c. Rotate injection sites.
   d. With EDTA observe for signs of hypocalcemia: tetany + convulsions.
   e. Provide for seizure precautions.
   f. Record accurate intake and output to evaluate kidney response to chelating agents.

DEATH AND CHILDREN

Assessment

A. Assess child's understanding of death.
1. Young child's concerns.
   a. Views death as temporary separation from parents, sometimes viewed synonymously with sleep.
   b. May express fear of pain and wish to avoid it.
   c. Child's awareness is lessened by physical symptoms if death comes acutely.
   d. Gradual terminal illness may simulate the adult process: depression, withdrawal, fearfulness and anxiety.
2. Older children's concerns.
   a. May identify death as a "person" to be avoided.
   b. May ask directly if they are going to die.
   c. Concerns center around fear of pain, fear of being left alone and leaving parents and friends.
3. Adolescent concerns.
   a. Recognize death as irreversible and inevitable.
   b. Often avoids talking about impending death and staff may enter into this "conspiracy of silence."
   c. Adolescents have more understanding of death than adults tend to realize.

B. Assess impact of death on child.
C. Assess parent's ability to cope with death of child.

Implementation

A. Always elicit child's understanding of death before discussing it with him or her.
B. Before discussing death with child, discuss it with child's parents.
C. Parental reactions include the continuum of grief process and stages of dying.
1. Reactions depend on previous loss experience.
2. Reactions also depend on relationship with the child and circumstances of illness or injury.
3. Reactions depend on degree of parental guilt.
D. Assist parents in expressing their fears, concerns, and grief so that they may be more supportive to the child.
E. Assist parents in understanding siblings' possible reactions to a terminally ill child.
1. Guilt: belief that they caused the problem or illness.
2. Jealousy: desire for equal attention from parents.
3. Anger: feelings of being left behind.

Appendix 1. DENTAL DEVELOPMENT

	Age at Eruption		Age at Shedding	
Deciduous Teeth	Maxillary	Mandibular	Maxillary	Mandibular
Central incisors	6 to 8 months	5 to 7 months	7 to 8 years	6 to 7 years
Lateral incisors	8 to 11	7 to 10	8 to 9	7 to 8
Cuspids	16 to 20	16 to 20	11 to 12	9 to 11
First molars	10 to 16	10 to 16	10 to 11	10 to 12
Second molars	20 to 30	20 to 30	10 to 12	11 to 13

	Age at Eruption	
Permanent Teeth	Maxillary	Mandibular
Central incisors	7 to 8 years	6 to 7 years
Lateral incisors	8 to 9	7 to 8
Cuspids	11 to 12	9 to 11
First molars	6 to 7	6 to 7
Second molars	12 to 13	12 to 13
First premolars	10 to 11	10 to 11
Second premolars	10 to 12	11 to 13
Third molars	17 to 22	17 to 22

Appendix 2. IMMUNIZATIONS

Age	Prevention
2 months	DPT*, TOPV†
4 months	DPT, TOPV
6 months	DPT, TOPV
12 months	Tuberculin test
15 months	MMR‡
1½ years	DPT, TOPV
4 to 6 years	DPT, TOPV
14 to 16 years	TD§, and thereafter every ten years

*DPT—diphtheria and tetanus toxoids and pertussis vaccine
†TOPV—trivalent oral polio virus vaccine
‡MMR—measles, mumps, and rubella vaccine; may be combined or separate
§TD—combined tetanus and diphtheria toxoids

Appendix 3. DRUG CONVERSION FOR CHILDREN

A. Clark's weight rule:
$$\text{Child's dose} = \frac{\text{Child's wt. in lbs.}}{150} \times \text{Adult dose}$$

B. Intravenous microdrip usually has 60 drops/cc.

C. Conversion of administration units:
- 1 tsp = 5 ml
- 1 tbl = 15 ml
- 1 ml = 16 minims
- 1 grain = 60 mg
- 1 gm = 1,000 mg
- 1 oz = 30 ml
- 1 dram = 4 ml

Appendix 4. PEDIATRIC DEVELOPMENTAL CHART

0–6 months

Gross Motor Development	Fine Motor Development	Language Development
Pulls self to sitting position	Brings hands or toys to mouth	Laughs aloud
Sits for short periods	Holds block in each hand	Begins babbling
Rocks	Reaches for objects beyond grasp	Vocalizes vowel sounds
Turns completely over, abdomen to back	Looks toward objects and sounds	Recognizes name
	Begins hand-eye coordination	

6–12 months

Gross Motor Development	Fine Motor Development	Language Development
Sits without support	Picks up objects fairly well	Speaks one or two words ("Mama," "Dada")
Pulls self to feet	Uses index finger and thumb to grasp	Understands several words and commands
Creeps and cruises	Holds own bottle or cup; feeds self	
Stands and walks holding on to objects	Transfers objects hand to hand	
	Follows rapid movements (vision is 20/200)	

12–18 months

Gross Motor Development	Fine Motor Development	Language Development
Stands and walks alone	Fine muscle coordination begins to develop	Uses jargon
		Understands simple commands
Climbs stairs with help	Explores environment	Is aware of expressive function of language
Throws a ball	Holds a spoon; holds cup with both hands	Has a vocabulary of 10–20 words
Weight triples at 12 months		
Anterior fontanel closes	Can release objects at will	Makes animal sounds
	Do not attempt to change from left to right hand	
	Vision conversion occurs	

Social Development	Play	Toys
Knows mother	Splashes in bath	Soft, colorful squeeze toys
Smiles at familiar people	Holds toys and rattles	Toys that don't have removable parts
Begins to recognize strangers	Responds to mobiles	Teething toys
Shows fear and anger	Plays sitting-up games	Metal cup and wooden spoon for banging
	Begins social games (pat-a-cake)	

Social Development	Play	Toys
Shows emotions: looks hurt, sad	Protect child from dangerous objects	New objects (blocks)
Is aware of environment: when unfamiliar, may be fearful	Loves to look at pictures	Toys that stimulate senses
Imitates gestures, facial expressions	Allow exploration outdoors	Containers
Entertains self		Bath toys
		Allow security toy

Social Development	Play	Toys
Indicates wants	Begins self-directed play rather than adult-directed	Pull and push toys
Likes an audience and will repeat performance		Balls; teddy bears
Shows anxiety about strangers	Requires safe environment (medications locked up and harmful items out of reach)	Pots and pans
Distinguishes self from others		Musical toys
		Telephone
Finds security in a blanket, favorite toy, or thumb sucking	Plays alone but near others (parallel play)	Sand box and fill toys
		Books and pictures
Show affection and encourage child to reciprocate	Can identify and play with geometric forms	

Appendix 4. PEDIATRIC DEVELOPMENTAL CHART (continued)

18 months to 2 years

Gross Motor Development	Fine Motor Development	Language Development
Walks up and down stairs	Uses a spoon without spilling	Speaks vowels correctly
Climbs on furniture	Builds tower of six cubes	Receptive vocabulary of 300 to 500 words
Walks and runs with a stiff gait	Fingerpaints	Begins to use short sentences
Kicks a ball in front of self	Eye accommodation well developed	100–200 word vocabulary
Daytime bladder and bowel control	Vision 20/40	Follows simple directions

2 to 3 years

Gross Motor Development	Fine Motor Development	Language Development
Balances on one foot	Copies horizontal and vertical strokes	Refers to self by pronoun "I"
Goes up and down stairs, alternating feet	Feeds self; uses fork	Asks questions about everything
Rides tricycle	Pours from pitcher	Uses "I", "me," "you" speech
Swings, climbs, jumps	Begins to use scissors	Has vocabulary of 900 words
	Vision is 20/30	Can remember and repeat three numbers

4 to 6 years

Gross Motor Development	Fine Motor Development	Language Development
Races up and down steps	Draws man with two to four parts	Asks abundant questions: What? Why? How?
Has good balance	Can button easily	Recites nursery rhymes
Skips, hops, performs stunts	Feeds self	Gives full name
Is agile and graceful	Brushes teeth	Has well-developed vocabulary
Begins to ride two-wheel bicycle	Exhibits small, well-controlled motor movements	Repeats sentence of ten syllables or more
Runs skillfully	Uses hands as manipulative tools in cutting, pasting, hammering	Talks constantly
Can catch a ball	Begins reading readiness	Defines words by use
Exhibits growth spurt	Vision now 20/20	Learns to read
Is very active, impulsive		Knows number combinations to ten

Social Development	Play	Toys
Has fear of parents leaving	Begins peer relationships—needs peers for play	Building blocks
Helps to undress; tries to button		Wagons
Wants to hoard, not share	Role-modeling for positive behavior is important	Pull toys
Begins to have feelings of autonomy	Self-directed play increases	Pounding toys, like a drum
Begins cooperation in toilet training		Books with pictures

Social Development	Play	Toys
Knows full name	Pushes and pulls large toys	Manipulative toys for muscle coordination
Displays negativism, temper tantrums	Able to entertain self for short periods	Crayons and paper
Is ritualistic	Engages in associative play	Simple games
Shows poorly developed judgment	Begins imaginative and make-believe play	Climbing apparatus
Wants to please		Tricycle
Begins to share		Record player
Uses toilet by self		

Social Development	Play	Toys
Shows interest in world about him	Alternate periods of active and quiet play	Books
Sees self as all-important	Explores environment	Puzzles
Begins to share; seeks peer relationships	Enjoys group play in small groups	Drawing
Is less negativistic	Encourage pretending, expressing self and imagination	Utensils
Does simple chores at home		Puppets
Still requires parental support	Needs guidance and limits	Games
Begins to accept authority outside home	Provide exercise to stimulate motor and psychosocial development	Bicycle

526

Appendix 4. PEDIATRIC DEVELOPMENTAL CHART (continued)

6 to 8 years

Gross Motor Development	Fine Motor Development	Language Development
Exhibits better coordination and control	Dresses self	Learns to read
Graceful body movements	Is capable of fine hand movements	Begins to tell time
Speed in movements	Writing improves	Vocabulary increases
Growth spurt	Eyes become fully developed	Defines words by use
		Begins cursive writing

8 to 10 years

Gross Motor Development	Fine Motor Development	Language Development
Arms grow long in proportion to body	Learns to use script	Increased capacity for logical thought.
Good timing and coordination of fine muscles	Demonstrates skill in manual activities because hand-eye coordination is developed	Vocabulary increases
Very active physically	Cares completely for own physical needs	Increased ability to discuss issues
Gains speed and strength		Grasps easy multiplication and division
		Understands money

Social Development	Play	Toys
Is more independent and competitive	Very active	Table games and card games
School is important	Group play is preferred	Magic tricks
Wishes to be like his friends; seeks out clubs and teams	Competitive games	Games that develop physical and mental skill
May have periods of shyness		

Social Development	Play	Interests
More self-assured in environment	Likes group projects, clubs	Games of skill
Increased modesty	Through play, learns new concepts: independence, competition, compromise, and cooperation	Competitive games
"Chum" stage occurs; has special friend in whom child confides		Team sports
Needs to be considered important by adults		Books
Questions regarding sex require simple, honest answers		Musical instruments
Lying and stealing may be problem		TV, records
		Organized clubs

Appendix 5. PEDIATRIC COMMUNICABLE DISEASES

Disease	Characteristics	Transmission	Nursing Care
Chickenpox (varicella)	Acute viral disease; onset is sudden with high fever; maculopapular rash and vesicular scabs in multiple stages of healing. Incubation is 10 to 21 days.	Spread by droplet or airborne secretions; scabs not infectious.	Isolate. Treat symptoms: fluids for fever, Tylenol. Prevent scratching. Observe for signs of complications.
Mumps	Acute viral disease, characterized by fever, swelling, and tenderness of one or more salivary glands. Potential complications, including meningoencephalitis.	Spread by droplet and direct and indirect contact with saliva of infected person. Most infectious 48 hours prior to swelling.	Prevent by vaccination. Isolate. Treat symptoms: ice pack to neck and force fluids, Tylenol. Watch for symptoms of neurological involvement: fever, headache, vomiting, stiff neck.
Measles (rubeola)	Acute viral disease, characterized by conjunctivitis, bronchitis, Koplik's spots on buccal mucosa. Dusky red and splotchy rash 3 to 4 days. Usually photophobia. Complications can be severe in respiratory tract, eye, ear, and nervous system. Incubation is 10 to 12 days.	Spread by droplet or direct contact.	Symptomatic: bedrest until cough and fever subside; force fluids, dim lights in room; tepid baths and lotion to relieve itching. Observe for signs of neurological involvement.
German Measles (rubella)	Viral infection. Slight fever, mild coryza and headache. Discrete pink-red maculopapules that last about 3 days. Incubation is 14 to 21 days.	Spread by direct and indirect contact with droplets. Fetus may contract measles in utero if mother has the disease.	Basically a benign disease. Symptomatic: bedrest until fever subsides.
Diphtheria	Local and systemic manifestations. Malaise, fever, cough with stridor. Toxin has affinity for renal, nervous and cardiac tissue. Incubation 2 to 6 days or longer.	Spread by droplets from respiratory tract or carrier.	Antitoxin and antibiotic therapy to kill toxin. Strict bedrest; prevent exertion. Liquid or soft diet. Observe for respiratory obstruction. Suctioning, oxygen, and emergency tracheotomy may be necessary.
Tetanus (lockjaw)	Acute or gradual onset. Muscle rigidity and spasms, headache, fever and convulsions. Death may result from aspiration, pneumonia or exhaustion. Incubation is 3 to 21 days.	Organisms in soil. Enter body through wound. Not communicable man to man.	Toxins must be neutralized. Bedrest during illness in quiet, darkened room. Avoid stimulation which can cause spasms. Observe for complications of laryngospasm and respiratory failure.
Pertussis (whooping cough)	Dry cough occurring in paroxysms. Dyspnea and fever may be present. Lymphocytosis. Incubation is 5 to 21 days.	Direct contact or droplet from infected person.	Symptomatic: rest, warm, humid air. Maintain nutritional status. Need to protect from secondary infections.

7

PSYCHIATRIC NURSING

This chapter emphasizes the principles of psychiatric nursing in the nursing process format. The material covers many important and recent developments in the field of psychiatric nursing. Nurse-client relationships and effective communication techniques, including interviewing and counseling skills, are fully explained to help students distinguish between therapeutic and nontherapeutic nursing approaches. Assessment, planning, implementation, and evaluation of major psychiatric disorders are described and organized according to the DSM III.

An overall review of psychotherapeutic techniques is provided, including how these techniques are applied in environmental, group, and family therapy. This chapter also contains special sections on child psychiatry, basic treatment modalities such as behavior modification, crisis intervention, and psychotropic drugs.

THE NURSE-CLIENT RELATIONSHIP

Definition: The nurse-client relationship is a therapeutic, professional relationship in which interaction occurs between two persons—the nurse, who possesses the skills, abilities, and resources to relieve another's discomfort, and the client, who is seeking assistance for alleviation of some existing problem.

Principles Underlying Relationship Therapy

A. The client's value as an individual must be acknowledged.
B. Awareness of the total client, including his or her physical needs, is important.
C. The nurse's understanding of self, motives, and needs is important in the therapeutic process.
D. Some degree of emotional involvement is required, but objectivity must be maintained.
E. Appropriate limits must be set, and consistency must be maintained.
F. Empathic understanding is therapeutic; sympathy is nontherapeutic.
G. Honest and open communication is basic to the therapeutic process.
H. Expression of feelings, within safe limits, should be encouraged.

Phases in Nurse-Client Relationship Therapy

A. Initiation or orientation phase.
    1. Establish boundaries of relationship.
    2. Identify problems.
    3. Assess anxiety levels of self and client.
    4. Identify expectations.
B. Continuation or active working phase.
    1. Promote attitude of acceptance of each other, which decreases anxiety.
    2. Use specific therapeutic and problem-solving techniques to develop working relationship.
    3. Continually assess and evaluate problems.
    4. Focus on increasing client's independence, and decreasing client's reliance on the nurse.
    5. Maintain the goal of client's confronting and working through identified problems.
C. Termination phase.
    1. Plan for the conclusion of therapy early in the development of relationship.
    2. Maintain initially defined boundaries.

3. Anticipate problems of termination.
    a. Client may become too dependent on the nurse. Encourage client to become independent.
    b. Termination may recall client's previous separation experiences, causing feelings of abandonment, rejection, and depression. Discuss client's previous experiences.
4. Discuss client's feelings about termination.

Assessment

A. Determine purpose of establishing a nurse-client relationship.
B. Assess the overall condition of the client to determine what benefits will be derived from a nurse-client relationship.
C. Observe what is happening with the client here and now.
D. Identify developmental level of client so relationship expectations will be realistic.
E. Determine whether client exhibits verbal or nonverbal communication patterns so the nurse can relate on the appropriate level.
F. Assess anxiety level of client.
G. Identify client expectations of a therapeutic relationship.
H. Examine your own feelings and expectations to evaluate potential impact on the relationship.

Planning and Analysis

A. The client will be assisted to meet own needs.
B. The client will experience the feeling of being accepted.
C. Mutual trust through consistent congruent behavior will be developed.
D. Increased self-esteem of client will be promoted.
E. A supportive environment for change will be provided.

Implementation

A. Assume the role of facilitator in the relationship.
B. Accept client as having value and worth as an individual.
C. Maintain relationship on a professional level.
D. Provide an environment conducive to client's experiencing corrective emotional experiences.
E. Keep interaction reality oriented, that is, in the here and now.
F. Listen actively.

G. Use nonverbal communication to support and encourage client.
  1. Recognize meaning and purpose of nonverbal communication.
  2. Keep verbal and nonverbal communication congruent.
H. Focus content and direction of conversation on client.
I. Interact on client's intellectual, developmental, and emotional level.
J. Focus on "how, what, when, where, and who" rather than on "why."
K. Teach client problem solving to correct maladaptive patterns.
L. Help client to identify, express, and cope with feelings.
M. Help client develop alternative coping mechanisms.
N. Recognize a high level of anxiety and assist client to deal with it.
O. Use therapeutic communication techniques.
  1. Use techniques to increase effective communication. (See Therapeutic Communication Techniques, Appendix 1.)
  2. Recognize blocks to communication and work to remove them. (See Blocks to Communication, Appendix 2.)

Evaluation

A. Client developed the ability to assess and meet own needs.
B. Expectations of both client and nurse were met.
C. Boundaries of the professional relationship were maintained.
D. Problem-solving ability of the client was improved.
E. Communication from client improved so that it was clearer, more explicit, and centered on problem areas.
F. A supportive environment was created so that client could reduce anxiety level and experience change.
G. Interactions with client were carried out on his or her intellectual, emotional, and developmental level.
H. Relationship was goal oriented.
I. Client was able to express feelings more effectively.
J. Client was able to develop more effective coping mechanisms.

K. Termination of the relationship was completed successfully.

THERAPEUTIC COMMUNICATION PROCESS

Definition: Communication is the process of sending and receiving messages by means of symbols, words, signs, gestures, or other action. It is a multilevel process consisting of the content or information of the message and the part that defines the meaning of the message. Messages sent and received define the relationship between people. *Therapeutic communication utilizes the principles of communication in a goal-directed professional framework.*

Characteristics

A. A person cannot *not* communicate.
B. Communication is a basic human need.
C. Communication includes verbal and nonverbal expression (also tone, pace, and manner of dress).
D. Successful communication includes:
  1. Appropriateness.
  2. Efficiency.
  3. Flexibility.
  4. Feedback.
E. Communication skills are learned as the individual grows and develops.
F. The foundation of the person's perception of him or herself and the world is the result of communicated messages received from significant others.
G. High anxiety in both nurse and client impedes communication.
H. Self-awareness during the interview facilitates honest communication.
I. Factors that affect communication:
  1. Intrapersonal framework of the person.
  2. Relationship between the participants.
  3. Purpose of the sender.
  4. Content.
  5. Context.
  6. Manner in which the message is sent.
  7. Effect on the receiver.
  8. Environment in which the interaction takes place.
J. Purpose of communication.
  1. To transfer ideas from one person to another.
  2. To create meaning through the process.

3. To reduce uncertainty, to act effectively, and to defend or strengthen one's ego.
4. To affect or influence others, one's physical environment, and one's self.

The Interview Process

Assessment

A. Determine purpose of the interview.
B. As the first step in therapeutic interviewing, assess the client's total condition—physical, emotional, spiritual, and social.
C. Observe accurately what is happening with client here and now.
D. Be aware of your own feelings, reactions, and level of anxiety.
E. Assess client's communication patterns, behavior, and general demeanor.
F. Determine life situation of client.
G. Assess environmental conditions that may affect nurse-client interaction.

Planning and Analysis

A. The interview will be goal-directed; that is, communication or transmission of facts, feelings, and meanings through words and gestures will accomplish a defined goal.
B. The environment will be conducive to the interview process.
C. Both nurse and client will make an agreement, implicit or explicit, to conduct the interview.
D. Purpose of interview will be accomplished.

Implementation

COMPONENTS OF INTERVIEW PROCESS

A. Provide a safe, private, comfortable setting if possible.
B. Encourage client to describe perceptions and feelings.
   1. Focus on communication but use indirect approach.
   2. Use minimal verbal activity.
   3. Encourage spontaneity.
C. Assist client to clarify feelings and events and place them in time sequence.
   1. Focus on emotionally charged area.
   2. Maintain accepting, nonjudgmental attitude.

D. Give broad openings and ask open-ended questions to enable client to describe what is happening with him or her.
E. Use body language to convey empathy, interest, and encouragement to facilitate communication.
F. Use silence as a therapeutic tool; it enables client to pace and direct his or her own communications. Long periods of silence, however, may increase client's anxiety level.
G. Define the limits of the interview: determine the purpose and structure the time and interaction patterns accordingly.
H. Never employ interviewing techniques as stereotyped responses during an interview.
   1. Use of such responses negates open and honest communication.
   2. Use of structured responses is counterproductive, as it presents nurse as a dishonest communicator.
   3. Interaction must be alive and responsive, not dependent on a technique for continuance.
   4. Use "I" messages rather than "you" messages. (For example, "I feel uncomfortable," not "you make me feel uncomfortable.")

COMPONENTS OF COUNSELING PROCESS

A. Be present and allow client to experience supportiveness.
B. Maintain consistency with flexibility to provide security.
C. Give information but not advice.
D. Assist client without persuading, admonishing, threatening, or compelling the client to change attitudes, beliefs, or behaviors.
E. Use the interviewing process to facilitate accomplishment of a goal.
F. Use active listening, therapeutic communication, and empathic understanding.
G. Set limits and determine goals.
H. Enable client to make fullest use of potential within his or her current experience to develop new ways of coping with life situations.
I. Assist client to build more effective coping mechanisms:
   1. Gather pertinent data.
   2. Define the problem.
   3. Mutually agree on working toward a solution.
   4. Set goals
   5. Select alternatives.
   6. Activate problem-solving behavior.

ANXIETY

Definition: Anxiety is an affective state subjectively experienced as a response to tensions. Anxiety is experienced as painful, vague uneasiness, or diffuse apprehension. It is a form of energy whose presence is inferred from its effect on attention, behavior, learning, and perception.

Characteristics

A. Anxiety is perceived subjectively by the conscious mind of the person experiencing it.
B. Anxiety is a result of conflicts between the personality and the environment or between different forces within the personality.
C. Anxiety may be a reaction to threats of deprivation of something biologically or emotionally vital to the person.
D. The causative conflicts and/or threats are undefined in the conscious mind of the person.
E. The amount or level of anxiety is related to the following factors:
  1. Degree of threat to the self.
  2. Degree to which behavior reduces anxiety.
F. Varying degrees of anxiety are common to all human beings at one time or another.
G. Anxiety is always found in emotional disorders.
H. Anxiety is easily transmitted from one individual to another.
I. Constructive use of anxiety is healthy; it is often an incentive for growth.
J. The more capacity to handle anxiety, the more control an individual has over his or her environment.

Assessment

A. A major assessment criterion for measuring the degree of anxiety is the person's ability to focus on what is happening to him or her in a situation.
  1. Mild anxiety: Client is able to focus realistically on most of what is happening within and to him or her.
  2. Moderate anxiety: Client is able to partially focus on what is happening; focus is limited.
  3. Severe anxiety: Client cannot focus on what is happening to him or her; focus is scattered.
B. Physiological reactions present in client.
  1. Increased heart rate.
  2. Increased or decreased appetite.
  3. Hyperventilation.
  4. Tendency to void and defecate.
  5. Dry mouth.
  6. Butterflies in stomach, nausea, vomiting, cramps, diarrhea.
  7. "Flight or fight" response.
  8. Tremors.
  9. Dyspnea.
  10. Palpitations.
  11. Tachycardia.
  12. Numbness of extremities.
C. Psychological reactions present in client.
  1. Lack of concentration on work.
  2. Feelings of depression and guilt.
  3. Harbored fear of sudden death or insanity.
  4. Dread of being alone.
  5. Confusion.
  6. Tension.
  7. Agitation and restlessness.
D. States of anxiety vary in degree and can be assessed as follows:
  1. Ataraxia (absence of anxiety).
    a. State is uncommon.
    b. Can be seen in persons who take drugs.
    c. Indicates low motivation.
  2. Mild.
    a. Senses are alert.
    b. Attentiveness is increased.
    c. Motivation is increased.
  3. Moderate.
    a. Perception is narrowed, and attention is selective.
    b. Degree of pathology depends on the individual.
    c. May be detected in complaining, arguing, teasing behaviors.
    d. Can be converted to physical symptoms such as headaches, low back pain, nausea, diarrhea.
  4. Severe.
    a. All senses are gravely affected.
    b. Behavior becomes automatic.
    c. Energy is drained.
    d. Defense mechanisms are used to control it.
    e. Cannot be used constructively by person.
    f. Psychologically extremely painful.
    g. Nursing action always indicated for this state.
  5. Panic.
    a. Individual is overwhelmed and feels helpless.

b. Personality may disintegrate.

c. Wild, desperate, ineffective behavior may be observed.

d. Client may do bodily harm to self and others.

e. Panic state cannot be tolerated very long.

f. Condition is pathological.

g. Immediate intervention is needed.

Planning and Analysis

1. Behavior and/or symptoms related to anxiety will be identified.

2. Anxiety will be decreased.

3. Nurse will intervene when client is unable to cope through implementation of specific treatment plan, i.e., chemotherapy, 1:1, seclusion, restraints, relaxation techniques, etc.

4. Identification and intervention into factors or persons which escalate the anxiety of client will be provided.

5. Some degree of insight will be gained into source of anxiety.

6. Tolerance for some degree of anxiety will be increased.

7. More effective coping mechanisms for handling anxiety will be developed.

8. Client will be assisted to channel the anxiety-produced energy into constructive behavior.

9. Client will be able to identify and modify lifestyle patterns that contribute to anxiety.

Implementation

A. Identify anxious behavior and the level of anxiety that determines degree of intervention.

B. Remain with an anxious client.

C. Recognize anxiety in self.

D. Maintain appropriate attitudes toward client.

1. Acceptance.

2. Matter-of-fact approach.

3. Willingness to listen and help.

4. Calmness and support.

E. Recognize if additional help is required for intervention.

F. Provide activities that decrease anxiety and provide an outlet for energy.

G. Establish person-to-person relationship.

1. Allow client to express his or her feelings.

2. Proceed at client's pace.

3. Avoid forcing client.

4. Assist client in identifying anxiety.

5. Assist client in learning new ways of dealing with anxiety.

H. Provide appropriate physical environment.

1. Nonstimulating.

2. Structured.

3. Designed to prevent physical exhaustion or self-harm.

I. Administer medication as directed and needed.

Evaluation

A. Intervention resulted in decrease of anxiety.

1. Overt anxious behavior is decreased.

a. Client is more attentive, more alert.

b. Client displays more control of own behavior, i.e., is able to sit with nurse rather than pace.

c. Client verbalizes rather than acts out thoughts.

2. Client is able to discuss anxious feelings.

a. Client identifies feelings of anxiety.

b. Client describes feelings of anxiety.

3. Client relates that physiological symptoms of anxiety decreased.

4. Tolerance level of anxiety is increased.

B. Client is able to learn new ways of coping with anxiety.

C. Client is able to identify and modify lifestyle patterns that contribute to anxiety.

Patterns of Adjustment (Defense Mechanisms)

Definition: Defense mechanisms are processes by which an individual relieves or decreases anxieties caused by uncomfortable situations that threaten self-esteem.

Characteristics

A. The purpose of defense mechanisms is to attempt to reduce anxiety and to reestablish equilibrium.

B. Adjustment depends on one's ability to vary responses so that anxiety is decreased.

C. Individuals use essentially the same mechanisms but may vary them.

D. Use of defense mechanisms may be a conscious process but usually takes place at the unconscious level.

E. Defense mechanisms are compromise solutions and include those listed in Appendix 3.

Assessment

A. Assess whether client evidences healthy adjustment in the way he or she uses defense mechanisms.
   1. Healthy adjustment is characterized by:
      a. Infrequent use of defense mechanisms.
      b. Ability to form new responses.
      c. Ability to change the external environment.
      d. Ability to modify one's needs.
   2. Healthy adjustment patterns may include mechanisms such as rationalization, sublimation, compensation, and suppression.
B. Assess whether client evidences unhealthy adjustment in the way he or she uses defense mechanisms.
   1. Unhealthy adjustment is characterized by:
      a. Undeveloped ability or loss of ability to vary responses.
      b. Retreat from the problem or reality.
      c. Frequent use of defense mechanisms, which may interfere with maintenance of self-image.
   2. Unhealthy adjustment patterns may include mechanisms such as regression, repression, denial, projection, and isolation.

Planning and Analysis

A. The extent of client's use of defense mechanisms and whether adjustment is healthy or unhealthy will be determined.
B. The degree to which anxiety is controlled by use of defense mechanisms will be evaluated.
C. Nurse will assist client to move from an unhealthy to a more healthy use of defense mechanisms by:
   1. Creating a safe, secure environment.
   2. Establishing a milieu where client will feel safe enough to examine source of anxiety and use of defense mechanisms.
   3. Assisting client to try out new healthier ways to handle anxiety.
D. Use of unhealthy defense mechanisms will be decreased and client's level of functioning will improve.

Implementation

A. Facilitate more appropriate use of defense mechanisms.

B. Remember that defense mechanisms serve a purpose and cannot be arbitrarily eliminated without being replaced.
C. Avoid criticizing client's behavior and use of adjustment mechanisms.
D. Help client explore the underlying source of the anxiety that gives rise to an unhealthy adjustment.
E. Assist the client in learning new or alternative adjustment patterns for healthier adaptation.
F. Use techniques to alleviate client's anxiety.
G. Use a firm supportive approach to explore any ineffective use of adjustment patterns.

Evaluation

A. Client's use of unhealthy defense mechanisms has decreased.
B. Nurse-client relationship has created a safe milieu, and client's anxiety level has decreased.
C. Client's level of functioning has improved.
D. Adjustment patterns have moved from unhealthy to a more healthy status.

ANXIETY DISORDERS

Definition: Anxiety disorders are those disorders in which the predominant disturbance is one of anxiety that is manifested as panic, generalized anxiety, phobias, or obsessive compulsive behavior.

Characteristics

A. Repression and projection are common defense mechanisms.
B. Patterns of behavior are used in a rather stereotyped way.
C. Client becomes more dependent as times goes on.
D. Client is almost always unaware of his or her behavior patterns.
E. The disorder that manifests is client's attempt to deal with anxiety.
F. Secondary gains become associated problems.
   1. Secondary gains are those social and psychological uses (fringe benefits) that the client may make of his or her symptoms.
   2. Client does not understand unconscious motivation.
   3. Secondary gains reinforce neurotic behavior.

G. Client has little difficulty talking, but conversation may be vague and unrevealing.

H. Low self-esteem is often observable in disorder.

I. Reality is not grossly distorted.

J. Personality is not grossly disorganized.

K. Attitude of martyrdom is common.

L. Client is highly amenable to suggestion.

Generalized Anxiety Disorder

Assessment

A. Client has diffuse persistent anxiety.

B. Client cannot control anxiety by defense mechanisms.

C. Psychological symptoms.
1. Lack of concentration on work.
2. Feelings of depression and guilt.
3. Harbored fear of sudden death or insanity.
4. Dread of being alone.
5. Confusion.
6. Rumination.
7. Agitation and restlessness—motor tension.
8. Impatience.

D. Physiological symptoms.
1. Tremors.
2. Dyspnea.
3. Palpitations.
4. Tachycardia.
5. Numbness of extremities.
6. Insomnia.

Planning and Analysis

A. Generalized anxiety level will be decreased.

B. Activities will be planned that reduce anxiety and increase self-esteem.

C. Sources of anxiety will be identified and explored.

D. Conscious awareness of anxiety will be developed, and measures to reduce it will be introduced.

E. Physiological symptoms that indicate presence of excessive anxiety will be eliminated.

F. More efficient coping mechanisms will be utilized by client.

G. Environment will be structured to decrease stimuli.

Implementation

A. Recognize behavior in client that denotes anxiety.

B. Maintain calm, serene approach because nurse's anxiety reinforces client's anxiety.

C. Help client to develop conscious awareness of anxiety.

D. Help client identify and describe feelings and source of anxiety.

E. Provide physical outlet for anxiety.

F. Remain with client.

G. Decrease environmental stimuli.

H. Avoid reinforcing secondary gains.

Evaluation

A. Interventions resulted in decrease in anxiety level as evidenced by changes in behavior.

B. Client learns to meet needs thus decreasing need for secondary gains.

C. Client's reliance on nurse is minimized.

D. Self-esteem is increased.

E. Environment supports client's efforts to change.

Phobic Disorders

Assessment

A. Fear is recognized by individual as excessive or unreasonable in proportion to reality.

B. There is a compelling desire to avoid subject or situation.

C. Client has unrealistic, irrational fear.

D. Client uses projection, displacement, repression, and sublimation.

E. Client transfers anxiety or fear from its source to a symbolic idea or situation.

F. Phobic disorders are classified into three types:
1. Agoraphobia—fear of being alone or in public places.
2. Social phobia—desire to avoid social situations in which individuals fear they will behave inappropriately.
3. Simple phobia—persistent or irrational fear other than the above.

Planning and Analysis

A. Fear and anxiety will be decreased so that client will be less fearful of object or situation.

B. Phobic behavior is gradually reduced and ultimately does not interfere with living experiences.

C. Client will utilize more effective coping mechanisms.

Implementation

A. Draw client's attention away from phobia.

B. Have client focus on awareness of self.

C. Do not force client into situation feared.

D. Slowly develop sound relationship with client.

E. Desensitize client to the phobia.

Evaluation

A. Client is less fearful of object or situation.

B. Client is desensitized to phobia.

C. Client's ability to participate in living experiences is increased.

Obsessive-Compulsive Disorder

Assessment

A. Client has anxiety associated with persistent, undesired ideas or thoughts that are experienced as senseless or repugnant.

B. Client releases anxiety through repetitive, stereotyped acts.

C. Personality characteristics.
   1. Insecure, guilt-ridden.
   2. Sensitive, shy.
   3. Straight-laced.
   4. Fussy and meticulous.

D. Client uses repression, isolation, and undoing to control anxiety.

E. Client is unable to control feelings of hostility and aggression.

F. Behavior interferes with social or role functioning.

G. Symptoms are distressing to client.

H. Most common obsessions are thoughts of violence, contaminations, and doubt.

I. Most common compulsions involve hand-washing, counting, checking, and touching.

Planning and Analysis

A. Obsessive thinking will be channeled into more appropriate acts.

B. Compulsive behavior will not interfere with activities of daily living.

C. More effective means of controlling anxiety will be developed by client.

D. Activities will be provided that will increase client's self-esteem.

Implementation

A. Avoid punishment or criticism.

B. Allow episodes of compulsive acts, setting limits only to prevent harmful acts.

C. Engage in alternative activities with client.

D. Limit decision-making for client.

E. Provide for client's physical needs.

F. Convey acceptance of client regardless of behavior.

G. Establish routine to avoid anxiety-producing changes.

H. Gear assignments to those which are routine and can be done with perfection such as straightening linen or cleaning.

I. Plan therapy, any change in routine or one-to-one contact after completion of a compulsive episode.

Evaluation

A. Client is able to focus more on activities of daily living than on compulsive acts.

B. Obsessive thoughts are decreased or eliminated.

C. Self-esteem is increased.

SOMATOFORM DISORDERS

Definition: Somatoform behaviors, also called psychosomatic disorders, are physical diseases that may involve any organ system, and whose etiologies are in part related to emotional factors.

Characteristics

A. An individual must adapt and adjust to stresses in life.
   1. The way a person adapts depends on the individual's characteristics.
   2. Emotional stress may exacerbate or precipitate an illness.

B. Psychosocial stress is an important factor in symptom formation.
   1. Stress imposes demands and requirements on the person.
   2. Symptoms reflect adaptive and coping patterns as well as the reaction of a particular organ system.
   3. The way an individual reacts to stress depends on his or her physiological and psychological make-up.

C. There is a synergistic relationship between repressed feelings and overexcited organs.

D. Any body system may be involved and result in a psychosomatic disorder.

E. Structural changes may take place and pose a life-threatening situation.

F. Defense mechanisms used include repression, denial, projection, conversion, and introjection.
G. Psychosomatic illness provides individual with coping mechanisms.
   1. Means of coping with anxiety and stress.
   2. Means of gaining attention in socially acceptable way.
   3. Means of adjusting to dependency needs.
   4. Means of coping with anger and aggression.
   5. Rationalization for failures.
   6. Means of punishing self and others.

Psychosomatic Disorders

Assessment

A. Assess which body system is involved that resulted in somatoform disorder.
   1. Gastrointestinal system.
      a. Peptic ulcer.
      b. Colic.
      c. Ulcerative colitis.
   2. Cardiovascular system.
      a. Hypertension.
      b. Tachycardia.
      c. Migraine headaches.
   3. Respiratory system.
      a. Asthma.
      b. Hay fever.
      c. Hiccoughs.
      d. Common cold.
      e. Hyperventilation.
   4. Skin—most expressive organ of emotion.
      a. Blushing.
      b. Flushing, perspiring.
      c. Dermatitis.
   5. Nervous system.
      a. Chronic general fatigue.
      b. Exhaustion.
   6. Endocrine.
      a. Dysmenorrhea.
      b. Hyperthyroidism.
   7. Musculoskeletal system.
      a. Cramps.
      b. Rheumatoid arthritis.
   8. Other.
      a. Diabetes mellitus.
      b. Obesity.
      c. Sexual dysfunctions.
      d. Hyperemesis gravidarum.
      e. Accident proneness.
B. Evaluate history for physical symptoms of several years' duration.
C. Observe closely and assess client's present condition.
   1. Collect data about physical illness—symptoms (multiple sources).
   2. Psychosocial adjustment.
   3. Life situation.
   4. Coping mechanisms that work for client.
   5. Strengths of client.
   6. Problem-solving ability.
D. Note if symptoms come and go.
E. Assess what kinds of things aggravate or relieve symptom.

Planning and Analysis

A. Origin of disorder will be identified readily so total treatment plan can be implemented.
B. Client will receive rest, and reduced stress will begin to alleviate symptoms.
C. Nurse-client relationship will facilitate change in behavior patterns.
D. Client will learn new alternative methods of handling anxiety-stress rather than somatizing.
   1. Verbalizing angry or frustrated feelings.
   2. Physical outlets for negative energy.
E. Holistic approaches to disorder will result in more healthy client behaviors.

Implementation

A. Provide restful, supportive environment.
   1. Balance therapy and recreation.
   2. Decrease stimuli.
   3. Provide activities that deemphasize the client's physical symptoms.
B. Care for the "total" person—physical and emotional.
C. Realize physical symptoms are real and that person is not faking.
D. Recognize that treatment of physical problems does not relieve emotional problems.
E. Reduce demands on client.
F. Develop nurse-client relationship.
   1. Respect the person and the person's problems.
   2. Help client to express his or her feelings.
   3. Help client to express anxiety and explore new coping mechanisms.

4. Allow client to meet dependency needs.
5. Allow client to feel in control.

G. Help client to work through problems and learn new methods of responding to stress.

Evaluation

A. Relief or decrease of physical symptoms has occurred by decreasing anxiety level.
B. Client identified stressors related to physical illness.
C. Client developed alternative coping mechanisms.
   1. Client verbalized feelings of anger, frustration, and resentment.
   2. Client channelled negative energy into positive outlets (i.e., verbalization exercise, relaxation methods).
D. Client follows medical regimen to minimize physical symptoms.

Conversion Disorder

Assessment

A. Establish psychosomatic origin by assessing physical condition and any organic basis for symptoms; i.e., neurological examinations, laboratory tests.
B. Identify conversion behavior/symptoms.
C. Evaluate client's attitude toward condition: "La belle indifference."
D. Identify primary gain.
   1. Keeps internal conflict or need out of awareness (repression).
   2. Symptom has symbolic value to client.
E. Identify secondary gain.
   1. Provides additional advantages such as avoidance, attention, or sympathy.
   2. Reinforces maladjusted behavior.
F. Assess whether symptoms disappear under hypnosis.

Planning and Analysis

A. Psychosomatic origin will be identified early so secondary gains are not reinforced by staff.
B. Anxiety level will be decreased.
C. Nurse-client relationship will not feed into secondary gains.
   1. Client will learn to function with symptom (disorder).
   2. Client will not become dependent on staff.

D. Client will learn new, alternative methods to handle stress or conflict rather than converting psychological pressure to a body symptom.

Implementation

A. Establish nurse-client relationship.
B. Reduce pressure on client.
C. Control environment.
D. Provide recreational and social activities.
E. Do not confront client with his or her illness.
F. Divert client's attention from symptom.
G. Do not feed into secondary gains through anticipating client needs.

Evaluation

A. Anxiety level is decreased.
B. Symptoms have been eliminated, and conflict is in client's awareness.
C. Client has developed alternative means to handling conflict and needs.
D. Need for secondary gains is decreased.
E. Client is more able to gain gratification from social situations.

Hypochondriasis

Assessment

A. Evaluate severe, morbid preoccupation with body functions or fear of serious disease.
B. Assess whether client shows lack of interest in environment.
C. Assess whether client shows severe regression.
D. Determine if client goes from doctor to doctor to find cure or enjoys recounting medical history.

Planning and Analysis

A. Client will learn to live with some organic discomfort or symptoms without becoming emotionally maladaptive.
B. Client will not focus all of his or her energy, attention, and awareness on physical functions.
C. Client will find new interests and gain satisfaction from them.
D. Client will develop more self-acceptance.
E. Client will not become so self-absorbed that client loses contact with reality.

Implementation

A. Accept client; recognize and understand that complaints are not conscious.

B. Provide diversionary activities in which client can succeed to build self-esteem.

C. Use friendly, supportive approach but do not focus on physical condition; i.e., avoid using "How are you today."

D. Help client to refocus interest.

E. Provide for client's physical needs; give correct information and correct any misinformation.

F. Assist client to understand how he or she uses illness to avoid dealing with life's problems.

G. Be aware of staff's negativity as it may lead to exacerbation of client's symptoms.

Evaluation

A. Anxiety level is decreased.

B. Hypochondriacal behavior no longer dominates client's existence.

C. Client gains more satisfaction from interests outside of self.

D. Client experiences increased self-esteem and is able to give up secondary gains from disorder.

EATING DISORDERS

Anorexia Nervosa

Definition: A syndrome of self-starvation with underlying emotional disturbance. The psychological aversion to food results in emaciation and physical problems.

Characteristics

A. Almost exclusively female (1 in 100 are males).

B. Most common in adolescent girls and young adults.

C. Often unnoticed in early stages; female "goes on diet to lose weight."

D. Dynamics of disorder.

1. History of a "model child." Becomes negative due to power struggles with family over pressure to eat.

2. Intense fear of obesity leads anorectic to report feeling fat.

3. Not a disturbance in appetite but distorted body image perceptions: related to disturbance in sense of self, identity, and autonomy.

4. Hormones altered—are they cause or effect of disorder?

5. Anorectics do not want treatment. Potentially lethal disease: mortality 15-20 percent.

6. Many anorectics have a single episode, then recover. Factors associated with positive prognosis include: onset of problem before age 15 and weight gain within two years.

Assessment

A. Assess weight: profound weight loss of 25 percent occurs with this disorder (old method of diagnosis).

B. New diagnostic criteria is no period for three months.

C. Assess for physical symptoms.

1. Malnutrition.

2. Fractures—calcium leached from bones.

3. Teeth enamel eroded and poor gums.

4. Hypotension.

5. Anemia.

6. Hypoproteinemia.

D. Monitor for potential complications.

1. Severe electrolyte imbalance (decreased K, kidney failure).

2. Heart failure and coma.

Implementation

A. Actions to improve nutritional status (to stabilize medical condition).

1. Diet.

a. High protein, high carbohydrate, especially amino acids.

b. Identify foods client prefers.

c. Small nutritious, attractive feedings.

2. Nasogastric feedings: if client refuses to eat, administer tube feedings as ordered.

B. Psychological care.

1. Care plan.

a. Formulate plan that all staff agree on. Do not allow manipulation. Do not engage in power struggle.

b. Do not focus on food, taste, recipes, etc.

c. Remain with client when eating or monitor when client eats with others.

d. Do not accept excuses to leave eating area (to vomit).

e. Set limits on amount client must eat. Reward when client adheres to plan.

f. Ensure that weight is taken same time every day with client dressed in only a hospital gown.

2. Therapy.
   a. Medications.
      (1) Antidepressants—cure lack of caring.
      (2) Antihistamins—cure hyperactivity.
   b. Focused on behavior therapy.
      (1) Set limits with positive and negative reinforcement.
      (2) Establish contract that specifies weight-gain privileges, restrictions.
   c. Insight-oriented therapy: correcting client's body perceptions and misconceptions about feelings, needs, self-worth, autonomy.
   d. Family therapy important focus as issues of control and autonomy connected to eating.

Bulimia

Definition: Eating disorder that involves binge eating, frequently followed by self-induced vomiting.

Characteristics

A. Etiology is unknown but this disorder is often accompanied by an underlying psychopathology.
B. More common in women than men.
C. Begins in adolescence or early adulthood and often follows a chronic course over many years.
D. Generally aware that eating patterns are abnormal (in contrast to anorectics).
E. Typically evidences impaired impulse control, low self-esteem, and depression.

Assessment

A. Assess degree of disruption in life caused by eating disorder.
B. Assess degree of depression: often due to guilt over eating binges. (New studies suggest link between bulimia and affective disorder.)
C. Assess weight fluctuation and potential danger of weight loss.

Implementation

A. Client is usually not hospitalized but does require therapy.
B. Behavior-modification and insight-oriented therapy used with limited success.
C. Care plan is similar to anorexia nervosa with focus on interrupting binge/purge cycle and altering attitudes toward food and self.

DISSOCIATIVE DISORDERS

Definition: This disorder is a sudden temporary alteration in the integrative functions of consciousness, identity, or motor behavior.

Characteristics

A. Client attempts to deal with anxiety through various disturbances or by walling off certain areas of the mind from consciousness.
B. Client remains in contact with reality.
C. Repression is used.
D. Manifestations.
   1. Amnesia: circumscribed, selective, generalized and continuous.
   2. Fugue or physical flight.
   3. Multiple personality.
   4. Depersonalization.

Assessment

A. Determine that symptoms are not of organic origin.
B. Assess what form the dissociative disorder is manifesting.
C. Evaluate degree of interference in lifestyle and interpersonal relationships.
D. Assess presence of accompanying symptoms such as depression, suicide ideation, etc.

Planning and Analysis

A. Client will return to state of integration and adaptive level of functioning.
B. Client will find alternative means of dealing with internal conflicts.
C. Client will experience increased self-esteem.

Implementation

A. Support therapeutic modality as established by treatment team.
B. Reduce anxiety-producing stimuli.
C. Redirect client's attention away from self.
D. Avoid sympathizing with client.
E. Increase socialization activities.

Evaluation

A. Condition has been recognized and evaluated, and appropriate intervention has been made.

B. If client is hospitalized, nurse-client relationship has created a safe environment for client to begin process of integration.

C. Client's self-esteem is enhanced.

PERSONALITY DISORDERS

Definition: A disorder in which individual does not adjust to life—exhibits behavioral problems, not symptoms.

Characteristics

A. Cannot adjust to demands of life situations.

B. Experiences inadequate interactions with society and individuals.
 1. Difficulty in forming loving and lasting interpersonal relationships.
 2. Difficulty with authority, laws and rules.

C. Assets are social skills—intelligence, charm and manipulation.

D. Experiences low tolerance for anxiety—will go to great lengths to avoid increased intellectual and emotional demands that raise anxiety.

E. Primary characteristic is manipulation—influencing others or events to meet own needs without regard for others' needs.

ASSESSMENT

Personality disorder types	Assess for specific profile Characteristics
A. Paranoid personality	1. Pervasive, unwarranted suspiciousness, and mistrust of people 2. Guarded, secretive, devious, and scheming 3. Puts blame on others for problems 4. Argumentative and exaggerates difficulties 5. Affectively restricted and cold 6. Lacks soft, sentimental, or tender feelings
B. Schizoid personality	1. Lack of social relationships 2. No warmth or tender feelings toward others—appears cold and aloof 3. Prefers to be alone and has few friends 4. Appears reserved, withdrawn, and seclusive 5. Flat affect—humorless and dull
C. Histrionic personality	1. Overly reactive, dramatic and intense 2. Disruptive relationships with others 3. Seeks attention and tends to exaggerate 4. May exhibit angry outbursts or tantrums 5. Immature, self-centered and dependent 6. Seductive and flirty with others
D. Narcissistic personality	1. Grandiose sense of self-importance 2. Preoccupation with fantasies of power, beauty, etc. 3. Exhibitionistic, with indifference or rage in response to criticism 4. Lack of empathy and exploits others
E. Borderline personality	1. Impulsiveness that is self-damaging, e.g., gambling, sex, spending, etc. 2. Pattern of unstable relationships 3. Explosive temper, affective lability, suicide gestures and acts of self-mutilation 4. Lack of self-identity 5. Chronic feeling of boredom and emptiness
F. Dependent personality	1. Passive, little sense of self-responsibility 2. Low self-esteem

Personality disorder types	Assess for specific profile Characteristics
	3. Sees self as stupid and helpless
	4. Dependent on others to meet needs
G. Compulsive personality	1. Restricted ability to express warmth toward others—cold, rigid
	2. Perfectionistic preoccupation with rules, orders, etc. Inflexible and stubborn
	3. Excessive devotion to work
	4. Indecisiveness but often high achiever
H. Passive-aggressive personality	1. Resists demands for adequate performance in job and relationships
	2. Procrastinates, dawdles and forgets
	3. Evidences intentional inefficiency
I. Antisocial personality	1. Intelligent, charming and self-centered, "con artist"
	2. Inability to feel guilt or learn from past experience
	3. Repeated lying and cheating, steals—diagnosis common in prisons
	4. Emotionally immature—lack of impulse control and low frustration tolerance
	5. Manipulation of others to fulfill wants and needs
	6. Resists authority, rules and laws
	7. Impulsive, lacks judgment
	8. Excessive use of drugs, alcohol, and sex
	9. Uses rationalization to justify behavior

Implementation

A. Recognize characteristics of manipulative behavior.
   1. Uses bargains, threats, demands or intimidation to get own way.
   2. Shows ability to identify and use other people's weaknesses for own benefit.
   3. Makes continuous, unrealistic demands.
   4. Pits one individual against one another, e.g., clients against staff.
   5. Pretends to be helpless and sorry for behavior.
   6. Lies to gain sympathy of staff or other clients.
   7. Acts out even when given acceptable behavioral alternatives.
   8. Keeps all relationships on a superficial level.
   9. Uses flattery, charm and excessive compliments to get needs met.
   10. Exploits the generosity of others.
   11. Identifies with staff or authority figure and acts as if he is not incarcerated.
   12. Finds a way around the unit rules and expectations.
   13. Uses sexuality to gain control over others. May approach the staff sexually too.
B. Interventions for manipulative behavior.
   1. Set clear and realistic limits. Be consistent and firm in setting behavioral expectations and limits.
   2. Confront client with his manipulative behavior. Do not try to outmanipulate—client is a master at it.
   3. Reinforce adaptive behavior through positive feedback and realistic praise.
   4. Do not be influenced by client's charming ways—all directed toward manipulating you.
   5. Do not be intimidated by client's behavior.
   6. Clearly and consistently communicate care plans and client's behavior to other staff. Present a united front.
   7. Accept no flattery, gifts or favors.
C. Form a therapeutic nurse-client relationship in which positive behavior is reinforced.

AFFECTIVE DISORDERS

Bipolar Disorders

Manic-Depressive Illness—Manic Episode

Definition: One manifestation of an affective disorder that involves mood swings of elation, euphoria, and grandiose behavior with or without a history of depression. Cyclothymic disorder is the second category of bipolar disorder and refers to a milder form of the same illness.

Characteristics

A. Specific etiology is unknown. May be related to a genetic predisposition to illness or to increased levels of dopamine in the brain. Attempts are now being made to discover why lithium is therapeutic in hopes of solving the mystery of manic illness.

B. Women experience this illness slightly more frequently than men. The lifetime risk of developing this illness is 1–2 percent of the population.

C. The first manic episode usually occurs before age 30 and, interestingly, is more common in the higher socio-economic group.

Assessment

A. Assess which stage of mania client is experiencing.

1. Mild elation: difficult to detect as it may not progress. Persons are often referred to as "hypomanics."

   a. Affect: feelings of happiness, freedom from worry, confidence, and noninhibition.

   b. Thought: rapid association of ideas but with little evidence of introspection.

   c. Behavior: increased motor activity (person always on the go); and increased sexual drives, with superficial relationship.

2. Acute manic episode: symptoms more intensified and observable. Client usually requires hospitalization.

   a. Mood disturbance and lability: mood is one of excessive euphoria. Expansive toward others, enthusiastic and intrusive. Mood may change to one of irritability, annoyance, and even rage and violence. Mood swings may last for hours or days.

   b. Hyperactivity: motor restlessness and overindulgence in recreational, sexual, and other activities. Engages in sexual indiscretions and poor money management. Client uses poor judgment in planning and starting projects and is over-optimistic and unrealistic. Evidences disturbed sleep patterns, often going without sleep for days.

   c. Flight of ideas and pressured speech: manic clients jump from one idea to another, using puns, jokes, and nuances in a continuous flow of loose and accelerated speech. Often, speech is loud, rapid, and appears to be pressured.

   d. Distractability: manic clients overly respond to environmental stimuli, switching focus rapidly from one stimulus to another.

   e. Distortion of self-esteem; grandiose perceptions of one's importance is common with an inflated self-esteem. Often this characteristic is manifested in delusions of grandeur (special relationship with God or the president).

3. Delirium: state of extreme excitement. Person is disoriented, incoherent, agitated, and frenetic.

   a. May experience visual or olfactory hallucinations.

   b. Exhaustion, dehydration, injury, and death are real dangers and must be prevented by the nurse.

B. Determine if client requires hospitalization (depends on range of symptoms).

C. Assess physical health.

1. Poor sleep habits and no apparent fatigue.

2. Poor nutrition.

3. Poor or even bizarre habits of grooming.

Planning and Analysis

A. Safe environment will be established to protect from self-injury (limits set).

B. Euphoric behavior will be reduced to within normal limits.

C. A trusting nurse-client relationship will be established.

D. Expression of feelings of depression, guilt, and hostility, which underlie euphoria, will be encouraged.

E. Physical health will be maintained to prevent further complications.

Implementation

A. Maintain a safe environment.

1. Reduce external stimuli: noise, people, and motion.

2. Avoid competitive activities. (Mild exercise, group singing, and swimming are examples of therapeutic activities.)

3. Redirect energy into short, useful activities.

B. Establish a nurse-client relationship.

1. Maintain accepting, nonjudgmental attitude and create conditions where trust can develop in the relationship.

2. Avoid entering into client's playful, joking activity.
3. Allow client to verbalize feelings, especially hostility.
C. Set realistic limits on behavior.
   1. Provide scope and limitations to behavior for a sense of security.
   2. Anticipate destructive behavior and set limits.
   3. Be firm and consistent.
   4. Involve client in setting own limits.
      a. Gives client sense of control.
      b. Client fears inability to control own behavior.
D. Give attention to physical needs.
   1. Provide a high calorie diet with vitamin.
   2. Ensure adequate rest and sleep.
E. Limit decision-making during acute phase.

Evaluation

A. Determine if client's manic behavior has diminished.
   1. Rate of talk (flight of ideas) has slowed down.
   2. Motor activity is decreased.
   3. Concentration is increased.
   4. Sexual indiscretions are diminished.
   5. Delusions are absent.
B. Dress has become more normalized, less bizarre and outlandish.
C. Client is able to set own limits.
D. Physical needs of client are met.
   1. Sleep pattern is normalized.
   2. Client's ability to sit and eat is normal.
E. Client is able to express feelings verbally.

Unipolar Disorders

Definition: Another manifestation of affective disorder; symptoms range from a disphonic, down mood that is mild and only slightly debilitating to a pathological condition of overwhelming intensity and long duration. This disorder may be chronic or episodic but it involves no episodes of elation.

Characteristics

A. The most common of all psychiatric illnesses, depression is a symptom probably experienced by 15 out of 100 adults in our society.

B. One cause is now thought to involve a genetic link; other possible causes are personality traits such as low self-esteem, neuro-chemical imbalances, and other biological factors.
C. Most acute depressive episodes are self-limiting and last from a few weeks (with treatment) to a few months.
D. More than half of those persons who experience a first episode go on to suffer a recurrence.
E. About 20–25 percent never return to their premorbid state of mental health.

Major Depressive Episode

A. General characteristics.
   1. Symptoms of a major depressive episode usually develop over a period of days to weeks.
   2. Episode may begin at any age and is twice as common in women.
   3. The clinical picture of depression varies considerably with no single symptom present in all clinical profiles.
B. Affective symptoms.
   1. Distinguished from grief reactions: normal, self-limited reactions to obvious loss is labeled grief. Grief reactions are usually brief and milder than pathological depression.
   2. Majority of depressed people experience prolonged periods of sadness, feeling down, gloomy, or unhappy. This depressed mood tends to color the whole of a person's life; it is pervasive and dominant.
   3. Loss of motivation: loss of interest in life and activities, feelings of hopelessness and helplessness, and suicidal thoughts.
      a. This is the most serious complication.
      b. One percent kill themselves within one year. In recurrent depression, 15 percent eventually commit suicide.
      c. The highest risk is the 6–9 month period after some improvement.
   4. Vegetative behavior: related to physical problems, these include loss of energy, loss of libido, psychomotor retardation, or agitation. Individual experiences sleep problems (insomnia is more common) and appetite disturbance, usually anorexia.
   5. Cognitive problems: persistent low self-esteem is present, difficulty in concentrating, poor memory, and apparent occupation with inner thoughts. A pervasive sense of guilt and worthlessness is also present.

6. Physical complaints: a series of bodily complaints often accompany this illness ranging from headaches and backaches to constipation and chest pain.

Major Depressive Episode Subtypes

A. Depression with melancholia.
   1. Predisposing factors appear to be dissatisfaction with accomplishments in life and loss of pleasure in the usual activities.
   2. Emphasis is on the vegetative signs and variation in mood (often called involutional melancholia).
   3. Common symptoms that accompany this disorder are a general depressed mood that is worse in the morning, psychomotor retardation, or agitation and anorexia which may result in weight loss.
B. Depression with psychotic symptoms.
   1. This subtype of depression is accompanied by an inability to test reality: delusions, hallucinations, and confusion.
      a. May also have severe impairment of personal and social functioning.
      b. May be severely withdrawn.
   2. Approximately 10 percent of those depressed have psychotic symptoms.
   3. Psychotic depressions are considered to be biologically based.

Table 1. AFFECTIVE ILLNESS

Depression Type	Distinguishing Feature
Bipolar Manic-depressive disorder Cyclothymic disorder	History of elation episodes with or without depression
Unipolar Major depressive disorder Depression with melancholia Depression with psychotic features Dysthymic disorder	History of depression without any history of elation

Dysthymic Disorder (Depressive Neurosis)

A. Symptoms of depression fluctuate and are less severe than with the major depressive disorder.
   1. Mild symptoms are present for at least two years.
   2. Depression may be episodic or constant.
B. Psychosis is not present.
C. Several of the following symptoms are usually present with this diagnosis.
   1. Low energy level.
   2. Loss of interest in pleasurable activities.
   3. Pessimistic attitude toward the future; thoughts of suicide.
   4. Tearful, crying demeanor.
   5. Feelings of low self-esteem.
   6. Decreased ability to concentrate.

Assessment

A. Assess mood level (affect is sad, gloomy, or unhappy), and establish diagnosis of depression.
B. Evaluate behavior (slowed actions, diminished purposeful movement, and neglect of personal appearance).
C. Assess thought processes (slowed down until there is a paucity of thinking).
D. Evaluate attitudes (pessimistic and self-denigrating; focus is on the problems and uselessness of life).
E. Assess physical symptoms:
   1. Usually a preoccupation with body and poor health.
   2. Weight loss.
   3. Insomnia.
   4. General malaise.
F. Determine social interaction patterns, which are reduced and inappropriate.
   1. Feelings of isolation.
   2. No contribution to interpersonal relationships.
G. Evaluate potential for suicide.

Planning and Analysis

A. Differential diagnosis will establish diagnosis of depression.
B. Client will be protected from self-injury by providing him or her a safe environment.
C. Client will achieve a more realistic and positive concept of him or herself so that feelings of self-esteem are enhanced.

D. Climate will be established where client may express feelings of anger and aggression outwardly rather than inwardly.

E. Physical needs will be met so that condition will not further deteriorate.

F. Client will be mobilized to prevent deeper depression.

Implementation

A. Provide a safe milieu and protect the client from self-injury (prevent suicide).

B. Provide a structured environment to mobilize the client.
 1. Allow time for daily activities.
 2. Stimulate recreational activity.
 3. Reactivate interests outside of the client's concerns.
 4. Motivate client for treatment.
 5. Introduce psychotherapy and occupational therapy.

C. Build trust through a one-to-one relationship.
 1. Employ a supportive, unchallenging approach.
 2. Use accepting, nonjudgmental attitude and behavior.
 3. Show interest; listen and give positive reinforcement.
 4. Redirect the client's monologue away from painful, depressing thoughts.
 5. Focus on the client's underlying anger and encourage expression of it.

D. Build the client's ego assets to increase his or her self-esteem.
 1. Lower standards to create successful experiences.
 2. Limit decision-making with the severely depressed.
 3. Support use of defenses to alleviate suffering.

E. Be attentive to the client's physical needs: provide adequate nutrition, sleep, and exercise.

Evaluation

A. Safe milieu was provided, and attempts at self-injury were prevented.

B. Structured plan of care assisted client to mobilize actions.

C. Nurse-client relationship was established and trust developed.

D. Client is more positive and realistic.

E. Client displays behavior that indicates increase in self-esteem.

Suicide

Definition: Suicide is an act or instance of intentionally killing oneself.

Characteristics

A. Suicide is the seventh most common cause of death for all ages in the United States today and the second cause of death among college students.

B. Suicide statistics are probably low because of unknown cases such as car accidents.
 1. Suicide ranks fourth as the cause of death in the fifteen to forty age group.
 2. For every successful suicide, it is believed that there are five to ten attempted suicides.
 3. Women make more suicide attempts than men. Four times as many men as women actually commit suicide.
 4. Suicide is increasing in the adolescent and elderly age group.

C. Factors that contribute to suicide attempts.
 1. The single most common cause is depression; alcohol is the second most common cause.
 2. Another common cause is that individuals feel overwhelmed by problems in living.
 3. A final cause may be the attempt to control others.

D. Depressed clients, when severely ill, rarely commit suicide.
 1. They do not have the drive and energy to make a plan and follow it through when severely depressed.
 2. Danger period occurs when depression begins to lift.

E. Eight out of ten known cases give warnings or messages through direct or indirect means.

F. Accompanying symptoms range from depression, disorientation, and defiance to intense dependence on another.

Assessment

A. Recognize level of depression and potential for suicide (when depression begins to lift).

B. Determine presence of suicide ideation.

C. Observe behavior closely as clues to potential suicide.

D. Listen to verbalization to determine what is meaningful for client.

E. Observe physical status so you can intervene if necessary (if client is not eating, sleeping, etc.)

F. Recognize ambivalence when client is considering suicide.

Planning and Analysis

A. Suicide attempt will be prevented by adequate assessment of suicide potential.
B. A viable nurse-client relationship is established to negate feelings of alienation, loneliness, non-acceptance, and self-denigration.
C. Good physical status is maintained.
D. A more realistic positive concept of self is enhanced.
E. Alternative means of handling feelings have been developed and these are more adaptive.

Implementation

A. Provide a safe environment to protect client from self-destruction.
B. Observe client closely at all times, especially when depression is lifting.
C. Establish a supportive relationship, letting client know you are concerned for his or her welfare.
D. Encourage expression of feelings, especially anger.
E. Ask relevant questions that relate to potential suicide ideation (ideas): "Do you wish you were dead?" "Did you think you might do something about it?" "What?" "Have you taken any steps to prepare?" "What are they?"
F. It is important to recognize a continued desire to commit suicide.
G. Focus on client's strengths and successful experiences to increase client's self-esteem.
H. Provide a structured schedule and involve client in activities with others.
I. Structure a plan for client to use as a means of coping when next confronted with suicide ideation.
J. Help client plan for continued professional support after discharge.

Evaluation

A. Potential suicide attempt has been recognized and intervention taken.
B. Suicide has been prevented.
C. Nurse-client relationship has provided groundwork for change in client's self-esteem, feelings of alienation, hopelessness, and loneliness.
D. Client has developed more adaptive alternatives to handling feelings.

E. Posthospitalization plans have been formulated and implemented.

SUBSTANCE ABUSE

Definition: Substance abuse includes any process by which an individual ingests any mind-altering, non-prescribed chemical that produces physiological and/or psychological dependence. Withdrawal symptoms are usually manifest when substance is not taken.

Characteristics

A. Psychological dependence: emotional dependence, desire, or compulsion to continue taking the substance or drug.
B. Tolerance: the gradual increase of the amount required to obtain the desired effect.
C. Physical dependence: physical need for the substance manifested by appearance of withdrawal symptoms when substance is withheld.

Alcoholism

Definition: The abuse of any alcoholic substance combined with physical and psychological addiction.

Characteristics

A. Alcohol consumption is permitted by law and supported by most people in our society as a recreational activity.
B. A fine line exists between the social drinker and the addicted or problem drinker.
C. The greatest difference involves the degree of compulsion to drink and the inability to survive the trials of everyday living without the ingestion of alcohol.
D. Alcoholism, the third largest health problem in the United States (heart disease and cancer rank first and second), affects 10 million people.
E. Alcoholism is involved in about 30,000 deaths and one-half million injuries (auto accidents) every year.
F. Alcoholism decreases life span 10 to 12 years.
G. Loss to industry caused by alcoholism is estimated at 15 billion dollars a year (affecting primarily the 35 to 55 age group).
H. Major U.S. social concern is the dramatic rise in teenage alcoholism, (estimated to affect 3 million adolescents).

Dynamics of Alcoholism

A. Alcoholic disease implies the consumption of alcohol to the point where it interferes with the individual's physical, emotional, and social functioning.
　1. The syndrome consists of two phases: problem drinking and alcohol addiction.
　2. Dependence on other drugs is very common.
B. No hereditary or organic basis for alcoholism has been proven to date.
C. Alcohol blocks synaptic transmission, depresses the central nervous system (CNS), and releases inhibitions. It acts initially as a stimulant but is actually a depressant.
　1. Chronic excessive use can lead to brain damage (sedative effect on CNS).
　2. High blood levels may cause malfunctions in cardiovascular and respiratory systems.
D. Blood level of 0.10% or more of alcohol is considered the level of intoxication.
E. Psychological effects of alcohol appear to be the gratification of oral impulses and the reduction of superego forces; abuse leads to shame and guilt and impaired ego function.
F. Alcohol may be said to be a defense against anxiety; therefore, the client needs to work on problems causing his or her anxiety.
G. Illnesses associated with alcoholism.
　1. Korsakoff's syndrome.
　2. Delirium tremens.
　3. Chronic gastritis.
　4. Poor nutritional intake resulting in beriberi, pellagra, cerebellar degeneration, and anemia.
　5. Laënnec's cirrhosis and hepatitis.
　6. Peripheral neuropathy.
　7. Osteoporosis.
　8. Individual is prone to infection.

Personality Characteristics of an Alcoholic

A. Dependent personality with resentment toward authority.
B. High self-expectations and low frustration tolerance.
C. Life usually characterized by patterns of failure.
D. False sense of success, power, and confidence from use of alcohol.
E. Apparent need to ease suffering, reduce anxiety, and cope with life stresses through use of alcohol.
F. Decreased ability to function intellectually, emotionally, and socially as need for alcohol increases.

G. Difficulty in interpersonal relationships.
H. Tendency to work, play, and engage in sex more than is normal.

Assessment

A. Assess inability to control alcohol consumption.
　1. Episodic drinking.
　2. Continuous excessive drinking.
　3. Sneaking drinks.
　4. Morning drinking.
　5. Blackouts.
　6. Arguments about drinking.
　7. Absence at work or school due to hangovers and drinking episodes.
　8. Difficulty with interpersonal relationships due to drinking habits.
　9. Alcohol related police record.
B. Recognize physical condition due to improper nutrition.
　1. Cirrhosis.
　2. Anemia.
　3. Peripheral neuropathy.
　4. Brain damage.
　5. Delirium tremens.
C. Evaluate accidents or physical injuries caused by intoxication.
D. Determine level of acute intoxication.
　1. Drowsiness, ataxia, nystagmus.
　2. Respiratory depression, stupor, possible coma, and death.
E. Assess alcohol withdrawal symptoms.
　1. Nausea.
　2. Insomnia.
　3. Anorexia.
　4. Anxiety.
　5. Hyperalertness.
　6. Restlessness.
　7. Delirium tremens: an acute condition usually manifested within 24 to 72 hours after the last ingestion of alcohol. May appear 7 to 10 days later during drinking periods when no food is ingested.
　　a. Marked tremors.
　　b. Hallucinations.
　　c. Paranoia.
　　d. Disorientation.
　　e. Tachycardia.
　　f. Tachypnea.
　　g. Diaphoresis.
　　h. Diarrhea.

i. Convulsions (grand mal).

j. Death (10 to 15 percent from cardiac failure).

Planning and Analysis

1. Self-destructiveness will be decreased.
2. Physical condition of client will improve.
3. Acute phase of detoxification will be closely monitored and complications prevented.
4. The environment will be conducive to client's realization of problem.
5. Rest and sleep will be promoted.
6. Client will be observed for impending delirium tremens.
7. Client's coping mechanisms will be increased.
8. Interventions will include medical, behavioral, social, and psychological aid.
9. Client's social recovery will be promoted.
10. Client will accept that he or she is an alcoholic and realize they will never be able to drink again.
11. Client will be assisted to restructure patterns of daily living.
12. Client will be assisted to increase his or her self-esteem and self-confidence.
13. The family will be assisted to focus on the needs and dynamics of the family unit.

Implementation

A. Nursing attitudes.
   1. Maintain a nonjudgmental attitude toward the alcoholic.
   2. Be firm and consistent in approach.
   3. Be accepting toward the individual, not his or her deviant behavior.
   4. Be supportive of attempts to change life patterns.
B. Acute treatment phase.
   1. Provide adequate diet and fluid intake.
   2. Provide vitamin therapy, especially vitamin B_6 and B complex.
   3. Administer some type of tranquilizers as ordered, usually Valium.
   4. Institute measures to control nausea and insomnia.
   5. Observe signs of infection or physiological problems.
   6. Promote rest.
   7. Control environment to decrease stimuli.
   8. Observe vital signs.

C. Long-term treatment phase.
   1. Set up a controlled and structured environment until client is able to manage his or her own circumstances.
      a. Set behavior limits and confront the client who is manipulative.
      b. Suggest group involvement for the client who experiences loneliness.
      c. Remember that client needs support, firmness, and a reality-oriented approach.
   2. Treatment techniques.
      a. Client must first go through detoxification—intensive care to avoid the toxic state and to return to a nonalcoholic state.
      b. Help client accept the fact that alcoholism is an illness.
      c. Help client accept that life must be managed without the support of alcohol.
      d. Provide psychotherapy techniques such as group and family therapy and nurse-client relationship therapy.
         (1) Focus on the underlying emotional problems.
         (2) Offer assistance in handling anxiety.
         (3) Focus on relieving feelings of inferiority and low self-esteem.
      e. Provide for rehabilitation or long-term supportive care.
         (1) Have client continue psychotherapy on an out-client basis.
         (2) Refer client to Alcoholics Anonymous.
         (3) Encourage client to continue taking prescribed medication such as Antabuse (alcohol-sensitizing drug that causes vomiting and cardiovascular symptoms if the person drinks alcohol).
         (4) Suggest social or vocational rehabilitation community programs that are available.

Evaluation

A. Individuals will evidence an increasing ability to behave in a self-constructive manner.
B. Client's coping mechanisms have increased.
C. Client shows interest in participating in therapies offered.
D. Client's physical condition has stabilized at optimal level within physical limitations.
E. Client evidences reduced social isolation.
F. Client's self-esteem has improved.

Drug Addiction

Definition: Drug addiction is state of dependency on drugs other than alcohol or tobacco that involve alteration of perception or mood and is produced by repeated consumption of drug.

Generalized personality characteristics

A. Difficulty forming intimate relationships.
B. Feelings of insecurity and inadequacy.
C. Rebellious toward authority.
D. Self-centered.
E. Copes through escapism.
F. Difficulty with sexuality and sexual identification.

Specific drug addictions

A. Narcotic addiction.
  1. The most common types of narcotics are heroin and morphine.
  2. Emotional dependence on the drug (to alter mood) occurs first, followed by physical dependence on the drug.
  3. Narcotics have a sedative effect on the CNS.
  4. Tolerance level increases, so greater amounts of the drug are necessary to produce pleasurable effects.
  5. Addiction tends to be chronic, with a high rate of relapse.
  6. Withdrawal symptoms.
     a. Anxiety.
     b. Nausea and vomiting.
     c. Sneezing, yawning, and watery eyes.
     d. Tremor and profuse perspiration.
     e. Stomach cramps and dehydration.
     f. Convulsions and coma.
B. Sedative hypnotics addiction.
  1. Common drugs include Librium, Valium, Quaalude, Equanil, Miltown, Seconal, Nembutal, and Sodium Amytal.
  2. Barbiturates have CNS sedative effect—danger of death from overdose and withdrawal.
  3. Psychological dependence occurs, followed by tolerance and physical dependence.
  4. Drug may have been prescribed for relief of chronic pain or sleeplessness.
  5. Individual usually has emotional problems and an anxious temperament.
  6. Sudden withdrawal of barbiturates may result in acute psychosis and seizures.

  7. Overdoses and acute withdrawal from barbiturates are medical emergencies and require hospitalization.
C. Amphetamines, Benzedrine, and Dexedrine.
  1. All effect or produce a "high."
  2. All are CNS stimulants, so overuse may result in brain damage, capillary bleeding and death.
  3. Large doses produce a hyperactive and agitated state.
  4. Amphetamines are emotionally addictive, especially for persons with insecure, inadequate personalities.
  5. Amphetamines affect individual's physical condition as the drug reduces appetite and awareness of body needs.
D. LSD, or "acid."
  1. LSD is a hallucinogenic drug and mimics hallucinations seen in psychoses.
  2. LSD produces changes in perception and logical thought processes.
  3. Drug not considered addictive per se, but individuals may become emotionally dependent on it.
  4. Experiences with LSD range from ecstasy to terror and the results are unpredictable.
E. Marijuana.
  1. Marijuana was considered to have low abuse potential but now most professionals agree that this is not the case.
  2. It produces a "dreamy" state and feelings of euphoria, hilarity, and well-being.
  3. Moods vary according to environmental stimuli.
  4. Marijuana changes perception of space and time which seem distorted and extendable.
  5. High dosage may produce hallucinations and delusions.
F. Cocaine.
  1. Cocaine is classified as a stimulant.
  2. Usual method of ingestion is by sniffing or IV.
  3. Use may cause strong psychological dependence.
  4. Most professionals believe use does develop physical dependence or tolerance.
G. PCP—"crystal," "elephant tranquilizer."
  1. PCP is usually smoked with marijuana. It may also be ingested or injected.
  2. Reactions vary from a sense of well-being to total disorientation and hallucinations.

3. PCP is considered an extremely dangerous "street" drug.
4. Psychological dependence may occur.
5. Cerebral cellular destruction and atrophy occur with even small amounts.
6. Overdoses or "bad trips" are characterized by erratic, unpredictable behavior; withdrawal symptoms; disorientation; self-mutilation; or self-destructive behavior.
7. Overdoses are treated with sedatives, decreased environmental stimuli and protecting client from harming self and others. Cannot be "talked down."

Assessment

1. Establish name and action of drug used.
2. Assess length of addiction or abuse.
3. Determine amount of drug used.
4. Determine other drugs used.
5. Assess physical condition of client by physical exam and blood and urine lab work.
6. Assess psychosocial network in which client lives.
7. Evaluate rehabilitative potential and support systems.

Planning and Analysis

1. Nurse will assist client through detoxification phase.
2. Client will recognize drug dependency needs.
3. Client will begin to make lifestyle changes.
4. Client will be directed to self-help groups.

Implementation

1. Support client during heroin withdrawal which is the first step in treatment and may be accomplished abruptly ("cold turkey") or gradually over a period of days.
2. Administer substitute drug (methadone) for heroin addiction if ordered to reduce the physical reaction to withdrawal.
3. Provide prolonged medical and psychiatric treatment for physical and emotional deterioration as part of convalescence.
4. Encourage client to take advantage of resocialization programs by professional or community resources.
5. Provide client with information concerning rehabilitation programs designed to help client reenter the mainstream of society.

a. Various self-help groups offer aid in rehabilitation.
b. Therapeutic communities and group therapy programs also provide rehabilitation.
6. Provide support to client during "bad trips," acute anxiety, and panic reactions to drug experience.
a. Place client in a quiet, safe, environment with a person to "talk them through" the experience for LSD.
b. Reassure client that this reaction is drug caused and of short duration.
c. Provide careful reality orientation by nurse.
d. Use nonthreatening, supportive approach.
e. Reassure client that he or she will not be allowed to harm himself or herself.
f. Refer client to drug counseling when the experience is over.

Evaluation

1. The individual is drug free through detoxification.
2. Client is able to discuss dependency needs and to describe feelings.
3. Client has learned new coping mechanisms for stress.
4. Client is involved in rehabilitative program after detoxification.

ORGANIC BRAIN SYNDROME

Definition: Organic brain syndromes are psychiatric disorders with organic etiology that may be reversible (delirium) or irreversible (dementia).

Delirium (Acute Brain Syndrome)

Characteristics

A. This syndrome is an organically caused disorder commonly referred to as acute brain syndrome.
B. Etiology.
1. Any acute disease or injury that interferes with cerebral function and often is temporary and reversible.
2. Includes infections, circulatory disturbances, metabolic and endocrine disorders, neoplasms, and tumors.

3. Injuries include brain trauma, invasive trauma.

4. Other causes are poisons, drugs, or systemic intoxication.

C. Characterized by global intellectual impairment with rapid onset.

D. Condition may last hours or weeks; usually resolves in a few days.

Assessment

A. Assess for clouding of consciousness—a cardinal symptom.

B. Assess for intellectual deficits.
   1. Memory loss.
   2. Poor abstract thinking.
   3. Poor problem-solving ability.

C. Assess for presence of hallucinations (visual most common), delusions, and confusion.

D. Assess for loss of contact with reality.
   1. Inattentive and distractable.
   2. Disorientation to time, place, and person.

E. Check for increased motor activity with no defined purpose.

F. Assess emotional stability.
   1. Reactions are blunted.
   2. Fearful.

G. Assess alterations in adjustment: tend to be worse at night, more fearful, etc.

Planning and Analysis

A. Specific etiology is established and treated vigorously.
   1. Physical problems of client assessed and evaluated.
   2. Cognitive, affective, and behavioral impairment determined.

B. Safe environment established to prevent accidents and self-injury.

C. Nutritional status reestablished.

D. Family included in treatment plan.

Implementation

A. Provide adequate nutritional and fluid intake as ordered by treatment plan.

B. Keep client in a quiet, structured environment.

C. Observe and monitor vital signs as necessary.

D. Keep siderails up and use restraints as necessary to protect client.

E. Implement treatment plan for elimination of causative factors.

F. Provide reality orientation approach with client.

G. Set limits on inappropriate behavior.

H. Express directions in a simple and concrete manner.

I. Observe client for signs of fever, shock, and increased intracranial pressure such as restlessness, acute anxiety, pain, and changes in vital signs.

J. Reassure and involve family as is appropriate.

K. Involve client in rehabilitation program as necessary.

Evaluation

A. Intervention resulted in decrease in cognitive, conative, affective and behavioral impairment.
   1. Client's orientation, memory, intellect, judgment, and affect improve.
   2. Vital signs stabilize.
   3. No hallucinations or delusions are evidenced.
   4. Causative organism is removed or eliminated.

B. Client is able to function without structure of hospital.

Dementia (Chronic Brain Syndrome)

Characteristics

A. Progressive degenerative condition characterized by irreversible brain damage and gradual destruction of neurons with functional loss in cognitive area.

B. Insidious onset but slow, progressive deterioration occurs.

C. Etiology is specifically unknown: results from wide variety of sources.
   1. Prenatal causes: congenital cranial anomaly, congenital spastic paraplegia.
   2. Infection: central nervous system, syphilis, meningeoencephalitis.
   3. Intoxication: drug or poison, alcohol.
   4. Trauma: brain trauma by gross force, brain surgery.
   5. Circulatory disorder: cerebral arteriosclerosis.
   6. Disturbance of innervation: convulsions.
   7. Disturbances of metabolism, growth, or nutrition.
      a. Senile brain disease: dementia.
      b. Glandular problems.
      c. Pellagra.
   8. New growths: brain neoplasm.

554

Degenerative Conditions

Alzheimer's Disease

A. Most common form of dementia: accounts for almost 50 percent of known cases.
B. Unknown etiology but diffuse atrophy of cerebral cortex occurs. Current speculation suspects abnormally high levels of aluminum in CNS.
C. Usually begins after age 60 but can be observed at 40.
D. Symptoms gradually and progressively worsen.
E. Clients may live for 10 years but progress to requiring total care.

Pick's Disease

A. Rare heredodegenerative process not associated with normal aging.
B. Becomes well advanced in 2–3 years.
C. Similar to Alzheimer's but involvement spares parietal lobes.
D. These clients act dull and lack initiative; otherwise, resemble Alzheimer's.

Huntington's Chorea

A. Genetically transmitted disorder caused by a single autosomal dominant gene.
B. Onset of symptoms after the age of 30–50 years.
C. Progressive mental and physical deterioration inevitable.
D. Characterized by personality changes with psychotic behavior, intellectual impairment, and, finally, total dementia.

Korsakoff's Syndrome

A. A disorder that occurs in chronic alcoholism and is often associated with Wernicke's encephalopathy.
 1. Wernicke's encephalopathy.
  a. Acute, life-threatening condition that can occur as a result of chronic alcoholism (inadequate diet leading to thiamine deficiency).
  b. Usual symptoms are cloudy consciousness, impaired mentation, ataxia, and polyneuropathy.
  c. Treatment is oral vitamin B complex and thiamine 100 mg IM STAT if client presents with the above symptoms and has a history of alcohol abuse.
 2. Korsakoff's is a chronic condition that remains after Wernicke's encephalopathy is treated.
B. Most important feature is recent memory impairment, especially in learning new information.
 1. Confabulation accompanies memory impairment.
 2. Memories for past events are not usually affected.
C. Syndrome improves with adequate diet (especially including vitamin B complex and thiamine) but only 25 percent recover fully.

Assessment

A. Assess onset which is generally slow.
B. Evaluate if illness is stabilized or in remission.
C. Assess for increasing deterioration.
D. Look for the following symptoms:
 1. Cognitive impairment.
  a. Disorientation.
  b. Severe loss of memory.
  c. Judgment impairment.
  d. Loss of capacity to learn.
  e. Perceptual disturbances.
  f. Decreased attention span.
  g. Paranoid ideation.
 2. Conative impairment.
  a. Decreased motivation, interests, and self-concern.
  b. Loss of normal inhibitions.
  c. Loss of insight.
 3. Affective impairment.
  a. Labile mood, irritableness, and explosiveness.
  b. Depression.
  c. Withdrawal.
  d. Anxiety.
 4. Behavioral impairment.
  a. Restlessness.
  b. Ritualistic, stereotyped behavior to deal with environment.
  c. Possible combativeness.
  d. Possible inappropriate and regressive behavior.
  e. Alterations in sexual drives and activity.
  f. Neurotic or psychotic behavior as client's defenses break down.
E. Assess psychological reactions to COB disorder.
 1. Change in self-concept.
 2. Anger and frustration as reactions to forced change in life role.

3. Denial used as defense.
4. Depression.
5. Acceptance of limitations.
6. Assumption of "sick" role by dependency and lack of motivation.

Planning and Analysis

A. Both physical and psychological needs will be met.
B. Client's contact with reality will be maintained as long as possible.
C. Client will be assisted to accept diagnosis.
D. Consistent staff interactions will reduce client's disorientation.
E. Therapeutic communication techniques will be used.
F. Safe, stable, consistent environment will be provided.
G. Goals within client's diagnosis and prognosis will be established.
H. Good nutrition will be maintained.
I. Rehabilitative potential will be assessed.
J. Plan will be developed to assist client to function at as high a level as possible for as long as possible.

Implementation

A. Meet client's physical needs.
   1. Avoid fostering dependence.
   2. Establish routine for activities of daily living.
B. Help client maintain contact with reality.
   1. Give feedback.
   2. Avoid small chatter.
   3. Personalize interaction.
   4. Supply stimulation to motivate client.
   5. Keep client from becoming bored and distracted.
C. Assist client in accepting the diagnosis.
   1. Be supportive.
   2. Maintain good communication.
   3. During denial phase, listen and accept; do not argue.
   4. Assist development of awareness.
   5. Help client develop the ability to cope with his or her altered identity.
D. Focus interactions with client and establish consistent contact.
   1. Have short, frequent contacts with client.
   2. Use concrete ideas in communicating with client.
   3. Maintain reality orientation by allowing client to talk about his or her past and to confabulate.
   4. Acknowledge client as an individual.
E. Provide activities that increase success of client.
   1. Social groups.
   2. Occupational therapy.
   3. Allow client, as interested, to do small chores around unit.
F. Provide supportive environment.
   1. Ensure a consistent staff and environmental structure.
   2. Do not change schedule suddenly.
   3. Provide handrails, walkers, wheelchairs, etc., as necessary.
   4. Ensure that the floor is not slippery, and that the environment is well lighted.
G. Assess client's disabilities and develop a nursing plan to deal with them.
   1. Update conferences with treatment team.
   2. Involve client in treatment planning as able.
   3. Communicate client needs to rehabilitation team.
H. Involve family and community in treatment and rehabilitation program.
   1. Plan visits by client to social community events.
   2. Encourage family involvement.
   3. Establish communication with family by using a friendly, warm approach.
   4. Encourage and arrange community groups (church groups, volunteer societies, and school groups) to visit on units.
I. Assist client to function at the highest level possible.
   1. Increase self-esteem.
   2. Avoid dependency.
   3. Allow and encourage personalization of client's room and environment.
   4. Dress client in his or her own clothing.
   5. Maintain client's cleanliness: clothes, hair, and person.
   6. Do not isolate client from others on the unit.

Evaluation

A. Client expresses interest in self and environment.
B. Client's disorientation is kept at minimal level.
C. Client is assessed by total treatment team on planned schedule.
D. Client is well nourished and neat in appearance.
E. Client is involved in unit activities.
F. Client accepts diagnosis.

SCHIZOPHRENIC DISORDERS

Definition: Schizophrenia is a psychiatric syndrome characterized by thought disturbance, withdrawal from reality, regressive behavior, ineffective communication, and severely impaired interpersonal relationships.

Characteristics

A. Schizophrenia may result from many possible factors: genetic constellation, the most current theory, individual adaptive patterns, lack of ego development, a deficit in cognitive development, or a biological origin.
B. Ego is weak and unable to function as mediator between the self and external reality.
C. Regression and repression are considered to be the primary mechanisms of schizophrenia.
D. Major maladaptive disturbances include impaired interpersonal relationships, inappropriate mental and emotional processes, and disturbances in overt behavior patterns.
E. Manifestations of the illness include acute psychosis involving the total personality or a group of symptoms circumscribed to one area of the personality.
F. The four "A's" provide clues to diagnosis.
  1. *Affect*—feelings or emotions minimal, i.e., flat, blunted, or inappropriate.
  2. *Associative looseness*—no connection between thoughts or ideas expressed.
  3. *Autistic thinking*—thoughts excessively involved with self; focused inward; unresponsive, mute with disintegrated thought processes.
  4. *Ambivalence*—two equally strong feelings (love and hate) neutralizing each other and immobilizing client.
G. Other important symptoms include the following:
  1. *Reality testing*—inability to distinguish between objective facts and wishes or fears.
  2. *Delusions* (fixed misinterpretation of reality)—false beliefs maintained despite evidence to the contrary.
  3. *Hallucinations* (unwilled sense perceptions with no basis in reality)—auditory, visual, olfactory, tactile, gustatory.
  4. *Withdrawal*—adoption of more satisfying regressive behavior; focus on internal world (autism).

  5. *Depersonalization*—feelings of estrangement or unconnectedness of body parts.
H. Schizophrenic subtypes.
  1. *Paranoid type.*
    a. Persecutory or grandiose delusions are prominent.
    b. Extreme suspiciousness and withdrawal are common manifestations.
  2. *Catatonic type.*
    a. Secondary symptoms of motor involvement are present.
      (1) Underactivity results in bizarre posturing.
      (2) Overactivity leads to agitation.
    b. Negativism: doing the opposite of what is asked.
      (1) Rigidity is the simplest form of negativism.
      (2) Mute behavior is another form of negativism.
  3. *Disorganized type.*
    a. Inappropriate affect: giggling and silly laughter. (formerly labeled hebephrenia.)
    b. Disorganization of speech.
    c. Regression.
    d. Absence of systematized delusions.
  4. *Undifferentiated type.*
    a. This type is characterized by a combination of symptoms, none of which discriminates a specific type of disorder.
    b. Flat affect and/or autism is usually present.
    c. Association disorders and thought disturbance, such as delusions or hallucinations, are usually present.
    d. This condition includes other behavioral maladaptations that cannot be otherwise classified.

Assessment

A. Assess any disturbance in thought processes.
  1. Client's thoughts are confused and disorganized, and ability to communicate clearly is limited.
  2. Client manifests tangential or circumstantial speech and has problems with symbolic meaning of certain words.
    a. May be very concrete in thinking and demonstrate an inability to think in abstract terms.

b. May live in a fantasy world, responding to reality in a bizarre or autistic manner, thereby having great difficulty in testing reality.

B. Assess any disturbance in affect.
1. Client has difficulty expressing emotions appropriately, and subjective emotional experience may be blunted or flattened.
2. Client has difficulty expressing positive or warm emotions; when they are expressed, it is often in an inappropriate manner.
3. While client's feelings may seem inappropriate to the thoughts expressed, they are appropriate to the client's inner experience and are meaningful to him.
4. Client's inappropriate affect makes it difficult to establish close relationships with others.

C. Assess any disturbance in behavior.
1. Client's behavior is often disorganized and inappropriate and apparently lacks a purposeful activity.
2. Client typically lacks motivation or drive for change in circumstances; general condition is one of apathy and listlessness.
3. Client's behavior may appear to be bizarre and extremely inappropriate to the circumstances.

D. Assess any disturbance in interpersonal relationships.
1. Client typically has great difficulty in relating to others.
a. Cannot build close relationships; probably has not experienced close, meaningful relationships in the past.
b. Has difficulty trusting others and experiences fear, ambivalence, and dependency that influence client's relationships with others.
c. Often learns to protect self from further hurt by maintaining distance, thus experiences lack of warmth, trust, and intimacy.
2. Client's relationships are impaired by the inability to communicate clearly and to react in an appropriate and empathic manner.

Planning and Analysis

A. Client will establish satisfying relationships with real people rather than imaginary ones.
B. Reality orientation will increase.
C. Thought disturbances will diminish.
D. Positive self-attitudes and concepts will increase.

E. Patterns of withdrawal will decrease.
F. Affect will be appropriate to situation.
G. Bizarre and inappropriate behaviors will be replaced by more adaptive behavior.
H. Appropriate medication will enhance adaptive behavior.
I. Personal hygiene habits will improve.
J. Client will participate more frequently in unit activities.
K. Milieu will be structured, safe and supportive.
L. Client will ask for assistance when he or she is getting out of control.
M. Self-destructive behaviors if present will be eliminated.

Implementation

A. General approaches.
1. Establish a nurse-client relationship.
a. Increase client's social contacts with others.
b. Build a positive and trusting relationship with client.
c. Provide client with a safe and secure environment.
2. Stress reality; help client to reality-test, to leave his or her fantasy world.
a. Involve client in reality-oriented activities.
b. Help client find satisfaction in the external environment.
3. Accept client as he or she is.
a. Do not invalidate disturbed thoughts or fantasies.
b. Do not invalidate client by inappropriate responses.
4. Use therapeutic communication techniques.
a. Encourage expression of emotions, negative or positive.
b. Encourage expression of thoughts, fears, and problems.
c. Attempt to fit nonverbal with verbal communications.
d. Focus on clear communications with the client.
5. Avoid fostering dependency relationship.
6. Avoid stressful situations or increasing client's anxiety.
7. Use real objects or activities (singing, for example) to distract or redirect client.
8. Decrease client's anxiety level.
9. Use warm, honest, matter-of-fact approach.

10. Recognize that the nurse and others influence client even if client appears unresponsive, remote, and detached at times.

B. Approaches to specific symptoms.

1. *Delusions.*
   a. Encourage client to recognize distorted views of reality.
   b. Focus on client's ego assets, strengths, etc.
   c. Provide a safe, nonthreatening milieu.
   d. Divert focus from delusional material to reality.
   e. Provide experiences in which client can feel success.
   f. Utilize specific nursing responses:
      (1) Avoid confirming or feeding into delusion.
      (2) Stress reality by denying you believe the client's delusion.
      (3) Respond to feelings. For example, validate the feelings of client by asking, "I sense you are afraid. Is this true?"

2. *Withdrawn behavior.*
   a. Assist client to develop satisfying relationships with others.
      (1) Initiate interaction.
      (2) Build a trusting relationship by being consistent in keeping appointments, in attitudes, and in nursing practice.
      (3) Be honest and direct in what is said and done.
      (4) Deal with therapist's feelings in relation to client's hostility or rejection.
   b. Help client to modify perception of self.
      (1) Do not structure situation in which client will fail.
      (2) Increase client's self-esteem by focusing on assets or strengths.
      (3) Relieve client from decision making until client is able to make decisions.
   c. Teach client renewal of social skills.
      (1) Increase social contacts with staff and other clients.
      (2) Increase social contacts with significant others when appropriate.
   d. Focus on reality situations.
      (1) Use nonthreatening approach.
      (2) Provide safe, nonthreatening milieu.
   e. Attend to physical needs, e.g., nutrition, sleep, exercise, occupational therapy.

3. *Hallucinations.*

a. Provide a safe, structured environment with routine activities.
b. Protect client from self-injury prompted by "voices."
c. Initiate short, frequent interactions.
   (1) Respond verbally to anything real that client talks about.
   (2) Avoid denying or arguing with client about the hallucinations he or she is experiencing.
   (3) Increase client's social interaction gradually from interaction with one person to interaction with small groups as tolerated by client.

C. Approaches to dealing with aggressive or combative behavior.

1. Observe client acutely for clues that client is getting out of control.
   a. Note rising anger—verbal and nonverbal behavior.
   b. Note erratic or unpredictable response to staff or other clients.
2. Intervene immediately when loss of control is imminent.
3. Use a nonthreatening approach to client.
4. Set firm limits on unacceptable behavior.
5. Maintain calm manner and do not show fear.
6. Avoid engaging in an argument or provoking client.
7. Summon assistance only when indicated; sudden involvement of many people will increase client's agitation.
8. Remove client from the situation as soon as possible.
9. Use seclusion and/or restraints only if necessary.
10. Attempt to calm client so that he or she may regain control.
11. Be supportive and stay with client.
12. Use problem-solving focus following outburst of aggressive or combative behavior.
    a. Encourage discussion of feelings surrounding incident.
    b. Attempt to look at causal factors of the behavior.
    c. Examine client's response to stimulus and alternative responses.
    d. Point out consequences of aggressive behavior.

Table 2. PROFILE DIFFERENTIATION

Schizophrenic	Non-Schizophrenic
Major ego impairment. Includes faulty reality testing, delusions, hallucinations (especially auditory).	No grave impairment of reality testing. No hallucinations or delusions.
Serious impairment of client's life, including social, vocational, and sexual.	Difficulty in relating, but interaction with others not prevented. Personality usually remains organized.
Little insight into problems and behavior. Client generally does not recognize he or she is ill.	Some awareness into problems. Keenly feels subjective suffering. Often unconsciously fights any changes in status (getting well).
Severe personality disorganization, e.g., poor judgment, memory, and perceptions.	Less severe disorganization. Can function but with decreased efficiency.
May be caused by both physiological or psychological factors.	Always a functional disorder; not organic in origin.
Usually requires hospitalization and long-term treatment.	Usually does not require hospitalization. May require long-term treatment.
Maladaptive adjustment mechanisms used in rigid, fixed way. May be seen as severe regression.	Suppression and repression used to handle internal conflicts; defenses are largely symbolic.
No secondary gain received.	Symptoms generally exploited for secondary gain.

     e. Discuss client's role of taking responsibility for his or her aggressive behavior.
D. Approaches to dealing with verbally abusive behavior.
  1. Do not respond in kind to abusive comments.
  2. Try not to take abuse personally.
  3. Interact with client on a therapeutic basis.
    a. Help client examine his or her feelings.
    b. Do not reject client.
    c. Give client feedback concerning your reactions to abusive comments.
    d. Teach alternative ways for client to express his or her feelings.

  4. Maintain a calm, accepting approach to client.
E. Approaches to dealing with demanding behavior.
  1. Do not ignore demands; they will only increase in intensity.
  2. Attempt to determine causal factors of behavior, e.g., high anxiety level.
  3. Set limits to response patterns when client is demanding.
  4. Control own feelings of anger and irritation.
  5. Teach alternative means to getting needs met.
  6. Plan nursing care to include frequent contacts initiated by the nurse.
  7. Alert the staff to try to give client the reassurance he or she needs.

Evaluation
A. Client established a satisfying relationship.
B. Thought disturbances decreased and appropriate communication patterns increased.
C. Withdrawn behavior diminished.
D. Reality orientation improved.
E. Self-esteem increased.
F. Client's personal hygiene improved.
G. Behavioral responses are appropriate to situations.
H. Affect became more appropriate and animated.
I. Client's participation in unit activities increased.
J. Client uses problem-solving approach when experiencing disturbing feelings.
K. Self-destructive behaviors are eliminated.
L. Need for medication is minimized and client is cooperative in taking medication.

PARANOID DISORDERS

Definition: Diagnosis of paranoid disorder is made when paranoid features dominate the personality. Other symptoms of maladaptive behavior may be absent.

Characteristics
A. Paranoia is characterized by extreme suspiciousness and withdrawal from all emotional contact with others.
B. The onset is usually gradual.
C. The onset of paranoid reactions may be precipitated by certain stressful events in client's life.
  1. Real or imaginary loss of a love object.

2. Experiences of failure with subsequent loss of self-esteem.
D. Behavioral manifestations of illness are seen with intense focus on hypochondriasis.
   1. Complaints of insomnia and weakness.
   2. Complaints of strange bodily sensations.
   3. The more common paranoid psychosis is manifested by delusional thoughts:
      a. The most common delusions are of persecution (people are out to harm, injure, or destroy).
      b. Other delusions may center around grandeur, somatic complaints, or delusions of jealousy.

Assessment

A. Determine client's degree of suspiciousness and mistrust of others.
B. Assess client's hostility toward others.
C. Determine if delusions are present. Delusions include: persecution, grandeur, and/or hypochondriasis.
D. Evaluate client's degree of insecurity, inadequate self-concept, and low self-esteem.
E. Assess anxiety level and its impact on disorder.

Planning and Analysis

A. Paranoid-suspicious behavior will be decreased through development of a trusting relationship.
B. Excessive energy will be channeled into satisfying activities.
C. Environment will be supportive and non-threatening.
D. Self-esteem and a more positive self-concept will be developed.
E. Feeling of success will be experienced.
F. Ability to test reality will be increased.
G. Healthy nutritional status is maintained by tube feeding if necessary.
H. Client will develop more appropriate outlets for expression of angry or hostile feelings.

Implementation

A. Establish a trusting relationship.
   1. Be consistent and friendly despite client's hostility.
   2. Avoid talking and laughing when client can see you but not hear you.
   3. If client is very suspicious, use a one-to-one relationship, not a group situation.
   4. Involve client in the treatment plan.
   5. Give support by being nonpunitive.
B. Reduce client's anxiety associated with interpersonal interactions.
   1. Avoid power struggles—do not argue with the client; arguing increases anxiety and hostility.
   2. Do not proceed too fast with nursing therapy. Remember that a paranoid client is suspicious and mistrustful of others.
   3. Be consistent and honest.
C. Help differentiate delusion from reality (refer to section on delusions).
   1. Do not explain away false ideas. Ideas are real to the client.
   2. Avoid any attempt to disagree with delusion as this action may reinforce it.
   3. Use reality-testing when possible.
   4. Focus on reality situations in the environment.
   5. Attempt to engage in activities that require concentration.

Evaluation

A. A trusting relationship is established.
B. Client's suspicious, extreme paranoid behavior is diminished.
C. Client is involved in unit activities that bring him or her satisfaction.
D. Client's self-concept has improved.
E. Client is reality oriented, and no delusional system is observed.
F. Client has encapsulated delusion and is able to function outside hospital environment. (It is not always possible for client to eliminate delusions—goal is to function in society in an adaptive manner.)
G. Expression of angry and hostile feelings is decreased; more adaptive alternatives for handling these feelings have been developed.

CHILD PSYCHIATRY

Emotionally Disturbed Child

Definition: Emotional disturbance in children encompasses any form of dysfunctional or maladaptive behavior. It can take as many forms as adult disturbance, ranging from healthy responses in situational or developmental crises to neurotic or psychotic disorders. Situational crises such as separation anxiety and developmental deviations are considered in the chapter on Pediatric Nursing.

Assessment

A. Assess for presence of somatic manifestations: enuresis or eating or sleeping difficulties.
B. Evaluate for evidence of withdrawn behavior.
C. Assess for presence of autistic behavior.
   1. Assess for bizarre responses, such as rocking, hand movements in the air, fecal smearing.
   2. Evaluate absent or inappropriate communication.
   3. Evaluate flat or inappropriate affect.
   4. Assess for tantrums of self-destructive behavior, such as head banging.
   5. Identify aggressive behavior toward persons or objects.
   6. Assess for absence of "self" image, e.g., inability to identify parts of the body.

Characteristics

A. Autism is complete self-involvement—withdrawal to an "inner world."
B. It occurs in infancy, and while the etiology is not known at this time, a physiological cause is suspected.
C. The Gesell Institute believes inherited cognitive abnormalities or brain damage at birth are possible causes.
D. It is generally thought that the autistic child manifests weak ego boundaries and fails to develop a separate concept of the "self."
E. The autistic child can neither distinguish him or herself from the world nor distinguish internal from external stimuli.
F. Autism is differentiated from childhood schizophrenia in which the child has more sense of self and views self as separate from mother.

Planning and Analysis

A. The nurse will be familiar with patterns of normal growth and development (Erikson and Piaget), basic principles of psychiatric intervention, communication techniques, and self-awareness.
B. The nurse will be able to assess the child's psychomotor skills, reactions to environment, interaction and communication patterns, emotional status, and body image.
C. The nurse will be able to establish some method of relating and/or communicating with the child.
D. Developmental tasks that were never completed are mastered.
E. Destructive or bizarre behavior will be handled.

Implementation

A. Establish a method of relating to the child, either verbal or nonverbal.
   1. Communication is essential for the development of a relationship.
   2. An effective relationship with a mute and/or withdrawn child may be difficult unless the nurse has mastered his or her own feelings.
   3. Genuine concern, warmth, and acceptance must be felt by the nurse toward the child in order for any interaction to be effective.
B. Teach and support the child in mastering beginning development tasks that were never completed.
C. Give good physical care and protect the child from self-destructive behavior.
D. Set firm limits and be consistent to provide a secure milieu.
E. Provide activities for participation, fun, and reeducation according to the developmental level of the child.

Evaluation

A. The nurse is educated, prepared and able to engage in a therapeutic relationship with a disturbed child.
B. A total profile of the disturbed child is put together and evaluated before treatment commences.
C. A therapeutic relationship between the nurse and child is established.
D. A method of communication, either verbal or nonverbal, is established.
E. Developmental tasks not achieved are beginning to be completed.
F. The child's bizarre, deviant or destructive behavior is diminished.
G. Physical status of the child is improved or maintained.

Adolescent Adjustment Problems

Definition: Adolescent emotional disturbances occur in adolescents when their behavior becomes maladaptive and adolescents cease to function effectively.

Characteristics

A. Adolescence is a period of ambivalence—dependence versus independence.
B. Influenced by peer group pressures, the adolescent may experience an identity crisis because his or her own identity has not yet been resolved.
C. The adolescent evidences an inability to resolve conflicts and to master developmental tasks (identity versus role diffusion). For a full discussion of Erikson's "Stages of Development," see Growth and Development.
D. Tasks of this stage of growth.
    1. Emotional separation from the parents.
    2. Foundations for an adult sense of self. One of the most difficult situations a parent must face is the arguing and the testing of limits in which their child engages in order to develop this.
    3. Sense of personal identity. Teenagers continue to need love, support, and consistency from the adults around them.
    4. Resolution of dependency and control issues.
E. Normal adolescent behavior can be bizarre at times, so abnormal behavior may not be so blatant. Families may become desensitized to abnormal behavior.

Assessment

A. Assess degree of maladaptation or adjustment problems.
B. Assess presence of confusion that may result in anxiety, depression, acting out, or antisocial behavior.
C. Observe for specific behaviors in adolescent maladjustment:
    1. Defiance and hostility, especially toward authority figures.
    2. Sullenness and withdrawal.
    3. Sexual deviations.
    4. Addiction to drugs or alcohol.
    5. Depression and self-destructive impulses.
    6. Acting out or testing.
D. Assess developmental level at which adolescent is functioning.
E. Assess skills in problem solving, motivation, and general attitude.
F. Assess if the client is in touch with his feelings; how does he see his relationship with his parents, other adults, people his own age?
G. Determine if client is in treatment willingly or because of a court order, parental insistence, etc.
H. Evaluate client's general communication skills and level of self-esteem.
I. Assess how client uses the problem behavior to meet needs.
J. Evaluate family structure.
    1. Assess whether the parents will join in treatment program.
    2. Ask how they believe the client's problems can be resolved. Determine the communication skills of each parent. Observe how the client's behavior meets the parents' needs. Assess other problems in the family (marital problems, other children with behavioral problems, financial worries, etc.).

Implementation

A. Provide the experience of a positive relationship.
    1. Encourage interaction when adolescent can share fears, problems, concerns.
    2. Reinforce authentic behavior from client.
    3. Encourage group interaction with peers.
B. Use behavior approach to therapy.
    1. Set firm limits and be consistent in approach.
    2. Confront maladaptive behavior and reinforce efforts to change it.
    3. Avoid being manipulated or supportive of acting-out behavior.
    4. Give verbal positive reinforcement for appropriate behaviors.
    5. Help client create alternate activities to use as substitutes for destructive behaviors.
    6. Assist client to notice when he returns to old patterns of behavior.
C. Use clear, open communication.
    1. Role model effective communication skills.
    2. Assist client to practice new styles of communicating; make use of role-playing, etc.
    3. Encourage exploration of feelings; provide safe environment for expression of feelings.
D. Assist adolescent to develop personal goals.
    1. Encourage client to set up personal goals, and provide encouragement and feedback.
    2. Assist client to identify steps in obtaining goal.

Table 3. ADOLESCENT BEHAVIOR CHART

Normal behavior	Dysfunctional behavior	Normal behavior	Dysfunctional behavior
Tends to be secretive and demands privacy from rest of family. Uses friends to ventilate feelings and concerns.	Secretive about experiencing severe emotional distress. Has no friends with whom he can communicate.	Parental discipline varies.	Extremes of parental discipline: too harsh or too permissive.
Varying degrees of loneliness; may feel loved but not understood.	Profound loneliness; feels total lack of loving; has no meaningful relationships. Danger of suicide.	Usually has few, infrequent major losses while growing up.	Many losses (parental love, frequent moves, etc.).
Experiences need for peer involvement; is very conscious of peer pressure.	May be friendless and does not socialize well; may act indifferent to making friendships.	Impulse control varies; usually has had consistent parental help to control behavior.	Poor impulse control, usually from no positive role model (lack of control can lead to drug abuse, violence, criminal behavior, suicide).
Varying levels of depression.	Long-standing depression may show as excessive passivity or agitation (agitated depression is seen as restless, hyperactive, bored, reckless, acting-out behavior). Danger of suicide.	Usually feels safe and cared for at home.	May feel unsafe and unwanted at home (child abuse, conflict with stepparent, sexual abuse in home).
Usually has at least one person who provides loving, supportive parenting.	Absence of parent or parents from home because of work or divorce. Emotional abandonment by parents. Conflict with stepparents. Alcoholic or abusive parents.	Self-esteem varies; struggles to find own identity; uses conflict with family as a vehicle to work out internal struggles.	Poor self-esteem; extreme difficulty in working out self-identity; cannot use conflict with family to work out internal struggles.
Families have varying degrees of conflict, overt or covert.	Adolescent views family as having severe, long-term conflict.	Develops personal goals.	Unable to develop personal goals.
Family moves several times while child is growing up.	Very frequent moves with little internal stability; may be accompanied by breakup of family.	May have vague physical ailments that come and go, especially when going through a high-growth period.	May present physical symptoms of chronic stress: frequent headaches, panic attacks, stomach ulcers, etc.
Usually has infrequent school changes; school achievement varies.	May have frequent school changes; poor school achievement.		

Family behaviors that foster adolescent dysfunction include:

   Scapegoating
   Child abuse
   Marital disharmony
   Parental indifference
   Unhealthy communication patterns—use of double messages

3. Encourage client to examine his family's rules and develop alternate rules for living.
4. Support client in sharing alternate rules with family and explore areas of negotiation.

Evaluation

A. Client's level of functioning has improved and maladaptive behavior has diminished.
B. Client's interpersonal relationships with nurse, staff, peers, and family have improved.
C. Client has demonstrated change in ability to handle life problems.
D. Client has experienced a positive relationship with the nurse.
E. Family support has been forthcoming and will continue after client is discharged.

PSYCHOTROPIC DRUGS

Definition: Psychotropic drugs are those used in psychiatry in conjunction with other forms of therapy to temporarily modify behavior.

Characteristics

A. Psychotropic drugs affect both the central and autonomic nervous systems.
B. These drugs affect behavior indirectly by chemically interacting with other chemicals, enzymes, or enzyme substrates.
   1. Changes in cellular, tissue, and organ functions occur.
   2. Drug effects vary from cellular activity to psychosocial interaction.

Antipsychotic Drugs

A. Drugs also known as ataractic or neuroleptic; introduced about 1953.
B. Most common are phenothiazine derivatives (Thorazine, Stelazine, Trilafon, Vesprin, and the long-acting phenothiazine, Prolixin).
C. Action: to alter the dopamine effect in the CNS and depress the reticular activating system.
D. Antipsychotic drugs can calm an excited client without producing a marked impairment of motor function or sleep.
E. Side effects.
   1. Blood dyscrasias.
      a. Agranulocytosis occurs in first 3–5 weeks of treatment. *Symptoms:* fever, sore throat.
      b. Leukopenia, preceded by altered white blood count.
   2. Extrapyramidal effects occur in 30 percent of clients, affecting the voluntary movements and skeletal muscles.
      a. Parkinsonism: symptoms occur 1–4 weeks; signs are similar to classic parkinsonism: rigidity, shuffling gait, pillrolling hand movement, tremors, dyskinesia, and mask-like face.
      b. Akathisia: very common; occurs 1–6 weeks; uncontrolled motor restlessness, foot-tapping, agitation, pacing.
      c. Dystonia: occurs early, 1-2 days; limb and neck spasms; uncoordinated, jerky movements; difficulty in speaking and swallowing, and rigidity and spasms of muscles.
      d. Tardive dyskinesia: develops late in treatment; estimated to occur in up to 50 percent of chronic schizophrenics. Antiparkinson drugs are of no help in decreasing symptoms. This is a permanent side effect; symptoms are shuffling gait, drooling, and general dystonic symptoms.
   3. Hypotension: orthostatic hypotension may occur. Monitor closely when client is elderly. Keep client supine for 1 hour and advise to change positions slowly.
   4. Anticholinergic effects: dry mouth, blurred vision, tachycardia, nasal congestion and constipation. Treat symptomatically.
F. Another common antipsychotic drug (classification—Butyrophenones) is haloperidol (Haldol).
   1. Less sedative than phenothiazines.
   2. Indicated for use with psychosis, Tourette's disorder and as an antiemetic.
   3. Incidence of severe extrapyramidal reactions.
   4. Other side effects include: leukocytosis, blurred vision, dry mouth, and urinary retention.
   5. Avoid alcohol and other CNS depressants.
G. Clozapine (Clozaril) is a new drug for management of psychotic symptoms in clients who do not respond to other antipsychotics.
   1. Side effects: similar to other antipsychotics; be aware of blood dyscrasias (leukopenia, neutropenia, agranulocytosis, esinophilia).
   2. Monitor monthly bilirubin, CBC, liver function studies.
H. Other classes of drugs are Thioxanthenes (Taractan and Navane) and Dibenzoxapines (Loxitane).

Antianxiety Drugs

A. These drugs induce sedation, relax muscles, and inhibit convulsions; major use to reduce anxiety.

B. These drugs are the most frequently prescribed drugs in medicine; demand is great for relief from anxiety and they are safer than sedative-hypnotics.

C. They potentiate drug abuse. Greatest harm occurs when combined with alcohol.

D. They are prescribed in neuroses, psychosomatic disorders, or functional psychiatric disorders, but do not modify psychotic behavior.

E. Drugs from two major classes. Benzodiazepines: safer and more common (Librium, Valium, Centrax, Serax, and Xanax—being tested for use in depression and panic disorders). Nonbenzodiazepines: Vistaril, Equanil, and Miltown.

F. Side effects.
  1. Drowsiness (avoid driving or working around equipment).
  2. Blurred vision, constipation, dermatitis, mental confusion, anorexia, polyuria, menstrual irregularities, and edema.
  3. Habituation and increased tolerance.
  4. Pancytopenia, thrombocytopenia, and agranulocytopenia.

Antidepressant Drugs

A. The tricyclics, the most commonly used antidepressants, include Elavil, Norpramin, Tofranil, Aventyl, and Vivactil.
  1. Anticholinergic: take 1–3 weeks to be effective. Produce antagonism of the parasympathetic system.
  2. Clients with morbid fantasies do not respond well to these drugs.
  3. Side effects.
    a. Anticholinergic effects: dry mouth, blurred vision, constipation, postural hypotension.
    b. CNS effects: tremor, agitation, angry states, mania.
    c. Cardiovascular effects: palpitations. Exert a quinidine-like effect on the heart so assess any patient with history of myocardial infarction.
  4. If client is switched from a tricyclic drug to an MAO inhibitor, a period of 1–3 weeks must elapse.

B. The monoamine oxidase inhibitors include Marplan, Niamid, Nardil, and Parnate.
  1. MAO inhibitors are toxic, potent, and produce many side effects.
  2. They should not be the first antidepressant drug used; effect is at best equal to a tricyclic and side effects more dangerous.
  3. Side effects.
    a. Most dangerous is hypertensive crisis.
    b. Drug interactions can cause severe hypertension, hypotension, or CNS depression.
    c. Postural hypotension, headaches, constipation, anorexia, diarrhea, and chills.
    d. Tachycardia, edema, impotence, dizziness, insomnia, and restlessness.
    e. Manic episodes and anxiety.
  4. All clients must be warned not to eat foods with high tyramine content (aged cheese, wine, beer, chicken liver, yeast), drink alcohol, or take other drugs, especially sympathomimetic drugs (amphetamines, L-Dopa, epinephrine).
  5. MAO inhibitors must not be used in combination with tricyclics.

C. Hypertensive crisis.
  1. Severe symptoms: headache, confusion, drowsiness, vomiting.
  2. Monitor for potential complications: encephalopathy, heart failure.
  3. Treatment.
    a. Drug of choice: Regitine, IV 5 mg with close monitoring; antihypertensive.
    b. Monitor vital signs, EKG and neurological signs; BP q5min.
    c. Norepinephrine is administered for severe hypotension.

D. Trazodone HCl (Desyrel) is a class of antidepressant drugs unrelated to the tricyclics.
  1. Inhibits the re-uptake of serotonin.
  2. Well-tolerated with minimal side effects (sedation and dizziness).
  3. Warning—this drug has been associated with priapism—persistent, abnormal erection. If symptom occurs, immediately discontinue drug.

E. Prozac, introduced in 1988, is chemically and pharmacologically distinct from other antidepressant drugs.
  1. A selective inhibitor of the uptake of serotonin.
    a. Studies suggest that increased serotonin in critical areas of the brain modifies certain affective behavior. Results in the increased

concentration of active serotonin in critical synaptic areas in the brain.

b. A number of neurochemical pathways can be affected by existing antidepressants—Prozac is highly selective for the serotonin pathway and exerts little or no effect on the uptake of other neurotransmitters or receptor sites.

2. Prozac exhibits less side effects than other antidepressant drugs.

a. Anticholingeric side effects such as dry mouth, constipation are fewer with Prozac.

b. Side effects observed are nausea, the most common, anxiety/nervousness, insomnia, drowsiness, and headache.

c. Co-administration of alcohol and Prozac is not recommended.

3. Recommended starting and maintenance dose is 20 mg per day—daily dose should never exceed 80 mg.

Antimanic Drugs

A. These drugs control mood disorders, especially the manic phase.

B. Before lithium therapy is begun, baseline studies of renal, cardiac and thyroid status obtained.

C. The most common form of drug is lithium carbonate, a naturally occurring metallic salt.

D. Drug must reach certain blood level before it is effective.

1. Stabilizing concentration occurs in 5–7 days; therapeutic effects 7–10 days.

2. Serum level can be simply and reliably measured in mEq/liter of blood.

E. Lithium is metabolized by the kidney.

1. Deficiency of sodium results in more lithium being reabsorbed thus increasing risk of toxicity.

2. Excessive sodium causes more lithium to be excreted and may lower level to a nontherapeutic range.

3. Normal dietary intake of sodium with adequate fluids to prevent dehydration.

4. Serum levels measured 2–3 times weekly (12 hours after last dose) in beginning of therapy; for long term maintenance therapy, every 2–3 months.

F. Drug concentration and side effects.

1. Therapeutic range of serum levels is 0.8–1.2 mEq/liter; for acute manic state, 1.2–1.5 mEq/liter.

2. Side effects occur at upper ranges, usually above 1.5 mEq/liter.

3. Gastrointestinal disturbances, metallic taste in mouth, muscle weakness, fatigue, thirst, polyuria, and fine hand tremors.

4. Hypothyroidism.

G. Lithium toxicity.

1. Appears when blood level exceeds 1.5–2.0 mEq/liter. May appear sooner depending on individual client.

2. Central nervous system is the chief target.

3. Initial symptoms include nausea, vomiting, drowsiness, tremors, slurred speech, blurred vision.

4. If drug is continued, coma, convulsions, and death may result.

5. Treatment for toxicity: gastric lavage, correction of fluid balance, drug (Mannitol) to increase urine excretion.

Antiparkinson Drugs

A. The term "extrapyramidal disease" refers to motor disorders often associated with pathologic dysfunction in the basal ganglia.

1. Clinical symptoms of the disease include abnormal involuntary movement, changes in tone of the skeletal muscles, and a reduction of automatic associated movements.

2. Reversible extrapyramidal reactions may follow the use of certain drugs.

3. The most common drugs are the phenothiazine derivatives.

B. Antiparkinson drugs act on the extrapyramidal system to reduce disturbing symptoms.

1. They are usually given in conjunction with antipsychotic drugs.

2. Two of the most common drugs are Artane and Cogentin.

3. Side effects are dizziness, gastrointestinal disturbance, headaches, urinary hesitancy, and memory impairment.

C. Benadryl, an antihistamine, is often given in place of Artane or Cogentin.

1. Controls the extrapyramidal side effects of phenothiazines.

2. Preferred because it does not cause as many untoward side effects as other antiparkinson drugs.

General Nursing Responsibilities

A. Give correct *drug* and *dose* at correct *time* to correct *client.*
B. Know specific actions and uses of drugs.
C. Be familiar with the side effects and precautions of major drug groups.
D. Observe client carefully for side effects.
E. Be aware that certain drug groups are not compatible.
F. Notify doctor of EPR side effects and lithium toxicity, and immediately implement nursing interventions.

See Drug Classification Chart, Appendix 5, and Chapter on Pharmacology.

TREATMENT MODALITIES

Electroconvulsive Therapy (ECT)

Definition: An electric current delivered to the brain to produce a convulsion.

A. Shock therapy has been negatively perceived by general public; in fact, it is one of most useful treatments for major depression.
B. Involves induction of grand mal seizure via an electric pulse through the brain.
C. Advantages.
  1. Works more quickly than antidepressants.
  2. Safer for elderly with history of cardiac illness than antidepressant medication therapy.
  3. Major depressive episode with vegetative aspects improvement rate of 80 percent.
D. Administration.
  1. Three types of medication administered: atropine, to block vagal stimulation so secretions are reduced; general anesthesia with a short-acting barbiturate, to make the client more comfortable; and a muscle relaxant, to reduce complications from the convulsion itself.
  2. Preparation: informed consent, medical history, and physical exam; lab work-up and education of client.
  3. Side effects: memory loss for recent events and difficulty learning new information—effects resolve in 6–9 months; headaches, muscle aches, weight gain, hypertension, and, occasionally, cardiac arrhythmias.

E. Nursing considerations.
  1. Prior to procedure.
    a. Explain to client about the procedure and how he will react upon awakening: confusion, disorientation.
    b. Keep NPO after midnight.
    c. Check to see if consent form is signed.
  2. Following procedure.
    a. Remain with client until alert.
    b. Monitor vital signs after general anesthesia.
    c. Reorient to unit.
    d. Reassure regarding memory loss and confusion.
    e. Assist to eat breakfast.

Behavior Modification

Definition: Behavior modification is a process for dealing with problematic, ineffective human behavior through planned, systematic interventions. It is a three-staged process involving behavior assessment, intervention, and evaluation.

Characteristics

A. Behavior modification assumes that maladaptive behaviors have been learned or acquired through life's experiences.
B. The process draws on learning theory as an approach to the modification of behavior.
  1. It involves stimulus-response type learning.
  2. Techniques are drawn from Pavlov, Skinner, or SOR.
  3. It has been labeled "behavior conditioning."
  4. It assumes that learned behavior is specifically connected with environmental reinforcers, e.g., American eating patterns.
  5. The appropriate location for behavioral intervention and change is the individual's environment.
C. Behavior cannot be thoroughly understood independent of events that precede or follow it.
D. The concept of contingency relationships is basic.
  1. The relationships occur between behavior and reinforcing events.
  2. Positive reinforcer is a desirable reward produced by a specific behavior; for example, salary is contingent on work: no work, no salary.

3. Negative reinforcer is a negative consequence of behavior; for example, a mother spanks a child for playing with matches.
4. Removal of a positive reinforcer; for example, a student is not allowed to watch TV until his or her homework is finished.
5. Removal of a negative reinforcer; for example, a mother threatens a child until the child cleans up his room. Removal produces avoidance behaviors.
6. Principle of extinction:
   a. Reduces the frequency of a behavior by disrupting its contingency with the reinforcement.
   b. Arranges conditions so that the reinforcing event, which has been maintaining the behavior, no longer occurs.
E. Goal is to arrange and manage reinforcement contingencies so that desired behaviors are increased in frequency and undesirable behaviors are decreased in frequency or removed.
F. Specific terminology.
   1. Behavior problem: condemned, excessive, or deficient behavior.
   2. Operant behavior: voluntary activities that are strongly influenced by events that follow them.
   3. Reinforcer: a reward that positively or negatively influences and strengthens desired behavior.
      a. A primary reinforcer is inborn.
      b. An acquired reinforcer is not inborn.
   4. Stimulus: any event impinging on, or affecting, an individual.
   5. Accelerating behavior: increase in frequency of a desired behavior.
   6. Decelerating behavior: decrease in frequency of an undesirable behavior.
   7. Target behavior: particular activities that the nurse wants to accelerate.

Principles of Implementation

A. The nurse can be the major treatment agent because she has the most significant number of contacts with the client and his environment.
B. The nurse may be in charge of designing and implementing the program.
C. The nurse may be in charge of supervising a program that another staff member is putting into effect.
D. Proximity to the client enables the nurse to identify any specifically maladaptive behavior.

Crisis Intervention

Definition: Crisis intervention is a form of therapy aimed at immediate intervention in an acute episode or crisis in which the individual is unable to cope alone.

Crisis Situation

A. An individual is typically in a state of equilibrium or homeostatic balance.
B. This state is maintained by behavioral patterns involving interchange between the person and his or her environment.
C. When problems arise, the individual uses learned coping mechanisms to deal with them.
D. When a problem becomes too great to be handled by previously learned coping techniques, a crisis situation develops.
   1. Result is major disorganization in functioning.
   2. In circumstances of inability to resolve crisis, the individual is more amenable to intervention, and the potential for growth increases.
E. Precipitant factors in a crisis.
   1. Threat to individual security which may be loss or threat of loss.
      a. Situational crisis: actual or potential loss (job, friend, mate, etc.).
      b. Developmental crisis: any change, i.e., marriage, new baby.
      c. Two or more severe problems arising concurrently.
   2. Precipitants typically occur within two weeks of onset of disorganization.

Stages of Crisis Development

A. Initial perception of problem occurs first.
B. Tension and anxiety rises; usual coping mechanisms are tried.
C. Usual situational supports are consulted.
D. Known methods prove unsuccessful and tension increases.
E. If new problem-solving methods are unsuccessful, the problem remains and cannot be avoided.
   1. Person's functioning becomes disorganized.
   2. Extreme anxiety is likely to be experienced.
   3. Perception is narrowed.
   4. Coping ability is further reduced.
F. Resolution usually occurs within six weeks with or without intervention.

Characteristics

A. Crisis is self-limiting, acute, and lasts one to six weeks.
B. Crisis is initiated by a triggering event (death, loss, etc.); usual coping mechanisms are inadequate for the situation.
C. Situation is dangerous to the person; he or she may harm self or others.
D. Individual will return to a state that is better, worse, or the same as before the crisis; therefore, intervention by the therapist is important.
E. Person is totally involved—hurts all over.
F. At this time the individual is most open for intervention; therefore, major changes can take place and the crisis can be the turning point for the person.

Assessment

A. Examine period of disorganization.
   1. Assess degree of disorganization.
   2. Assess length of time situation has existed.
   3. Determine level of functioning.
B. Determine precipitant event.
   1. Determine problem that triggered crisis.
   2. Evaluate significance of the event to the individual.
C. Assess past coping mechanisms.
   1. Check history or past experiences of similar situations.
   2. Assess past history in coping with similar situations.
D. Evaluate situational supports.
   1. Ask about significant others in individual's life.
   2. Check available agencies.
E. Determine alternative coping mechanisms.
   1. Assess new coping alternatives.
   2. Assess uses of situational supports.

Planning and Analysis

A. Individual will be assisted to return to precrisis level.
B. Immediate intervention will be implemented because the time period for intervention is limited to six weeks.
C. Accurate assessment of the problem will be made.
D. Intervention will prevent crisis from developing further.
E. Individual will find relief and move out of crisis period.

Implementation

A. Focus on immediate problem.
B. Use reality-oriented approach.
C. Stay with "here and now" focus.
D. Set limits.
E. Stay with client or have significant persons available if necessary.
F. Explore available coping mechanisms.
   1. Develop strengths and capitalize on them.
   2. Do not focus on weakness or pathology.
   3. Help explore the available situational supports.
G. Clarify the problem and help the individual understand the problem and integrate the events in his life.
H. When the above steps are completed, some plans for future support should be worked out by the therapist and the client.

Evaluation

A. Client coped with crisis and returned to precrisis level of functioning.
B. Intervention was made within six-week period.
C. Client's level of functioning and ability to cope increased.
D. Alternative ways to handle crises were explored.

Rape Intervention

Definition: Rape is a sexual assault on a person that is basically an act of violence; only secondarily considered a sex act.

Assessment

A. Physical data.
   1. Assist with a complete physical examination.
   2. Carefully assess and document all physical damage.
      a. Injuries.
      b. Signs of physical entry.
B. Emotional data.
   1. Degree of emotional trauma.
   2. Presence of symptoms.
C. Crisis response.
   1. Acute: shock, crying, high anxiety, hysterical, incoherent, agitated, fearful, volatile, poor problem-solving ability.
   2. Beginning to cope: denial, appears calm and controlled, withdrawn, fearful, begins to talk about feelings, expresses anger, makes decisions.

3. Resolution: realistic attitudes, able to express feelings, controlled anger, acceptance of facts.

Planning and Analysis

A. To set priorities according to client's needs (physical injuries require immediate attention).
B. To provide accepting environment that will reduce trauma and anxiety.
C. To provide the resources whereby the victim will return to physical and emotional health without subsequent sexual maladaptation.

Implementation

A. Treatment focus.
  1. Emotional: crisis counseling and call Women Against Rape.
  2. Medical: immediate medical care; assess assault and degree of trauma.
  3. Legal: do not bathe, douche, or change clothes; gather evidence.
B. Guidelines for care.
  1. Recognize that the assault of rape is a humiliating and violent experience and that the victim is experiencing severe psychological trauma.
  2. Accept the fact that the victim was indeed raped and that the victim is to be supported, not treated as the "accused."
  3. Understand that the victim's behavior might vary from hysterical crying and/or laughing to very calm and controlled.
C. Interventions
  1. Provide immediate privacy for examination.
  2. Choose a staff member of the same sex to be with the victim.
  3. Remain with the victim.
  4. Administer physical care.
    a. Do not allow client to wash genital area or void before examination; these actions will remove any existing evidence such as semen.
    b. Keep client warm.
    c. Prepare client for complete physical examination to be completed by physician (same sex as client if possible).
    d. Physical exam includes:
      (1) Head-to-toe exam.
      (2) Pap smear.
      (3) Saline suspension to test for presence of sperm.
      (4) Acid-phosphatase to determine recency of attack.
    e. Physical treatment may include:
      (1) Prophylactic antibiotics.
      (2) Tranquilizers.
  5. Provide emotional support.
    a. Demonstrate a nonjudgmental and supportive attitude.
    b. Express warmth, support, and empathy in relating to the victim.
    c. Listen to what the victim says and document all information.
    d. Encourage the victim to relate what happened, having her tell you in her own words if it appears that she would like to talk about the experience.
    e. Do not insist if client chooses not to talk; allow the victim to cope in her own way.
    f. During the interview, continue to be sensitive to the victim's feelings and degree of control. If, in relating the attack, she becomes hysterical, do not continue questioning at this time.
  6. Provide beginning follow-up care.
    a. Assess ability to cope when client leaves hospital (suicide potential).
    b. Explore support system and resources.
    c. Encourage victim to arrange follow-up visits with a counselor.
    d. Involve in planning and support decisions.
  7. Termination of crisis relationship.
    a. Counsel client to receive repeat test for sexually transmitted diseases in three weeks or sooner if symptoms appear.
    b. Help reestablish contact with significant people.
    c. Refer to appropriate community resource for follow-up care.
    d. Keep accurate records, as they may be important in future legal proceedings.

Post-traumatic Stress Disorder

Definition: Characterized by a set of symptoms that occur from re-experiencing a traumatic and/or stressful event. The individual is not able to adjust to the event that occurred outside the range of normal experience (e.g., rape, airplane crash, military combat).

Assessment

A. Assess for symptoms of anxiety and depression.
 1. Emotional instability.
 2. Feelings of detachment or guilt.
 3. Nightmares.
 4. Withdrawal and isolation.
 5. Self-destructive behavior.
B. Aggressive or acting-out behavior.
 1. Explosive or unpredictable behavior.
 2. Impulsive behavior; change in life-style.

Implementation

A. Recovery process follows four stages.
 1. Recovery—reassure client that he is safe following experience of the traumatic event.
 2. Avoidance—client will avoid thinking about traumatic event; support client.
 3. Reconsideration—client deals with event by confronting it, talking about it and working through feelings.
 4. Adjustment—client rehabilitates and adjusts to environment following event; functions and is able to view future positively.

Environmental Therapy

Definition: Environmental therapy is a broad term that encompasses several forms and mechanisms for treating the mentally ill.

Community Mental Health Act

A. The Community Mental Health Act of 1964 provides for the establishment of mental health centers to serve communities across the country.
B. Each community must provide full service for its population.
C. Services include in- and out-patient treatment services, long-term hospitalization if necessary, emergency service, and consultation and educational services.

Characteristics

A. Hospitalization may be provided by private or public psychiatric hospitals or in psychiatric units of general hospitals.
B. Day-night hospitals provide structured treatment programs for a specified part of each day, after which the client returns to his or her family.
C. Half-way houses provide live-in facilities with guidance and treatment available for clients who are not quite ready to return to the community and function independently.
D. Therapeutic communities provide milieu therapy, a therapy involving the total community (or unit). The staff formulates and, together with the clients, implements the treatment program. Emphasis is often on group therapies and group techniques.

Group Therapy

Definition: Group therapy refers to the psychotherapeutic processes that occur in formally organized groups designed to effect improvement in symptoms or behavior through group interactions.

Types of Groups

A. Structured group: group has predetermined goals and leader retains control. Group has directed focus, factual material is presented, and format is clear and specific.
B. Unstructured group: responsibility for goals is shared by group and leader; leader is nondirective. Topics are not preselected, and discussion flows according to concerns of group members. Often emphasis is more on feelings than facts, and decision making is part of the group process.

Phases of Group Therapy

A. Initial phase: group is formed; goals are clarified and expectations expressed; members become acquainted; superficial interactions take place.
B. Working phase: problems are identified; confrontation between members occur; problem-solving process begins; group cohesiveness emerges.
C. Termination phase: evaluation occurs; fulfillment of goals is explored; support for leave-taking is undertaken.

Principles Underlying Group Work

A. Support: members gain support from others in group via sharing and interaction.
B. Verbalization: members express feelings, and group reinforces appropriate (versus inappropriate) communication.
C. Activity: verbalization and expression of feelings and problems are stimulated by activity.
D. Change: members have opportunity to try out new, more adaptive behaviors in group setting.

Methods of Focusing Group Therapy

A. Focus on here and now versus there and then. Group members are helped to express inner experiences occurring right in the present rather than in the past. The past cannot be altered; the person can only report on it.

B. Focus on feelings versus ideas. Abstract or cognitive focus directs group away from dealing with here and now feelings and experiences and allows no opportunity for exploring and coping with feelings.

C. Focus on telling versus questioning. Focus on the individual's reporting about self rather than on questioning of others, which is artificial and a defensive posture.

D. Focus on experience versus "ought" or "should." "Should" systems, which focus on judgmental and critical content rather than on supportiveness, should be avoided.

Leader Functions and Roles

A. Determine structure and format of group sessions.

B. Determine goals and work toward helping group achieve these goals.

C. Establish the psychological climate of group, e.g., acceptance, sharing, and nonpunitive interactions.

D. Set limits for the group and interpret group rules.

E. Facilitate group process to promote flow of clear communication.

F. Encourage participation from silent members and limit participation of monopolizers.

G. Exert leadership when group flounders; always maintain a degree of control.

H. Act as resource person and role model.

Advantages of Group Therapy

A. Economy in use of staff is possible.

B. Increased socialization potential in group setting leads to increased interaction between clients.

C. Feedback from group members occurs.
   1. Increases reality testing mechanisms.
   2. Builds self-confidence and self-image.
   3. Can correct distortions of problem, situation, or feelings by group pressure.

4. Gives information about how one's personality and actions appear to others.

D. Reduction in feelings of being alone with problem and being the only one experiencing despair.

E. Opportunity for practicing new alternative methods for coping with feelings such as anger and anxiety.

F. Increased feelings of closeness with others, thus reducing loneliness.

G. Potential development of insight into one's problems by expressing own experiences and listening to others in group.

H. Therapeutic effect from attention to reality, from focus on the here and now rather than on own inner world.

Family Therapy

Definition: Family therapy is a form of group therapy based on the premise that it is the total family rather than the identified client that is dysfunctional.

Basic Assumptions

A. An identified client is not ill; rather, the total family is in need of and will benefit from treatment.

B. An identified client reflects disequilibrium in the family structure.

C. Family therapy focuses on exploration of patterns of interaction within the family rather than on individual pathology.

D. Conjoint family therapy (Virginia Satir) treats the family as a group. It was originally developed as a method of treatment for schizophrenics.

Therapist Behaviors

A. Models role of clear communicator.
   1. Clarifies and validates communication.
   2. Points out dysfunctional communication.

B. Acts as resource person.

C. Observes and reports on congruent and incongruent communications and behaviors.

D. Supports entire family as members attempt to change inappropriate patterns of relating and communicating with one another.

E. In general, follows the same therapeutic approaches as in nurse-client relationship therapy.

Appendix 1. THERAPEUTIC COMMUNICATION TECHNIQUES

Listening	The process of consciously receiving another person's message. Includes listening eagerly, actively, responsively, and seriously.
Acknowledgment	Recognizing the other person without inserting your own values or judgments. Acknowledgment may be simple and with or without understanding. For example, in the response "I hear what you're saying," the person acknowledges a statement without agreeing with it. Acknowledgment may be verbal or nonverbal.
Feedback	The process the receiver uses to relay to the sender the effect the message has had, which either helps keep the sender on course or alters his course. It involves acknowledging, validating, clarifying, extending, and altering. *Nurse to client:* "You did that well."
Mutual Fit or Congruence	Harmony of verbal and nonverbal messages. For example, a client is crying, and the nurse says, "I want to help," and puts her hand on the client's shoulder.
Clarification	The process of checking out or making clear either the intent or hidden meaning of the message, or of determining if the message sent was the message received. *Nurse:* "You said it was hot in here. Would you like to open the window?"
Focusing or Refocusing	Picking up on central topics or "cues" given by the individual. *Nurse:* "You were telling me how hard it was to talk to your mother."
Validation	The process of verifying the accuracy of the sender's message. *Nurse:* "Yes, it is confusing with so many people around."
Reflection	Identifying and sending back a message acknowledging the feeling expressed or reflecting back last few words of the message. (Conveys acceptance and great understanding.) *Nurse:* "You distrust your doctor?"
Open-ended Questions	Asking questions that cannot be answered "Yes" or "No" or "Maybe," generally requiring an answer of several words in order to broaden conversational opportunities and to help the client communicate. *Nurse:* "What kind of job would you like to do?"
Nonverbal Encouragement	Using body language to communicate interest, attention, understanding, support, caring, and/or listening in order to promote data gathering. *Nurse:* Nods appropriately as someone talks.
Restatement	Restating what the client says. *Nurse:* "You said that you hear voices."
Paraphrase	Summarizing or rewording what has been said. *Nurse:* "You mean you're unhappy."
Neutral Response	Showing interest and involvement without saying anything else. *Nurse:* "Yes. . . ." "Uh hm. . . ."
Incomplete Sentences	Encouraging client to continue. *Nurse:* "Then your life is. . . ."
Minimum Verbal Activity	Keeping your own verbalization minimal and letting the client lead the conversation. *Nurse:* "You feel. . . .?"
Broad Opening Statements	Opening the communication by allowing the client freedom to talk and to focus on himself. *Nurse:* "How have you been feeling?"

Appendix 2. BLOCKS TO COMMUNICATION

Internal Validation	Making an assumption about the meaning of someone else's behavior that is not validated by the other person (jumping to conclusions). The nurse finds the suicidal client smiling and joking and tells the staff he's in a cheerful mood.
Giving Advice	Telling the client what to do. Giving your opinion, or making decisions for the client, implies client cannot handle his or her own life decisions and that you are accepting responsibility for client. *Nurse:* "If I were you. . . ."
Changing the Subject	Introducing new topics inappropriately, a pattern that may indicate anxiety. The client is crying and discussing her fear of surgery, when the nurse asks, "How many children do you have?"
Social Response	Responding in a way that focuses attention on the nurse instead of the client. *Nurse:* "This sunshine is good for my roses. I have a beautiful rose garden."
Invalidation	Ignoring or denying another's presence, thoughts, or feelings. *Client:* "Hi, how are you?" *Nurse:* "I can't talk now. I'm on my way to lunch."
False Reassurance Agreement	Using clichés, pat answers, "cheery" words, advice, and "comforting" statements as an attempt to reassure client. Most of what is called "reassurance" is really false reassurance. *Nurse:* "It's going to be all right."
Overloading	Talking rapidly, changing subjects, and giving more information than can be absorbed at one time. *Nurse:* "What's your name? I see you're forty-eight years old and that you like sports. Where do you come from?"
Underloading	Remaining silent and unresponsive, not picking up cues, and failing to give feedback. *Client:* "What's your name?" *Nurse:* Smiles and walks away.
Incongruence	Sending verbal and nonverbal messages that contradict one another; two or more messages, sent via different levels, seriously contradicting one another. The contradiction may be between the content, verbal, nonverbal, and/or content (time, space). This contradiction is a *double message. Client:* "I like your dress." *Nurse:* Annoyed, frowns and looks disgusted.
Value Judgments	Giving one's own opinion, evaluating, moralizing or implying one's own values by using words such as "nice," "good," "bad," "right," "wrong," "should," and "ought." *Nurse:* I think Dr. Ross is a very good doctor."

Appendix 3. EGO-DEFENSE MECHANISMS

Compensation	Covering up a lack or weakness by emphasizing a desirable trait, or making up for a frustration in one area by overemphasis in another area. This is learned early in childhood and may be easily recognized in adult behavior; for example, the physically handicapped individual who is an outstanding scholar.
Denial	Refusal to face reality. The ego protects itself from unpleasant pain or conflict by rejecting reality. Denial of illness is a common example; people wait to see a doctor because they don't want to know the truth. A more subtle example is the individual who avoids reality by getting "sick."
Displacement	Discharging pent-up feelings from one object to a less dangerous object. A fairly common mechanism; for example, your supervisor yells at you, you yell at your husband.
Fantasy	Gratification by imaginary achievements and wishful thinking; for example, children's play. Sometimes, in order to satisfy a need, one relieves the tension by anticipating the pleasure of gratification.
Fixation	The persistence into later life of interests and behavior patterns appropriate to an earlier age.
Identification	The process of taking on the desirable attributes in personalities of other people one admires. Identification plays an important role in the development of a child's personality; for example, the child who mimics mother or daddy. A kind of satisfaction can be derived from sharing the success or the experience of others, such as the nurse who feels sick watching a traumatic procedure on a client.
Insulation	Withdrawal into passivity, becoming inaccessible in order to avoid further threatening circumstances. Sometimes the individual appears cold and indifferent to his surroundings. Insulation may be used harmlessly at times, but becomes very serious if used so much it interferes with interaction with others.
Isolation	Excluding certain ideas, attitudes, or feelings from awareness. Isolation is separating the feelings from the intellect by putting emotions concerning a specific traumatic event into a lock-tight compartment; for example, the individual talks about a significant situation such as an accident or death without a display of feelings. This pattern can be positive if used temporarily to protect the ego from being overwhelmed.
Introjection	A type of identification in which there is a symbolic incorporation of a loved or hated object, belief system, or value into the individual's own ego structure; there is no absolute assimilation as in identification.
Projection	Placing blame for difficulties on others or attributing one's own undesirable traits to someone else; for example, the child who says to a parent, "You hate me," after the parent has spanked the child. In an adult, this mechanism is a predominant indicator of paranoia. The paranoid client projects hate for others by saying that others are out to get client.
Rationalization	The mechanism that is almost universally employed to prove or justify behavior. It is face saving to give a reason that is acceptable rather than the real reason, as in remarks such as, "It wasn't worth it anyway," "It's all for the best." This mechanism relieves anxiety temporarily and helps the person avoid facing reality.

Appendix 3. EGO-DEFENSE MECHANISMS (continued)

Reaction-Formation	Prevention of dangerous feelings and desires from being expressed by exaggerating the opposite attitude—a kind of denial. The overly neat, polite, conscientious individual may have an unconscious desire to be untidy and carefree. The behavior becomes pathological when it interferes with tasks or produces anxiety and frustration.
Regression	Resorting to an earlier developmental level in order to deal with reality. Regression is an immature way of responding, and it is frequently seen during a physical illness. It is sometimes used to an extreme degree by the mentally ill, who may regress all the way back to infancy.
Repression	The unconscious process whereby one keeps undesirable and unacceptable thoughts from entering the conscious. This repressed material may be the motivation for some behavior. The superego is largely responsible for repression; the stronger, more punitive the superego, the more emotion will be repressed. The child who is frustrated and downtrodden by a parent may rebel against authority in later life.
Sublimation	The mechanism by which a primitive or unacceptable tendency is redirected into socially constructive channels. This adjustment is at least partly responsible for many artistic and cultural achievements, such as painting and poetry.
Substitution	The replacement of a highly valued unacceptable object with an object that is more acceptable to the ego.
Suppression	The act of keeping unpleasant feelings and experiences from awareness.
Symbolization	Use of an idea or object by the conscious mind to represent another actual event or object. Sometimes the meaning is not clear because the symbol may be representative of something unconscious. Children use symbolization in this way and have to learn to distinguish between the symbol and the thing being symbolized. Examples include obsessive thoughts or behavior (hand washing, cleansing) and the incoherent speech of the schizophrenic (by the time the painful thoughts reach the surface, they are so jumbled that they lose their painfulness).
Undoing	Closely related to reaction-formation—performance of a specific action that is considered to be the opposite of a previous unacceptable action. This action is felt to neutralize or "undo" the original action; for example, when Lady MacBeth rubbed and washed her hands.

Appendix 4. DRUG CLASSIFICATION CHART

Antipsychotics	Method of Administration	Daily Dose
Thorazine	Tablets, concentrate, syrup, IM, IV, suppositories	20–1500 mg
Sparine	Tablets, concentrate, syrup, capsules, IM, IV	50–100 mg
Mellaril	Tablets, concentrate	100–800 mg
Serentil	Tablets, concentrate, IM	30–400 mg
Trilafon	Tablets, concentrate, syrup, IM, suppositories	6–64 mg
Prolixin decanoate	Concentrate, IM, SC	2.5–10 mg
Prolixin Permitil	Tablets	12.5–25 mg
Stelazine	Tablets, concentrate, IM	2–50 mg
Compazine	Tablets, capsules, syrup, concentrate, IM, IV, suppositories	15–150 mg
Taractan	Tablets, concentrate, IM	30–600 mg
Navane	Capsules, concentrate, IM	6–60 mg
Haldol	Tablets, concentrate, IM	2–40 mg
Loxitane	Capsules, concentrate, IM	10–50 mg
Clozaril	Tablets	300–450 mg

Antianxiety Drugs

Atarax	Tablets, syrup	50–400 mg
Vistaril	Capsules, suspension IM only	50–400 mg 50–100 mg
Librium, Librax	Tablets, capsules, IM, IV	10–100 mg
Valium	Tablets, IM, IV	2–40 mg
Serax	Capsules, tablets	30–120 mg
Meprobamate (Equanil, Miltown)	Tablets, capsules, suspension	400–1200 mg

Antidepressants (Mood Elevators)

MAO Inhibitors

Marplan	Tablets	10–30 mg
Niamid	Tablets	125–200 mg
Nardil	Tablets	15–75 mg
Parnate	Tablets	20–30 mg

Appendix 4.   DRUG CLASSIFICATION CHART

Antidepressants (Mood Elevators)

Tricyclics

Tofranil	Tablets, IM	75–300 mg
Elavil	Tablets, IM	50–200 mg
Norpramin	Tablets	75–150 mg
Aventyl	Capsules, liquid	20–100 mg
Vivactil	Tablets	15–60 mg
Sinequan	Capsules	25–300 mg

Miscellaneous

Desyrel	Tablets	100–300 to 600 mg
Ludiomil	Tablets	50–75 to 300 mg
Prozac	Tablets	20–80 mg

Antimanic Drugs

Lithium carbonate	Tablets, capsules	600–1800 mg
Lithane, Litho-Tabs		
Lithonate		

Antiparkinson Drugs

Cogentin	Tablets, IM	1–6 mg
Artane	Tablets, elixir, capsules	1–10 mg
Akineton	Tablets, IM, IV	1–8 mg
Kemadrin	Tablets	6–15 mg

Appendix 5. MENTAL ASSESSMENT SUMMARY

General appearance, manner and attitude.
Assess *physical appearance.*

Note *grooming,* mode of dress, and *personal hygiene.*

Note *posture.*

Note speed, pressure, pace, quantity, volume, and diction of *speech.*

Note relevance, content, and organization of *responses.*

Expressive aspects of behavior
Note *general motor activity.*

Assess *purposeful movements* and gestures.

Assess style of *gait.*

Consciousness
Assess level of *consciousness.*

Thought processes and perception
Assess coherency, logic, and relevance of *thought processes.*

Assess *reality orientation:* time, place, and person.

Assess *perceptions* and reactions to stimuli.

Thought content and mental trend
Ask questions to determine general themes that identify *degree of anxiety.*

Assess *ideation* and *concentration.*

Mood or affect
Assess prevailing or variability in mood by observing behavior and asking questions such as "How are you feeling right now?" Check for presence of abnormal *euphoria.*

If you suspect *depression,* continue questioning to determine depth.

Memory
Assess *past and present memory* and *retention* (ability to listen).

Assess *recall* (recent and remote).

Judgment
Assess *judgment* and interpretations.

Insight
Assess *insight,* the ability to understand.

Intelligence and fund of information
Assess *intelligence.*

Assess *fund of information.*

Sensory ability
Assess the five *senses.*

Developmental level
Assess client's *developmental level.*

Addictive patterns
Identify *addictive patterns.*

Coping devices and defense mechanisms
Identify *defense-coping mechanisms* and their effect.

MENTAL-SPIRITUAL ASSESSMENT

The mental assessment is completed throughout the physical assessment and history-taking time frame. It is not generally considered a separate entity. Mood, memory, orientation, and thought processes can be evaluated while obtaining the health history. A spiritual assessment can be obtained as a part of the health history, although specific sociocultural beliefs may need to be ascertained separately. Nutritional preferences and restrictions can be accomplished as a part of a client care plan and may or may not be included in the general client assessment.

The purpose of a spiritual assessment is to facilitate the client adapting to the hospital environment and help the staff understand stressors the client may be experiencing as a result of belief systems.

The purpose of a mental status assessment is to evaluate the present state of psychological functioning. It is not designed to make a diagnosis; rather, it should yield data that will contribute to the total picture of the client as he or she is functioning at the time the assessment is made.

The specific rationale for completing a mental status assessment is:

- To collect baseline data to aid in establishing the etiology, diagnosis, and prognosis.
- To evaluate the present state of psychological functioning.
- To evaluate changes in the individual's emotional, intellectual, motor, and perceptual responses.

- To determine the guidelines of the treatment plan.
- To ascertain if some seemingly psychopathological response is, in fact, a disorder of a sensory organ (i.e., a deaf person appearing hostile, depressed, or suspicious).
- To document altered mental status for legal records.

The initial factors that the nurse must consider in completing a mental status assessment are to correctly identify the client, the reason for admission, record of previous mental illness, present complaint, any personal history that is relevant, (living arrangements, role in family, interactional experience), family history if appropriate, significant others and available support systems, assets, and interests.

The actual assessment process begins with an initial evaluation of the appropriateness of the client's behavior and orientation to reality. The assessment continues by noting any abnormal behavior and ascertaining the client's chief verbalized complaint. Finally, the evaluation determines if the client is in contact with reality enough to answer particular questions that will further assess the client's condition.

MENTAL STATUS ASSESSMENT

ASSESSMENT	NORMAL	ABNORMAL
GENERAL APPEARANCE, MANNER AND ATTITUDE		
Assess **physical appearance**	General body characteristics, energy level, sleep patterns	Inappropriate physical appearance, high or low extremes of energy, poor sleep patterns
Note **grooming**, mode of dress, and **personal hygiene**	Grooming and dress appropriate to situation, client's age, and social circumstance Clean	Poor grooming Inappropriate or bizarre dress or combination of clothes Unclean
Note **posture**	Upright, straight, and appropriate	Slumped, tipped, or stooped Tremors
Note speed, pressure, pace, quantity, volume, and diction of **speech**	Moderated speed, volume, and quantity Appropriate diction	Accelerated or retarded speech and high quantity Poor or inappropriate diction
Note relevance, content, and organization of **responses**	Questions answered directly, accurately, and with relevance	Inappropriate responses, unorganized pattern of speech Tangential, circumstantial or out-of-context replies
EXPRESSIVE ASPECTS OF BEHAVIOR		
Note **general motor activity**	Calm, ordered movement appropriate to situation	Overactive, e.g., restless, agitated, impulsive Underactive, e.g., slow to initiate or execute actions
Assess **purposeful movements** and **gestures**	Reasonably responsive with purposeful movements, appropriate gestures	Repetitive activities, e.g., rituals or compulsions Command automation Parkinsonian movements
Assess style of **gait**		Ataxic, shuffling, off-balance gait

ASSESSMENT	NORMAL	ABNORMAL
CONSCIOUSNESS		
Assess **level of consciousness**	Alert, attentive, and responsive Knowledgeable about time, place, and person	Disordered attention; distracted, cloudy consciousness Delirious Stuporous Disoriented in time, place, and person
THOUGHT PROCESSES AND PERCEPTION		
Assess **coherency**, **logic**, and **relevance** of thought processes by asking questions about personal history, e.g., "Where were you born?" "What kind of work do you do?"	Clear, understandable responses to questions Attentiveness	Disordered thought forms Autistic or dereistic (absorbed with self and withdrawn); abstract (absent-mindedness); concrete thinking (dogmatic, preaching)
Assess **reality orientation**: time, place, and person awareness	Orderly progression of thoughts based in reality Awareness of time, place, and person	Disorders of progression of thought: looseness, circumstantial, incoherent, irrelevant conversation, blocking Delusions of grandeur or persecution: neologisms, use of words whose meaning is known only to the client Echolalia (automatic repeating of questions) No awareness of day, time, place, or person
Assess **perceptions** and reactions to personal experiences by asking questions such as "How do you see yourself now that you are in the hospital?" "What do you think about when you're in a situation like this?"	Thoughtful, clear responses expressed with understanding of self	Altered, narrowed, or expanded perception Illusions Depersonalization
THOUGHT CONTENT AND MENTAL TREND		
Ask questions to determine general themes that identify **degree of anxiety**, e.g., "How are you feeling right now?" "What kinds of things make you afraid?"	Mild or 1 + level of anxiety in which individual is alert, motivated, and attentive	Moderate to severe (2 + to 4 +) levels of anxiety
Assess **ideation** and **concentration**	Ideas based in reality Able to concentrate	Ideas of reference Hypochondria (abnormal concerns about health) Obsessional Phobias (irrational fears) Poor or shortened concentration

ASSESSMENT	NORMAL	ABNORMAL
MOOD OR AFFECT		
Assess prevailing or **variability in mood** by observing behavior and asking questions such as "How are you feeling right now?" Check for presence of abnormal **euphoria**	Appropriate, even mood without wide variations high to low	Cyclothymic mood swings; euphoria, elation, ecstasy, depressed, withdrawn
If you suspect **depression**, continue questioning to determine depth and significance of mood, e.g., "How badly do you feel?" "Have you ever thought of suicide?"	May be sad or grieving but mood does not persist indefinitely	Flat or dampened responses Inappropriate responses Ambivalence
MEMORY		
Assess **past and present memory** and **retention** (ability to listen and respond with understanding or knowledge); ask client to repeat a phrase, e.g., an address	Alert, accurate responses Able to complete digit span Past and present memory appropriate	Hyperamnesia (excessive loss of memory); amnesia; paramnesia (belief in events that never occurred) Preoccupied Unable to follow directions
Assess **recall** (recent and remote) by asking questions such as "When is your birthday?" "What year were you born?" "How old are you?"	Good recall of immediate and past events	Poor recall of immediate or past events
JUDGMENT		
Assess **judgment, decision-making ability** and interpretations by asking questions such as "What should you do if you hear a siren while you're driving?" "If you lost a library book, what would you do?"	Ability to make accurate decisions Realistic interpretation of events	Poor judgment, poor decision-making ability, poor choice Inappropriate interpretation of events or situations
AWARENESS		
Assess **insight**, the ability to understand the inner nature of events or problems, by asking questions such as "If you saw someone dressed in a fur coat on a hot day, what would you think?"	Thoughtful responses indicating an understanding of the inner nature of an event or problem	Lack of insight or understanding of problems or situations Distorted view of situation

ASSESSMENT	NORMAL	ABNORMAL
INTELLIGENCE		
Assess **intelligence** by asking client to define or use words in sentences, e.g., recede, join, plural	Correct responses to majority of questions	Incorrect responses to majority of questions indicates possible severe psychiatric disorders
Assess **fund of information** by asking questions such as "Who is President of the United States?" "Who was the President before him?" "When is Memorial Day?" "What is a thermometer?" (Consider client's cultural and educational background)	Correct responses to majority of questions	Deteriorated or impaired cognitive processes
SENSORY ABILITY		
Assess the **five senses**, e.g., vision, hearing, tasting, feeling, and smelling abilities	Able to perceive, hear, feel, touch appropriate to stimulus	Lack of response Suspicious, hostile, depressed Kinesthetic imbalance
DEVELOPMENTAL LEVEL		
Assess client's **developmental level** as compared to normal	Behavior and thought processes appropriate to age level	Wide span between chronological and developmental age Mentally retarded
LIFE-STYLE PATTERNS		
Identify **addictive patterns** and effect on individual's overall health	Normal amount of alcohol ingested Smoking habits Prescriptive medications Adequate food intake for physical characteristics	High quantity of alcohol taken frequently Heavy smoker Addicted to illegal drugs Habituative medication; user of over-the-counter or legal medications Anorexic eating patterns Obese or overindulgence of food
COPING DEVICES		
Identify **defense-coping mechanisms** and their effect on individual	Conscious coping mechanisms used appropriately such as compensation, fantasy, rationalization, suppression, sublimation or displacement Mechanisms effective, appropriate, and useful	Unconscious mechanisms used frequently such as repression, regression, projection, reaction-formation, insulation or denial Mechanisms inappropriate, ineffective, and not useful

GLOSSARY

Abreaction vivid recall of a painful experience with the expression of emotion appropriate to the original situation.

Abuse an act that injures, damages, or corrupts.

Acceptance favorable reception; basic acknowledgment.

Acrophobia fear of high places; a common phobia.

Acting out expression of unconscious emotional conflicts of hostility or love in actions that the person does not consciously know are related to such conflicts of feelings.

Activities of daily living actions or skills needed to function independently.

Adaptive reaction a response in which the person attempts to improve or alter his condition in relation to the environment.

Adolescence the developmental stage that occurs from age 11–19, during which time various developmental tasks are mastered to prepare the individual for adult tasks.

Affect generalized feeling, tone, or mood.

Aggression any verbal or nonverbal activity that may be forceful abuse of self, another person, or thing.

Agitation excessive restlessness; increased mental and especially physical activity.

Agoraphobia fear of crowds, open places.

Alcohol hallucinosis a withdrawal syndrome from alcohol where the client experiences hallucinations.

Alcohol withdrawal the physiological process the body goes through as the client is withdrawing from dependence on alcohol.

Alcoholism dependence, either physical or emotional, on alcohol with the inability to get through the stress of living without turning to alcohol.

Alleviate to make more bearable; reduce (pain, grief, or suffering).

Ambivalence the simultaneous existence of contradictory and contrasting emotions toward a person or object, that is, love and hate.

Amnesia the individual experiences a loss of memory because of physical or emotional trauma.

Anger a feeling of extreme displeasure, hostility, indignation, or exasperation toward someone or something.

Angina a sense of suffocation with symptoms of severe, steady pain and a feeling of pressure in the region of the heart.

Anorexia loss of appetite occurring from a variety of possible reasons.

Anorexia nervosa a disorder in which the person refuses to eat due to a psychological disturbance of body image.

Anxiety a troubled or apprehensive feeling; experiencing a sense of dread or fear.

Apathy pathological indifference.

Apprehension a fearful or uneasy anticipation of the future; dread.

Arrhythmia irregular rhythm.

Ascribed role a role in life that the person is given by viture of age, sex, etc.

Assistance aiding, helping, or giving support.

Ataraxia a state of complete mental calm and tranquility.

Attention the focus of mental activity on an object.

Attitude a state of mind or feeling with regard to some matter; disposition.

Autism detachment from reality when self-preoccupation and involvement are predominant.

Autogenic training a method of deep muscle relaxation that enables one to reduce the stress response, regain homeostasis, and prepare to handle additional stress.

Autoimmunization immunity produced by an attack of the disease or by processes occurring within the body.

Autonomic nervous system the part of the nervous system that regulates the functioning of internal organs and glands; it controls such functions as digestion, respiration, and cardiovascular activity.

Autonomy independent control over a part of one's life, work situation, etc.

Behavior the actions or reactions of persons under specified circumstances.

Behavior modification changing behavior through the application of principles of learning theory (reinforcement).

Biofeedback a training technique that utilizes monitoring instruments to assist people to control stress-related disorders through self-regulation of internal functions.

Bipolar affective disorder the form of an affective disorder that is characterized by swings from manic episodes to depression.

Blocking a gap or interruption in speech that is related to distracted or absent thoughts.

Body image the picture a person has about himself; both conscious and unconscious attitudes.

Body language the message sent to another through body movement or body position.

Bradycardia slowed heart action, below 60 beats/minute.

Bulimia eating disorder characterized by excessive binges of eating followed by vomiting.

Cardio prefix pertaining to the heart.

Cardiovascular pertaining to the heart and blood vessels.

Catatonic a form of schizophrenia characterized by immobile, mute behavior with bizarre posturing.

Catatonic excitement the opposite of mute, withdrawn behavior when the client becomes severely agitated and out of control.

Catharsis emotional release that occurs when a client expresses his thoughts and emotions to another person.

Cathexis term used by Freud to denote psychic energy that is attached to an object.

Cerebral cortex the extensive outer layer of grey tissue of the cerebral hemispheres (brain) responsible for higher nervous functions.

Child abuse physical, emotional, or sexual injury to a child, usually occurring within a family.

Clarify to make clear or easier to understand.

Claustrophobia fear of enclosed places.

Cliché stereotyped response; a trite or overused expression or idea.

Client-centered therapy the form of therapy designed by Carl Rogers that states as its primary thesis that the client can cure himself if the therapist provides a safe and supportive environment in which change can occur.

Cognition the mental process or faculty by which knowledge is acquired.

Cohesive a force that attracts; when referring to a group, the cement that holds the group together and helps the members to feel a sense of belonging.

Coitus sexual intercourse with a person of the opposite sex.

Commitment the legal process of admitting a client to the hospital because he is a danger to self or others or he cannot care for himself.

Communication the exchange of thoughts, information, or messages.

Compensation a mechanism that attempts to keep the personality in balance; the lack of gratification in one area is made up by increased gratification in another area.

Compulsion an irresistible urge to repeat an act that must be carried out to avoid anxiety.

Concreteness being very specific and definitive rather than abstract and intellectual, especially when discussing feelings or behavior.

Confabulation filling in a memory gap with a made-up response in order to protect one's self-esteem when a memory is lost.

Confer to hold a conference; to compare views or consult together.

Confidentiality a term used in psychiatric nursing to denote maintaining the client's privacy of information with the exception of disclosure to appropriate staff.

Conflict a struggle between two or more opposing forces.

Confrontation a term that refers to the process of pointing out perceived maladaptions in behavior so that the client may become aware of unacceptable behavior.

Confusion disorder; jumble; distraction; bewilderment.

Congruence agreement; conformity.

Consensual validation the agreement of two or more persons on the meaning of behavior.

Consent to agree; to be of the same mind.

Context the setting in which an interaction or event occurs.

Conversion reaction expression of a psychological conflict as a physical symptom; an unconscious attempt to deal with anxiety.

Convey to communicate or make known; to impart.

Cope to contend with, strive, or handle.

Coping mechanism means by which an individual adjusts or adapts to a threat or a challenge; actions that assist in maintaining homeostasis.

Counseling to give support or to provide guidance.

Counter transference the emotional reaction of a therapist that is inappropriate to the client or situation.

Covert hidden; below the surface.

Crisis a crucial point or situation in the course of anything; turning point.

Crisis intervention a form of therapy in which the client's crucial problem is immediately addressed in order to obtain relief.

Cyclothymia alterations in mood from high to low.

Data base all the information dealing with a client from which his problem can be determined.

Defense mechanism an activity originally identified by Anna Freud by which the ego defends itself by not allowing unacceptable thoughts or feelings to come into awareness to cause anxiety.

Delirium an organic mental disorder that is characterized by a loss of conscious awareness, usually with an acute onset.

Delirium tremens a symptom of alcohol withdrawal characterized by tremors, anxiety, insomnia, paranoia, etc.

Delusion a false belief maintained in spite of facts or evidence to the contrary.

Delusion of grandeur false belief that one is in a position of power, wealth, and prominence; usually associated with paranoid disorder.

Delusions of persecution false beliefs that one is

586

being pursued, followed, or intimidated by an opposing power.

Dementia the medical diagnostic term denoting an organic mental disorder that involves the destruction of neurons in the brain; usually irreversible.

Denial refusal to grant the truth of a statement or allegation.

Depersonalization the feeling or subjective experience of separateness or alienation from oneself; the state in which the client cannot distinguish self from others and which involves disintegration of the ego.

Depression an unshakable feeling of sadness accompanied by feelings of hopelessness, worthlessness, and bleakness regarding the future.

Detoxification removal of toxic substances from the body, as in alcohol withdrawal.

Deviant noncompliance with an accepted social norm or form of behavior.

Diaphoresis profuse sweating.

Disorientation a condition where the individual manifests loss of ability to recognize or locate himself in respect to time, place, or other persons.

Displacement behavior toward one object which is unconsciously motivated toward another, more acceptable object.

Dissociation the exclusion of memories or experiences that are painful from one's conscious awareness.

Double message two conflicting messages given simultaneously (as in a verbal message that contradicts a nonverbal message).

Double bind the end result of receiving double messages; the receiver has no escape when he receives two conflicting messages, for he will be wrong whatever message he responds to.

Drug abuse the use of any chemical substance that is not prescribed for treatment.

Dynamics of homeostasis danger or its symbols, whether internal or external, resulting in the activation of the sympathetic nervous system and the adrenal medulla. The organism prepares for flight or fight.

Dystonia the side effect of muscle spasms caused by the administration of an antipsychotic, such as a phenothiazine drug.

Echolalia a condition where the individual constantly repeats what is heard.

Echopraxia a condition where the individual mimics what is done.

Ego a Freudian term denoting that aspect of the psyche which is conscious and most in touch with external reality; the "I" part of the person. Also, the part of the personality that makes decisions, is

conscious, and represents the thinking-feeling part of a person.

Ego boundaries the perception of the dividing line between one's perception of self and the external world.

Ego state role behaviors of adult, parent, or child that one assumes in a situation, according to the theory of transactional analysis.

Electroshock a medical procedure of applying electric current to certain areas in the brain. Used in the treatment of certain psychiatric disorders (especially depression).

Emesis the end result of vomiting.

Emotion any strong feeling, as of joy, hate, sorrow, love.

Emotional affected by strong feelings, as of joy and sorrow.

Empathy ability to readily comprehend the feelings, thoughts, and motives of another person.

Encounter therapy the application of confrontation therapy in a group setting; the focus of this form of therapy is here and now with direct feedback as to how one perceives another's interactions.

Endorphins a naturally occurring body chemical similar to morphine but many times stronger.

Enkephalins peptides that occur naturally in the central nervous system and react similarly to opiates on the body.

Environmental therapy a form of therapy that focuses on the modification of the environment in order to provide the client with a natural, social surrounding.

Esteem to consider as of a certain value; regard; respect.

Ethic an accepted standard of behavior that is followed or accepted by a group.

Etiology the cause or causes of disease.

Euphoria a feeling of elation or joy.

Evaluate to examine and judge, appraise.

Exhibitionism nonadherence to socially acceptable behavior such as the exposure of one's sexual organs to public view.

Existentialism a philosophy that focuses on the immediate experiences of man and the belief that man creates his own reality.

Expression to manifest or communicate; make known.

Extinction the process of extinguishing an unwanted piece of behavior through reinforcement.

Extrapyramidal effect side effects that occur as a result of the administration of an antipsychotic medication, and that resemble the symptoms of Parkinson disorder: tremors, drooling, uneven gait, etc.

Family therapy the form of therapy that involves the entire family and takes as a premise that the family is disturbed, rather than an identified client. Therapy focuses on the communication and interaction between family members to identify the context in which an observable problem is recognized.

Fear response to an actual situation or person posing danger.

Fight or flight one's immediate response to stress; although archaic and often inappropriate, this response is part of our central nervous system biological heritage.

Fixation a stage in development when there is an abnormal attachment; inability to move on to later developmental tasks.

Flight of ideas pattern of speech characteristic of the manic client in which one idea rapidly generates another in sequence.

Free association a technique associated with Freud's psychoanalytic therapy; the client is encouraged to relate all of his thoughts as rapidly as possible to prevent censoring of the ideas as they come into conscious awareness.

Frustration a feeling that may contain elements of anger, hopelessness, or defeat. It occurs when goals set by perceived needs are blocked.

Fugue a condition experienced as a transient disorientation—client is unaware that he has physically escaped or run to another place.

Functional used in psychiatry to denote mental illness existing without known physical cause or structural changes.

Gastro term that denotes the stomach.

Gastrointestinal pertaining to the stomach and the intestine.

General adaptation syndrome a general theory of stress response formulated by Dr. Hans Selye; describes the action of stress response in three stages—the alarm reaction, the stage of resistance, and the stage of exhaustion.

-Genic suffix indicating generation or production.

Genuine the quality of a relationship that is characterized by openness, honesty, and sincerity; an essential trait if the client is to trust the nurse in relationship therapy.

Geriatrics the treatment of diseases that occur as a result of old age.

Grief intense mental anguish, deep remorse, sorrow, or the like.

Group maintenance functions carried out by a group to maintain group integrity; usually oriented toward satisfaction of the members' emotional needs.

Hallucination a false perception having no relation to reality and not accounted for by external stimuli.

Health the state of physical, psychological, and sociological well-being.

Helping relationship an interaction of individuals that sets the climate for movement of the participants toward common goals.

Helplessness the feeling that one is unable to function by oneself and that no one will come to the rescue.

Holistic a way of looking at individuals and organisms as a whole rather than a sum of the parts.

Homeostasis the maintenance of a constant state in the internal environment through self-regulatory techniques that preserve an organism's ability to adapt to stress.

Hostility feelings of anger and resentment, usually directed toward another person.

Hyperactivity excessively active with much movement and action; usually associated with the state of mania.

Hypertension a condition in which the client has a higher blood pressure than judged to be normal.

Hypochondriasis a state of morbid concern about one's body or health for which there is no physical evidence.

Hypomania a state that is similar to but not as severe as a manic episode; clinically, a hypomanic usually does not require hospitalization.

Hysteric involves elements of both conscious and unconscious exaggerated reaction, often in a dramatic manner, to some stimuli.

Id a Freudian term denoting a division of the psyche from which comes blind, instinctual impulses that lead to immediate gratification of primitive needs, dominated by the pleasure principle.

Idealization to regard as ideal; to make or regard someone or something as absolute perfection.

Ideas of reference a distortion of reality where a person believes that activities of others have a personal reference to him.

Identity the organizing view of the personality that provides for unity and consistency of the individual; the awareness that one is unique and that the "self" is the result of all previous experiences and perceptions of the whole.

Illness a state characterized by the malfunction of the biopsychosocial organism.

Illusion distorted perceptual experience where the individual misinterprets actual data from the environment. Examples: a mirage on the desert; seeing a lake when it is only light refraction.

Implementation the fourth step in the nursing process that denotes action or carrying out of the plan that involves intervention.

Impulsive act of driving onward with sudden force.

Incongruence   the discrepancy in messages between the verbal and nonverbal levels of communication.

Insight   an individual's understanding of the origin and mechanisms of his attitudes and behavior.

Insomnia   inability to sleep; difficulty with sleeping.

Interpersonal   that which exists between two or more persons.

Intrapersonal   that which exists within one person.

Introjection   the mechanism whereby the client incorporates the values or behavior of another person. Individual may release these qualities in the future because they never become integrated into the personality, as with identification.

Ischemic   local and temporary anemia due to obstruction of the circulation to a part.

La belle indifference   a French term used to describe the client's lack of concern or indifference toward his physical symptom; this is a clue that the symptom is a result of hysteria, rather than an organic basis.

Labile   frequent alterations in mood levels, as a rapid change from happiness to sadness.

Latent   a trait that manifests below the surface of awareness.

Latency   the stage of development that occurs between ages 6 and 12 where the major task is to develop a sense of competency.

Learning   the process of gaining knowledge, comprehension or awareness through experience or study.

Lethality   in terms of the choice of method used, this term refers to the probability that a person who attempted suicide will try again; the more lethal the method, the higher the probability.

Libido   one's psychic energy; a term coined by Freud.

Lifestyle   the manner in which one is accustomed to living.

Limit setting   the process of establishing firm limits with an individual as well as the sanctioning of behavior if the client does not comply with the limits.

Loose associations   when one thought does not connect to another or does not make any logical sense; frequent manifestation of schizophrenia.

Malingering   deliberate manufacturing of an illness in order to prolong hospitalization.

Manipulation   the process by which one individual influences another individual to function in accordance with his needs without regard to the other's needs or goals.

Maturational crises   transitional periods of a person's life when he experiences a crisis condition related to a specific developmental period when certain tasks need to be mastered.

Meditation   the act of reflecting upon or pondering; contemplation.

Memory   the recall of past events or experiences.

Mental retardation   a term for mental deficiency or lack of normal development of intelligence.

Mental status   the level of a client's mental functioning in relation to a set of norms of intellectual processes, behavior, mood, degree of insight, level of awareness, etc.

Milieu   the total environment, emotional as well as physical.

Monoamine oxidase inhibitor (MAO)   antidepressant medications that inhibit the production of monoamine oxidase and are mood elevators.

Mood   an emotional state or feeling that influences one's personality and functioning.

Mourning   a time when one experiences the loss of another; when the mourning period is completed, the loss is resolved.

Multiple personality   dissociative reaction in which the client develops several personality systems, complete and separate from the other or primary personality. Requires long-term reintegrative therapy.

Musculo   pertaining to the muscles.

Musculoskeletal   pertaining to the muscles and the skeleton.

Narcissism   the love of one's self excessively in a childish or infantile fashion.

Narcotics   the group of drugs that have analgesic and euphoria-producing qualities; usually addictive.

Nausea   inclination to vomit, usually preceding emesis.

Negative reinforcement   the process of removing or extinguishing a particular behavior by the application of a negative stimulus.

Negativism   a strong resistance to suggestions coming from others.

Neologism   a term that refers to the coining of a new word, as seen in schizophrenia.

Neurotic disorders   now termed anxiety disorders; the individual experiences a high level of anxiety that results in maladaptive behaviors with no distortion of reality.

Noncompliance   failure of the client to adhere to the prescribed treatment or plan of care.

Nonverbal communication   communication of a message without the use of words; may involve gestures, body position, movement, actions, etc.

Nurse Practice Act   the state law that defines and limits the practice of nursing; the components of the law must be followed by all licensed nurses in that state.

Nursing diagnosis the judgment of a professional nurse in terms of administering nursing care to a designated client; a statement of the nursing problem which may or may not be the same as the medical diagnosis.

Nursing process the problem-solving or decision-making process used by nurses as their primary unifying framework for nursing knowledge; includes the five-step process of assessment, analysis, planning, implementation and evaluation.

Obsession a persistent repetitive and unwanted thought.

Operant conditioning modification of behavior through the application of learning theory principles, antecedents and consequences.

Organic based on structural alterations, gross or microscopic.

Orientation the process of relating the self to time, place, person, and situation.

Overt discernible; out in the open.

Pain a sensation in which a person experiences discomfort, distress, or suffering.

Panic the extreme level of anxiety where a person may experience disintegration of the personality and complete loss of control.

Paranoia feelings of suspicion and persecution; unconscious mechanism of projection where client projects own thoughts to others.

Parapsychology study of experiential and alternative psychology; often considered outside the five senses and paranormal.

Parasympathetic nervous system a division of the autonomic nervous system that regulates acetylcholine and conserves energy expenditure; it slows down the system.

Parataxic a term coined by Sullivan to mean distorted perception.

Passive-aggressive the covert or indirect expression of hostility or anger.

Perception the process of receiving and interpreting sensory impressions.

Perspective subjective evaluation of relative significance; a view.

Phenothiazines a group of antipsychotic medications used to control the manifestations of schizophrenia.

Phobia the dread of an object, an act, or a situation that is not realistically dangerous but that has come to represent a danger.

Premorbid personality the status of an individual's personality (conflicts, defenses, strengths, weaknesses) before the onset of clinical illness.

Pressure the act of bearing down; exerting force against.

Primary gain the decrease of anxiety that results from certain measures the client uses to cope with high anxiety level.

Primary thought process unconscious thought processes kept from awareness through repression.

Professional an individual who acts in a prescribed manner according to accepted doctrines that are mastered as a result of advanced study or specialization in a field.

Projection the defense mechanism by which one transfers impulses, thoughts or wishes that belong to oneself to another person.

Psyche a term meaning the mind or the mental and emotional "self."

Psychogenic originating within the psyche or mind. Sometimes used to describe physical disorders that are believed to stem from the emotions.

Psychosis major impairment of ego functioning, especially reality-testing; grave maladjustment to everyday life.

Psychosomatic pertaining to phenomena that are both physiological and psychological in origin.

Rape defined legally as the forcible perpetration of the act of sexual intercourse on the body of a woman.

Rapport a feeling of mutual trust and harmony experienced by persons in a satisfactory relationship.

Rationalization justification of behavior by a reason that person believes will be socially approved and will be more advantageous.

Reality testing a function of the ego that determines the reality of experience; validation of what is objectively there.

Refer to send or direct someone for action or help.

Regression reverting to types of behavior characteristic of an earlier level of development.

Relationship an interaction of individuals over a period of time.

Relaxation a lessening of tension or activity in a part of the body.

Resistance a mechanism an individual employs to prevent certain ideas or feelings from coming into consciousness.

Resolution the state of having made a firm determination; a course decided upon.

Restitution a return to a former status.

Role playing assuming roles and acting out a particular situation to increase one's understanding and insight into that situation.

Schizoid a term used to describe a form of personality disorder characterized by an unsocial, withdrawn, shy type of personality.

Schizophrenia the form of psychotic disorder that manifests by the person losing touch with reality, becoming withdrawn, acting inappropriately and manifesting disordered thought processes.

Seclusive a term describing persons who are unsociable, reserved, secretive, and adverse to interacting with people.

Secondary gain advantages that occur as the result of particular behaviors that do not have to do with the primary gain of a decrease in anxiety; attention and sympathy from others.

Self-actualization the process of developing and fulfilling one's potential.

Self-concept the picture one holds of himself that encompasses his beliefs, attitudes, and convictions about himself.

Self-esteem a sense of pride in oneself or self-love.

Senility refers to impaired intellectual functioning in the aged; a nonspecific and nonmedical term that is usually derogatory.

Separation anxiety anxiety that occurs in children when they are separated from their parents and experience a loss.

Shock a term used to designate a clinical syndrome with varying degrees of disturbances of oxygen supply to the tissues.

Social involvement with communities and other persons.

Soma a term meaning body.

Somatic referring to the body.

Somatic delusion the false belief that something is wrong with one's body or body part.

Stamina constitutional energy; strength; endurance.

Stress a nonspecific response of the body to any internal or external event or change that impinges on a person's system and creates a demand.

Stressor a specific demand that gives rise to a coping response.

Substance abuse the use of any agent that alters the mind or body to the extent that it interferes with daily functioning.

Suicide death inflicted by oneself.

Suicide attempt any action an individual takes that has as its goal his own death.

Superego a Freudian term referring to a system within the total psyche that is developed by incorporating parental standards such as moral values; the two components of superego are *conscience* and *ego ideal*.

Support to lend strength or give assistance to.

Suppression the conscious elimination from one's awareness of thoughts that are uncomfortable.

Sympathetic nervous system a division of the autonomic nervous system that controls energy expenditure and mobilizes for action when confronted with a threat.

Synergistic the reaction between two or more substances that enhance the effect of both agents on the body.

Tachycardia abnormal rapidity of heart action, above 100 beats/minute.

Tangential speech a manner of speaking that is off target or off the original point.

Tardive dyskinesia side effect of antipsychotic medication; involves unfocused movement of the extremities and contractions of the muscles.

TENS a noninvasive method to relieve pain that involves stimulation to the skin via a mild electric current.

Therapeutic having medicinal or healing properties; a healing agent.

Touch a tactile sense.

Tranquilizer a drug that acts to reduce tension and anxiety without interfering with normal mental activity.

Transference the unconscious process of attributing feelings toward the therapist that originally belong to a significant person in the client's past life.

Tricyclics a group of drugs that act as antidepressants on the body.

Unconscious a Freudian term that refers to the part of the mind where mental activity is always going on, although not on a conscious level.

Understanding to perceive and comprehend the nature and significance of; to know.

Undoing a defense mechanism aimed at removing a painful memory.

Unique being the only one of its kind.

Validate to substantiate or verify.

Value clarification the method of discovering and exploring one's own values.

Values concepts that a person believes in and holds worthy; developed from past experience.

Verbal communication the transmission of a message through spoken or written means.

Voluntary admission the form of admission to a psychiatric hospital where the person signs himself in and agrees to receive treatment.

Waxy flexibility a condition associated with catatonic schizophrenia, where a posture is maintained for long periods of time.

Wellness a state of physical, psychological, and sociological well-being of a whole person. Synonym for health.

Withdrawal to pull back or away.

Word salad communication characterized by jumbled words; no coherent message.

8

GERONTOLOGICAL NURSING

This chapter presents fundamental material on the aging segment of our population. In the 1990's, this group will increase to over 30 million and most members will require some form of medical and nursing care. This chapter covers general concepts of aging and demographics including health care costs; how the body systems age; diseases common to the aged; and the most common medical-nursing problems that the elderly experience. The focus is on nursing assessment and implementaton.

GENERAL CONCEPTS OF AGING

General Concepts

A. Aging is an *individual* process.
B. Most older persons view their health as a positive state.
C. Coping with life has been successful because the person has "survived" to be old.
D. "Normal" aging may be confused with disease process in aging persons.
   1. Illness is frequently misdiagnosed as "normal" aging.
   2. Because of "decline" due to "normal" aging, symptoms are neglected by family and medical personnel.
   3. Older persons under-report symptoms of illness as they interpret symptoms as "growing older."
E. Most older persons have more than one chronic disease.

Definitions Relating to the Elderly

A. Gerontology: Scientific study of the process of aging; examining the changes that occur as a person ages; study of the needs of the elderly.
B. Aging: Process of growing older; physiological changes in body systems as the person grows older; a biological/physiological process influenced by emotional state and social context.
C. Life span: Maximum potential for survival of a species.
D. Life expectancy: Amount of time lived from birth to death.
E. Frail old: Person 75 years of age or older with some impairment in ability to provide functional self-care.
F. Gerontological nursing: Use of the nursing process in caring for the physiological, psychological, and sociological needs of the aging person.

Classification of Aging

A. Middle age: 40–61 years of age.
B. Young old: 61–70 years of age.
C. Middle old: 70–80 years of age.
D. Very old: 80–90 years of age.
E. Old old: 90+ years of age.

Demographics

A. There are predicted to be 28 million persons (13 percent of the U.S. population) over the age of 65 by the turn of the century.
   1. The post-World War II "baby boom" babies will reach senior status around the year 2010.
   2. The number of persons over 65 years of age is projected to double by 2030.
B. Average life expectancy in 1986 has increased to 74.9, over 74.7 years of age in 1985.
   1. White females live approximately 7.5 years longer than white males.
   2. Black females live approximately 14 years longer than black males.
   3. White females live approximately 5.5 years longer than black females.
C. Human potential life span is estimated to be 115 years.
D. Increased life expectancy due to:
   1. Advanced health care.
   2. Decreased infant/child mortality.
   3. Improved nutrition and sanitation.
   4. Increased infectious disease control.
E. Median income for an older female was $6,425 in 1986.
F. Most live in urban or rural settings.
G. About 50 percent are high school graduates.
H. About 50 percent have convenient access to senior service centers, but a low number use these centers.
I. 2–10 percent are alcohol abusers.

Health Care Costs

A. Government spending for health care of the elderly has doubled in the last twenty years.
   1. Health care services are used more by the aged person.
   2. The older the age of the person, the longer the stay in the hospital.
   3. Older persons personally pay one-fourth of the cost of the health care they utilize.
B. 5–6 percent of the aged live in nursing homes.
   1. 22 percent over age 85 are in nursing homes.
   2. Before death, 20–27 percent of the aged use institutional care.
C. Nursing home residents have an average of 3.9 diseases.
   1. Over 40 percent have more than one illness.
   2. Diseases may be multiple and chronic.

D. 18 percent of the elderly die at home.

E. Institutional placement most often results from a lack of social support as families become exhausted with caregiving.

Morbidity and Mortality

A. Causes of death (in order of frequency): heart disease, cancer, stroke, COPD, pneumonia/flu, diabetes, suicide.

B. Three out of four elderly people die of heart disease, cancer, or stroke.
  1. Heart disease is leading cause of death, although it has declined since 1968.
  2. Death rates from cancer continue to rise, especially lung cancer.
  3. Death statistics for people in the 65–74 age group:
     a. Heart disease accounted for 38 percent.
     b. Cancer, 30 percent of deaths.

C. Leading chronic conditions for elderly.
  1. Arthritis 44%
  2. Hypertensive disease 39%
  3. Heart conditions 27%
  4. Hearing impairments 28%
  5. Visual impairments.
  6. Dementia.

D. Objectives to maintain vitality and independence of people age 65 and older (1989 Year 2000 Objectives, U.S. Department of Health and Human Services).
  1. Increase average active life expectancy.
  2. Reduce proportion of noninstitutionalized people age 65 and older.
  3. Reduce incidence of adverse drug reactions.
  4. Reduce suicide deaths.
  5. Reduce hip fractures.
  6. Reduce influenza-associated deaths.
  7. Reduce pneumonia-related days of restricted activity.
  8. Reduce certified heat-related deaths.

Theories on Aging

A. Biological.
  1. Cellular. As cells are damaged there is instability in the body.
     a. Free Radical. Oxidation releases chemicals that affect the cell membrane and DNA replication.
     b. Cross-Link. Chemical bondage of elements that are generally separated.
     c. Doubling/Biological Clock. A cell has a genetically predetermined number of replications (Hayflick's theory).
     d. Stress. Homeostatic imbalance causes wear and tear on the organism.
     e. Error Catastrophic. Transcription errors in the RNA and DNA leading to cell mutation which is perpetuated.
  2. Immunity. The thymus and bone marrow become less functional so the body is less protected.

B. Psychological.
  1. Adaptation to stress. Genetic make-up and personal learning to deal with life crisis.
  2. Life experience.
     a. Disengagement. The person and society let go of each other.
     b. Dependence. Reliance on others for satisfaction of physical and emotional needs.

C. Sociological.
  1. Cultural and role expectation. Relates to adaptation/dependence when defining level of activity/behavior/wellness.
  2. Environment: toxins and pollutants.

NURSING PROCESS IN CARING FOR THE AGED PERSON

Systems Assessment

A. Priority—determine individual's capacity for safe, functional self-care.

B. Utilize multidimensional approach to provide basis for individualized care plan.
  1. Physiological.
     a. Structural changes, normal and abnormal.
     b. Signs of chronic illness.
     c. Signs of medication effects.
  2. Psychological.
     a. Mentation.
     b. Motivation.
     c. Needs.
  3. Sociological.
     a. Usual and preferred living arrangements.
     b. Status of social network and caregiving.

C. Assess altered presentation of data.
  1. Complex interrelationship between aging,

chronic, and acute illness.

   2. Signs and symptoms of illness—atypical or lacking.

Systems Analysis

A. Differentiation of normal aging vs disease process.

B. Differentiation of depression vs dementia.

C. Differentiation between real vs imagined social isolation.

Systems Planning

A. Safe environment.

B. Maximize functional self-care capacity.

C. Safe procedures for the frail elderly.

D. Set priorities.
   1. Client may be content with situation as it is.
   2. Encourage change, but do not force it.
   3. Safety is a major concern.

E. Inform client of plan of care.
   1. Afford adequate time for input.
   2. Write out all plans and schedules.

F. Needs of client and family.
   1. Involve the client and his family in planning.
   2. Enlist cooperation of other health care professionals.

Systems Implementation

A. Perform and/or supervise needed care.

B. Support level of self-functioning to maintain independence.

C. Maintain safety precautions.
   1. Siderails when in bed.
     a. Watch for disorientation when awakens.
     b. Prevent falls, due to weakened muscles.
     c. Prevent orthostatic hypotension.
   2. Bed in low position when not giving direct client care.
   3. Handrails in bathrooms and halls.
   4. Uncluttered rooms and floors.
   5. Adequate, nonglare lighting.
   6. Restraints when necessary.

D. Provide psychosocial care.
   1. Encourage psychological activity to aid sense of normality.
   2. Encourage verbalization about the past.
   3. Assist in selecting and attending activities.
   4. Foster touching, which is a very useful tool in establishing trust.
   5. Provide dignity and the feeling of worth.
   6. Foster the wellness approach to life.

E. Teach family how to help/cope.

Systems Evaluation

A. Client maintains functional and independent lifestyle.

B. Consistent nursing actions prevent further problems and promote health.

THE AGING BODY

Physiological Implications

A. Physical changes.
   1. Decrease in physical strength and endurance.
   2. Decrease in muscular coordination.
   3. Tendency to gain weight.
   4. Loss of pigment in hair and skin.
   5. Increased brittleness of the bones.
   6. Greater sensitivity to temperature changes with low tolerance to cold.
   7. Degenerative changes in the cardiovascular system.
   8. Decreased sensory faculties.
   9. Decreased resistance to infection, disease, and accidents.

B. Intellectual impairment.
   1. Estimated 10 percent of Americans over age 65 suffer impairment.
   2. 3 million diagnosed as senile.
   3. 20 percent of these, condition can be reversed.
   4. Drugs and poor nutrition contribute to this deterioration.

Psychological Implications

A. Fears about losing job—focus for living.

B. Competition with younger generation.

C. Relationships change.
   1. Loss of nurturing functions within family.
   2. Role change within and outside of family.

D. Loss of spouse, particularly females.

E. Realization that person is not going to accomplish some of the things that he or she wanted to do may lead to depression.

F. Physiological changes in body.

G. Changes in body image.

H. Illness.

I. Fears of approaching old age and death.

Developmental Tasks of the Elderly

A. Maintains ego integrity versus despair (Erikson).
   1. Integrity results when an individual is satisfied with his or her own actions and lifestyle, feels life is meaningful, remains optimistic, and continues to grow.
   2. Despair results from the feeling that he or she has failed and that it is too late to change.

B. Continues a meaningful life after retirement.

C. Adjusts to income level.

D. Makes satisfactory living arrangements with spouse.
   1. Adjusts to loss of spouse.
   2. Maintains social contact and responsibilities.

E. Faces death realistically.

F. Provides knowledge and wisdom to assist those at other developmental levels to grow and learn.

G. Developmental process retrogresses.
   1. Increasing dependency.
   2. Concerns focus increasingly on self.
   3. Interests may narrow.
   4. Needs tangible evidence of affection.

Sociological Implications

A. Major fears of the aged.
   1. Physical and economic dependency.
   2. Chronic illness; high percentage of elderly have chronic problems.
   3. Loneliness.
   4. Boredom resulting from not being needed.

B. Major problems of the aged.
   1. Economic deprivation.
      a. Increased cost of living on a fixed income.
      b. Increased need for costly medical care.
      c. Poverty rate for persons age 65 and over is 12.4 percent.
         (1) Women, blacks, Hispanics, and those who live alone are poorest.
      (2) Major source of income is social security (35 percent).
      d. Median income of couples age 65 and older is $22,000 (1986 statistics).
   2. Chronic disease and disability.
   3. Loneliness and social isolation.
      a. Suffer losses of friends.
      b. Men die earlier, so many women are on their own.
         (1) Five times more women than men are widowed.
         (2) Half of older women are widows.
   4. Blindness.
   5. Organic brain changes.
      a. Not all persons become senile.
      b. Most people have memory impairment.
      c. The change is gradual.

C. Death in the life cycle.
   1. In American culture death is not considered a positive process.
   2. Elderly may see death as an end to suffering and loneliness.
   3. Death is not feared if the person has lived a long and fulfilled life, having completed all developmental tasks.
   4. Religious beliefs and/or philosophy of life important.

D. Elderly may provide knowledge and wisdom from their vast experiences, which can assist those at other developmental levels to grow and learn.

E. Approximately 30 million people will be over the age of 65 in the United States by 1990.

General Physiological Changes

A. Cells.
   1. Fewer in number.
   2. Larger in size.
   3. Decreased total body fluid due to decreased intracellular fluid.

B. The ear.
   1. Presbycusis (sensorineural hearing loss).
      a. Progressive hearing loss in inner ear.
      b. High frequency tones are lost first.
      c. Sounds are distorted; difficulty understanding words when other noises in background.
      d. Present in 50 percent of those over age 65.
   2. Tympanic membrane atrophic, sclerotic.
   3. Cerumen accumulates; may become impacted

due to increased amount of keratin.
C. The eye.
1. Presbyopia—vision impairment caused by diminished power of accommodation from loss of elasticity of lens.
2. Pupil sphincter sclerosis with loss of light responsiveness.
3. Cornea more spherical.
4. Lens more opaque.
5. Increased light perception threshold.
   a. Adapt to darkness more slowly.
   b. Difficulty seeing in dim light.
6. Loss of accommodation.
7. Decreased visual field; less peripheral vision.
8. Decreased color discrimination on blue/green end of scale.
9. Distorted depth perception.
10. Glare intolerance.
11. Reduced lacrimation.
D. Vital Signs.
1. Increased systolic blood pressure.
2. Increased diastolic blood pressure.
3. Heart rate remains unchanged.
4. Respiratory rate unchanged.
5. Core temperature unchanged.
6. Prone to hypothermia.
E. Mood.
1. Multiple losses.
2. Neurological changes.
3. Loss of environment and interpersonal stimuli.
4. Defense mechanisms less effective.

Baseline Assessment

A. Temperature.
1. May be as low as 95°F.
2. Sublingual most accurate.
3. Easily dehydrated with increased temperature.
B. Pulse.
1. Rate, rhythm, volume.
2. Apical, radial, pedal, other sites as indicated by disorder.
C. Respirations.
1. Rate, rhythm, depth.
2. Irregularity common.
D. Arterial blood pressure.
1. Lying, sitting, standing.
2. Postural hypotension common.
3. Hypertension (160/95 or greater).

E. Weight—gradual loss in late years.
F. Orientation level.
G. Memory.
H. Sleep pattern.
I. Psychosocial adjustment.
1. Depression.
2. Paranoia.
3. Loneliness.
4. Increasing dependency.
5. Concerns focus increasingly on self.
6. Displays narrower interests.
J. Immunization history.
K. General appearance.
1. Gray and thinning hair.
2. Wrinkled, pigmented, and thin skin.
3. Eyes slightly sunken.
4. Ears/nose appear slightly larger.
5. Respond more slowly to questions and directions.
6. Recent memory impaired; slower recall.
7. Trunk thicker; thinner arms and legs.
8. Gait slower and less steady.
9. Slower movements.
10. Possible slight tremor.
11. Flexion of spine/limbs.

Neurological System

Physiological Age Changes

A. Decreased speed of nerve conduction.
B. Delay in response and reaction time, especially with stress.
C. Diminution of sensory faculties.
1. Decreased vision.
2. Loss of hearing.
3. Diminished sense of smell and taste.
4. Greater sensitivity to temperature changes with low tolerance to cold.

Assessment

A. Facial symmetry.
B. Poor reflex reactions.
C. Level of alertness—presence of organic brain changes.
1. Not all persons become senile.
2. Most people have memory impairment.
3. Change is gradual.
4. Potential for accidents, falls.
D. Malnutrition—dehydration.

E. Eyes: movement, clarity, presence of cataracts.
  1. Level of blindness.
  2. Pupils: equality, dilation, construction.
  3. Visual acuity—decreases with age.
      (a) Do not test vision while client is facing window.
      (b) Use hand-held chart.
      (c) Check condition of glasses.
F. Sensory deprivation—understimulation.
G. Hypothermia.
H. Hearing acuity
  1. Hearing aid.
  2. Tinnitus.
  3. Cerumen in outer ear—do not clean.
I. Presence of pain.

Implementation

A. Maintain safety precautions.
  1. Evaluate reflex reactions to protect against accidents.
  2. Evaluate level of alertness.
B. Monitor dietary intake and fluid intake.
C. Provide adequate lighting.
  1. Natural lighting best.
  2. Avoid glare.
  3. Night light at all times in bathrooms, halls.
D. Encourage sensory stimulation.
  1. Large print books.
  2. Changes in environment.
  3. Colors client can see.
E. Maintain reality orientation.
  1. Calendars.
  2. Clocks.
  3. One-to-one visits.
F. Keep client warm—prevent hypothermia.

Cardiovascular System

Physiological Age Changes

A. Mitral and aortic valves thicken and become rigid.
B. Cardiac output decreases one percent per year after age 20 due to decreased heart rate and stroke volume.
C. Vessels lose elasticity.
  1. Less effective peripheral oxygenation.
  2. Position change from lying-to-sitting or sitting-to-standing can cause blood pressure to drop as much as 65 mm Hg.
D. Increased peripheral vessel resistance.

  1. Blood pressure increases: systolic may normally be 170, diastolic may normally be 95.
  2. Smooth muscle in arteries is less responsive.
E. Blood clotting increases.

Assessment

A. Peripheral circulation, color, warmth.
  1. Apical pulse.
  2. Jugular vein distention.
B. Orthostatic hypotension
  1. Dizziness.
  2. Fainting.
C. Edema.
D. Activity intolerance.
  1. Weakness.
  2. Fatigue.
E. Dyspnea.
F. Transient Ischemic Attacks (TIA's)
G. Anemia.

Implementation

A. Monitor vital signs—pulse, blood pressure.
B. Monitor medications—digitalis, diuretics, etc.
C. Maintain dietary restrictions (low salt).
D. Change position slowly, especially from horizontal to vertical, to prevent hypotensive reaction.
E. Maintain circulatory homeostasis.
  1. Encourage activity to increase circulatory stimulation.
  2. Provide warmth by applying blankets and clothing.
  3. Use gentle friction during bath.
  4. Avoid tight/restrictive clothing.

Respiratory System

Physiological Age Changes

A. Respiratory muscles lose strength and become rigid.
B. Ciliary activity decreases.
C. Lungs lose elasticity.
  1. Residual capacity increases.
  2. Larger on inspiration.
  3. Maximum breathing capacity decreases; depth of respirations decreases.
D. Alveoli increase in size, reduce in number.
  1. Fewer capillaries at alveoli.
  2. Dilated and less elastic alveoli.
E. Gas exchange is reduced.

1. Arterial blood oxygen PaO_2 decreases to 75 mm Hg at age 70.
2. Arterial blood carbon dioxide $PaCO_2$ unchanged.

F. Coughing ability is reduced—less sensitive mechanism.

G. Decline in immune response.

H. More dependent on the diaphragm for breathing.

I. System less responsive to hypoxia and hypercardia.

Assessment

A. Chest excursion.

B. Lung/breath sounds.

C. Quality of cough, if present; sputum.

D. Rib cage deformity.

E. Dyspnea, hypoxia, and hypercarbia.

F. Need for oxygen therapy.

G. Activity intolerance.

H. Anxiety.

Implementation

A. Manage airway clearance.
  1. Clean nares if nasal passages are clogged.
  2. Postural drainage, if necessary.

B. Monitor hydration status.

C. Promote respiratory activity with exercises.
  1. Deep breathing.
  2. Forced expiration.
  3. Coughing.

D. Monitor oxygen therapy.
  1. Caution: check for carbon dioxide narcosis.
  2. Symptoms: confusion, profuse perspiration, visual disturbance, muscle twitching, hypotension, cerebral dysfunction.

Gastrointestinal System

Physiological Age Changes

A. Tooth loss.
  1. Periodontal disease is major cause of loss after 30 years of age.
  2. Other causes include poor dental health, poor nutrition.

B. Taste sensation decreases.
  1. Chronic irritation of mucous membranes.
  2. Atrophy of up to 80 percent of taste buds.
  3. Lose sensitivity of those on tip of tongue first: sweet and salt.
  4. Lose sensitivity of those on sides later: salt, sour, bitter.

C. Esophagus dilates, decreased motility.

D. Stomach.
  1. Hunger sensations decrease.
  2. Secretion of hydrochloric acid decreases.
  3. Emptying time decreases.

E. Peristalsis decreases and constipation is common.

F. Absorption function is impaired.
  1. Body absorbs less nutrients due to reduced intestinal blood flow and atrophy of cells on absorbing surfaces.
  2. Decrease in gastric enzymes affects absorption.

G. Hiatal hernia common (40–60 percent of elderly).

H. Diverticulitis (40 percent over age 70).

I. Liver.
  1. Fewer cells with decreased storage capacity.
  2. Decreased blood flow.
  3. Enzymes decrease.

J. Impaired pancreatic reserve.

K. Decreased glucose tolerance.

Assessment

A. Tooth loss—poor dentition, inadequate chewing, poor swallowing reflex.

B. Condition of teeth, gums, buccal cavity.

C. Dietary intake—malnutrition.
  1. Anorexia; nausea and vomiting.
  2. Regurgitation.
  3. Anemia.

D. Indigestion, heartburn, pain, indications of possible hiatal hernia.

E. Bowel problems.
  1. Constipation.
  2. Distention, impaction.
  3. Diarrhea.

F. Drug toxicity.

Implementation

A. Stimulate appetite.
  1. Small, frequent feedings of high quality.
  2. Attractive meals, wine if allowed.
  3. Female, 1600 calories; male, 2200.
  4. Preferred foods if possible; ethnic choices.

B. Lessen/prevent indigestion.
  1. Fowler's position for meals.
  2. Antacids contraindicated.
  3. Plan meals.
    a. Smaller meals without gas formers.
    b. Low fat.

    c. Avoid chocolate, cola, coffee—foods that cause distress.

    4. Adequate fluids.

C. Prevent constipation.

    1. Ensure adequate bulk and fluid in diet.

    2. Encourage activity.

    3. Ensure regular and adequate time for bowel movement.

    4. Provide privacy and normal positioning.

    5. Administer laxative or suppository if above not effective.

Genitourinary System

Physiological Age Changes

A. Kidneys.

    1. Smaller due to nephron atrophy.

    2. Renal blood flow decreases 50 percent.

    3. Glomerular filtration rate decreases 50 percent.

    4. Tubular function diminishes.

        a. Less able to concentrate urine; lower specific gravity.

        b. Proteinuria 1 + is common.

        c. Blood urea nitrogen, BUN, increases to 21 mg%.

    5. Renal threshold for glucose increases.

B. Bladder.

    1. Muscle weakens.

    2. Capacity decreases to 200 ml or less, causing frequency.

    3. Emptying is more difficult, causing increased retention.

C. Prostate enlarges to some degree in 75 percent of men over age 65; hypertrophy.

D. Menopause occurs by mean age of 50.

E. Perineal muscle weakens.

F. Vulva atrophies.

G. Vagina.

    1. Mucous membrane becomes dryer.

    2. Elasticity of tissue decreases, so surface is smooth.

    3. Secretions become reduced, more alkaline.

    4. Flora changes.

H. Sexuality.

    1. Older people continue to be sexual beings with sexual needs.

    2. No particular age at which a person's sexual functioning ceases.

    3. Frequency of genital sexual behavior (inter-course) may tend to decline gradually in later years, but capacity for expression and enjoyment continue far into old age.

Assessment

A. Dehydration, fluid intake and output.

B. Drug toxicity.

C. Urine: appearance, color, odor.

D. Bladder: frequency, urgency, hesitancy.

    1. Distention.

    2. Incontinence.

E. Nonspecific signs: fever, vomiting, dysuria, lower abdominal discomfort, hematuria for possible asymtomatic urinary tract infection.

F. Sexuality.

    1. Vaginal irritation.

    2. Painful coitus.

Implementation

A. Adequate fluid intake: 2000-3000 ml daily.

B. Incontinence prevention.

    1. Offer opportunity to void every two hours.

    2. Keep night light in bathroom to prevent falls.

    3. Schedule diuretics for maximum effect during daylight hours.

    4. Limit fluids near and at bedtime.

C. Sexuality.

    1. Provide counseling if desired.

    2. Provide opportunity for desired sexual expression.

    3. Encourage touching and companionship, which are important for older people.

Musculoskeletal System

Physiological Age Changes

A. Contractures.

    1. Muscles atrophy, regenerate slowly.

    2. Tendons shrink and sclerose.

B. Range of motion of joints decreases.

    1. Lack of adequate joint motion, ankylosis.

    2. Slight flexion of joints.

C. Mobility level.

    1. Ambulate with or without assistance or devices.

    2. Limitations to movement.

    3. Muscle strength lessens.

    4. Gait becomes unsteady.

D. Kyphosis.

E. Intervertebral discs narrow.

F. Trunk length decreases by 1.2 cm.

G. Redistribution of subcutaneous fat to abdomen/hips.

H. Bone changes.
   1. Loss of trabecular bone.
   2. Lose density/fat content.
   3. Become brittle.

I. Degeneration of the extrapyramidal tract.

Assessment

A. Backward tilt of head (kyphosis).

B. Hips, knees, and wrists more flexed.

C. Decreased height (thinning discs).

D. Decreased movement; impaired mobility.

E. Muscle cramps and/or tremors.

F. Pain.

G. Stiff and enlarged joints.

H. Frequent falls.

Implementation

A. Ambulate within limitations.

B. Alter position every two hours; align correctly.

C. Prevent osteoporosis of long bones by providing exercises against resistance.

D. Provide active and passive exercises.
   1. Rest periods necessary.
   2. Paced throughout the day.

E. Provide range-of-motion exercises to all joints three times a day.

F. Educate family that allowing the client to be sedentary is not helpful.

G. Encourage walking, which is best single exercise for the elderly.

Integumentary System

Physiological Age Changes

A. Skin less effective as barrier.
   1. Decreased protection from trauma.
   2. Less ability to retain water.
   3. Decreased temperature regulation.

B. Skin composition changes.
   1. Dryness (osteotosis) due to decreased endocrine secretion.
   2. Loss of elastin.
   3. Increased vascular fragility.
   4. Thicker and more wrinkled on sun exposed areas.
   5. Melanocyte cluster pigmentation.

C. Sweat Glands.
   1. Decreased number and size.
   2. Decreased function of sebaceous glands.

D. Hair.
   1. General hair loss.
   2. Decreased melanin production.
   3. Facial hair increases in women.

E. Nails more brittle and thick.

Assessment

A. Skin.
   1. Temperature, degree of moisture, dryness.
   2. Intactness, open lesions, tears, decubiti.
   3. Turgor, dehydration.
   4. Pigmentation alterations, potential cancer.
   5. Pruritus—dry skin most common cause.

B. Bruises, scars.

C. Condition of nails (hard and brittle).
   1. Presence of fungus.
   2. Overgrown or horny toenails; ingrown.

D. Condition of hair.

E. Infestations (scabies, lice).

Implementation

A. Bathing can minimize dryness.
   1. Have client take complete bath only twice a week.
   2. Use superfatted soap or lotions to aid in moisturizing.
   3. Use tepid, not hot, water.
   4. Apply emollient (lanolin) to skin after bathing.

B. Clip facial hairs for female clients if desired.

C. Handle gently to prevent skin tears.

D. Cut toenails unless contraindicated.
   1. Mycosis of nails.
   2. Certain medical/surgical conditions, such as diabetics, may require special order.

Endocrine System

Physiological Age Changes

A. Production of most hormones is reduced.

B. Parathyroid function and secretion are unchanged.

C. Pituitary decreases in weight and changes in cell type proportion. Significance is undetermined.
   1. Growth hormone present, but in lower blood levels.
   2. Reduced ACTH, TSH, FSH, LH production.

D. Reduced thyroid activity.
   1. Decreased basal metabolic rate.

2. Reduced I_{131} uptake.
E. Reduced aldosterone production.
F. Reduced gonadal secretion of progesterone, estrogen, testosterone.

DISEASES COMMON IN THE AGED

Dementia

Definition: An impairment in cognitive function manifested by long- and short-term memory loss with impaired judgment, abstract thinking, and behavior, resulting in self-care deficit.

Characteristics

A. Etiology is unknown.
B. Incidence is 1.2 million in the U.S. over age 65; 10–20 percent of the population.
C. Leading cause of institutionalization in older people. Of 1.3 million nursing home residents, one-half to two-thirds have some form of cognitive impairment.
D. A leading cause of death (120,000 annually).
E. Cost to society is $30 billion annually.
F. 10–21 percent of dementias are pseudodementia-reversible.
G. Possible causes of false senility.
   1. Drug side effects: most common are lithium, barbiturates, atropine, bromides.
   2. Depression.
   3. Nutritional deficiency.
   4. Toxins: air pollution and alcohol.
   5. Heavy metals: lead and mercury.
   6. Diseases, e.g., metabolic disorders, multiple sclerosis, hyperthyroidism, anemia, hypoglycemia.
H. Irreversible dementia: gradual onset with a progressive course.
   1. 50–70 percent are Alzheimer type (most common).
   2. 15–25 percent are multi-infarct or vascular type.
   3. Other types include Parkinson's disease, alcohol abuse.

Diagnosis

A. Diagnostic criteria—must meet one criteria numbered 1 through 5.

1. Sufficiently severe loss of intellectual abilities that interfere with social or occupational functioning.
2. Memory impairment, usually short-term memory.
3. Impairment of abstract thinking or impaired judgment; disturbance of higher cortical function or personality change.
4. Cloudy state of consciousness.
5. Presence of a specific organic etiology or presumed presence.
B. Onset slow, insidious, unrelated to specific situation.
C. Gradual degeneration.
D. Mental status examination shows poor reality orientation, confusion, lack of understanding, etc.
E. History reveals symptoms.
   1. Onset slow, progressive decline.
   2. Personality changes, withdrawn.
   3. Confusion noted by others but not by client.
   4. Early in the disease will attempt to find the right answer; later will not understand question.
   5. Unaware of memory loss.
      a. Begins with recent memory loss.
      b. Later there are problems with coding and retrieving information.
   6. Oblivious to failures.
F. Possible predisposing factors: genetic, familial history of Down's Syndrome, enzyme deficiency, immune system deficiency, aluminum toxicity, acetylcholine deficiency (a neurotransmitter).

Assessment

A. Adequate physical health; usually not affected.
B. Intellectual impairment.
   1. Alertness.
   2. Orientation.
   3. Appropriate responses to questions.
   4. Aphasia, may produce words but not sentences.
   5. Does not recognize staff or family.
C. Behavior.
   1. Performance of grooming and hygiene tasks gradually diminish.
   2. Cooperative.
   3. Distracted.
   4. Agitated.
   5. Paranoid, delusions.
   6. Restless.
   7. Wandering behavior (stimulus, "sundowners").
D. Motor responses.
   1. Stability of gait (motor ability declines).

2. Functional position of limbs/joints.
E. Condition of skin.
F. Bowel and bladder function—incontinent.

Implementation

A. Provide safe environment to prevent falls, unsafe wandering.
B. Monitor medications.
   1. Give lowest dose of antipsychotic (one-fourth the dose of a middle-aged adult).
   2. Evaluate effect of antipsychotic, antidepressant, anti-anxiety medication.
C. Use clear, verbal communication techniques.
   1. Short words, simple sentences, verbs, and nouns.
   2. Call client by name and identify yourself.
   3. Speak slowly, clearly; wait for response.
   4. Ask only one question, give one direction at a time.
   5. Repeat, do not rephrase.
D. Use nonverbal communication.
   1. Approach in a calm, friendly manner.
   2. Use gestures, move slowly.
   3. Stand directly in front of client, maintain eye contact.
   4. Move or walk with client; do not try to stop.
   5. Listen actively; show interest.
   6. Chart all phrases and nonverbal techniques used and use those that "work."
E. Monitor activities of daily living.
   1. Orient to environment and activity on a "here and now" basis.
   2. Provide consistent routine with activities.
   3. Remind how to perform self-care activities as dressing, eating, toileting.
   4. Avoid tasks that tax the memory.
   5. Give tasks that distract and occupy as listening to music, coloring, watching TV.
F. Maintain the client's physical activity within limits of safety.
   1. Walk outside if grounds are fenced, alarmed, or if accompanied.
   2. Dance.
   3. Exercises with simple commands.
   4. Active games.
   5. Balance activities.
   6. Activities of daily living.
G. Provide mental stimulation.
   1. Simple hobbies.
   2. One-to-one contact.

3. Reality orientation.
4. Play word, number games.
H. Use consistent staff to provide care; change is frightening.
I. Encourage self-care, give cues. Pantomime brushing teeth instead of brushing client's teeth.
J. Put families in touch with support groups such as Alzheimer's Disease and Related Disorders Assoc., Inc., chapters (ADRDA).

Depression

Definition: A mood disorder dominated by sadness, gloomy attitude, hopelessness, and a lack of pleasure in life.

Characteristics

A. 13 percent of older generation are depressed; 1–2 percent suffer from major depression.
B. Most commonly ignored disorder in the elderly.
C. 15 percent of the elderly suffer from this problem (double the normal population).
D. Often mistaken for "hardening of the arteries" or other type of dementia.
E. Depression leads to other major problems, increasing the susceptibility to disease.
   1. Undernourishment.
   2. Dehydration.
   3. Inactivity.
   4. Self-neglect.

Assessment

A. History of depression.
   1. Loss of interest in life.
   2. Sense of hopelessness and sadness.
   3. Difficulty sleeping.
   4. Weight loss due to loss of interest in food.
   5. Fatigue.
   6. Reduced sexual desire.
B. History of multiple losses.
   1. Death of a spouse, friends.
   2. Loss of job-related challenges and focus.
   3. Loss of normal physical functioning.
   4. Loss of social interaction and contacts; isolation.
   5. Loss of self-esteem.
C. Complaints of memory loss.
D. Complaints of physical pain.
E. Drug side-effects.

F. Potential suicide risk—high incidence in the older population.
 1. With depression comes high risk for suicide.
 2. Number in men is 46 per 100,000 (1986 statistics).
 3. Most significant risk factor is recent loss of significant relationship.
 4. Assess for specific cues related to suicide.
  a. Hopeless talk about the future.
  b. Hints: "Things will change soon."
  c. Relates plan for ending life.

Implementation

A. Implement safety precautions for suicide risk (see section on Depression in Psychiatric Nursing chapter).
B. Establish daily activities to reinforce positive experiences.
 1. Give some area of control or power to person.
 2. Provide variation in daily schedule but not too many changes, as change is anxiety-producing for the elderly.
C. See specific nursing interventions for depression in Psychiatric Nursing chapter.

Hip (femoral neck) Fracture

Definition: Fracture at femoral neck can result in avascular necrosis; death of the bone due to insufficient blood supply–occurs most frequently in elderly women.

Characteristics

A. Usually results from a fall in the elderly.
B. Directly related to loss of bone strength due to osteoporosis.
C. People over 65 account for 87 percent of hip fracture cases.
 1. More than 249,000 occur each year.
 2. Most are women.
D. One in five hip fracture clients dies of complications.
E. Personal and social consequences for the elderly.
 1. Restriction of daily activities can result in depression, complications, etc.
 2. Hospitalization adds financial burden, dependence.

Assessment

A. Assess for pain, tenderness or muscle spasm over fracture site or in groin.
B. Assess for lateral rotation and shortening of leg with minimal deformity.
C. Degree of disability.
D. Elimination problems.
E. Nutritional status.
F. Emotional reaction to immobility.
G. Degree of support from family.

Implementation

A. Operative Procedure.
 1. Femoral head replacement–surgical fixation with nails, pins, or screws.
 2. Occasional total hip replacement.
B. Preoperative Care.
 1. Provide care as given to clients in skin traction.
 2. Observe for elimination regularity.
 3. Teach coughing and deep breathing. Encourage isometric exercises and use of overhead trapeze.
 4. Maintain proper positioning—splinting injured leg with pillows on unaffected side.
 5. Assist client with eating; nourishing diet essential for healing process.
C. Postoperative Care.
 1. Turn client from unaffected side to back as routine, turn every two hours; a physician's order is required to turn from side to side.
 2. Turn client with hip prosthesis by always placing pillows between legs to avoid adduction.
 3. Elevate head, may be limited to 30 to 40 degrees to avoid acute hip flexion.
 4. Introduce quadricep and gluteal setting muscle exercises; encourage use of overhead trapeze for assistance in moving.
 5. Take measures to protect client when moving from bed to chair (client not to bear weight on affected leg).
 6. Provide routine postoperative measures to ensure client's comfort.
 7. Take measures as necessary to prevent complications.
  a. Avascular necrosis of femoral head.
  b. Nonunion.
  c. Pin complications.
  d. Dislocation of prosthesis.

Urinary Incontinence

Definition: Involuntary release of urine of such

severity as to have social and/or hygienic consequences.

Characteristics

A. 10 million adults are incontinent—over half the residents of nursing homes and one-third of elderly living at home are affected.
B. Prevalence rises with age.
C. This condition is not a normal consequence of aging; it is a symptom signaling the presence of other problems.
D. Types.
 1. Stress incontinence—result of sudden increase in intra- abdominal pressure which pushes urine out of the bladder.
 2. Urge incontinence—leakage of urine before one reaches the toilet usually caused by uncontrolled contraction of the bladder.
 3. Overflow incontinence—constant dribble of urine results when bladder is not completely emptied during voiding.
 4. Functional incontinence—nonorganic; impaired mobility, depression, and dementia can prevent client from reaching bathroom.

Treatment

A. Pelvic floor muscle exercises (Kegel exercises) and behavioral training (biofeedback).
B. Drug therapy.
 1. Anticholinergic (Pro-Banthine).
 2. Antispasmodic (Ditropan) inhibit bladder contractions.
C. Surgery to strengthen pelvic muscles, repair a damaged urethra, remove an obstruction.

Assessment

A. Assess pattern of problem—see types of incontinence.
 1. Decreased bladder tone/volume.
 2. Muscle tone—urgency and frequency.
B. Presence of other problems, disease states, or change in physical health.
 1. Congestive heart failure.
 2. Urinary tract infection.
 3. Pneumonia.
 4. Stool impaction.
C. Effects of medication(s).
D. Environmental problems.
 1. Access to toilet.
 2. Restraints.
 3. Privacy.
 4. Response of staff/family.
E. Skin condition.
F. Emotional coping in relation to the problem.

Implementation

A. Provide appropriate skin care.
B. Establish toileting schedule.
 1. Easy access.
 2. Appropriate clothing, client's own, if possible.
C. Assist client to learn Kegel exercises.
 1. Will help to control stress and urge for incontinence.
 2. Steps are to contract pubococcygeus muscle, hold contraction for 10 seconds, relax for 10 seconds. Work up to 25 repetitions 3 times a day.
D. Provide protection-plan for accidents.
 1. Accidents are embarrassing and often limit excursions and social activities.
 2. Prevent problems and avoid disrupting client's life.
E. Devise ways to build client's self-esteem.
 1. Positive reinforcement.
 2. Plan activities that client can enjoy.

Impaired Mobility-Disability

Definition: The elderly can suffer impaired mobility and disability due to decreased physical function and/or accidents.

Characteristics

A. Nearly 23 percent of older people living in the community have some degree of disability.
 1. Those 85 and older constitute a disproportionate share of those who are dependent in physical functioning.
 2. Those 85 and older constitute 27 percent of those who have impaired mobility.
B. Impaired mobility can lead to many subsequent problems: depression, negative self-image, dependent behavior, loss of independence, etc.
C. Effects of disability.
 1. Impact upon the individual's body image.
 a. Physical appearance.
 b. Bodily sensations.
 2. Behavior during reaction period.
 a. Appears confused and disorganized.
 b. Denies disability exists.

c. Overreacts to situations and physical condition.
d. Assumes false positive attitude.
e. Becomes self-centered.
f. Becomes depressed.
g. Mourns loss of function or body part.
3. Adaptation and adjustment.
a. Revises body image by modifying former picture of self.
b. Reorganizes values.
c. Accepts degree of dependency.
d. Accepts limitations imposed by disability.
e. Begins to develop realistic goals.

Assessment

A. Specific source of disability or impaired mobility.
B. Presence of accompanying disease state: arthritis, stroke, dementia, diabetes, CHF, COPD.
C. Strength and function of limbs and joints.
D. Stability of gait.
E. Presence of pain.
F. Condition of skin.
G. Drug effects—sedation, incontinence, orthostatic hypotension.
H. Motivation for rehabilitation.
I. Nutritional status.
J. History of falls.

Planning

A. Strive for optimal function.
B. Prevent further injury or complications.
C. Restore normal function.
D. Accept philosophy underlying rehabilitative nursing.
1. Rehabilitation begins with initial contact.
2. Every illness has intrinsic threat of disability.
3. Principles of rehabilitation are basic to care of all clients.

Implementation

A. Develop nursing care plan to meet client's needs.
B. Focus on disability or impaired mobility.
C. Establish supportive relationship.
D. Teach activities of daily living.
1. Activities which must be accomplished each day for individual to care for own needs and be as independent as possible.
2. Ascertain best assistive aid for client.
3. Demonstrate and encourage individual to

practice.
4. Increase activities as individual progresses and is able to assume activity.
5. Give positive reinforcement for all effort expended.
E. Prevent deformities and complications.
1. Turn and position in good alignment.
a. Prevent contractures.
b. Stimulate circulation.
c. Prevent thrombophlebitis.
d. Prevent decubiti.
2. Prevent edema of extremities.
3. Promote lung expansion.

Types of Exercise for Rehabilitation

A. Passive.
1. Carried out by the therapist or nurse without assistance from client.
2. Purpose—retain as much joint range of motion as possible, and maintain circulation.
B. Active assistive.
1. Carried out by the client with assistance of therapist or nurse.
2. Purpose—encourage normal muscle function.
C. Active.
1. Accomplished by the individual without assistance.
2. Purpose—increase muscle strength.
D. Resistive.
1. Active exercise carried out by the individual working against resistance produced by manual or mechanical means.
2. Purpose—provide resistance in order to increase muscle power.
E. Isometric or muscle setting.
1. Performed by the individual without assistance.
2. Purpose—maintain strength in a muscle when a joint is immobilized.
F. Range of Motion (ROM).
1. Movement of a joint through its full range in all appropriate planes.
2. Purpose–maintain joint mobility and increase maximal motion of a joint.
3. Nursing care.
a. Assess general condition of client.
b. Establish extent of ROM before present condition.
c. Discontinue ROM at point of pain.
4. Deterrents to ROM exercises: fear and pain.

Use of Aids/Devices

A. Cane.
   1. Purpose.
      a. Provide greater stability and speed when walking.
      b. Relieve pressure on weight-bearing joints.
      c. Provide force to push or pull body forward.
   2. Safety factors.
      a. Handle at level of greater trochanter.
      b. Elbow flexed at 25 to 30 degree angle.
      c. Light-weight material.
      d. Rubber suction tip.
   3. Techniques for walking with cane.
      a. Hold cane close to body.
      b. Hold in hand on unaffected side.
      c. Move cane at same time as affected leg.
B. Crutches.
   1. Purpose—provide support during ambulating when lower extremities unable to support body weight.
   2. Safety factors.
      a. Measure $1\frac{1}{2}$ to 2 inches from axillary fold to floor (4 inches in front and 6 inches to side of toes).
      b. Hand piece adjusted to allow 30 degree elbow flexion.
      c. Rubber suction tips on crutches.
      d. Well-fitting shoes with nonslip soles.
   3. See gait sequence on page 265.
C. Tilt table.
   1. Board or table that can be tilted gradually from a horizontal to a vertical position.
   2. Purpose.
      a. Assist individual to gradually adjust to upright position.
      b. Start weight-bearing activities.
      c. Increase standing tolerance.
      d. Prevent disuse syndrome.
      e. Prevent demineralization of bones.
D. Prosthesis—artificial replacement for a missing body part.
E. Brace—support that protects or supports weakened muscles.

Infections in the Elderly

A. Older clients more susceptible to infection—diminished resistance.
B. Important to recognize high risk clients.
C. Diseases that contribute to high risk.
   1. Diabetes mellitus.
   2. Congestive heart failure.
   3. Malignancy—double risk due to chemotherapy depressing the immune system.
   4. Renal failure.
D. Conditions that make clients prone to infection.
   1. Dehydration.
      a. Fluid depletion—skin more penetrable by pathogens.
      b. Thick mucosal secretions—coughing more difficult.
      c. Monitor fluid intake—1,500–2,500 cc daily.
   2. Bed confinement.
      a. Increases risk of renal infection by causing urine backflow through ureters up into kidneys.
      b. Voiding while bedridden increases pressure on bladder, adds to risk of urinary tract infection.
      c. To minimize risk, assist client to sit when voiding, if possible.
   3. Poor skin turgor; less effective as barrier to trauma.
      a. Less resistance to friction increases risk of decubitus ulcers.
      b. Maintaining nutrition and fluid intake lessens risk.
   4. Bowel problems lower resistance.
      a. Constipation may lead to intestinal obstruction and perforation.
      b. Prevention—fiber rich fruits and vegetables, whole grain breads and cereals.
E. When infection develops.
   1. Older person may not show fever (baseline may be low so slight increase is not noted).
      a. Take baseline rectal temperature.
      b. Before insertion, thermometer must register below 95°F, 35°C.
   2. Lower temperature only when it goes above 104°F.
      a. Fever inhibits bacterial and viral growth; new studies indicate fever is curative until it reaches seizure or delirium level—105°F.
      b. Evaluation of antibiotic therapy (fever drops) is more accurate without antipyretic.
   3. Older clients more susceptible to adverse effects of antibiotics.
      a. Hearing loss—especially with isoniazid and amnioglycosides.

b. Vertigo with amnioglycosides.

c. Monitor BUN and creatinine levels to check for nephrotoxicity.

d. Diarrhea (ampicillin, tetracycline, chloramphenicol)—leads to electrolyte imbalance.

COMMON PROBLEMS FROM IMMOBILITY

Pressure Ulcers

Definition: Localized areas of necrosis of skin and subcutaneous tissue due to pressure.

Characteristics

A. Cause—pressure exerted on skin and subcutaneous tissue by bony prominence and the object on which body rests.

B. Predisposing factors.
 1. Malnutrition.
 2. Anemia.
 3. Hypoproteinemia.
 4. Vitamin deficiency.
 5. Edema.

C. Common sites: bony prominence of body such as sacrum, greater trochanter, heels, elbows, etc.

Assessment

A. Stage of ulcer.

B. Identify if infection is associated with decubitus ulcer.

C. Effectiveness of ulcer treatment.

D. Healing process of the ulcer.

E. Other bony prominence for potential formation of decubiti.

F. Presence of conditions that inhibit wound healing.

Implementation

A. Prevention.
 1. Relieve or remove pressure.
 2. Stimulate circulation.
 3. Keep skin dry.

B. Positioning.
 1. Encourage client to remain active.
 2. Change position frequently.

C. Maintain good skin hygiene; inspect frequently.

D. Provide for active and/or passive exercises.

E. Use alternating air pressure mattress, etc.

F. Use sheepskin padding.

G. Provide for adequate nutritional intake.

External Rotation of Hip

Definition: Outward rotation of hip joint.

Characteristics

A. Cause—lying for long periods of time on back without support to hips.

B. Incorrect positioning in bed.

Implementation

A. Trochanter roll extending from crest of ilium to midthigh when positioned on back.

B. Frequent change of position.

C. Proper positioning.

Footdrop

Definition: Tendency for foot to plantar flex.

Characteristics

A. Causes.
 1. Prolonged bed rest.
 2. Lack of exercise.
 3. Weight of bed clothing forcing toes into plantar flexion.

B. Complications.
 1. Individual will walk on his toes without touching heel on ground.
 2. Unable to walk.

Implementation

A. Prevention.
 1. Position feet against footboard.
 2. Use footcradle to keep weight of top linen off toes.
 3. Provide range of motion exercises.

B. Check that soles of feet are against footboard to prevent permanent footdrop.

Contractures

Definition: Abnormal shortening of muscle, tendon, or ligament so joint cannot function properly.

Characteristics

A. Cause—improper alignment, lack of movement.

B. Result is decrease in mobility and joint movement.

Implementation

A. Proper alignment at all times.
 1. Use pillows.
 2. Provide supportive splints.
B. Provide for range of motion exercises.

Bladder Dysfunction

Definition: When an individual is unable to void and the reflex act of micturition (urination) cannot occur.

Characteristics

A. Causes.
 1. Disease process.
 2. Lack of innervation.
 3. Lack of motivation.
B. Treatment will involve bladder retraining, surgery, drugs.

Implementation

A. Bladder training—purpose.
 1. Prevent urinary tract infection and preserve renal function.
 2. Keep individual dry and odor free.
 3. Help individual maintain social acceptance.
B. Procedure.
 1. Set up specific time to empty bladder.
 2. Give measured amounts of fluids.
 3. Position in normal voiding position.
 4. Instruct how to Credé bladder.
 5. Keep record of amount and time of intake and output.
 6. Encourage client to wear own clothing, particularly underwear.

Bowel Dysfunction

Definition: Normal elimination does not occur due to a structural problem or disease state.

Characteristics

A. Cause.
 1. Disease process.
 2. Inadequate intake.
 3. Poor prior habits.
B. Treatment involves surgery, dietary modifications, or drugs.

Implementation

A. Identify purpose of bowel training.
 1. Develop regular bowel habits.
 2. Prevent fecal incontinence, impaction, and/or irregularity.
B. Implement nursing procedure.
 1. Establish specific time.
 2. Provide for adequate roughage and fluid intake.
 3. Use normal posture.
 4. Instruct to bear down and contract abdominal muscles.
 5. Provide privacy and time.
 6. Provide exercise.

Hypostatic Pneumonia

Definition: Inflammatory process in the lungs in which alveoli fill with exudate.

Characteristics

A. Incidence.
 1. Very young, very old.
 2. Debilitated.
 3. Immobile.
B. Cause—stasis of secretions in lungs.

Implementation

A. Prevention.
 1. Assess lung function.
 2. Encourage deep breathing, coughing.
 3. Turn every two hours.
 4. Ensure adequate hydration.
B. Provide for postural drainage, if indicated.
C. Administer oxygen, as ordered.
D. Monitor antibiotic therapy.

PROBLEM AREAS FOR ELDERLY CLIENTS

Sensory Impairment

A. Elderly experience loss of function in the senses.
 1. Ability to taste declines after age 40; taste buds are fewer in number and there is less saliva flow.
 2. Ability to smell declines.
 3. Hearing fades, especially in high frequency ranges.

4. Regulation of body temperature in less efficient.

B. Major diseases or degeneration of organs occurs.
   1. Vision loss—see section on page 133 for Nursing Implications.
      a. Glaucoma—increased pressure causes damage to optic nerve, leading to blindness.
      b. Cataracts—clouding of the lens leading to blurred vision.
      c. Retinal detachment.
   2. Hearing loss—see section on page 134 for Nursing Implications.
      a. Otosclerosis requiring a stapedectomy.
      b. Hearing loss due to accumulation of ear wax—requires periodic irrigation of auditory canal.

Nutrition

A. Physiological requirements do change (decrease) with age.
   1. Nutrition intake must meet two major demands.
      a. Normal structural repair.
      b. Energy production for functional needs.
   2. Met by protein and amino acids and adequate calorie intake.
B. Many elderly are deficient in nutrients, especially protein, B vitamins, Vitamins A and C, iron, and calcium.
   1. Change in diet often responsible.
      a. Sense of taste and smell decreases, thus less conscious of hunger.
      b. Teeth in poor condition or dentures don't work properly.
      c. Physical disabilities or lack of mobility, unable to buy groceries.
      d. Loss of interest in eating.
      e. Limited income affects buying nutritious food.
   2. System cannot assimilate nutrients as well as when younger.
      a. Reduced hydrochloric acid, reduced stomach activity.
      b. Decreased salivary flow.
C. Health status affects nutritional state.
   1. Chronic diseases: heart disease, cancer, diabetes, gastro-intestinal problems, etc.
   2. Drugs: antacids, antidepressants, anticonvulsants, cathartics, diuretics, antimicrobials, etc.
D. Decreased physical activity and metabolic changes reduce caloric needs.
E. Financial resources, emotional, and physical state affect nutritional status.

Assessment

A. Hydration status, body weight, edema.
B. Anemia.
C. Appetite.
D. Ability to feed self—physical and mental.
   1. Dentition.
   2. Mastication.
   3. Swallowing.
   4. Desire to eat.
E. Fatigue, energy reserve.
F. Constipation.
G. Compliance to special diets.
H. Effects of drugs on nutrition.
   1. Gastrointestinal irritation.
   2. Food-drug interactions.
   3. Some drug side effects are nausea and vomiting.
I. Skin and mucous membrane condition.

Implementation

A. Offer/give oral fluids in small amounts every hour.
B. Plan diet to be high in nutrients.
   1. Give foods with high fiber.
   2. Balance of vitamins and minerals.
   3. Use lemon, vinegar, herbs on foods (rather than salt) to stimulate appetite.
C. Devise tools and plates which assist self-feeding.
D. Serve meals with others present to reduce isolation.

Medications

A. 25 percent of all prescriptive drugs are used by the elderly, and this does not include over-the-counter drugs.
B. 80 percent of people age 65 and over have at least one chronic medical problem that requires medications (one-third have three or more chronic problems).
C. Typical elderly American takes between 4 and 7 prescription drugs each day in addition to over-the-counter drugs.
D. Elderly (13 percent of the population) suffer 50 percent of all drug side effects (estimated 17 per 100,000 population).
   1. Increased risk for drug toxicity.
      a. Renal excretion altered—kidneys cannot process drugs as well.
      b. Liver enzymes altered.
      c. Diminished blood circulation to liver.
      d. Receiving multiple drugs that compete for

binding and interact.

  e. CNS more sensitive to drugs.
    (1) Drugs interfere with neurotransmitters (chemicals) that regulate brain function.
    (2) Side effects result in confusion in elderly.
  f. Altered body mass and ratio of fat to muscle.
 2. Iatrogenic illness can be caused by drug therapy.
 3. Most commonly abused drugs by the elderly.
    a. Tranquilizers most frequently abused.
    b. Sleeping pills.
    c. Medications to control pain.
    d. Laxatives.
E. Major problems with prescriptive drugs in the elderly.
 1. Drug interactions—people who use multiple physicians and pharmacies run risk of taking drugs that interact to cause adverse reactions.
 2. Medication errors—the more medications a person takes, the greater the risk of medication error (people over age 75 take an average of 17 prescriptions annually).
 3. Noncompliance—not taking right dose at right time or discontinuing drug without consultation; common due to lack of understanding about reason to take drug and general knowledge base of drug action.
 4. Unpredictable drug action—physiological changes in the elderly associated with age and disease may alter effects of the drugs.
 5. Drug side effects not recognized—elderly not aware or do not understand potential dangerous side effects of drugs.
 6. Inadequate monitoring—elderly often alone or not monitored consistently so drug problems are not identified.
 7. Cost of drugs—multiple medications are costly for many elderly, so they stop taking drugs.

Administration of Medications

A. Oral route.
 1. Check for mouth dryness.
    a. Drug may stick and dissolve in mouth.
    b. Drug may irritate mucous membrane.
 2. Place client in sitting position.
 3. Crush tablets if they are very large.
 4. Do not open capsules.
 5. Do not crush enteric-coated tablets.
 6. Check with pharmacy for liquid preparations if

client has difficulty swallowing tablets.
B. Suppository.
 1. Position for comfort.
 2. May take longer to dissolve due to decreased body core temperature.
 3. Do not insert suppository immediately after removing from refrigerator.
C. Parenteral.
 1. Site may ooze medication or bleed due to decreased tissue elasticity.
 2. Do not use immobile limb.
 3. Danger of overhydration with IV.
D. Self-administration.
 1. Check compliance with amounts and times.
 2. Color code to facilitate proper administration.

Assessment

A. Changes in mental status.
B. Vital signs.
 1. Orthostatic blood pressure.
 2. Apical pulse.
C. Urine production, retention.
D. Hydration and appetite.
E. Visual disturbances.
F. Swallowing ability.
G. Evaluate effects of drug.
 1. Laboratory studies.
 2. Signs and symptoms for toxic/interaction effects of drugs.
H. Bowel function.
I. Effects of nutrition and foods on drug response.

Implementation

A. No alcohol or alcohol based elixirs when receiving benzodiazepines or antihistamines.
B. Method of administering drugs.
 1. Deep breathing and relaxation to reduce use of analgesic drugs.
 2. Position client sitting with head slightly flexed to reduce chance of aspiration.
C. Administering tablets.
 1. Do not crush time-released or enteric-coated tablets.
 2. Crush large tablets if not contraindicated.
 3. Give with textured foods (nectar, applesauce) if not contraindicated.
D. Stroke victim—give drug on functional side of mouth.

Drug-Food Interactions for Elderly

A. Foods and vitamin-minerals can interfere with therapeutic effects of drugs.
   1. Reduce absorption of drug.
   2. Interfere with cellular action.
B. Medication regimen affected by nutrition may put client at risk.
   1. Important to assess client's diet.
   2. Monitor potential vitamin/drug interactions.
C. Review client's prescriptive and over-the-counter drugs.
   1. Review in relation to normal dietary intake.
   2. Consider vitamin-mineral intake and supplements in terms of decreasing effect of medications.
   3. Check lab values for problems.
D. Document findings so health-care team is informed of diet-drug plan.
E. Food sources of vitamins and minerals.
   1. Folic acid sources: liver, kidney, fresh vegetables.
   2. Niacin sources: yeast, meat, fish, milk, eggs, green vegetables, and cereal grains.
   3. Pantothenic acid sources: meat, vegetables, cereal grains, legumes, eggs, milk, fish, and fruit.
   4. Pyridoxine hydrochloride (Vitamin B_6) sources: cereal grains, legumes, vegetables, liver, meat, and eggs.
   5. Cyanocobalamin (Vitamin B_{12}) sources: animal foods, liver, kidney, fish, shellfish, meat, and dairy foods.
   6. Ascorbic acid (Vitamin C) sources: fresh fruits and vegetables.
   7. Vitamin A sources: eggs, milk, cream, butter, organ meats, fish.
   8. Vitamin D source: activated in body by sunlight.
   9. Vitamin E sources: vegetables oils, whole grains, animal fats, eggs, and green vegetables.
   10. Vitamin K sources: green leafy vegetables, spinach, broccoli, cabbage, and liver.

Lab Values in the Elderly

Urinalysis

A. Protein.
   1. Normal 0–5 mg/100 ml—rises slightly.
   2. May reflect changes in kidney or subclinical urinary tract infection.
B. Glucose.
   1. Normal 0–15 mg/100 ml—declines slightly.
   2. May reflect changes in kidney.
C. Specific gravity.
   1. 1.032—decline to 1.024 by age 80.
   2. 30–50 percent decline in number of nephrons affects ability to concentrate urine.

Hematology

A. Hemoglobin.
   1. Men 13–18 g/100 ml—drops 10–17 g/100 ml.
   2. Women 12–16 g/100 ml—no change.
B. Hematocrit.
   1. Men 45–52 percent—no change.
   2. Women 37–48 percent—no change.
C. Leukocytes.
   2. 4,300–10,800/cu mm—drops to 3,100–9,000/cu mm.
   2. As bone marrow diminishes, hematopoiesis declines.
D. Lymphocytes.
   1. 500–2,400/cu mm—T-lymphocytes fall.
   2. 50–200/cu mm—B-lymphocytes fall.
E. Platelets, prothrombin time (PT) and partial thromboplastin time (PTT) no change.

Blood Chemistry Tests that Change with Age

A. Blood urea nitrogen (BUN).
   1. Men 10–25 mg/100 ml—increases, may be as high as 69 mg/100 ml.
   2. Women 8–20 mg/100 ml—increases.
   3. Renal function decreased due to decline in cardiac output, renal blood flow, and glomerular filtration rate.
B. Creatinine.
   1. 0.6–1.5 mg/100 ml—increases as high as 1.9 mg/100 ml in men and women.
   2. Endogenous creatinine production as lean body mass shrinks.
   3. Drugs excreted by urinary system may cause toxicity if creatinine level too high.
C. Creatinine clearance.
   1. 104–125 ml/min.
   2. Referenced interval: men's formula for age: 140 − age × Kg body weight divided by 72 × serum creatinine.
D. Glucose tolerance.
   1. One hour: 160–170 mg/100 ml.

Two hours: 115–125 mg/100 ml.

Three hours: 70–110 mg/100 ml.

2. With age, results rise more quickly in first two hours, then drop to baseline more slowly.

3. Alcohol, MAO inhibitors, and beta blockers can all cause a rapid fall in glucose.

E. Thyroxine (T_4) 4.5–13.5 mcg/100 ml and triiodothyronine (T_3) 90–220 mg/100 ml both decrease by 25 percent.

Prescription for Long Life and Good Health

A. Regular exercise—elderly must continue to exercise regularly to maintain health (can increase function by 50 percent through exercise).

B. Nutritious diet—intake of adequate nutrients and calories to maintain body.

1. Malnutrition in elderly contributes to high incidence of chronic disease.

2. Obesity contributes to increased health risks (heart disease, hypertension).

3. Diet adequate to maintain normal body weight, low-fat and include all four food groups for minimal nutrients, vitamins and minerals.

C. No smoking—smokers die earlier than nonsmokers and have a higher incidence of heart disease, heart attack, cancer and chronic lung disease.

D. Moderate alcohol intake; high alcohol intake is a health risk that leads to liver disease, nervous system damage, gastrointestinal problems.

E. Prevention of health problems—yearly physical examinations are important for the elderly to diagnose early disease process.

1. Check warning signs of cancer, heart disease (hypertension).

2. Pap smear and mammogram for women as precaution against cancer.

F. Managing stress–stress is associated with increased incidence of heart disease, hypertension, cancer and other diseases.

G. Maintain contact with friends for support; studies show that isolated elders have more health problems and die earlier than people who have close attachments.

Gerontological References

A Profile of Older Americans. American Association of Retired Persons. Washington, DC, 1987.Calkins, Evan, et al. *The Practice of Geriatrics*. Philadelphia: W.G. Saunders Company, 1986.Burnside, Irene. *Nursing and the Aged Roman*. New York: McGraw-Hill Book Company, 1988.Carnevali, Doris, et al. *Nursing Management for the Elderly*. Philadelphia: J.B. Lippincott Company, 1979.Eliopoulos, Charlotte. *Gerontological Nursing*. Philadelphia: J.B. Lippincott Company, 1987.Kane, Robert, et al. *Essentials of Clinical Geriatrics*. New York: McGraw-Hill Book Company, 1984.Matteson, Mary-Ann, et al. *Gerontological Nursing*. Philadelphia: W.B. Saunders Company, 1988.

9

LEGAL ISSUES IN NURSING

This chapter reviews important legal issues in nursing. Topics covered include the Nurse Practice Act, clients' rights, nurses' liability, key legal terms, drugs and the nurse, and grounds for professional misconduct. While the provisions of the Nurse Practice Acts are quite similar from state to state, it is imperative that the nurse knows the licensing requirements and the grounds for license revocation as defined by the state in which he or she works.

Legal and ethical standards for nurses are complicated by a myriad of federal and state statutes and the continually changing interpretation of them by the courts of law. Nurses are faced today with the threat of legal action based on malpractice, invasion of privacy, and other grounds. For self-protection, the nurse should remain alert to legal and ethical implications during the daily performance of nursing responsibilities.

NURSE PRACTICE ACT

Definition: A series of statutes enacted by each state legislature to regulate the practice of nursing in that state. Subjects covered by the Nurse Practice Acts include definition of scope of practice, education, licensure, grounds for disciplinary actions, and related topics. The Nurse Practice Acts are quite similar throughout the United States, but the professional nurse is held legally responsible for the specific requirements for licensure and regulations of practice as defined by the state in which he or she is working.

The Practice of Nursing

A. Professional nursing.
1. Responsibilities.
   a. Performance, for compensation, of a defined range of health care services including assessment, planning, implementation, and evaluation of nursing actions as well as teaching and counseling.
   b. Administration of medications and treatments as prescribed by a licensed physician or other designated licensed professional.
   c. Supervision of other nursing personnel.
2. Requirements: specialized skills taught by and acquired at an accredited nursing school.
B. Major functions of registered nurses.
1. Direct and indirect client care services.
2. Performance of basic health care, testing, and prevention procedures.
3. Observation of signs and symptoms of illness, treatment reactions, and general physical or mental conditions.
4. Documentation of nursing care.

Board of Registered Nursing (BRN)

A. Each state has a Board of Registered Nursing (or its equivalent) organized within the executive branch of the state government. Primary responsibilities of the BRN include administration of the state Nurse Practice Act as applied to registered nurses.
B. Functions of state Boards of Registered Nursing.
1. Establishing educational and professional standards for licensure.
2. Conducting examinations, registering, and licensing applicants.
3. Conducting investigations of violations of statutes and regulations.
4. Issuing citations and holding disciplinary hearings for possible suspension or revocation of licenses.
5. Imposing penalties following disciplinary hearings.
6. Formulating regulations to implement the Nurse Practice Act.

Authorization to Practice Nursing

A. To legally engage in the practice of nursing, an individual must hold an active license issued by the state in which he or she intends to work.
B. The licensing process.
1. The applicant must pass a licensing examination administered by the state Board of Registered Nursing, or the BRN may grant reciprocity to an applicant who holds a current license in another state.
2. The applicant for R.N. licensure examination must have attended an accredited state school of nursing, must be a qualified related nursing professional or para-professional, or must meet specified prerequisites if licensed in a foreign country.
3. Boards of Registered Nursing contract with the National Council of State Boards of Nursing, Inc., for use of the National Council Licensure Examination.

PROFESSIONAL MISCONDUCT AND POTENTIAL PENALTIES

Grounds for Professional Misconduct

A. Licensed professional nurses are regulated and disciplined by the state in which they work.
B. The practicing nurse should know how his or her state defines professional misconduct.
C. Common grounds for professional misconduct.
1. Obtaining R.N. license through fraudulent methods.

2. Practicing in an incompetent and/or negligent manner.
3. Practicing when ability to practice is impaired by mental or physical disability, drugs, or alcohol.
4. Being habitually drunk or being dependent on or a habitual user of drugs.
5. Conviction of or committing an act constituting a crime under federal or state law.
6. Refusing to provide health care services on the grounds of race, color, creed, or national origin.
7. Permitting or aiding an unlicensed person to perform activities requiring a license.
8. Practicing nursing while license is suspended.
9. Practicing medicine without a license.

Penalties for Professional Misconduct

A. Each state Board of Registered Nursing has the authority to impose penalties for professional misconduct.
B. Types of discipline include:
   1. Probation.
   2. Censure and reprimand.
   3. Suspension of license.
   4. Revocation of license.

NATURE OF THE LAW

Definition: A system of principles and processes by which people who live in a society deal with their disputes and problems. Laws are rules of human conduct.

Types of Laws

A. Criminal.
   1. The harm is against society and guilt requires proof beyond a reasonable doubt.
   2. Punishment may be a fine or imprisonment.
B. Civil.
   1. The harm is against another individual and guilt requires proof by a preponderance of the evidence.
   2. Punishment is generally the payment of monetary compensation.

Elements for Liability

A. There must be a legal basis such as statutory law for finding liability.
B. A causal relationship must exist between the harm experienced by the client and the act or omission to act by the nurse.
C. There must be some damage or harm sustained by the client.

Table 1. NURSING LIABILITY

Civil Law	Criminal Law
Contract	Assault and Battery
Unintentional Tort	Homicide
Intentional Tort	Murder
Negligence	Manslaughter

KEY LEGAL TERMS

Negligence

A. The key elements of negligence are based on:
   1. The duty of the nurse to provide clients with due care.
   2. A breach of that duty which is the cause of a compensatory injury to the client.
B. Malpractice is negligence on the part of a nurse, physician, or other health care professional.
C. Classifications of malpractice: criminal, civil, and ethical.

Liability

A. A nurse has a personal, legal obligation to provide a standard of client care expected of a reasonably competent professional nurse.
B. Professional nurses are held responsible (liable) for harm resulting from their negligent acts, or omissions to act.

Respondeat Superior

A. Legal doctrine that holds an employer liable for negligent acts of employees in the course and scope of employment.
B. Physicians, hospitals, clinics, and other employers may be held liable for negligent acts of their employees.
C. This doctrine does not support acts of gross negligence or acts that are outside the scope of employment.

Table. 2. CLASSIFICATIONS OF LAW RELATED TO NURSING

Classification	Example
Constitutional	Clients' rights to equal treatment
Administrative	Licensure and the state BRN
Labor Relations	Union negotiations
Contract	Relationship with employer
Criminal	Handling of narcotics
Tort	
Medical Malpractice	Reasonable and prudent client care
Product Liability	Warranty on medical equipment

RISK AREAS

Definition: Certain areas of practice that increase the risk of potential liability for the nurse because of increased nursing involvement, potential hazards involved in the nurse's functions and/or an increased social awareness on the part of clients and their families and associates.

Client's Rights

A. A right or claim may be moral and/or legal.
   1. A legal right can be enforced in a court of law.
   2. Within the health care system, all client's retain their basic constitutional rights such as freedom of expression, due process of law, freedom from cruel and inhumane punishment, equal protection, and so forth.
B. Client rights may conflict with nursing function.
   1. Key elements of a client's rights with which nurses should be thoroughly familiar include consent, confidentiality, and involuntary commitment.
   2. The client's right may be modified by his or her mental or physical condition as well as his or her social status.

Consent to Receive Health Services

A. Consent is the client's approval to have his or her body touched by a specific individual (such as doctor, nurse, laboratory technician).
   1. Types of consent: expressed or implied—verbal or written.
   2. Informed consent: prior to granting a consent, the client must be fully informed regarding treatment, tests, surgery, etc., and must understand both the intended outcome and the potentially harmful results.
   3. The client may rescind a prior consent verbally or in writing.
B. Authority to consent.
   1. A mentally competent adult client must give his or her own consent.
   2. In emergency situations, if the client is in immediate danger of serious harm or death, action may be taken to preserve life without the client's consent.
   3. Parents or legal guardians may give consent for minors.
   4. Court-authorized persons may give consent for mentally incompetent clients.
C. Voluntary admission.
   1. A person freely consents to enter an institution for purposes of receiving psychiatric care and treatment.
   2. Clients who enter on a voluntary basis may leave at will.
D. Involuntary admission.
   1. An individual may legally be admitted to an institution without his or her own consent when that individual does not have the mental

capacity or competency to understand his or her own acts.

2. Occurs when the client is judged by a court of law to be mentally ill or dangerous to him or herself and others, and to require admission to a psychiatric ward or center.

E. Nurse's liability.

1. The nurse who asks a client to sign a consent form may be held personally liable if the nurse knows or should know that the client has not been fully informed by the physicians, hospital staff, or others regarding potentially harmful effects of treatments, tests, surgery, and other acts.

2. Nurses must respect the right of a mentally competent adult client to refuse health care; however, a life-threatening situation may alter the client's right to refuse treatment.

Client's Right to Privacy

A. Confidential information.

1. Clients are protected by law (invasion of privacy) against unauthorized release of personal clinical data such as symptoms, diagnoses, and treatments.

2. Nurses, as well as other health care professionals and their employers, may be held personally liable for invasion of privacy as well as other torts should litigation arise from unauthorized release of client data.

3. Nurses have a legal and ethical responsibility to become familiar with their employers' policies and procedures regarding protection of client's information.

4. Confidential information may be released by consent of the client.

5. Information release is mandatory when ordered by a court or when state statutes require reporting child abuse, communicable diseases, or other incidents.

B. Client care: nurses have an ethical responsibility to protect the client's personal privacy during treatment or hospitalization by means of gowns, screens, closed doors, etc.

C. Medical records.

1. As the key written account of client information such as signs and symptoms, diagnosis, treatment, etc., the medical record fulfills many

functions both within the hospital or clinic and with outside parties.

a. Documents care given the client.

b. Provides effective means of communication among health care personnel.

c. Contains important data for insurance and other expense claims.

d. May be utilized in court in the event of litigation.

2. Nurses have a strong ethical and legal obligation to maintain complete and timely records, and to sign or countersign only those documents which are accurate and complete.

DRUGS AND THE NURSE

Definition: In their daily work, most nurses handle a wide variety of drugs. Failure to give the correct medication or improper handling of drugs may result in serious problems for the nurse due to strict federal and state statutes relating to drugs. (See Chapter Two for legal issues in drug administration.)

Regulation

A. The Comprehensive Drug Abuse Prevention Act of 1970 provides the fundamental regulations (federal) for the compounding, selling, and dispensing of narcotics, stimulants, depressants, and other controlled items.

B. Each state has a similar set of regulations for the same purpose.

Violation

A. Each state pharmacy act provides standards for dispensing drugs.

B. Noncompliance with federal or state drug regulations can result in liability.

C. Violation of the state drug regulations or licensing laws are grounds for BRN administrative disciplinary action.

LEGAL ISSUES IN PSYCHIATRIC NURSING

Note: Legal rights for both the psychiatric client and the community at large are an important aspect of psychiatric nursing.

Statutes of Protection

A. Laws of certain states protect individuals from themselves.
   1. These laws require that such persons be evaluated by competent psychiatric personnel.
   2. The laws protect the client's rights and civil liberties by not allowing psychiatric clients to be hospitalized inappropriately.
B. Laws also protect family members and the general community from persons who are dangerous or severely disturbed.

Admission Procedures

A. There are voluntary and involuntary admissions for psychiatric clients.
B. Voluntary admission occurs when an individual recognizes that he or she needs treatment and signs into a hospital.
   1. After admission, the client is *not* free to leave before a specified period of time.
   2. Such a client may leave the hospital against the physician's advice if the client gives notice of such intent at least one or two days prior to leaving.
   3. If the physician feels the client is too ill, he can legally assign the client to involuntary status.
   4. A voluntary client loses none of his or her civil rights.
C. Involuntary status occurs when the client is psychiatrically evaluated to be too ill to function outside the hospital.

   1. When a client is committed, he or she cannot leave the hospital against medical advice.
   2. Family members, a physician, a law officer, or a community member can institute commitment proceedings.
   3. Clients are permitted to leave only when psychiatric evaluation indicates they are able to care for themselves or are not dangerous to themselves or others.

NURSING MANAGEMENT: DELEGATION OF ACTIVITIES

A. Be familiar with the nurse practice act in your state.
   1. The nurse practice act is different in each state.
   2. Determined by state legislature.
B. The RN is legally responsible for client care.
   1. The LVN works with the RN, who initiates the nursing care plan; LVN may update care plan.
   2. RN validates assessment changes noted by LVN.
   3. RN is responsible for Nursing Assistant client care; RN assigns, directs, monitors, and evaluates care performed by NA.
C. Intravenous administration parameters vary by state.
   1. RN may initiate IVs and add medications.
   2. LVNs, depending on each state's standards, may not add medications to an IV, do IV push, or administer piggy-back solutions.
   3. LVNs may add vitamins and minerals in most states.
   4. LVN may initiate IV after completing IV course.
D. RN initiates client teaching and evaluates result.
   1. LVN may not initiate client teaching with exception of using standard care plan.
   2. LVN may reinforce client teaching.

SIMULATED NCLEX-RN CAT TEST

1. Ken White, age 86, has a fractured hip and his physician has applied Buck's traction preoperatively. Your assessment to ensure that there is adequate countertraction will include

(1.) Weights hanging freely off the floor and bed.
2. Ropes knotted to prevent them from moving through the pulleys.
3. Checking that the client is pulled down on the bed, using the end board as a foot rest.
4. Checking that the foot of the bed is elevated to provide countertraction.

2. You are supervising a student nurse giving an IM injection to a client with right hip arthroplasty. You will know the SN requires further instruction if she

1. Administers the injection in the left deltoid muscle.
(2.) Turns the client on her right hip to administer the injection.
3. Keeps the abduction pillow in place and turns the client 10 degrees to administer the injection on the unaffected side.
4. Administers the injection after turning the client to her left thigh, keeping the abduction pillow in place.

3. Suzie Whiting, age 14, will receive a Milwaukee Brace to correct for scoliosis, 24° curve. Reviewing her discharge instructions, you will know Suzie does not require more teaching when she says she will

(1.) Wear the brace all day and remove it only to bathe.
2. Wear the brace after school and at night.
3. Put the brace on a minimum of 1 hour 3 times per day.
4. Take off the brace if her skin gets sore or starts to break down.

4. You are the nurse assigned to Robin as her induction of labor is begun. After 20 minutes of the Pitocin infusion, you observe a contraction that does not relax after 90 seconds. Your first action is to

1. Notify the physician.
2. Turn the client on her left side.
3. Start oxygen by mask.
(4.) Discontinue the Pitocin infusion.

5. You are the RN in the emergency room that admits a 20-year-old woman who has been raped and suffered severe lacerations. Initially, your assessment should focus on the client's

1. Mental status.
(2.) Physical injuries.
3. Degree of crisis.
4. Ability to recount the incident.

6. John Andrews is scheduled for electroconvulsive therapy (ECT). You will do the client teaching. One important principle is to tell Mr. Andrews that

1. He will receive three types of medication.
(2.) When he wakes up, he may have some short-term memory loss for recent events.
3. This procedure will help his depression.
4. He will recover rapidly from the effects of the procedure.

7. A common test used to determine fetal status in the presence of preeclampsia is the NST (nonstress test). If this test is "reactive," it means that

1. It was normal, showing an increased fetal heart rate (FHR) with fetal movement.
2. It was normal, showing no change in FHR with fetal movement.
3. It was abnormal, indicating a need for an immediate Oxytocin challenge test (OCT).
4. Ultrasound is indicated to determine fetal habitat and placental placement.

8. You are assisting a client to choose a meal that follows his dietary orders of high calorie, high protein, decreased sodium, and low potassium. You will know he understands his dietary guidelines when he chooses

1. Crab, beets and spinach, baked potato, and milk.
2. Halibut, salad, rice, and instant coffee.
3. Sirloin steak, salad, baked potato with butter, and chocolate ice cream.
4. Salmon, rice, green beans, sourdough bread, coffee, and ice cream.

9. You are caring for a client who has had an Addisonian crisis. The priority goal of care should focus on

1. Keeping the client quiet.
2. Reestablishing fluid and electrolyte balance.
3. Monitoring vital signs.
4. Preventing infection.

10. The physician orders Meperidine hydrochloride IM q4h prn for a client in labor. Which phase of labor is the safest for the nurse to administer this medication?

1. Early active phase.
2. Active phase.
3. Transition phase.
4. Expulsion phase.

11. A nurse friend of yours is in her 1st trimester of pregnancy. While working in the hospital, you know that she should avoid

1. Any client with an infection.
2. A 3-month-old infant with a generalized rash.
3. A child with a fever and upper respiratory disorder.
4. A client who has just been diagnosed with lupus erythematosus.

12. Assessing reflexes of a 6-week-old infant, you would expect to find which of the following reflexes present?

1. Babinski's sign, neck righting reflex.
2. Moro's reflex, rooting reflex.
3. Sucking reflex, walking reflex.
4. Kernig's reflex, Moro's reflex.

13. Mrs. Tabber arrives in the emergency room. An initial assessment indicates that crowning is occurring. The first nursing action is to

1. Apply gentle perineal pressure to prevent rapid expulsion of the head.
2. Notify the physician.
3. Ask the client to push according to your instructions.
4. Instruct the client to take short shallow breaths to improve fetal oxygenation.

14. A client with Wernicke's encephalopathy is brought into the emergency room. The first physician's order you expect to carry out is

1. Thiamine 100 mg IM stat.
2. IV glucose.
3. IV glucose with vitamin B complex supplement.
4. IV Valium.

15. Using Leopold's maneuvers, the nurse assesses the presence of a firm round prominence over the pubic symphysis, a smooth convex structure on the client's right side, irregular structures on the left side and a soft roundness in the fundus. The nurse concludes that the fetal position is

1. Left occiput anterior—LOA.
2. Left occiput posterior—LOP.
3. Right occiput posterior—ROP.
4. Right occiput anterior—ROA.

16. You are the RN responsible for administering a thiazide medication to Mr. Barton. His recent lab reports are K⁺ 3.0 and NA⁺ 140. The correct intervention is to

1. Administer the thiazide drug.
2. Notify the physician.
3. Withhold the drug and report both lab results to the physician.
4. Withhold the drug and report K⁺ level to the physician.

17. In planning an elderly, senile client's schedule, it is most important that the daily activities

1. Are changed each day to meet the need for variety.
2. Provide many opportunities for making choices to stimulate involvement and interest.
3. Are highly structured to reduce anxiety.
4. Involve physically limited activity, as the client tires easily.

18. Your client is receiving an antineoplastic drug. An important safety intervention in administering this drug is to

1. Monitor the vital signs before administering.
2. Check the drug with another nurse before administration.
3. Wear surgical latex gloves and a disposable gown for administration.
4. Request a special nurse to administer the drug.

Mr. Martin, a 39-year-old engineer, has been admitted to the hospital with clinical manifestations indicating acute renal failure. A precipitating factor seems to be a viral infection of the upper respiratory tract.

19. You are the nurse assigned to complete a physical assessment on Mr. Martin. From his diagnosis, you would expect to observe

1. Urine output of 400 cc/day, dyspnea, neck vein distention.
2. Anuria, bradycardia, tachypnea.
3. Urine specific gravity of 1.010, decreased creatinine levels, hypokalemia.
4. Hypomagnesemia, nausea, vomiting, weakness.

20. Evaluating Mr. Martin's knowledge of dietary restrictions, you will know he understands a therapeutic diet if he says

1. "I should restrict protein foods to those containing complete amino acid composition."
2. "Protein should be restricted only before dialysis, as the procedure itself removes protein end products."
3. "I should have a low-calorie diet because I cannot process complex carbohydrates."
4. "I should eat foods such as fruits, juices, bananas, and green leafy vegetables and no protein."

Mr. Mirren awakens with severe substernal chest pressure and dyspnea. He takes two nitroglycerin tablets without relief. In five minutes, he takes two more without relief. He calls his physician who instructs him to go directly to the hospital.

21. Understanding the rationale for the physician's instructions, the nurse knows that sudden death (outside the hospital) in association with coronary artery disease is most often due to

1. Acute myocardial infarction.
2. Pump failure accompanied by pulmonary congestion.
3. Arrhythmias.
4. Papillary muscle dysfunction.

22. After a few days, Mr. Mirren is recovering. While eating his evening meal he states that the food is "tasteless." As his nurse, you explain that he has been placed on a cardiac diet which is

1. Low in unsaturated fats—shellfish, spinach, rice.
2. Usually bland—cheese sandwich, chips, milk.
3. Low in salt—halibut, rice, green salad.
4. Clear liquid without spices—chicken, peas, baked potato.

23. The next afternoon Mr. Mirren requests a snack. Considering his dietary restrictions, you will know he understands them if he chooses

1. Fresh fruit.
2. A turkey sandwich.
3. Ice cream.
4. A seafood salad.

---

24. The set of formal guidelines for governing an RN's professional action is called

1. Patient's Bill of Rights.
2. Nurses' Code of Ethics.
3. Professional responsibility.
4. Accountability.

25. The best rationale for introducing yourself to a blind client and telling him exactly what you are doing is that these actions

1. Illustrate the principle of open communication.
2. Decrease the client's anxiety and fear of the unknown.
3. Are the accepted procedure for beginning a nurse-client relationship.
4. Encourage and utilize clear communication.

26. Sitting down at the client's bedside to talk with the client will convey a sense of

1. Sympathy.
2. Communication.
3. Empathy.
4. Encouragement.

27. Mr. Betman is admitted to the CCU with a diagnosis of anterior myocardial infarction. Shortly after admission, he states that he might as well have died because now he won't be able to do anything. Your best response is

1. "Don't worry about it, Mr. Betman. Everything will be all right."
2. "You shouldn't be thinking about that because you are doing so well now."
3. "What do you mean about not being able to do anything, Mr. Betman?"
4. "Take life one day at a time, Mr. Betman."

28. While assessing a client who has orders for a hot-water bottle, heating pad, or hot compress, the first sign of possible thermal injury is

1. Tingling sensation in the extremities.
2. Redness in the area.
3. Edema.
4. Pain.

29. When charting the procedure for applying restraints to a client, you will include

1. What the client says about the restraint.
2. Procedure for applying the restraint.
3. Physician's orders regarding the restraint.
4. Condition of the extremity following application.

Jon Stevens is 11 years old and has type A hemophilia. He is brought to the emergency room after being knocked down in a touch football game. This condition is accompanied by frequent bruising and persistent bleeding from even minor injuries.

30. In type A hemophilia, a child is deficient in the clotting factor of

1. VIII. —TYPe A
2. IX. —Type B
3. XI.
4. XII.

31. Jon's mother is in the emergency room with him. She says to you, "This never would have happened if I had watched him more closely." Your most appropriate response is to say

1. "Hemophiliac children should not be allowed to play contact sports."
2. "I understand how you feel, but at some point Jon is going to have to accept responsibility for monitoring his own activities."
3. "All mothers of chronically ill children feel this way, but it doesn't accomplish anything."
4. "It is difficult not to feel guilty, particularly when you could have watched him more closely."

32. Jon has been transferred to the pediatric unit. In your nursing care plan for Jon, you would include

1. Immobilization of the joint.
2. Passive exercises to the affected limb.
3. Traction of the affected limb.
4. Active exercises to the affected limb.

---

33. Mary Lynn Larson is brought to the maternity unit by her husband. She went into labor at home and the contractions are four minutes apart and regular. Mary Lynn's membranes rupture spontaneously. All of the following actions are appropriate; the first nursing intervention is to

1. Check the fetal heart rate (FHR).
2. Check the color of fluid.
3. Assess the quantity of fluid.
4. Notify the physician.

34. Mrs. Blair is to be discharged and she wishes to walk outside. You explain that the reason clients are discharged in a wheelchair is for

1. Comfort.
2. Convenience.
3. Safety.
4. Rehabilitation.

Mr. Hoffmeyer, a 32-year-old man, was admitted to the locked unit of the psychiatric hospital because he was caught slashing his neighbors' tires. He states that he "knew they were out to get him." You are assigned to complete a physical examination.

35. Considering Mr. Hoffmeyer's mental state, the most immediate nursing intervention is to

1. Explain the need for the physical examination.
2. Postpone the examination until Mr. Hoffmeyer is calmer.
3. Place Mr. Hoffmeyer in a protected environment that will help him control his behavior.
4. Give Mr. Hoffmeyer a chance to calm himself down and then approach him about the examination.

36. The most appropriate intervention for a client such as Mr. Hoffmeyer, who has a potential for violence, is to

1. Arrange for distraction by exposure to constant stimuli.
2. Stay close to the client so that he does not feel people are afraid of him.
3. Remove stimuli that appear to frighten the client.
4. Place the client in four-point restraints.

37. To perform the skill, "turning to the side-lying position," you would lower the head of the bed, elevate bed to working height, move client to your side of the bed, and flex client's knees. The next intervention would be to

1. Roll the client on his side.
2. Reposition client.
3. Place one hand on client's hip and other on shoulder.
4. Reposition client's arms so they are not under his body.

38. Julie Monroe had a fairly long and difficult labor but finally delivered a 3.4 kg baby girl. On the first postpartum day, Julie asks you to bathe and change the baby. Your best response is

1. "I'd be glad to."
2. "Don't you remember how from your last baby?"
3. "How does it feel to have a new baby to care for?"
4. "It's better if you care for the baby."

39. Your client insists on being discharged from the hospital against medical advice. From a legal standpoint, the most important nursing action is to

1. Notify the supervisor and hospital administration.
2. Determine exactly why the client wants to leave.
3. Put all appropriate forms in the client's chart before he leaves the hospital.
4. Request that the client sign the against medical advice (AMA) form.

40. Mrs. Susman returns to the clinic on postpartum day four. You find on your physical exam that her fundus is five finger breadths below the umbilicus, her lochia is scant and serosa, her breasts are full and dripping milk. Your analysis of the findings leads you to

1. Alert the physician.
2. Observe her again in about 30 minutes for changes.
3. Do nothing. The findings are normal.
4. Place her under constant observation.

41. You are moving the client from the bed to a chair. The first appropriate intervention is to

1. Dangle the client at his bedside.
2. Put nonslip shoes or slippers on client's feet.
3. Rock the client and pivot.
4. Position client so that he is comfortable.

42. An indication or signal of impending violent and assaultive behavior could be

1. Foul language.
2. Hallucinations that are threatening, new, and commanding in nature.
3. Sudden withdrawal and refusal to speak.
4. Increased tendency to approach people and make physical contact, such as touching faces.

43. Justin Brey, a client on your unit with a diagnosis of simple schizophrenia, is given an antipsychotic drug, Trilafon. After two days his behavior appears calmer. Two weeks later he approaches you and complains of sore throat, fever, and fatigue. With these symptoms, you suspect Mr. Brey may be developing

1. The flu.
2. Agranulocytosis.
3. Akathisia.
4. German measles.

44. Sarah White, a 24-year-old married female comes to the maternity clinic of a local hospital because she suspects that she is pregnant. Upon examining Sarah, the physician finds that Chadwick's sign is present. Chadwick's sign is

1. Wavy streaks that appear on the abdomen, breast, and thighs during pregnancy.
2. Thin yellowish fluid present in the breasts during pregnancy.
3. Separation of the muscles due to abdominal distention during pregnancy.
4. Deep reddish or purplish discoloration of the vagina due to increased vascularity.

45. Louise Stead is five months pregnant and comes to the clinic for a check-up. You instruct her to immediately report any visual disturbances. The best rationale for this instruction is that this

1. Is a symptom of preeclampsia.
2. Indicates increased intracranial pressure.
3. Means Louise needs more protein in her diet.
4. Indicates a deficiency in iron.

46. Following an angry outburst the previous evening, Todd says, "I'm feeling calmer now. I don't know what got into me. You all must think I'm crazy." The best response to Todd's statement would be

1. "That's all right. We're here to help you."
2. "Why would you think that?"
3. "You think your behavior was crazy?"
4. "How were you feeling last evening?"

47. Instructing a new mother-to-be about her nutritional needs during her pregnancy, you tell her that she should increase her intake of

1. Calories.
2. Fat.
3. Carbohydrates.
4. Vitamin B.

48. The primary purpose of client education is to

1. Collect client data.
2. Determine readiness to learn.
3. Assess degree of compliance.
4. Increase client's knowledge that will affect health status.

49. Mrs. Foster gave birth to a 7 pound baby boy with a cleft lip. You will feed this infant with a

1. Gavage tube.
2. Nipple on the side with the cleft.
3. Nipple on the side without the cleft.
4. Rubber-tipped medicine dropper placed on the side without the cleft.

Mr. Rudy Olsen, aged 32, is married and has no children. His mother lives with him and his wife. He has been experiencing abdominal pain for several months and his physician suspects a duodenal ulcer.

50. Assessing the symptoms described by Mr. Olsen, you will chart that the pain will be

1. Constant over the epigastric area when eating.
2. Experienced about two to three hours after eating.
3. Experienced about one-half hour after eating regardless of the diet.
4. Intermittent with no correlation between food intake and when the pain occurs.

51. The nursing care plan will include observations for possible complications associated with duodenal ulcer disease. An indication of a serious complication is

1. Constipation of several days duration.
2. Severe diarrhea.
3. Bright-red bloody stools.
4. Tarry stools.

52. During visiting hours, a client you are caring for becomes very agitated and angry with his visitor. The most effective nursing approach to this client is to

1. Restrict his visitor from coming to the hospital for a few days.
2. Approach your client in a warm, supportive manner and assist him to explore his feelings.
3. Confront your client and tell him that talking about his feelings is therapeutic.
4. Ask your client if he would like his prn sedative in order to rest.

53. Your initial instruction to a client on the use of crutches to move upstairs should be to

1. Start with crutches and the unaffected leg on the same level.
2. Start with crutches and the affected leg on same level.
3. Place crutches on the step after the affected leg is moved up the stair.
4. Place crutches on the stair and then move the affected leg to the stair.

54. When a client experiences a severe anaphylactic reaction to a medication, your initial action is to

1. Start an IV.
2. Assess vital signs.
3. Place the client in a supine position.
4. Prepare equipment for intubation.

55. The client with gastric pain is advised to take antacids to relieve pain. You will teach him that the antacid that is contraindicated for this condition is

1. Aluminum hydroxide.
2. Amphojel.
3. Maalox.
4. Soda bicarbonate.

Thirty-month-old Brian is admitted to the hospital with severe diarrhea. He is running a slight temperature and appears dehydrated.

56. Upon admission, the most important nursing assessment is to

1. Weigh the child.
2. Take his apical-radial heart rate.
3. Check the condition of his skin.
4. Check his hydration status.

57. Planning Brian's care, the toy most suitable to provide for him is

1. Play dough.
2. A stuffed animal.
3. A box of jacks.
4. A mobile.

58. Brian's parents are unable to "room in" because of other responsibilities at home. During painful hospital procedures, you notice that Brian becomes very quiet and never cries. Based on your knowledge of growth and development, you should interpret Brian's behavior as evidence that he

1. Has given up fighting and has become despondent and hopeless.
2. Was well prepared by his parents for the separation and hospitalization.
3. Has been taught not to misbehave in front of strangers.
4. Does not feel well.

59. You are assigned a client with a diagnosis of diabetes. His physician has ordered short and long acting insulin. When administering two types of insulin, you will

1. Withdraw the long acting insulin into the syringe before the short acting insulin.
2. Withdraw the short acting insulin into the syringe before the long acting insulin.
3. Draw up in two separate syringes, then combine into one syringe.
4. Administer the two types of insulin separately.

Mr. Buford a 58-year-old vice-president of a bank, began having intermittent chest discomfort. After evaluation, a diagnosis of angina pectoris due to atherosclerotic heart disease was made. Nitroglycerin was prescribed to control Mr. Buford's attacks.

60. When instructing Mr. Buford on how to adjust to his condition, it should be emphasized that angina may be brought on by many things, but the most common cause is

1. Stress.
2. Sudden change in position.
3. Physical exertion.
4. Constant activity.

61. As Mr. Buford's nurse, you teach him that nitroglycerin should be taken

1. Every two to three hours during the day.
2. Before every meal and at bedtime.
3. At the first indication of chest pain.
4. Only when chest pain is not relieved by rest.

---

62. Hyperalimentation has been ordered for Tony Speno, age five. This is a method of

1. Providing the necessary fluids and electrolytes to the body.
2. Providing complete nutrition by the intravenous route.
3. Tube feeding that provides necessary nutrients to the body.
4. Blood transfusion.

Mr. Marsh, age 60, is admitted to the hospital for a possible low intestinal obstruction. His preoperative work-up indicates vital signs of BP 100/70, P 88, R 18, and temperature of 96.4°F.

63. You are assessing Mr. Marsh to formulate a nursing care plan. Listening to bowel sounds, you expect to find

1. Absence of bowel sounds.
2. Gurgling bowel sounds.
3. Hyperactive, high-pitched sounds.
4. Tympanic, percussion sounds.

64. With a complete bowel obstruction, you would expect the drainage and amount to be

1. Green and yellow with 2000 ml/day.
2. Yellow and fecal-smelling and scant amount.
3. Clear and scant amount.
4. Clear with 2000–3000 ml/day.

---

65. You are assigned a client whose orders include heparin therapy. When you are administering heparin, the substance you will keep at the bedside as the antidote is

1. Magnesium sulfate.
2. Vitamin K.
3. Protamine sulfate.
4. Calcium gluconate.

Marsha Whiting was admitted to the psychiatric unit of the hospital with a diagnosis of obsessive-compulsive disorder. The admission history describes Marsha as having difficulty adjusting to situations, having a low tolerance for anxiety, and exhibiting compulsive personality traits.

66. Your understanding of this disorder is that the primary purpose for compulsive behavior is an attempt to

1. Reduce anxiety.
2. Gain control of the environment.
3. Influence others.
4. Avoid anxiety.

67. Mrs. Whiting's compulsive behavior involves folding her bed sheets and blankets in a particular pattern every morning. This activity takes at least an hour and Mrs. Whiting usually misses breakfast. The most appropriate nursing intervention in this situation would be to

1. Allow Mrs. Whiting to eat in her room after completing the compulsive activity.
2. Interrupt the activity for breakfast and then allow her to finish it.
3. Get her up early so that she has time to finish the activity before breakfast.
4. Let Mrs. Whiting choose whether to finish the activity and miss breakfast or to postpone the activity until she has had breakfast.

68. Mr. Sacco, age 68, has an external shunt placed in preparation for hemodialysis. Your nursing care plan will include

1. Observing for blood going through the shunt to identify possible clotting that may occur immediately following the dialysis run.
2. Listening for a bruit over the shunt area; if bruit is heard, then shunt may be clotted.
3. Testing the shunt to determine if it is cool to the touch, like that of the forearm, which signifies patency.
4. Observing for dark spots in the shunt that may represent clot formation.

69. To understand the procedure of hemodialysis, your analysis will include the principle that

1. Diffusion of dissolved particles can move across a semipermeable membrane.
2. Pore size of the membrane permits passage of high molecular weight substances.
3. Water being a large molecule, is unable to move freely through the membrane.
4. Plasma proteins are large and, therefore, can move easily through the membrane.

70. On the third postoperative day, Mr. Kandee develops thrombophlebitis. Your assessment of this condition will reveal

1. Bluish discoloration along the vein.
2. Pain in the area.
3. Varicosities.
4. Surrounding area cool to the touch.

71. You would determine that a thrombus is present by testing for

1. Doll's sign.
2. Kernig's sign.
3. Hegar's sign.
4. Homan's sign.

72. Marge Gallo is brought to the hospital by her husband who says she is highly anxious and spends half the morning doing rituals. As part of her treatment plan, Marge will join a daily group therapy session at 10:30 in the morning. The rationale for choosing this time of day is

1. Anxious clients are more relaxed in the morning.
2. Mornings are better for group therapy because clients have the rest of the day to work through problems that come up during the sessions.
3. Most groups are planned for the morning when physicians are on the unit.
4. Mrs. Gallo will have just completed her ritualistic activity.

73. Jamie Kern has just returned from a myelogram when he complains of itching and dyspnea. You observe that his face is flushed. The first intervention is to

1. Place him in low-Fowler's position.
2. Administer oxygen at 6L/min.
3. Call the physician.
4. Start an IV with normal saline.

74. Renata Gordon, age 32, is in her 37th week of pregnancy and is showing early signs of preeclampsia. Your nursing care plan will include assessment for further signs of this condition. Indications of progression of preeclampsia to a more severe state would be the presence of

1. Severe hypertension, glycosuria, polyuria.
2. Hyperreflexia, oliguria, epigastric pain.
3. Hypertension, weight loss, diuresis.
4. Hypertension, convulsions, polyuria.

Brittany, a 4-year-old black girl, lives in San Francisco with her mother and father. Her mother brought her to the clinic where an initial diagnosis of sickle cell anemia was made.

75. Brittany experiences her first thrombic crisis. Based on your knowledge of this disease, you know that a thrombic crisis is the result of

1. Pooling of the blood in the spleen.
2. Occlusion of small blood vessels.
3. Hemarthrosis.
4. Injury to the joints.

76. While Brittany is hospitalized, her mother, Angie, learns that she is pregnant. When Angie comes to visit Brittany, she asks you if her new baby will also get sickle cell anemia. The best answer is

1. "No, since only you have the trait and not your husband, the chances are fifty-fifty that the new baby will not have the disease."
2. "It depends upon whether both you and your husband have the disease."
3. "It is possible, because in order for Brittany to have the disease, both of you must at least carry the trait."
4. "Yes, since you have one child with the disease, all of your children will have sickle cell anemia."

June Blanchard, now at 40 weeks' gestation, is in labor, and has been admitted to the hospital. She is 4 cm dilated and having strong contractions every four minutes lasting 40 seconds.

77. June complains of much back discomfort and an urge to bear down during the contraction. These signs lead you to conclude that

1. She is fully dilated.
2. The baby is in a posterior position.
3. She needs analgesic medication.
4. She should get up and walk around.

78. A nursing action that will provide the best source of relief for June's back pain is to

1. Direct her attention to the TV or to talk with her.
2. Have her walk around.
3. Give her a narcotic analgesic.
4. Apply counterpressure to her sacral area.

79. Mrs. Franc is given a blood transfusion. She begins to wheeze and her skin is flushed with hives. These symptoms are characteristic of a(n)

1. Allergic reaction.
2. Hemolytic reaction.
3. Thrombic crisis.
4. Transfusion reaction.

80. If a blood transfusion reaction occurs, the first intervention is to

1. Place the client in high-Fowler's position.
2. Call the physician.
3. Slow the rate of infusion to "keep open" rate.
4. Shut off the transfusion.

Mrs. Newman is admitted to the hospital as a terminal client. She has been a client on the oncology unit for two months and has become a favorite with the staff. Although her condition is deteriorating, she remains cheerful and pleasant.

81. Mrs. Newman is in a great deal of pain but it is controlled with PCA—patient-controlled IV analgesia. The rationale for using this method is that it

1. Allows nurses to care for more clients.
2. Enables clients to administer medication when pain is experienced.
3. Results in less pain medication used by client.
4. Programs medication to remain within acceptable limits.

82. Mrs. Newman's condition is critical, and you are assigned to care for her. Of the following tasks, the one with the highest priority is to

1. Attend to her physical needs and assess the situation for changes.
2. Contact the family and give them needed support.
3. Encourage Mrs. Newman to express her fears of dying.
4. Contact a priest so she can have last rites.

---

83. The correct action for instilling eye drops is to instill the drops

1. At the outer canthus of the eye.
2. Over the conjunctiva.
3. Directly on the cornea.
4. Into the center of conjunctival sac.

84. A client with advanced cirrhosis of the liver will most likely be ordered a diet of

1. No protein, low potassium.
2. Low protein and sodium.
3. Fat controlled, low potassium and sodium.
4. Low protein and fat, low carbohydrate.

85. Ben Rother, 18, fell off a ladder while painting his parent's home. He has been brought to the hospital by ambulance. You are assigned to complete an initial assessment. An indication of increased intracranial pressure (ICP) that you will observe for is a

1. Pulse rate of 96.
2. Respiratory rate of 18 and irregular.
3. Blood pressure of 160/80.
4. Temperature of 100°F orally.

86. One day a client with terminal cancer says to you, "Well, I've given up all hope. I know I'm going to die soon." The most therapeutic response you could make is to say

1. "Now, one should never give up all hope. We are finding new cures every day."
2. "We should talk about dying."
3. "You've given up all hope?"
4. "You know, you doctor will be here soon. Why don't you talk to him about your feelings."

Mrs. Brynes, a 50-year-old with a chronic respiratory problem, comes into the emergency room complaining of fever, cough, chest pain, and tachycardia. An arterial blood gas panel is obtained with a repeat test one hour later; oxygen via nasal prongs at 6 liters/minute is started. Following are the ABG results:

	FIO$_2$	pH	pCO$_2$	HCO$_3$	pO$_2$
ABG 1:	21%	7.35	50	27	48
ABG 2:	6 liters	7.20	75	29	140

87. Assessing these symptoms would lead you to identify the nursing diagnosis of

1. Airway Clearance, Ineffective.
2. Respiratory Function, Alterations in: Ineffective Breathing Patterns.
3. Cardiac Output, Alterations in: Decreased.
4. Respiratory Functions, Alterations in: Ineffective Gas Exchange, Impaired.

88. The acid-base abnormality demonstrated with ABG 1 in the values listed above is

1. Respiratory acidosis.
2. Respiratory alkalosis.
3. Metabolic acidosis.
4. Metabolic alkalosis.

89. After analyzing the data base, you would be alert to the complication of

1. Increased cyanosis.
2. Acid-base imbalance.
3. Fluid and electrolyte imbalance.
4. Somnolence and coma.

David Benezra, after an automobile accident in which he sustained a head injury, has been scheduled for a craniotomy.

90. The preoperative preparation will probably include physician's orders of

1. Giving a soapsuds enema.
2. Hydrating with 3000 cc's IV fluid.
3. Administering steroids.
4. Inserting a nasogastric tube.

91. Analyzing David's immediate postoperative needs, your care plan will include

1. Keeping his temperature below 97°F to decrease metabolic needs.
2. Placing him in supine position.
3. Maintaining fluid and electrolyte balance by administering at least 3000 cc D5 Lactated Ringer's every 24 hours.
4. Obtaining serial blood and urine samples.

Sandy King is a 9 year old who has been admitted to the hospital for hematological studies. Following the initial tests, her parents are informed that Sandy has acute lymphocytic leukemia.

92. The King's initial reaction to the diagnosis is to say to the nurse, "I think you have made a mistake and have mixed up the lab results." The best response would be to say

1. "I will recheck the results and the hospital numbers to verify that the blood tested was Sandy's."
2. "Did you question the physician regarding this point?"
3. "Why do you think we've made a mistake?"
4. "We can sit down and talk about the results and your feelings about it."

93. Assessing Sandy, you would expect to find the common early signs of leukemia, such as

1. Fatigue, mouth lesions, hepatomegaly.
2. Pallor, lethargy, anorexia, fever.
3. Fatigue, pallor, alopecia, hemorrhage.
4. Lethargy, petechiae, splenomegaly, headache.

94. Sandy is to receive Cytoxan. The most important nursing intervention when caring for a child receiving Cytoxan is to

1. Observe for ulceration of the oral mucosa.
2. Give large quantities of fluids prior to and following drug administration.
3. Observe for signs of gastrointestinal disturbance.
4. Observe for changes in mental alertness.

---

95. Assessing a client for hypovolemic shock, the sign that you would expect to note if this complication occurs is

1. Hypertension.
2. Cyanosis.
3. Oliguria.
4. Tachypnea.

96. Harriet Saunders is 75 years old and is a resident of the Westbrook Nursing Home. Her diagnosis is organic brain syndrome. In planning Mrs. Saunders' daily schedule, it is important for the nurse to understand that Mrs. Saunders

1. May have moderate-to-severe memory impairment and short periods of concentration.
2. Will be more comfortable with a rigid daily schedule.
3. Is more likely to be able to remember current experiences than past ones.
4. Can usually be trusted to be responsible for her daily care needs.

97. When evaluating the client's understanding of a low potassium diet, you will know he understands if he tells you that he will avoid

1. Pasta.
2. Raw apples.
3. Dry cereal.
4. French bread.

98. Irrigating a nasogastric tube should be carried out using which one of the following protocols?

1. Gently instill 20 cc normal saline and then withdraw solution.
2. Instill 30 cc sterile water and then withdraw solution.
3. Instill 30 cc sterile saline, forcefully if necessary, and allow fluid to flow into basin for return.
4. Gently instill 20 cc sterile water and then allow fluid to flow into basin for return.

99. Paralytic ileus is a frequent complication of postoperative abdominal surgery. According to the physician's orders and your own assessment, a planned intervention would be to

1. Administer PO fluids only.
2. Insert a nasogastric tube.
3. Listen for bowel sounds.
4. Insert a rectal tube.

Mr. Cassidy, age 50, is admitted to the hospital for a gastric resection. Following surgery Mr. Cassidy arrives in the recovery room in stable condition. His vital signs are BP 132/80, P 80, R 20.

100. One hour postoperatively, Mr. Cassidy's urine is 40 cc/hr and he has a CVP reading of 4–5. His BP is 100/40, P 88, and R 24. Based on this data, your initial intervention is to

1. Place him in Trendelenburg's position.
2. Administer intravenous fluids as ordered to maintain a CVP reading of 5 to 9 cm of water pressure.
3. Place several blankets over him to increase his body temperature.
4. Administer vasodilator drugs as ordered.

101. A week later, with Mr. Cassidy much improved, his family is making plans for discharge. His further recovery will be most influenced by

1. His wife's clear understanding of his dietary needs.
2. The amount of emotional support he receives from his family.
3. His understanding of the causes of his illness.
4. His expectations of himself to get back to work as soon as possible.

Mrs. Forrest, 65, falls and is transported to the hospital for x-rays. It is found that she has a fractured right hip that is only slightly displaced. Mrs. Forrest is scheduled for hip surgery.

102. Following total hip replacement, immediately postoperatively you will formulate a goal to include

1. Head of bed elevated to 45° angle.
2. Operative leg maintained in abduction.
3. Buck's traction until hip can be put through range of motion.
4. Turn on operative side only immediately postoperatively.

103. The morning of the second postoperative day, Mrs. Forrest is to be ambulated. Your first intervention is to

1. Get her up in a chair.
2. Use a walker when getting her up.
3. Have her put minimal weight on the affected side.
4. Practice getting her out of bed by slightly flexing her hips.

104. You are assigned a client who has just had a nasogastric tube inserted postoperatively. During your evaluation of his status, you will check for

1. Electrolyte imbalance.
2. Gastric distention.
3. Ulcerative colitis.
4. Infection.

105. Before administering a nasogastric feeding, you aspirate the stomach contents and obtain 50 cc of residual. Your next action is to

1. Discard aspirate and begin tube feeding.
2. Replace aspirate and begin tube feeding.
3. Discard aspirate and hold the tube feeding.
4. Replace aspirate and hold the tube feeding.

106. You are assigned to a client with a central vein IV infusing hyperalimentation solution. The most important nursing intervention is

1. Preparing the next bottle of solution prior to use.
2. Maintaining the exact amount of solution administered hourly by adjusting the flow rate.
3. Checking urine specific gravity, sugar, and acetone every four hours.
4. Changing the IV filter and tubing with each bottle change.

107. If your client has an injury to the seventh cranial nerve, your assessment will identify an abnormality in

1. Closing the eyelid.
2. Trapezius muscle movement.
3. Hearing.
4. Tongue control.

Lorraine Sacs gave birth to baby Jennifer after a normal labor and delivery. Jennifer weighed only five pounds and is considered premature.

108. One of the most important principles in providing nutrition to Jennifer is to

1. Use a regular nipple with a large hole.
2. Feed every 4–6 hours.
3. Use a premie nipple for bottle feeding.
4. Use milk high in fat for the formula.

109. Lorraine visits her baby every day. One day the nurse asks Lorraine if she would like to feed Jennifer. She says, "Oh, no, you do it so well. I want my child to be well cared for." You interpret this reply as a(n)

1. Compliment to the nurse's ability.
2. Sign that the mother is still tired from the delivery and is not yet ready to care for the child.
3. Expression of her sense of inadequacy in caring for her own child.
4. Admission of her inexperience in dealing with premature infants.

110. The nurse's most appropriate response to Lorraine is

1. "I'll feed him today. Maybe tomorrow you can try it."
2. "It's not difficult at all. He is just like a normal baby, only smaller."
3. "You can learn to feed him as well as I can; I wasn't good when I first fed a premature infant either."
4. "It's frightening sometimes to feed an infant this small, but I'll stay with you to help."

Ellen, a 16-year-old high school student, is brought into the hospital by her mother, who is worried about Ellen's lack of interest in anything, loss of weight, somatic complaints, and constant tiredness.

111. Ellen continues to verbalize feeling sad and hopeless, and is not mixing well with the other clients on the unit. As you formulate a nursing plan of care, an important consideration is to

1. Allow Ellen to keep to herself until she feels like mixing with others.
2. Assign Ellen to several groups so she will begin to mix.
3. Formulate a structured schedule so Ellen will not have time to contemplate her feelings.
4. Counsel her family that family therapy is indicated.

112. Ellen, her mother, and you are having a predischarge conference. Ellen's mother asks for some guidance in helping Ellen when she returns home. Counseling Ellen's mother, you tell her that parents will have fewer conflicts with their adolescent children if they

1. Formulate a very strict disciplinary code.
2. Try to remember their own adolescence.
3. Allow the adolescent to solve some of his or her own problems.
4. Continuously evaluate the adolescent.

---

113. Bill Tolliver has an order for nasogastric feedings. After insertion of a nasogastric tube, you will evaluate the position of the tube by checking

1. Regular intermittent bubbling when the tube is submerged in water.
2. Hearing a rush of air from the stomach after injecting 1 cc of air into the tube.
3. Aspirating gastric contents and checking to see if the pH is acidic.
4. Checking that no coughing or choking occurs when the tube is inserted.

Mrs. Maria Garcia, a 50-year-old woman, was admitted to the medical unit for a breast biopsy. Following the results, Mrs. Garcia was scheduled for a modified mastectomy.

114. Mrs. Garcia says to the nurse, "I don't know why you are all so concerned; I'm not that sick." The defense mechanism she is using is

1. Denial.
2. Rationalization.
3. Projection.
4. Regression.

115. Following her modified mastectomy, Mrs. Garcia's care plan should provide for her to be positioned

1. On her operative side.
2. On her unoperative side.
3. In semi-Fowler's with her affected arm flat on bed.
4. In semi-Fowler's with her affected arm elevated.

116. You will know that Mrs. Garcia understands her dietary guidelines if she tells you that she avoids eating

1. Cheese, chicken, shrimp, nuts, raw fruit.
2. Beef, pork, bread, cooked vegetables.
3. Lunch meat, canned soups, tomatoes, yellow vegetables.
4. Milk, eggs, canned vegetables, fish.

---

117. Jane has been ordered to have blood work drawn for serum electrolytes. She is on bedrest and has an IV in the vein of the right forearm. The most appropriate site for blood withdrawal is

1. Left upper arm (brachial vein).
2. Right forearm (radial vein).
3. Foot (greater saphenous vein).
4. Left forearm (median cubital vein).

118. You are talking to a client whose physician has ordered the antidepressive drug, Elavil. She asks you which side effects she should watch for when taking Elavil. You tell her that she

1. Should not eat certain foods such as wine, cheese, beer, or chicken livers.
2. Should try to drink a lot of fluid, as this drug depletes fluid balance.
3. Will probably have to take Cogentin to reduce the extra-pyramidal effects.
4. Should watch for hypertension, drowsiness, fatigue, and tremors.

119. Laurie is 39 and just recently learned she is pregnant. While discussing this pregnancy, she says to you, "It just can't be; I'm too old. I'm not sure my husband and I want a baby now." Your best response is

1. "Was this pregnancy planned?"
2. "Would you like to talk to the social worker?"
3. "You are having a normal reaction. Let's talk about being pregnant."
4. "I understand. Would you like the number of the counseling clinic?"

120. Mr. Robert Anders is being treated with chemotherapy and radiation therapy as an out-patient in the clinic. The client teaching that should be included in the initial discussion before radiation therapy begins is that

1. Radiation therapy can cause pneumonitis.
2. Radiation ionizes atoms in the chemical systems of the cells and causes side effects.
3. Radiodermatitis may occur three to six weeks after the start of therapy.
4. Radiation therapy causes cell damage that may be permanent.

121. Following several radiation treatments you observe that a client's skin appears wet and weeping. According to clinic protocol, your intervention is to

1. Not give the treatment and explain not to bathe the skin until the weeping is stopped.
2. Give the treatment and make a note on the record concerning the skin condition.
3. Not give the treatment and notify the physician.
4. Give the treatment and instruct the client to use antibiotic lotion on the lesions.

Karl Korngold has been diagnosed as having a right side retinal detachment. He is admitted to the hospital and scheduled for surgery later that day.

122. The most important nursing intervention in the preoperative hours is to position Mr. Korngold

1. With the head of his bed flat.
2. On his right side.
3. So that the area of the detachment is dependent.
4. With the head of his bed elevated.

123. Mr. Korngold asks to go to the bathroom. The most appropriate response to his request is to tell him that he

1. Must remain on strict bedrest.
2. May get up with assistance.
3. May briefly get up, but he should keep the area dependent.
4. May get up as long as he does not bend his head down.

124. Postoperatively, Mr. Korngold will receive routine care. In sequence, you will first assess for

1. Nausea and vomiting, shock, sudden eye pain, and ability to deep breathe.
2. Hemorrhage, nausea and vomiting, sudden eye pain, and postoperative position.
3. Shock, sudden eye pain, restlessness, and nausea and vomiting.
4. Hemorrhage, restlessness, shock, and nausea and vomiting.

125. You have been assigned to Mrs. Franks, who needs to have a sterile urine specimen sent to the laboratory for a culture and sensitivity. After inserting the catheter, you find that urine is not flowing. Your next action is to

1. Remove the catheter, check the meatus, and reinsert the catheter.
2. Obtain a new, larger sized catheter and insert it.
3. Reassess if the catheter is in the vagina; if so, remove it and reinsert into meatus.
4. Insert the catheter a little farther, wait a few seconds, and if urine does not flow, reassess placement.

126. When the urine begins to flow through Mrs. Frank's catheter, your next action is to

1. Inflate the catheter balloon with sterile water.
2. Place the catheter tip into the specimen container.
3. Connect the catheter into the drainage tubing.
4. Place the catheter tip into the urine collection receptacle.

Charlie Wells, two years old, lives with his mother, who is divorced, and her boyfriend. Charlie likes to explore cupboards and is constantly into everything. One day Charlie opens a cupboard and eats half a bottle of ferrous sulfate tablets.

127. Charlie's mother calls the hospital. As the nurse who answers the telephone, you should first advise her to

1. Bring Charlie to the hospital immediately.
2. Give Charlie 15 ml of ipecac.
3. Give Charlie burned toast with milk.
4. Not do anything, because vitamins are not poisonous.

128. Since Charlie has had one poison ingestion, statistically he is nine times more likely to have poisoning episode within the year. To prevent further poisoning incidents, the most important information to tell Charlie's mother is to

1. Keep purses out of Charlie's reach.
2. Never give medications to others in front of Charlie.
3. Keep all cabinets locked at all times.
4. If poisoning occurs, do as the label on the bottle recommends.

---

129. Amniocentesis would *not* be performed on a woman if you assess that she

1. Were carrying twins.
2. Would not consider an elective abortion.
3. Were a Ashkenazic Jew.
4. Had a family history of genetic disorders.

130. You are counseling a woman who has just learned she is pregnant. She says she does not want to gain too much weight because her husband likes her "thin." Your best response is

1. "It's best for the baby is you don't try to stay too thin."
2. "If you are careful about the foods you eat, especially those high in calories, you will not gain too much."
3. "Let's talk about the importance of good nutrition and weight gain in pregnancy."
4. "Why don't you have your husband come to the clinic next time, and we can all talk about nutrition."

131. A three year old, brought to the emergency room for a broken arm, has bruises all over his body. The nurse asks Mike's mother how he got the bruises. She replied that he is always falling down and hurting himself. The next action the nurse should take is to

1. Report the suspected child abuse to the authorities.
2. Continue evaluating the circumstances.
3. Ask the psychiatrist to talk with Ms. Potter.
4. Ask Ms. Potter to bring her boyfriend in for a conference.

132. If it is suspected that a child is abused, the legal responsibility of the staff who evaluated the case is that

1. The nurse is legally responsible for reporting a suspected child abuse.
2. The doctor, not the nurse, is legally responsible for reporting child abuse.
3. Both the doctor and the nurse are legally responsible for reporting child abuse.
4. Neither the doctor nor the nurse is legally responsible for reporting child abuse.

Joan Clous, a 32-year-old mother of three has come to the OB clinic where you are a nurse. Her last menstrual period (LMP) was eight weeks ago (1/21/94). The results of her tests indicate that she is pregnant.

133. According to Nägele's Rule, Joan's expected date of confinement (EDC) would be

1. 10/28/94.
2. 10/14/94.
3. 11/21/94.
4. 10/1/94.

134. If Joan did not have a LMP date to go by, the sign most useful in calculating her EDC is

1. Appearance of linea nigra.
2. Ultrasound examination.
3. Estriol level at 12 weeks.
4. Detection of Goodell's sign.

135. Mr. Cody's physician has ordered a cholecystogram. The intervention most important as a part of the preparation for this procedure is

1. Assessing for shellfish allergy.
2. Giving the client a high-fat meal.
3. Administering an enema.
4. Allowing a light breakfast.

136. For a client to whom you are assigned, a diagnosis of carcinoma is confirmed. While making morning rounds the day before surgery, you observe the client crying. An appropriate response would be to

1. Ignore the crying, as you realize she may not want to talk.
2. Acknowledge her by saying, "Good morning," as you pass the door and observe if she seems to wish to talk.
3. Go in the room and ask her why she is crying.
4. Go in the room, sit down, and stay quietly with her.

Susan Medieras, an obese 14 year old, is admitted to the adolescent unit with a tentative diagnosis of type I diabetes mellitus.

137. In preparing a care plan for Susan, you know that her admission to the hospital may cause her to experience fears of

1. Being displaced.
2. Separation.
3. Loss of independence.
4. The unknown.

138. Adolescent diabetics such as Susan frequently have more difficulty than diabetics in other age groups because

1. The disease is usually more severe in adolescents than in younger children.
2. Adolescents as a group have poor eating habits.
3. Adolescents have a difficult time with long-acting insulin.
4. Adolescents have difficulty regulating their insulin.

---

139. Following surgery, a client is returned to your unit with a T-tube in place. To ensure optimal functioning, the principle to consider is that the

1. Client is positioned to prevent backflow of bile into the liver.
2. Client is positioned in a prone position to promote bile drainage.
3. T-tube is connected to the drainage bottle at the level of the bed to prevent bile backflow.
4. T-tube is not to be clamped.

Kate Benning, a 30-year-old mother of two, was brought to the hospital by her husband. Her husband complained that Kate could not manage the house, was easily distracted, and was constantly in motion. The admitting diagnosis is manic episode.

140. The nurse noticed that Kate is unable to converse rationally and changes the subject frequently. This is most clearly an example of

1. Delusions.
2. Associative looseness.
3. Flight of ideas.
4. Echolalia.

141. Kate manifests an excess of energy, and it is difficult for her to sit still. The most useful activity for Kate that the nurse might suggest would be to

1. Play volleyball outside.
2. Engage in occupational therapy and group exercises.
3. Empty wastebaskets on the unit.
4. Deliver linen to the rooms.

142. Kate frequently exhibits bizarre and inappropriate behavior. Such behavior may be best explained by which one of the following statements?

1. The purpose of the behavior is to attract attention.
2. Kate has little or no control over her impulsive behavior.
3. Kate's behavior is a method of expressing herself in a symbolic way.
4. Kate's behavior is caused by a genetic imbalance.

143. Mrs. Green's surgeon orders a Foley catheter to be inserted. Of the following interventions, the one you would carry out first is to

1. Clean the perineum from front to back.
2. Check the catheter for patency.
3. Explain the procedure to Mrs. Green and tell her that she will feel slight, temporary discomfort.
4. Arrange the sterile items on the sterile field.

144. Lawrence Jones is being given Sucralfate (Carafate), ordered by his physician for treating his peptic ulcer. Before he leaves the hospital, you will review the discharge orders. An important instruction for Mr. Jones is that he should take the medication

1. With meals, on a full stomach.
2. At bedtime only.
3. One hour before or after meals on an empty stomach.
4. One hour before or after meals and at bedtime.

145. Mrs. Harrington's physician orders a nasogastric tube to be inserted. During the insertion of the NG tube you will position the client in

1. Low-Fowler's with head tilted back.
2. High-Fowler's with head bent forward.
3. Right side-lying with head straight up.
4. High-Fowler's with neck hyperextended.

146. Gerry Swanson came into the emergency room in respiratory distress. The physician gave her theophylline to relax the smooth muscle of the bronchi. You will monitor the effects of this medication by checking

1. Respiratory rate.
2. Blood pressure.
3. Heart rate and rhythm.
4. Pulse rate.

147. You are assigned to care for a client who is just completing the last cycle of peritoneal dialysis. Two liters of fluid were infused and there was one liter of fluid returned. The appropriate nursing intervention is to

1. Chart the discrepancy and report to the head nurse.
2. No other intervention is necessary.
3. Flush the catheter with normal saline.
4. Insert a needle into the drainage system air vent.

148. Mrs. Kerwin is a 42-year-old client diagnosed as a chronic schizophrenic. Assessing Mrs. Kerwin, the nurse keeps in mind that a diagnosis of schizophrenia involves

1. Inability to concentrate.
2. Loss of contact with reality.
3. Guilt feelings.
4. Feelings of worthlessness.

149. Clients are assigned to a chronic schizophrenic group therapy session. The best rationale for this form of treatment is that it

1. Is the most economical—one staff member can treat many clients.
2. Is not psychoanalytically based, but deals with unconscious material.
3. Enables clients to become aware that others have problems and that they are not alone in their suffering.
4. Provides a social milieu similar to society in general, where the client can relate to others.

After falling down the basement steps in his house, Mr. Thomas is brought to the emergency room. His physician confirms that his leg is fractured.

150. Following application of a leg cast, you will first check Mr. Thomas' toes for

1. Increase in temperature.
2. Change in color.
3. Edema.
4. Movement.

151. Mr. Thomas is unable to feel you apply pressure on his toes and complains of tingling. These signs indicate

1. Pressure on a nerve.
2. Phantom pain syndrome.
3. Overmedication of an analgesic.
4. Improper alignment of the fracture.

152. From your knowledge of the casting procedure, you understand that a wet cast should be

1. Placed on a firm surface for the first few hours.
2. Handled only with the palms of the hands.
3. Left alone to set for at least three hours.
4. Petaled to lessen chance of irritation to the client.

153. After application of the cast, it takes 24 to 48 hours to dry. When the cast is completely dry, the surface will

1. Appear dull.
2. Appear pitted and irregular.
3. Have a shiny appearance.
4. Feel warm when touched.

---

154. A client on lithium carbonate is instructed to return to the clinic to have her blood checked in a week. Your rationale for emphasizing this teaching is that the

1. Serum level of lithium must be kept below 1.6 mEq/liter.
2. Serum level of lithium is important to test to determine if the level present is controlling symptoms but not toxic.
3. Toxic range appears only at levels exceeding 2.0 mEq/liter.
4. Central nervous system is the chief target, so the serum level must be kept stable, not fluctuating.

155. When the client returns to the clinic, her lithium level is only slightly higher than the previous week but she complains of blurred vision and ataxia. Your first intervention is to

1. Withhold the next dose.
2. Instruct her to watch for signs of toxicity.
3. Notify the physician.
4. Suggest she drink more fluid.

156. Mrs. Culley has otosclerosis and is scheduled for a stapedectomy. This condition chiefly involves the

1. Auditory canal.
2. Tympanic membrane.
3. Ossicle.
4. Auditory nerve.

157. Which of the following skin cancers has the poorest prognosis because it metastasizes so rapidly and extensively via the lymph system?

1. Basal cell epithelioma.
2. Squamous cell epithelioma.
3. Malignant melanoma.
4. Sebaceous cyst.

Jane Bruning delivered a 32-week, 5 lb. female infant. The infant demonstrates nasal flaring, intercostal retraction, expiratory grunt, and slight cyanosis.

158. Blood gases and electrolyte studies of the baby are ordered immediately to assess the infant's

1. Leukocyte count.
2. Oxygen, carbon dioxide, and pH levels.
3. Antibody titer for RH.
4. Blood glucose level.

159. Baby Bruning was placed in a heated isolette because

1. The infant has a small body surface for her weight.
2. Heat increases the flow of oxygen to extremities.
3. Her temperature control mechanism is immature.
4. Heat within the isolette facilitates drainage of mucus.

---

160. Planning the premature infant's care, you will make careful note of the oxygen level in the isolette because it could

1. Produce kernicterus.
2. Cause retrolental fibroplasia.
3. Cause peripheral circulatory collapse.
4. Contribute to cardiac damage.

161. Thirty-year-old Jim Brown has burns on the front and back of both his legs and arms. The approximate percentage of his body that has been involved is

1. 27 percent.
2. 36 percent.
3. 45 percent.
4. 54 percent.

162. During a retention catheter insertion or bladder irrigation, the nurse must use

1. Sterile equipment and wear sterile gloves.
2. Clean equipment and maintain surgical asepsis.
3. Sterile equipment and maintain medical asepsis.
4. Clean equipment and technique.

163. At 10 months of age, Alissa can stand alone but has not taken any steps. Her mother is upset because she has been told by a friend that many babies walk by 10 months of age. You can respond by saying

1. "Your friend is exaggerating."
2. "Children never walk before one year."
3. "Perhaps Alissa hasn't had enough experience crawling."
4. "Each child develops at his or her own rate."

164. Care for a client following a bronchoscopy will include

1. Withholding food and liquids until the gag reflex returns.
2. Providing throat irrigations every four hours.
3. Having the client refrain from talking for several days.
4. Suctioning frequently, as ordered.

165. Which of the following statements best explains why premature infants are more likely to develop hyperbilirubinemia?

1. Liver enzymes are immature.
2. Antibody formation is immature.
3. Premature infants receive few antibodies from the mother.
4. White blood cells are immature.

166. Reviewing the lab tests of a client scheduled for surgery, you find that the white blood cell count is 9800/cu mm. The most appropriate intervention is to

1. Call the operating room and cancel the surgery.
2. Notify the surgeon immediately.
3. Take no action as you recognize that it is a normal value.
4. Call the lab and have the test repeated.

Mrs. Overbrook, 45 years old, has just been admitted to the hospital for an abdominal hysterectomy. She is quite fearful and dreads the operation, but states she will be glad to get it over with since she has been experiencing long painful periods and the doctor has recently found fibroid tumors in her uterus.

167. Nursing responsibilities for the preoperative period include notifying the physician if the

1. Erythrocyte count is 6 million/cc mm.
2. Temperature is 99.6°F orally.
3. Hemoglobin is 14 gm/100 ml.
4. Urine report indicates ketonuria.

168. While you are orienting Mrs. Overbrook to her surroundings, she states she is afraid of what will happen the next day. The most appropriate response is to

1. Assure her that the surgery is very safe and problems are rare.
2. Let her talk about her fears as much as she wishes.
3. Explain that she has an excellent doctor and she has nothing to worry about.
4. Explain that worrying or anxiety has been proven to prolong her hospitalization.

169. The milliliters of drug that should be used to give 0.5 gm if the label on the bottle reads 5 gm in 10 ml is

1. 2.0 ml.
2. 1.0 ml.
3. 0.5 ml.
4. 5.0 ml.

170. One year ago, Mrs. Brown lost her husband to whom she had been married for ten years. They had had a stormy marriage, punctuated by frequent disagreements and several separations. Mrs. Brown is experiencing intense grief, which she seems unable to work through. To understand this behavior, the nurse should know

1. The longer the marriage, the more intense the grief.
2. The more dependent the relationship, the more difficult the grief process.
3. The more ambivalent the relationship, the more intense the grief.
4. It is too soon to expect Mrs. Brown to have worked through the grief process.

171. Jane failed her psychology final exam and spent the entire evening berating the teacher and the course. This behavior is an example of

1. Reaction-formation.
2. Compensation.
3. Projection.
4. Acting out.

172. Following abdominal surgery, a client complaining of "gas pains" should be positioned on his

1. Left side, recumbent.
2. Left side, Sims'.
3. Right side, semi-Fowler's.
4. Left side, semi-Fowler's.

173. After removing the fecal impaction, the client complains of feeling light-headed and the pulse rate is 44. Your priority intervention is to

1. Monitor vital signs.
2. Place in shock position.
3. Call the physician.
4. Begin CPR.

Margaret Samuels, 42 years old, complains of pain in her stomach radiating to her right shoulder. Her doctor suspects cholelithiasis.

174. Gathering information from Ms. Samuels, the nurse should be alert to her complaints of

1. Chronic pain in her lower right abdomen.
2. Chronic pain in her lower left abdomen.
3. Fatty food intolerance while eating.
4. Fatty food intolerance several hours after eating.

175. Ms. Samuels' biliary pain will best be controlled by administering the medication

1. Thorazine.
2. Codeine.
3. Morphine.
4. Demerol.

176. Surgery is scheduled for Ms. Samuels. It should be anticipated that the major postoperative complication following a cholecystectomy is

1. Paralytic ileus.
2. Thrombophlebitis.
3. Pneumonia.
4. Hemorrhage.

177. The most appropriate breakfast for Ms. Samuels on her third postop day following a cholecystectomy is

1. Cocoa, cereal with half and half, grapefruit, toast and jelly.
2. Tea, boiled eggs, sausage, toast and butter.
3. Coffee, oatmeal with cream, scrambled egg, toast and butter.
4. Tea, banana, boiled egg, toast and jelly.

---

178. Which one of the following statements is most correct regarding colostomy irrigations?

1. The solution temperature should be 100°F.
2. 1000 cc is the usual amount of solution for the irrigation.
3. The solution container should be placed 10 inches above the stoma.
4. The irrigation cone is inserted in an upward direction in relation to the stoma.

179. The steps in preparing for clean moist compresses include gathering the material, taking baseline vital signs, and lubricating the skin. The next step is to

1. Inspect the skin for possible complications from the heat treatments.
2. Place the compress material in a warming solution.
3. Wring out the compresses.
4. Put on sterile gloves.

180. When administering a tepid bath, a client begins to shiver. Your intervention is to

1. Continue with the bath, as this helps dissipate the heat.
2. Stop the bath for a few minutes and place a warm blanket on the client to stop shivering.
3. Stop the bath, as the body is attempting to produce heat.
4. Warm the solution, continue the bath, and change the location of cloth placement.

181. A person with a diagnosis of diabetes should understand the symptoms of a hyperglycemic reaction. You will know this client understands if she can tell you these symptoms are

1. Thirst, polyuria, and decreased appetite.
2. Flushed cheeks, acetone breath, and increased thirst.
3. Nausea, vomiting, and diarrhea.
4. Weight gain, normal breath, and thirst.

182. A client calls the diabetic hot-line and tells you that she has flu-like symptoms with no fever, but has been vomiting and has had diarrhea since 4:00 A.M. She is taking NPH insulin. You determine that she will probably need

1. No insulin.
2. Her regular dose of NPH insulin.
3. A smaller dose of her NPH insulin.
4. An increased dose of her NPH insulin.

183. Mr. Bayliss has been taking Thorazine for two days and is beginning to develop extrapyramidal effects. The drug you would expect the physician to order for these side effects is

1. Xanax.
2. L-dopa.
3. Cogentin.
4. No medication will resolve symptoms; the drug must be discontinued.

184. As part of preoperative teaching, you inform the client of postoperative measures to prevent atelectasis. The intervention that will best accomplish this goal is to

1. Have the client turn, cough, and deep breathe every two hours.
2. Put pillows under the client's knees to decrease pressure on the incision, thereby increasing her willingness to take deep breaths.
3. Apply a scultetus binder as soon as the client is fully awake to assist with deep breathing.
4. Closely observe the client's intake of fluids to liquefy secretions.

185. Before a client goes to surgery, it is necessary for him to sign an operative permit. The most appropriate sequence for having him sign the permit is to

1. Have the client sign the permit as soon as he is admitted so he knows what surgery he will be having.
2. Prepare the client for surgery, give the preoperative narcotics, and have him sign the permit before he goes to sleep.
3. Ensure that the surgeon has explained the surgery to the client, answer his questions, have him sign the permit, and then complete the final preparations for surgery.
4. Have the client sign the operative permit and then notify the physician that the permit has been signed.

Tommy Fitzgerald, a 9 year old, is hospitalized to undergo evaluation. His history indicates that he has frequent severe respiratory infections. A tentative diagnosis of cystic fibrosis is made.

186. You expect that Tommy will have a test used for the diagnosis of cystic fibrosis called

1. Sweat chloride.
2. Blood glucose.
3. Sputum culture.
4. Stool specimen for fat content.

187. Tommy has greatly improved and is about to be discharged. Knowing that children with cystic fibrosis often develop pneumonia secondary to colds, the self-care principle it is important to teach Tommy before discharge is the

1. Need for protein enzymes in his diet to protect him from colds.
2. Exercise restrictions he must adhere to after discharge to prevent sweating and catching a chill.
3. Breathing exercises he should do to develop lung potential.
4. Need for high-protein, moderate-fat diet to improve nutritional status.

188. Helping Mrs. Fitzgerald plan for Tommy's care at home, the type of diet most appropriate is

1. High caloric, high protein, low fat.
2. Low carbohydrate, high protein, high fat.
3. Low caloric, low fat, low protein.
4. High carbohydrate, high fat, high protein.

189. Tommy will take pancreatic enzymes three times a day. You will know Mrs. Fitzgerald understands the purpose of these enzymes if she says

1. "They should be taken at intervals of eight hours with a large glass of milk."
2. "They should be given following breakfast, lunch, and dinner."
3. "Tommy can take them at any time from six to eight hours apart depending on the family schedule."
4. "Tommy should take them prior to meals."

190. Negative nitrogen balance can occur following surgery. You will evaluate for the clinical manifestation most indicative of this state, which is

1. Dehydration leading to poor skin turgor.
2. Edema or ascites of the abdomen and flank.
3. Jaundice.
4. Diarrhea.

191. As you are administering daily care, the client suddenly coughs and an evisceration of the wound occurs. Your priority intervention is to

1. Apply butterfly tape to the wound edges.
2. Apply an abdominal binder to the incision.
3. Obtain vital signs.
4. Place the client in a supine position.

192. Young Kenny Crew weighs 10 kilograms and the adult dose of a medication is 10 mg. The closest correct dosage to give the child is

1. 1.0 mg.
2. 1.5 mg.
3. 2.5 mg.
4. None of the above.

193. In which situation would gloves not be necessary when caring for an AIDS client?

1. When in contact with urine.
2. When suctioning clients.
3. Changing an ostomy pouch.
4. Monitoring an IV infusion.

194. When performing naso-oral suctioning, the correct action is to

1. Insert the catheter 6 to 8 inches into nares.
2. Apply suction while inserting the catheter into the bronchus.
3. Apply continuous suction as the catheter is removed during the procedure.
4. Suction for 30 seconds and then allow a three minute rest period.

Barney Johns, aged 18, is admitted to the ICU following a car accident. He is unconscious and has multiple injuries. His most serious injury is a flail chest, which has resulted in hypoventilation.

195. Barney was brought to the hospital by the paramedics. To begin treatment the hospital staff must

1. Attempt to obtain parental consent.
2. Obtain a court order.
3. Wait for Barney to regain consciousness.
4. Immediately begin treatment without consent.

196. If Barney continues to hypoventilate, you will evaluate for a consequence of this condition,

1. Respiratory acidosis.
2. Respiratory alkalosis.
3. Metabolic acidosis.
4. Metabolic alkalosis.

You are assigned to care for Len Royce, a 20-year-old who has just had chest tubes inserted.

197. An important intervention is to

1. Place a hemostat nearby in case of an air leak.
2. Check the chest tubes every two hours for air leaks.
3. Coil the tubes carefully to prevent kinking which could result in an air leak.
4. Keep Len flat to avoid leaks in the tubing.

198. Nursing goals to be included in the care plan for Len while he has chest tubes in place will be to

1. Keep the chest tubes free of kinking by attaching them to the bed.
2. Keep the bottles below bed level to prevent backflow.
3. Check that water fluctuation is continuous in the trap bottle.
4. Check that the amount of pressure does not exceed 5 cm water in the pressure chamber.

---

199. Bill Geary, age 10, has just completed chelation therapy for lead poisoning. As you assess his condition, you observe that he is experiencing tetany. This is caused by

1. Increased sodium (NA+).
2. Decreased calcium (Ca++).
3. Decreased magnesium (Mg++).
4. Decreased potassium (K+).

200. Brian Woodlin is admitted to the hospital with a diagnosis of portal cirrhosis—late stage. He has generalized edema and ascites. He has difficulty sleeping and asks you to get him something to help him sleep. The doctor orders phenobarbital (Luminal) 100 mg H.S. or prn. The nursing intervention is to

1. Hold the dose until he asks for it during the night.
2. Give the dose as ordered at bedtime.
3. Question the drug that was ordered.
4. Question the dose of the drug.

201. You observe that signs of hypoxia occur during a tracheostomy suctioning procedure. The step in the procedure that will prevent hypoxia is to

1. Ensure that the catheter is no more than three quarters the diameter of the tube.
2. Limit suction time to 30 seconds.
3. Hyperinflate lungs with 100% oxygen prior to suctioning.
4. Suction no more than three consecutive times before administering oxygen.

202. If a client needs oxygen therapy, you would be alert for the sign or symptom of

1. Yawning.
2. Bradycardia.
3. Hypercapnia.
4. Rosy lips.

Marie Simmons fell from a horse and sustained a head injury.

203. As Marie's nurse, you will consider all of the following goals. The one to receive first priority is to

1. Control her pain and restlessness.
2. Maintain an open airway.
3. Maintain her fluid-electrolyte balance.
4. Monitor her neurological status, including vital signs.

204. The most sensitive indication of Marie's clinical condition following her head injury is

1. Pupillary changes.
2. Level of consciousness.
3. Blood pressure and pulse.
4. Motor function.

205. You are assigned to work with a highly anxious client who is difficult to work with and occasionally you find yourself getting irritated. The attitude important to maintain in working with this client is

1. A matter-of-fact and down-to-earth approach.
2. Willingness to help her in everything.
3. Calm and supportive.
4. Light and amusing.

206. Lucy Greenburg has diabetes and she asks you what will happen to her insulin requirements during her pregnancy. The best response is

1. "Because your case is so mild, you are not likely to need much insulin during your pregnancy."
2. "As the pregnancy progresses to term, you will need increased insulin."
3. "Every case is individual so there's really no way to say."
4. "If you follow the diet well and don't gain too much weight, your insulin needs should stay about the same."

207. A new mother asks you how her diabetes relates to breast feeding. The most accurate statement is that it is

1. Contraindicated because insulin is passed to the infant through the milk.
2. Contraindicated because the diabetic's milk production mechanism is faulty.
3. Contraindicated because it puts too much stress on the mother's body.
4. Not contraindicated.

208. For a client who requires the highest possible concentration of oxygen, the delivery system you will use is a

1. Nasal cannula.
2. Venturi mask.
3. Face tent.
4. Mask with reservoir bag.

209. The most important nursing intervention for clients on IPPB therapy is to

1. Make the client comfortable in a supine position during the treatment.
2. Monitor blood pressure, pulse, and respirations before and after the treatment.
3. Instruct the client to inhale, and then cover mouthpiece with mouth and exhale into the machine.
4. Instruct the client to breathe at the rate of 20 times per minute.

210. While assessing a client in skeletal traction, you observe the distal extremity to be pale with slow capillary refill and palpated at a 1+ pulse. Your initial action is to

1. Assess the client every 15 minutes for changes.
2. Observe for ecchymosis or signs of infection.
3. Remove the traction.
4. Notify the physician.

211. Kevin is 18 months old. You counsel his mother that the best procedure to follow if her child swallows something poisonous is to first

1. Telephone the local poison control center.
2. Bring the child to the emergency room.
3. Give the child syrup of Ipecac to drink to induce vomiting.
4. Ascertain what substance the child swallowed.

212. You are eating in a restaurant and someone yells, "Help! My husband is choking." Knowing first aid, the first thing you should do is

1. Give an abdominal thrust.
2. Give a back blow.
3. Establish an airway.
4. Ask the victim, "Can you talk?"

213. On duty in the emergency room, you are concerned when a client continues to bleed from severe lacerations even after applying direct pressure. Your next action is to

1. Apply ice to lower the body temperature.
2. Monitor closely for signs of shock.
3. Elevate her upper extremities and apply blankets to raise her body temperature.
4. Maintain a patent airway and prevent vomiting.

214. The IV is placed on a controller to maintain the flow rate. If the alarm sounds on the controller, which of the following actions will you not perform?

1. Ensure that the drip chamber is full.
2. Assess that height of IV container is at least 30 inches above venipuncture site.
3. Ensure that the drop sensor is properly placed on the drip chamber.
4. Evaluate the needle and IV tubing to determine if they are patent and positioned appropriately.

215. Mrs. Edison asks why the medication erythromycin is put in her baby's eyes. You explain that it is placed in the baby's eyes to prevent

1. Gonorrheal infection.
2. Retrolental fibroplasia.
3. Blindness.
4. Transferral of AIDS virus.

216. As part of your newborn assessment, you know that signs of hypoglycemia in the infant include

1. Restlessness, whining cry.
2. Stuporlike behavior, no cry.
3. High-pitched cry.
4. Weak, soft cry.

Mr. Hurd, an obese man of 54, came into the emergency clinic complaining of a painful, tender big toe. His admitting diagnosis was gout.

217. Mr. Hurd was put on colchicine medication. You explain to Mr. Hurd that the primary action of this medication is to

1. Reduce inflammation.
2. Alleviate pain.
3. Decrease uric acid level.
4. Alkalinize urine.

218. You are preparing Mr. Hurd's discharge plan. You will know he understands his dietary requirements if he chooses

1. Liver, fried onions, potatoes, and cauliflower.
2. Cheese omelet, wheat toast, and broiled tomato.
3. Broiled chicken, potato, gravy, and green beans.
4. Salmon, rice, broccoli, and milk.

219. Marjorie, age 16, is admitted with a diagnosis of anorexia nervosa because she refused to eat at home. A history that includes certain signs or symptoms is used for diagnosis of this disorder. The most definitive signs and symptoms are

1. Significant weight loss and heart failure.
2. Weight loss of 25 percent and broken bones due to calcium leaching.
3. Hypotension and anemia.
4. Weight loss of 25 percent and no menstrual period for three months.

220. Mrs. Peterman, a diabetic, gave birth to a healthy 8 lb. baby. For the second feeding, Baby Peterman was given glucose water. The next most important nursing action is to

1. Observe for hyperbilirubinemia.
2. Administer formula, preferably breast milk.
3. Monitor is infant's respiratory status.
4. Monitor glucose levels in the infant with Dextrostix.

ANSWERS AND RATIONALE

The correct answer for each question is indicated in parentheses. The rationale explains why that answer is correct and often provides additional background information to reinforce your understanding of the subject. The code that follows each rationale defines the NCLEX Test Plan categories. A description of these categories can be found in the introduction to the book. The categories are as follows:

NP   Nursing Process
    AS   Assessment
    AN   Analysis
    PL   Planning
    IM   Implementation
    EV   Evaluation

CN   Client Need
    SE   Safe, Effective Care Environment
    PH   Physiological Integrity
    PS   Psychosocial Integrity
    HM   Health Promotion and Maintenance

CA   Clinical Area
    ME   Medical Nursing
    SU   Surgical Nursing
    MA   Maternity Nursing
    PE   Pediatric Nursing
    PY   Psychiatric Nursing

1. (1) Weights must hang freely off floor and bed to ensure countertraction. Ropes should be securely knotted, but they must move freely through pulleys. The client should not be pulled down in bed, since this position will negate the traction. NP–AS; CN–SE; CA–SU

2. (2) Since the most common complication of total joint replacement is dislocation, correct positioning is important. Turning the client on either side without keeping the abduction pillow in place could lead to dislocation of the new prosthesis. NP–EV; CN–HM; CA–ME

3. (1) It is important that the brace remain on at all times except for bathing. It will also be important to teach her to use good skin care in the area where the brace touches her skin. NP–EV; CN–HM; CA–SU

4. (4) If a contraction lasts longer than 90 seconds, the safe and correct first action is to turn off the Pitocin. Prolonged contractions can result in a ruptured uterus. The nurse may also administer oxygen and call the physician. NP–IM; CN–SE; CA–MA

5. (2) Initially, physical injuries will take precedence over other aspects of care. They need to be assessed, treated and documented for possible legal action. Crisis treatment will be the next goal of care. NP–AS; CN–PH; CA–PY

6. (2) Mr. Andrews needs to be prepared for short-term memory loss and told that it will resolve in six to nine months. While it is true that he will receive three medications, he needs more specific information about their action. NP–IM; CN–PS; CA–PY

7. (1) Reactive = good outcome. Increased FHR with movement indicates normal reaction and adequate CNS integration. NP–AN; CN–PH; CA–MA

8. (4) The best choice of meal is fish (not halibut or cod, both high in potassium), rice, and green beans. Bread and ice cream will add calories and protein. Instant coffee is high in potassium, and beets and spinach are high in sodium. NP–EV; CN–HM; CA–ME

9. (2) While all of the actions should be carried out, the priority of care is to restore fluid and electrolyte balance. This condition may lead to death from shock, vascular collapse or hyperkalemia. NP–PL; CN–PH; CA–ME

10. (2) The safest phase is at 4 to 5 cm dilatation or the active phase. Given too early, this medication will decrease or stop labor; given later in labor, it will depress the infant's respirations. NP–PL; CN–PH; CA–MA

11. (2) German measles or rubella, if contracted in the 1st trimester of pregnancy, may result in a child with congenital malformations of the heart, eye and ear, as well as mental retardation. NP–AN; CN–HM; CA–MA

12. (2) Moro's and rooting reflexes are present at birth and disappear at about 4 months. Neck righting reflex evolves at 4 months and disappears at 9 to 12 months. Kernig's sign is present with meningeal irritation. NP–AS; CN–HM; CA–PE

13. (1) The first action is to support the perineum to prevent tears and rapid delivery. The nurse will ask the client to take short breaths (following instructions) but to prevent pushing; the nurse will also send someone for the physician. NP–IM; CN–SE; CA–MA

14. (1) Wernicke's is a life-threatening condition that occurs as a result of chronic alcoholism with inadequate nutrients, especially thiamine. It must be treated by thiamine stat. An IV glucose with B-complex vitamins will also be initiated. NP–PL; CN–SE; CA–PY

15. (4) The head is down, the back is on the right side, legs on left, and fetus' bottom in the fundus indicate the position of ROA. NP–AN; CN–PH; CA–MA

16. (4) The appropriate intervention is to withhold the thiazide medication until you receive further orders and report K^+ level to the physician. Normal K^+ is 3.5 to 5.5 mEq/l. His NA^+ level is normal (range 135 to 145 mEq/l). NP–IM; CN–SE; CA–ME

17. (3) Elderly senile clients are often anxious, especially in an unfamiliar environment. Structure decreases anxiety. Making choices and constantly changing activities will increase anxiety. Their activity should not necessarily be limited. NP–PL; CN–PS; CA–PY

18. (3) An important safety guideline issued by the Occupational Safety and Health Administration (OSHA) is to wear surgical gloves and a disposable gown. The nurse will need special training but there is not a special nurse assigned to give the drug, nor are these drugs checked with a second nurse.
NP–IM; CN–SE; CA–ME

19. (1) These signs are indicative of fluid overload due to decreased ability to excrete urine. When the end products of metabolism cannot be excreted in sufficient amounts, they will accumulate in the body. Resultant blood samples will indicate higher levels of creatinine, potassium, and magnesium, not lower levels. When fluid overload occurs due to decreased urine output, the intravascular compartment becomes overloaded with fluids causing tachycardia and neck vein distention. NP–AS; CN–PH; CA–ME

20. (1) Complete amino acid proteins break down into end products of protein that are removed by the dialysis procedure. There should only be adjustment, not full restriction, to maintain positive nitrogen balance and replace protein lost in dialysis. A high-calorie diet should be encouraged with sodium and potassium restricted. Foods in answer (4) are high in potassium. NP–EV; CN–HM; CA–ME

21. (3) About 50 percent of the people who do die outside the hospital have a fatal arrhythmia, usually shortly after experiencing the onset of symptoms. NP–AN; CN–PH; CA–ME

22. (3) In order to maintain blood volumes which do not overwork the heart muscle, low sodium diets are recommended. Unsaturated fats are recommended for clients with coronary artery disease, as they do not seem to contribute to atherosclerosis formation. Bland diets are used for clients with gastrointestinal diseases who cannot tolerate roughage and spices. A clear liquid diet is used in some centers for clients with myocardial infarctions; this is done to reduce the risk of aspiration and to decrease the workload of the heart. NP–IM; CN–HM; CA–ME

23. (1) Fresh fruit is the lowest in sodium of the foods listed. Turkey, bread, and mayonnaise contain larger amounts of sodium. Ice cream contains sodium, and seafood salad may contain salty, seasoned sauces. NP–EV; CN–HM; CA–ME

24. (2) The Code of Ethics assists the nurse to problem solve where judgment is required. It encompasses professional responsibility and accountability. NP–AN; CN–SE; CA–PY

25. (2) Blind clients become anxious when they hear someone enter the room without talking. NP–PL; CN–PS; CA–ME

26. (3) Nonverbal action conveys acceptance, openness to listen, and empathy. It assists the client to verbalize feelings. NP–IM; CN–PS; CA–PY

27. (3) By keeping the lines of communication open, Mr. Betman may be able to discuss his fears and concerns. If he can verbalize these issues, he can begin to cope with his condition and continue in the rehabilitative process. The other responses close off communication. NP–IM; CN–PS; CA–PY

28. (2) Redness, or erythema, is the first sign of possible injury. This is an important observation to prevent a burn injury. NP–AS; CN–SE; CA–ME

29. (4) Evaluation of the effects of the restraint is important to chart. Procedure is not relevant and what the client says may or may not be appropriate. Physician orders are already charted so you would not chart them again. NP–EV; CN–SE; CA–PY

30. (1) Type A is a factor VIII deficiency; type B, a IX deficiency; and type C, a factor XI deficiency. NP–AN; CN–PH; CA–PE

31. (2) The nurse acknowledges the mother's feelings, but at the same time identifies a factor that must be dealt with as the child grows older and demands more independence. NP–IM; CN–PS; CA–PE

32. (1) The immediate action would be to immobilize the joint. Passive range of motion exercises should be started 48 hours following immobilization. NP–PL; CN–PH; CA–PE

33. (1) The FHR needs to be checked first to determine whether the cord is prolapsed. The cord has an increased possibility of prolapsing when the membranes rupture. NP–IM; CN–SE; CA–MA

34. (3) Transportation by wheelchair can prevent falls and injury; therefore, safety is the important issue. NP–IM; CN–SE; CA–ME

35. (3) The client who is out of control and physically strikes out needs to have his behavior immediately controlled by the nursing staff. The client must not be allowed to injure himself or others. NP–IM; CN–PS; CA–PY

36. (3) The first goal for the nurse is to prevent loss of control. Removing stimuli that may be frightening to the client would be the first intervention. NP–PL; CN–PS; CA–PY

37. (3) Before rolling client on his side, your hands must be in the correct position to turn. Answer (4) would be the final intervention. NP–IM; CN–SE; CA–ME

38. (3) It is important to find out how Julie feels about baby care. She may just be tired, she may be afraid, or she may have some other reason for her request that you need to assess further. NP–AS; CN–PS; CA–MA

39. (4) All of the above actions would be appropriate to carry out. Legally, signing the against medical advice (AMA) form is most important. NP–IM; CN–HM; CA–ME

40. (3) These are normal physical findings for postpartum day four. If Mrs. Susman is breast feeding, it may be time for the baby to nurse. If she is not breast feeding, she should have on a tight, well-fitted bra. Ice packs may be applied to the breasts. NP–PL; CN–PH; CA–MA

41. (1) Before moving the client, dangling at the bedside is important. This procedure stabilizes the client and allows you time to assess whether he develops vertigo from a drop in blood pressure. NP–IM; CN–SE; CA–SU

42. (2) Violent behavior often occurs as a response to a real or imagined threat. Hallucinations can be threatening in nature. NP–AN; CN–PS; CA–PY

43. (2) These are symptoms of a blood dyscrasia, agranulocytosis, which indicates the immune system is depressed. Akathisia is a side effect that also occurs with an antipsychotic drug, but it is an extrapyramidal effect. NP–AN; CN–PH; CA–PY

44. (4) With pregnancy, there is an increased vascularity and blood supply to the vaginal area causing tissue to appear deep red or purplish in color. NP–AN; CN–PH; CA–MA

45. (1) Visual disturbance is a symptom of preeclampsia and the client must immediately be put under a physician's care to prevent further development of eclampsia. NP–EV; CN–HM; CA–MA

46. (4) Todd is encouraged to express his feelings. This may lead to further discussion of the client's reactions to his own feelings when he feels threatened. Answers (2) and (3) are incorrect and focus on the intellectual aspect of this reaction. Answer (1) is incorrect because it does not encourage Todd to express his feelings and explore his behavior. NP–IM; CN–PS; CA–PY

47. (1) During pregnancy, there is an increased need for calories, protein, and iron. A high fat, high carbohydrate diet is not recommended because it may cause excessive weight gain and fat deposits, which are difficult to lose after pregnancy. NP–IM; CN–HM; CA–MA

48. (4) The primary purposes of client education include increasing knowledge, increasing self-esteem, improving client's ability to make decisions, and facilitating behavioral changes. NP–AN; CN–HM; CA–PY

49. (3) A nurse should use a soft or regular nipple with a slightly enlarged hole and feed the infant on the side opposite the cleft. NP–PL; CN–SE; CA–PE

50. (2) Pain is reduced upon eating when the client has a duodenal ulcer. When the duodenum is empty, about two to three hours after eating, the pain recurs. NP–AS; CN–PH; CA–ME

51. (4) Bleeding is a more severe complication than either constipation or diarrhea. Bright-red stools indicate a bleeding problem low in the gastrointestinal tract. A bleeding duodenal ulcer would have tarry stools, as the blood has been digested by the action of the intestinal juices. NP–EV; CN–PH; CA–ME

52. (2) This approach would help decrease your client's anxiety and assist him in gaining insights. Answers (1) and (4) deny the problem and (3) is not as conducive to open communication. NP–AN; CN–PS; CA–PY

53. (1) The crutches and unaffected leg start on the same level; then, the unaffected leg is moved to the step, followed by the crutches and affected leg. NP–IM; CN–HM; CA–SU

54. (3) The shock position is necessary to maintain vital signs. The other interventions may be carried out, but are not initial actions. NP–IM; CN–PH; CA–ME

55. (4) Soda bicarbonate is absorbed into the system and destroys acid balance; it can lead to alkalosis. NP–IM; CN–HM; CA–ME

56. (4) While all the objectives listed in the answers are important, assessment of his hydrational status is the most critical. NP–AS; CN–SE; CA–PE

57. (2) A stuffed animal would not be harmful and it would be comforting. Play dough is more appropriate for older children. Jacks are not safe for an infant; they will go immediately into the infant's mouth. NP–PL; CN–HM; CA–PE

58. (1) A toddler who passively accepts aggressive painful intrusions into his or her life has usually given up any sense of hope and is suffering from separation anxiety. He is depressed and requires specialized care from the staff and parents. NP–AN; CN–HM; CA–PE

59. (2) Short acting insulin is withdrawn first in order to prevent possible contamination of the short acting insulin bottle by the longer acting insulin. NP–PL; CN–SE; CA–ME

60. (3) Exertion increases myocardial oxygen needs and is the most common cause of angina. Constant activity and stress will also increase the need for oxygen but it will not be as dramatic. NP–AN; CN–PH; CA–ME

61. (3) Nitroglycerin should be taken whenever the client feels a full, pressure feeling or tightness in his or her chest, and not wait until chest pain is severe. It can also be taken prophylactically to prevent an anginal attack before engaging in an activity known to cause angina. NP–IM; CN–HM; CA–ME

62. (2) This is a method that involves infusion of a solution of protein, glucose, electrolytes, vitamins, and minerals—complete nutrition by the intravenous route. NP–AN; CN–PH; CA–PE

63. (3) You will note these sounds with an obstruction. Paralytic ileus has no bowel sounds or gurgling. Gastric distention will have tympanic sounds. NP–AS; CN–PH; CA–ME

64. (4) A complete bowel obstruction will have clear drainage and may approach 3000 ml/day. A small bowel obstruction will have yellow and fecal-smelling drainage. NP–AN; CN–PH; CA–ME

65. (3) Protamine sulfate is the antagonist for Heparin. Answer (2), Vitamin K, is the antagonist for Coumadin. Answer (4) is the antagonist for magnesium sulfate. NP–PL; CN–SE; CA–ME

66. (1) The primary purpose for the compulsive activity is an attempt to reduce the anxiety level. If anxiety is increased, the client may extend the compulsive behavior or develop a new compulsion—all in an attempt to reduce anxiety. NP–AN; CN–PS; CA–PY

67. (3) The most appropriate nursing goal is to arrange the schedule so that Mrs. Whiting is up in time to complete the activity so that she will eat with the other clients. It is not therapeutic to interrupt the activity or to force Mrs. Whiting to make a choice because these actions will only raise her anxiety level. NP–IM; CN–PS; CA–PY

68. (4) Shunts should be inspected several times each day for presence of possible clotting. Dark spots will

quickly be followed by separation of the sera and cells if clotting becomes complete. When dark spots appear, clients should be instructed to immediately seek treatment for declotting. NP–PL; CN–SE; CA–SU

69. (1) The principle underlying the way dialysis works is the ability of fluid to move between compartments across a semipermeable membrane. When blood moves through the dialysate, the waste products, such as urea, are removed because they are low weight molecules and can be diffused through the membrane; water is able to move across the membrane.
NP–AN; CN–PH; CA–SU

70. (2) Pain is the only symptom that would occur with thrombophlebitis. The surrounding area would be warm to the touch, and red, indicating an inflammatory response. There is no relationship between varicosities and thrombus formation.
NP–AS; CN–PH; CA–ME

71. (4) On dorsiflexion of the foot, the client will experience upper posterior pain in the calf if a clot is present. This is termed Homan's sign.
NP–EV; CN–PH; CA–ME

72. (4) It is best to plan any activity, particularly therapy, to follow the compulsive activity because anxiety is lowest at this time. NP–PL; CN–PS; CA–PY

73. (1) Low-Fowler's position promotes optimal perfusion and adequate ventilatory exchange. Oxygen administration is the second nursing intervention.
NP–IM; CN–SE; CA–ME

74. (2) Hyperreflexia occurs with increased CNS irritation. Epigastric pain is usually due to edema or bleeding into the liver capsule and oliguria. Other signs include edema and hypertension.
NP–EV; CN–PH; CA–MA

75. (2) Thrombic crises are the result of occlusion of small blood vessels. Sequestration crises are the result of pooling of blood in the spleen. Hemarthroses occurs in hemophilia. NP–AN; CN–PH; CA–PE

76. (3) Answer (1) is wrong because Brittany could not have the disease if only one parent has either the trait or the disease. Answer (2) is wrong because one parent could have the disease, one parent the trait, or both parents have the trait. Answer (3) is correct.
NP–IM; CN–PH; CA–PE

77. (2) A posterior position often causes severe back pain and a bearing-down sensation during the contraction. NP–AN; CN–PH; CA–MA

78. (4) Counterpressure provides much pain relief by supporting the sacrum as the head is driven down by the contraction. Also try positional changes—knee-chest often provides pain relief. It is too early for any analgesics. NP–IM; CN–SE; CA–MA

79. (1) These signs, in addition to laryngeal edema, are characteristic of an allergic reaction which is, less specifically, a transfusion reaction. Chills, increased temperature, and pain in the kidney region are indications of a hemolytic reaction. NP–AN; CN–PH; CA–ME

80. (4) If the nurse suspects an allergic reaction, the blood should be shut off immediately, then the physician should be notified and the client placed in a position to facilitate breathing. NP–IM; CN–SE; CA–ME

81. (2) PCA works more effectively to control pain for the client with no significant difference in the amount of medication used. It is less time consuming for the nurse, but this is not the essential rationale. NP–AN; CN–PS; CA–ME

82. (1) Since Mrs. Newman's condition is terminal, the highest priority is to attend to her physical needs and continue assessment. Contacting her family and supporting them is part of your role as a professional nurse, but contacting the priest is inappropriate without Mrs. Newman or the family specifically requesting it. NP–PL; CN–PH; CA–ME

83. (4) Drops instilled in the center of the sac will assist in distributing the medication over the entire surface of the conjunctiva and anterior eyeball.
NP–PL; CN–SE; CA–ME

84. (2) This diet will control the end products of protein metabolism and prevent ammonia buildup, as well as decrease fluid accumulation. A small amount of protein is needed for tissue repair.
NP–PL; CN–HM; CA–ME

85. (3) Blood pressure is increased with a wide pulse pressure (the difference between the systolic pressure and the diastolic pressure). The cerebrospinal fluid pressure may cause elevated blood pressure by reducing oxygen supply to the hypothalamic vasomotor center. The excess of carbon dioxide which then forms will

stimulate the center and cause an increase in the blood pressure. NP–AS; CN–PH; CA–ME

86. (3) This reflective response will open up communication and enable the client to express whatever concerns or feelings she has without confining her to a discussion of dying (answer 2). NP–IM; CN–PS; CA–PY

87. (4) Mrs. Brynes' drive to breathe is hypoxia. When she was given an FIO_2 to return her arterial pO_2 level to above normal, the peripheral chemoreceptors no longer could respond to hypoxia. NP–AN; CN–PH; CA–ME

88. (1) Respiratory acidosis (hypercarbia or increased CO_2) exhibits the following manifestations: headache, dizziness, confusion, tremor, somnolence. Respiratory alkalosis (hyperventilation or decreased CO_2) exhibits the following manifestations: paresthesias, tetany, anxiety, tachycardia. NP–AS; CN–PH; CA–ME

89. (2) The central chemoreceptors had been dulled over the years by the constant increased CO_2 level, so they did not respond to an increasing pCO_2 level. Hypercarbia (increased pCO_2) exhibits symptoms of somnolence and coma in the acute situation. NP–EV; CN–PH; CA–ME

90. (3) Steroid administration is frequently ordered to decrease edema and prevent inflammation. Enemas are usually not administered as they tend to cause straining, which can lead to increased intracranial pressure. A nasogastric tube, if inserted, is done under sedation to prevent increased intracranial pressure. IV fluids are usually limited so as not to increase fluid volume, hence increasing ICP. NP–PL; CN–SE; CA–SU

91. (4) Serial blood and urine samples are collected, because sodium regulation disturbances frequently accompany head injury. The temperature should be kept at normal to avoid increasing metabolic needs. At 97°F, the client would probably shiver, causing not only increased intracranial pressure but also increased metabolic rate. Fluids are kept at a minimum to prevent overhydration, which can lead to cerebral edema. NP–PL; CN–PH; CA–SU

92. (4) The Kings are denying the disease. In most circumstances this will pass, as it is a coping mechanism that shields them partially from the grief of the situation. Now they need to feel free to discuss their feelings and to grieve. NP–IM; CN–PS; CA–PE

93. (2) Though all these symptoms may occur during the course of leukemia, every answer except (2) includes one symptom that occurs as a late sign as the disease continues, or as a result of therapy. NP–AS; CN–PH; CA–PE

94. (2) A serious side effect of Cytoxan is hemorrhagic cystitis, and fluids would help prevent this from occurring. NP–IM; CN–SE; CA–PE

95. (3) In shock, there is decreased blood volume through the kidneys. This is evidenced by a decrease in the amount of urine excreted. The body has numerous compensatory mechanisms that assist in keeping the blood pressure normal for a short time. NP–EV; CN–PH; CA–ME

96. (1) It is important to remember that OBS clients usually have some memory and concentration impairment. The degree depends upon the individual and is influenced by the basic personality structure and the cause of the problem. NP–PL; CN–PS; CA–PY

97. (2) Raw apples are high in potassium, while white-enriched and French bread, dry cereal, and pasta are foods low in potassium. NP–EV; CN–HM; CA–ME

98. (1) Gentle pressure is necessary when irrigating a nasogastric tube to prevent damage to the stomach wall. Saline prevents electrolyte imbalance. NP–PL; CN–SE; CA–ME

99. (3) The client will not be fed until bowel sounds are present, abdominal distention relieved, and flatus is passed. Answer (3) would be the first intervention, followed by (2) and (4) if necessary. NP–IM; CN–SE; CA–SU

100. (2) Your first intervention is to increase IV fluids to maintain a CVP reading of 5–9 cm water pressure. Vasodilators will be administered to reduce peripheral resistance to blood flow and to increase capillary perfusion after the intravascular space has been expanded. NP–IM; CN–SE; CA–SU

101. (2) Answers (3) and (4) are important, but the emotional support of his family is vital. Intellectual understanding may not affect an improvement in his condition inasmuch as it may be used to avoid the underlying feelings and conflicts. NP–EV; CN–PS; CA–PY

102. (2) The leg must be kept in abduction. This position prevents dislocation of the new hip until range of

motion can be instituted. Buck's traction is no longer used following total hip replacement. Physicians now order that the client may be turned on either side postop. NP–PL; CN–PH; CA–SU

103. (2) Postoperative hip replacement clients may get up the first day, but need to use a walker for balance. They should not bear any weight on the affected side or sit in a chair, flexing their hips. Positions with 60° to 90° flexion should be avoided. NP–IM; CN–SE; CA–SU

104. (1) Nasogastric intubation can lead to the complication of electrolyte imbalance because of removing the gastric contents by suctioning. Large amounts of sodium and potassium are lost through the suctioning and, if not replaced via IV fluids, can lead to serious electrolyte imbalance. NP–EV; CN–PH; CA–SU

105. (2) The aspirate contains electrolytes and hydrochloric acid; therefore, it must be replaced to prevent an imbalance. With a residual of 50 cc, the usual action is to administer the tube feeding. NP–IM; CN–PH; CA–ME

106. (3) Checking the urine for glucose and acetone is essential to prevent a hyperosmolar condition. Insulin may have to be administered according to rainbow coverage. Notify physician for urine glucose over 2+ and positive acetone. NP–IM; CN–PH; CA–ME

107. (1) The seventh cranial nerve supplies both motor and sensory function. The eyelid closure is a result of the motor function. NP–AS; CN–PH; CA–ME

108. (3) A regular nipple is too hard and will make it difficult for the infant to suck, causing unnecessary fatigue. A premie soft nipple should be used. NP–PL; CN–SE; CA–PE

109. (3) This comment reflects her feelings of inadequacy because the infant is so small, implying that she does not feel capable of caring for her own child. NP–AN; CN–PS; CA–PY

110. (4) The nurse, while recognizing and accepting this mother's apprehension, assures her that she will have assistance. NP–IM; CN–PS; CA–PY

111. (3) Ellen's history and behavior indicate that she is depressed. The most important interventions for a depressed person are to mobilize and activate

them. A structured schedule will accomplish this objective. NP–PL; CN–PS; CA–PY

112. (3) Adolescents want to be independent most of all, so it is important for them to make their own decisions. NP–IM; CN–HM; CA–PY

113. (3) The safest method, other than x-ray, is to test the contents of the stomach. If the pH is below 3, acid is present and placement is confirmed. While hearing the rush of air in the stomach is an indicator that proper tube placement has occurred, it is not safe because lung inspiration may be confused with the rush of air in the stomach. Though answer (4) is partially correct, it does not definitely indicate that the tube is in the correct position. NP–EV; CN–SE; CA–ME

114. (1) The client is refusing to accept the implications of the diagnosis to protect herself from the unpleasant reality. Denial is a stage of the grief process. NP–EV; CN–PS; CA–PY

115. (4) Semi-Fowler's position will aid in lymphatic and venous drainage of fluid in the affected arm. NP–PL; CN–SE; CA–SU

116. (1) These foods are difficult to digest and can be irritating to the GI tract. They can lead to additional GI symptoms. NP–EV; CN–HM; CA–ME

117. (4) Blood should be drawn from the most peripheral vein to preserve the integrity of the vein for future lab work. With an IV in the right forearm, this site would be unacceptable for blood withdrawal. NP–AS; CN–SE; CA–ME

118. (4) These are the normal side effects of Elavil. Answer (1) refers to MAO inhibitors. Elavil does not deplete fluids (answer 2), and answer (3) refers to the phenothiazines that cause extrapyramidal effects. NP–IM; CN–HM; CA–PY

119. (3) Ambivalence about being pregnant is common in early pregnancy. Your role as her nurse is to provide reassurance that her response is normal and to help her express her concerns. The task of the first trimester is acceptance of the pregnancy. NP–IM; CN–PS; CA–MA

120. (4) The client's initial symptoms usually are related to skin problems and client teaching is important. He should not be told about pneumonitis but

could be told about reporting any unusual symptoms. Answer (2) is too technical and not necessary for client understanding of the disease process. NP–PL; CN–HM; CA–ME

121. (3) During the time the reaction occurs, the protocol states that clients are taken off radiation therapy and instructed to use antibiotic lotion and steroid cream to prevent infection. NP–IM; CN–SE; CA–ME

122. (3) It is important to position Mr. Korngold so that the area of detachment is dependent; this will prevent blindness. All of the other responses are incorrect, as the position totally depends on the area of detachment. NP–PL; CN–SE; CA–ME

123. (1) He must remain on strict bedrest to prevent further damage and to keep the retina attached to the choroid until surgery. Both (3) and (4) are incorrect, as getting up would not keep the retina approximated to the choroid. NP–IM; CN–PH; CA–ME

124. (2) The most common complication with this surgery is hemorrhage; therefore, you would assess for this first. Next you would assess for nausea and vomiting because straining can cause hemorrhage. Sudden eye pain is also indicative of complications. Finally, postoperative position should be flat or low-Fowler's to prevent complications. NP–AS; CN–PH; CA–SU

125. (4) Check if catheter is inserted far enough into urethra or if it is in vagina. If in vagina, leave in place as a landmark, obtain new sterile set-up, and insert new catheter. NP–IM; CN–SE; CA–SU

126. (2) When urine begins to flow, the catheter tip is placed into the specimen container. When the specimen is collected, the catheter tip is placed into the collection receptacle until urine flow ceases. NP–IM; CN–SE; CA–ME

127. (2) Treatment for poisoning should begin at home with syrup of ipecac so Charlie will throw up the tablets from his stomach. Then the nurse should instruct Charlie's mother to bring him into the hospital. NP–IM; CN–SE; CA–PE

128. (3) Answers (1) and (2) are also necessary information but keeping cabinets locked is critical. Not all labels include sufficient information. Charlie's mother should be given the telephone number of a poison control center. NP–IM; CN–HM; CA–PE

129. (2) The test is done primarily to determine fetal trisomy 21 (Down's syndrome) in pregnant women over 35 years of age. If the fetus is defective and the woman or couple do not wish to have an elective abortion, the procedure would probably not be performed due to its potential risk (though small) to the woman. Answer (3) is not correct as Ashkenazic Jews have a high incidence of Tay-Sachs disease. Although more difficult, amniocentesis may be performed on women carrying twins. NP–AS; CN–PS; CA–MA

130. (3) Adequate nutrition and weight gain in pregnancy are directly related to decreased mortality and morbidity in the newborn. Helping the client understand the role of nutrition and weight gain will help her then explore the best way to talk to her husband about his concerns. NP–IM; CN–HM; CA–MA

131. (2) The nurse doesn't have enough data or information to report Mike's case as child abuse, so she should continue the assessment. NP–IM; CN–HM; CA–PE

132. (3) Both the nurse and doctor, independently, are legally responsible to report a suspected battered child to the proper authorities. NP–EV; CN–PS; CA–PE

133. (1) Nägele's Rule is to subtract three months and add seven days. Using this formula, Joan's EDC would be 10/28/94. NP–PL; CN–HM; CA–MA

134. (2) Fetal age is detected by ultrasound (usually BPD or length of femur). Another gestational age determinant is quickening, which is first perceived between 17 to 19 weeks' gestation. NP–AS; CN–HM; CA–MA

135. (1) If Mr. Cody is allergic to shellfish, he most likely will be allergic to the dye used for the cholecystogram. Answers (3) and (4) might be carried out, but they are not the most important. NP–AS; CN–SE; CA–ME

136. (4) The most effective communication technique in this case would be silence; support the client nonverbally, accept her, and open up the opportunity for an expression of feelings. NP–IM; CN–PS; CA–PY

137. (3) Adolescents, having recently achieved some measure of independence, have a fear of losing it. Fear of being displaced occurs in the school-age child and fear of separation occurs in the very young. NP–AN; CN–HM; CA–PE

138. (2) As young adults start spending more time with their peer groups, they frequently adopt eating habits of this group which are often not appropriate for diabetics. NP–AN; CN–HM; CA–PE

139. (1) Clients are positioned in a semi-Fowler's position to assist in drainage. The T-tube can be clamped before meals to accumulate enough bile for digestion. The drainage bottle is positioned below the level of the bed to facilitate drainage. NP–AN; CN–PH; CA–SU

140. (3) The symptom is a characteristic flow of ideas in which one idea rapidly triggers another. The difference between this symptom and associative looseness is that in the latter ideas are not clear or sensible and one idea does not connect to another.
NP–AN; CN–PS; CA–PY

141. (4) This activity would channel her energy, but not increase the external stimuli as the group activities would do. NP–PL; CN–PH; CA–PY

142. (2) Kate, in a manic state, can exert little control over her behavior. She is impulsive, uses poor judgment, and has difficulty making decisions. While gaining attention (answer 1) and finding a way to express herself symbolically (answer 3) may play a part in understanding the underlying reason for Kate's behavior, they are not the most complete or the best answers. NP–EV; CN–PS; CA–PY

143. (3) Giving the client an adequate explanation for the procedure will result in less anxiety and more cooperation. NP–IM; CN–PS; CA–ME

144. (4) Carafate stimulates the release of prostaglandins and stimulates the mucosal barrier so it is important to take the drug on an empty stomach, one hour before or after meals and at bedtime. The duration of drug action is five hours. NP–IM; CN–HM; CA–ME

145. (2) The preferred position is Fowler's with the head flexed forward to assist the tube to move into the esophagus. You would never ask the client to hyperextend the neck, as this might open the airway and cause the tube to enter the trachea. NP–IM; CN–SE; CA–ME

146. (3) Since this drug can cause tachycardia and arrhythmias, it is important to assess the heart rate and rhythm. It may also cause hypotension and GI distress. NP–EV; CN–PH; CA–ME

147. (4) If drainage is stalled, inserting a needle into the air vent will provide an airway in the bag. This will assist drainage by allowing the escape of air from the system, facilitating drainage of dialysate. Another intervention would be to move the client from side to side to stimulate drainage. NP–IM; CN–SE; CA–ME

148. (2) Loss of contact with reality is a symptom of schizophrenia. All of the other symptoms are indicative of depression. And, while schizophrenia may be accompanied by depression, these symptoms will not usually be observed. NP–AS; CN–PS; CA–PY

149. (4) Since many people's problems occur in an interpersonal framework, the group setting is a way to correct faulty perceptions as well as work on ineffective ways of relating to others. The remaining answers are all accurate, but they do not fit the requirement of best rationale. NP–AN; CN–PS; CA–PY

150. (2) A cast is rigid and used to maintain alignment. If it is too tight, it will press on blood vessels. The color of the toes will change first, then temperature, when blood supply is decreased. As the blood flow slows through the walls of the vessels, edema will occur. NP–EV; CN–SE; CA–ME

151. (1) Since the client cannot feel sensory stimuli, a blockage of the nerves between the central nervous system and the peripheral system would be indicated. NP–AS; CN–PH; CA–ME

152. (2) If a wet cast is handled with the fingers, indentations in the cast will occur. This can cause pressure on the skin and cause weakness in the cast. NP–PL; CN–SE; CA–ME

153. (3) One of the methods of determining when a cast is dry and may be moved is when the surface turns from a dull to a shiny appearance.
NP–EV; CN–SE; CA–ME

154. (2) Lithium needs to be monitored to determine if it both controls symptoms and is not in the toxic range. Blood level fluctuates so it needs to be consistently monitored. Side effects may occur at levels above 1.6 mEq/liter but toxicity usually does not occur below 2.0 mEq/liter. Toxicity may occur even with an acceptable level of lithium in the blood. NP–EV; CN–HM; CA–PY

155. (1) These are symptoms of toxicity and you must withhold the next dose. You would then notify the

physician. Kate needs to maintain a normal fluid level to prevent toxicity but this may not be the cause. NP–IM; CN–SE; CA–PY

156. (3) The stapes and ossicle in the middle ear become fixed and immovable. NP–AN; CN–PH; CA–SU

157. (3) Basal cell epithelioma and squamous cell epithelioma are both superficial, easily excised, slow-growing tumors. A sebaceous cyst is a benign (nonmalignant) growth. NP–AN; CN–PH; CA–ME

158. (2) Blood gases are drawn to determine if the oxygen, carbon dioxide, and pH levels are within normal range. The treatment given to the infant depends to a great extent on these results. For example, if the blood pO_2 level is down and the pCO_2 is elevated, the concentration of oxygen the infant is receiving will be increased and the infant may be placed on CPAP or PEEP to increase residual capacity and improve oxygenation. Drugs such as sodium bicarbonate may be given to correct acidosis or a low pH. Normal values: pH 7.35–7.45; pO_2 40–60; pCO_2 35–45.
NP–AS; CN–PH; CA–PE

159. (3) The premature infant has poor body control of temperature and needs immediate attention to keep from losing heat. Reasons for heat loss include little subcutaneous fat and poor insulation, large body surface for weight, immaturity of temperature control, and lack of activity. NP–AN; CN–PH; CA–PE

160. (2) High blood levels of oxygen cause spasms of the retinal vessels, and the destruction of these vessels can cause retrolental fibroplasia and blindness. NP–PL; CN–PH; CA–PE

161. (4) Mr. Brown's burns cover approximately 54 percent of his body surface. Each arm is 9 percent (18 percent) and each leg is 18 percent (36 percent). NP–AN; CN–PH; CA–ME

162. (3) To prevent introduction of pathogens into the urinary tract, sterile equipment is used and its sterility maintained. NP–PL; CN–SE; CA–ME

163. (4) One of the principles of growth and development is that children develop at different rates. NP–IM; CN–HM; CA–PE

164. (1) Until the gag reflex returns, the client cannot handle foods or liquids, and may aspirate. Suctioning is not usually ordered. NP–EV; CN–SE; CA–ME

165. (1) Immaturity of the liver is responsible for hyperbilirubinemia and white cell count would be related to potential infection. NP–AN; CN–PH; CA–PE

166. (3) The normal WBC is 4500 to 11,000/cu mm. If the results were abnormally high, the surgeon would have to be notified and the surgery may be canceled. Tests with abnormal results are not routinely repeated unless the results are grossly abnormal. NP–IM; CN–SE; CA–SU

167. (4) All the other reports are within normal range. The ketonuria indicates a probable diabetic complication or other metabolic condition. NP–IM; CN–SE; CA–SU

168. (2) Allowing the client to express her fears results in a decrease in anxiety and a more realistic and knowledgeable reaction to the situation. NP–IM; CN–PS; CA–PY

169. (2) Dose on hand is in 10 ml, so multiply answer of dose desired divided by dose on hand by 10 ml. Example: 0.5 divided by 5 and multiplied by 10 equals 0.1, then multiplying by 10 equals 1 ml. NP–AN; CN–SE; CA–ME

170. (3) When both positive and negative feelings are felt toward the deceased, the grief process is more difficult to resolve because of guilt arising from the negative feelings. NP–AN; CN–PS; CA–PY

171. (3) Jane is projecting her own inadequacies on the teacher and not taking responsibility for her own behavior. NP–EV; CN–PS; CA–PY

172. (1) The left side position assists in easy insertion of the tube due to the anatomical position of the rectum. NP–PL; CN–PH; CA–SU

173. (2) The client requires treatment for shock. Vital signs are monitored after placing the client in the shock position; then the physician is called for orders. NP–IM; CN–SE; CA–ME

174. (4) Pain is due to contraction of the gallbladder, which has stones present. The gallbladder empties when fat is present in the stomach. The gallbladder is located in the upper right side of the abdomen along the side of the liver. NP–AS; CN–PH; CA–ME

175. (4) If narcotics are used, such as morphine, they can cause biliary colic; therefore, Demerol would be

the drug of choice for pain. Thorazine is used to control anxiety or nausea. NP–PL; CN–PH; CA–ME

176. (3) Clients with high abdominal incisions tend to splint and do not like to cough and deep breathe because of the resulting pain. NP–EV; CN–PH; CA–SU

177. (4) This breakfast has the lowest total grams of fat. The egg will provide some of the daily allotment of protein necessary for tissue building. Fat in the diet should be avoided for at least several weeks postoperatively. NP–IM; CN–PH; CA–SU

178. (2) The same amount of irrigating solution is used for both an enema and a colostomy irrigation. The principles for both interventions are basically the same. NP–AN; CN–SE; CA–SU

179. (3) The next step is to wring out the compress. Inspecting the skin and placing compresses in the warming solution are done prior to taking vital signs. Sterile gloves are not necessary. NP–IM; CN–SE; CA–ME

180. (3) Stop or modify the bath to prevent shivering. Shivering is a method of producing body heat. NP–IM; CN–PH; CA–ME

181. (2) All the other choices have one wrong answer or symptom: (1) hunger, not decreased appetite; (3) pain in abdomen, not diarrhea; (4) breath odor acetone, not normal. Answers such as this are tricky, for you have to pick out the wrong answers from amongst several right answers. NP–EV; CN–HM; CA–ME

182. (3) Although she is unable to eat, the client still needs some insulin for body metabolism processes. If fever is not present, insulin is not increased. NP–PL; CN–PH; CA–ME

183. (3) Cogentin is an antiparkinson drug and will reduce these side effects. Xanax is an antianxiety drug. L-dopa is given to clients with Parkinson's disease but is not useful for dystonic effects; answer (4) is not treatment of choice, since the client needs Thorazine to control her symptoms. NP–PL; CN–PH; CA–PY

184. (1) Atelectasis is collapse of alveoli caused by mucus plugs in the small bronchioles due to inadequate ventilation. Turning, coughing, and deep breathing improve ventilation and help prevent the collapse. Liquefying secretions is important but answer (1) is more critical. NP–IM; CN–SE; CA–SU

185. (3) Informed consent by a client who is mentally competent is required in order to have an operative permit signed. This means the doctor must talk to the client and the client must not be under the influence of narcotics. The operative permit does not have to be witnessed. NP–PL; CN–SE; CA–SU

186. (1) Cystic fibrosis children produce abnormally high levels of sodium chloride in their sweat. Though answers (3) and (4) might be used during the diagnostic workup, they do not definitively diagnose the disease. NP–PL; CN–PH; CA–PE

187. (3) Cystic fibrosis children typically evidence a shallow breathing pattern which does not utilize lung potential and may contribute to frequent infections. Instruction in breathing exercises would be an important part of the teaching for Tommy. NP–PL; CN–HM; CA–PE

188. (1) The client should receive a balanced diet including increased carbohydrate and protein and decreased fat. Good nutrition is essential. NP–PL; CN–HM; CA–PE

189. (4) The purpose of the pancreatic enzymes is to replace the enzymes unavailable in the child's system that assist with the digestion of fats. Therefore, they should be taken prior to the ingestion of food. NP–EV; CN–HM; CA–PE

190. (2) Edema is due to insufficient nitrogen for synthesis which then leads to a change in the body's osmotic pressure, resulting in oozing fluids out of the vascular space. This phenomenon results in the formation of edema in the abdomen and flanks. NP–EV; CN–PH; CA–SU

191. (4) The client's wound opens and the bowel contents protrude when an evisceration occurs. Intra-abdominal pressure changes create a shock state; thus the supine position is required. NP–IM; CN–SE; CA–SU

192. (2) The adult dose is multiplied by the child's weight in *pounds*, so kilograms must first be changed to pounds. Then this number is divided by 150. NP–AN; CN–SE; CA–PE

193. (4) The first three situations could result in transmission of the HIV virus. Starting an IV would require gloves, but monitoring an infusion, a closed system, would not. NP–AN; CN–SE; CA–ME

194. (1) The catheter is inserted through the nares without applying suction. Suctioning is limited to fifteen seconds, and suction on the catheter is released intermittently during the procedure. NP–IM; CN–SE; CA–ME

195. (1) In most states age 18 is still considered to be minor status. Because this is an emergency situation, the staff will initiate treatment if they cannot immediately contact Barney's parents. NP–AS; CN–SE; CA–ME

196. (1) Respiratory acidosis represents an increase in the acid component, carbon dioxide, and an increase in the hydrogen ion concentration (decreased pH) of the arterial blood. NP–EV; CN–PH; CA–ME

197. (1) The most important safety measure is to tape a hemostat nearby to use in case of an air leak. Chest tubes should be checked periodically, but not necessarily every two hours. Len should be in semi-Fowler's position to increase lung expansion. NP–IM; CN–SE; CA–SU

198. (2) The bottles must be kept below bed level to facilitate drainage. Answer (1) is not incorrect, but more specifically, the tubes need to be coiled loosely, then attached to the bed. Answers (3) and (4) are inaccurate. NP–PL; CN–SE; CA–SU

199. (2) Tetany is caused by hypocalcemia due to the chelation process which carried the calcium, as well as the lead, out of the body. NP–AN; CN–PH; CA–PE

200. (3) It is appropriate and good nursing judgment to question the order because with late stage cirrhosis, the ability to detoxify the medication by the liver is limited. As a result, barbiturates or sedatives are not ordered for these clients. NP–IM; CN–SE; CA–ME

201. (3) Hyperinflation of lungs with oxygen prevents hypoxia during suctioning procedure in clients requiring frequent treatments. Catheter should be no longer than one-half the diameter of the trach tube; suctioning time is 5–10 seconds; and client should be oxygenated between each suctioning. NP–PL; CN–SE; CA–ME

202. (1) Hypoxia results in yawning, restlessness, shortness of breath, and tachycardia. NP–AS; CN–SE; CA–ME

203. (2) A patent airway is always a priority need, particularly in a client with a head injury, because hypoxia and hypercapnia cause cerebral edema with increasing intracranial pressure. NP–PL; CN–PH; CA–ME

204. (2) Even though Marie is unconscious, the nurse should be aware that highly specialized tissue in the cerebral cortex is most sensitive to lack of oxygen; thus, level of consciousness is the most sensitive index of the client's clinical condition. NP–EV; CN–PH; CA–ME

205. (3) The most important attitude and demeanor to maintain is calmness, for anxiety is easily transmitted and exacerbated. Support is also important for an anxious client. The other attitudes do not contribute to a therapeutic friendship. NP–AN; CN–PS; CA–PY

206. (2) Because of the diabetes and normal changes caused by pregnancy, there is usually an increased insulin need in the 2nd and 3rd trimesters. NP–IM; CN–HM; CA–MA

207. (4) Insulin does not cross into the milk. The mother's calorie intake needs to be adjusted with an increase in protein intake. Insulin must be adjusted and care must be exercised during weaning. NP–PL; CN–HM; CA–MA

208. (4) A mask with a reservoir bag provides 70–100% oxygen at flow rates of 8–10 liters. NP–PL; CN–PH; CA–ME

209. (2) Alterations in vital signs could be an indication of nebulizer medication side-effects. NP–IM; CN–SE; CA–ME

210. (4) There is a circulatory compromise and thus the physician needs to be notified immediately. The other actions, except removing traction, will be carried out later. NP–IM; CN–SE; CA–SU

211. (4) It is important that the mother know what the child swallowed since the emergency treatment will depend on the type of substance consumed. The next action is to call the local poison control center who will tell her what to do. NP–IM; CN–HM; CA–PE

212. (4) By asking, "Can you talk?" you can establish that the victim has something in his airway. If the victim is able to answer, he is not choking because a victim is unable to talk when choking. Following this assessment, you may use the Heimlich maneuver. NP–IM; CN–SE; CA–ME

213. (2) Blood loss results in shock; therefore, close monitoring of vital signs and shock symptoms is essential. NP–IM; CN–SE; CA–ME

214. (1) The drip chamber should be only one-third full so that the sensor can "pick up" the drops. NP–PL; CN–SE; CA–ME

215. (3) Every newborn receives silver nitrate, 1%, or more commonly, a broad spectrum antibiotic in the eyes to prevent blindness caused by the mother having a sexually transmitted disease, such as chlamydia or gonorrhea. NP–IM; CN–SE; CA–MA

216. (3) Infants with signs and symptoms of hypoglycemia usually have a high-pitched cry. NP–AS; CN–HM; CA–MA

217. (1) Colchicine is an anti-inflammatory drug that is taken at the first sign of joint pain. Pain will be alleviated as a secondary factor. The drug Allopurinol decreases uric acid level, and sodium bicarbonate alkalinizes urine. NP–IM; CN–HM; CA–ME

218. (2) Mr. Hurd should be on a low purine diet and should recognize the restricted foods: gravy, fish, fowl, and organ meats. Eggs, cheese, breads, fat, and most vegetables are allowed. NP–EV; CN–HM; CA–ME

219. (4) The new diagnostic criteria is no menstrual period for three months. A loss of 25 percent of normal body weight was the original method of diagnosis, and it is still used. The other symptoms occur, but are not used for diagnosis. NP–AS; CN–PH; CA–PY

220. (4) Dextrostix results yield data about blood glucose level; this is essential data for monitoring hypoglycemia in the infant of a diabetic mother. NP–IM; CN–SE; CA–MA

INDEX

Computer Disk
for
Simulated NCLEX/CAT Test

A vinyl envelope containing a computer disk is attached inside the back cover of this book. This 3.5" disk, which will operate on IBM and IBM-compatible personal computers, contains the same questions that are printed at the back of the book. After completing the questions on the disk, you can obtain your Performance Summary in terms of Nursing Process, Client Needs, and Clinical Area. You will also be able to obtain a list of questions you answered incorrectly. We recommend that you refer to the rationales printed at the back of the book to understand the principles underlying the answers for all of the practice questions.

Please Note: This book is not returnable if the vinyl disk holder has been opened or removed from the book.